Clinical Pediatric Neurology

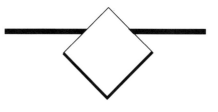

Clinical Pediatric Neurology

A Signs and Symptoms Approach

SECOND EDITION

GERALD M. FENICHEL, M.D.

Professor and Chairman, Department of Neurology
Vanderbilt University School of Medicine
Nashville, Tennessee

W.B. SAUNDERS COMPANY

Harcourt Brace Jovanovich, Inc.
Philadelphia   London   Toronto   Montreal   Sydney   Tokyo

W. B. SAUNDERS COMPANY

Harcourt Brace Jovanovich, Inc.

The Curtis Center
Independence Square West
Philadelphia, Pennsylvania 19106

Library of Congress Cataloging-in-Publication Data

Fenichel, Gerald M.

Clinical pediatric neurology : a signs and symptoms approach /
Gerald M. Fenichel.— 2nd ed.

  p. cm.
  Includes bibliographical references.
  Includes index.
  ISBN 0-7216-6463-6
  1. Pediatric neurology. 2. Nervous system—Diseases—Diagnosis.
  I. Title. [DNLM: 1. Nervous System Diseases—diagnosis. 2. Nervous
  System Diseases—in infancy & childhood. WS 340 F333c]

  RJ486.F46   1993   618.92′8—dc20

  DNLM/DLC   92-3860

Clinical Pediatric Neurology: ISBN 0-7216-6463-6
A Signs and Symptoms Approach
2nd Edition

Printed in Mexico.

Last digit is the print number: 9   8   7   6   5   4   3   2   1

To my mother, Sarah Fenichel, and
my grandson, Aaron Michael Simon

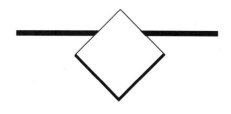

Preface

In this second edition of *Clinical Pediatric Neurology* the format of the text is unchanged. The first edition was well accepted, and I saw the need for a 5-year update rather than a change in format. Patients still present with complaints rather than diseases, and a symptom-based text remains more practical than any other format.

Several disorders are included in this edition that were inadvertently omitted from the first edition or that have been described only during the past 5 years. Some sections, such as AIDS encephalopathy and Lyme disease, have been expanded. Approximately one third of the references in the second edition are new. References were selected because they are recent and easily accessible rather than "first descriptions." The text remains a manual of practical information, much derived from my own experience, for physicians caring for children.

I am grateful to the following colleagues who provided counsel: Kathryn Edwards (infectious disease), Mark T. Jennings (neuro-oncology), Patrick J.M. Lavin (neuro-ophthalmology), Kathleen Shannon (movement disorders), and Noel Tulipan (neurosurgery). I am also grateful to Mrs. Lester Tilley, who keeps my office running so that I have the opportunity to write.

GERALD M. FENICHEL, M.D.
Nashville, Tennessee

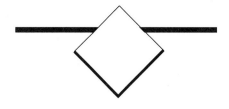

Contents

Paroxysmal Disorders

Paroxysmal events are routinely suspected of being seizures and usually prompt neurologic consultation. Despite 30 years of pediatric neurology practice, I am still confronted regularly with descriptions of "spells" that are unlike anything in my experience. Detailed questioning fails to clarify the nature of the spell, and like a car that only runs well when taken to the mechanic, the child will not have a spell in the office. Since observation of the spell is critical to diagnosis, the solution is a video camera. "Spells" seldom remain unexplained after being viewed. Most families either own or can borrow a video camera; even if purchased, the camera is more cost effective than brain imaging studies, and at least the family has something useful to show for the expenditure.

In children the most common causes of sudden and recurrent episodes of neurologic dysfunction that clear completely are epilepsy, syncope, and migraine. Less common causes are movement disorders, psychogenic disturbances, and some metabolic disorders. Episodic symptoms that last only seconds and cause no abnormal signs are unlikely to be explained and do not warrant laboratory investigation. The differential diagnosis of paroxysmal disorders varies considerably from the newborn to infancy, childhood, and adolescence and is best presented by age groups.

◆ Paroxysmal Disorders of Newborns

Seizures are the major paroxysmal disorder of the newborn. The challenge for the clinician is to differentiate seizure activity from normal neonatal movements and from pathologic movements caused by other mechanisms (Table 1–1).

APPROACH TO DIAGNOSIS
Seizure Patterns

Seizures in newborns, especially those who are premature, are poorly organized and difficult to distinguish from normal activity. Newborns with hydranencephaly or atelencephaly are capable of generating the full variety of neonatal seizure patterns. This supports the notion that seizures may arise from the brainstem as well as the hemispheres (Danner et al, 1985). Seizures arising in the brainstem may be confined there by the absence of myelinated pathways for propagation. For the same reason, seizures originating in one hemisphere are unlikely to spread beyond the contiguous cortex or to produce secondary bilateral synchrony.

Table 1–2 lists clinical patterns that have been associated with epileptiform discharges in newborns. This classification is useful but does not do justice to the rich variety of patterns actually observed or take into account that 79% of prolonged epileptiform discharges on the electroencephalogram (EEG) are not associated with visible clinical changes (Clancy et al, 1983). Generalized tonic-clonic seizures do not occur. Most newborns suspected of having generalized tonic-clonic seizures are actually *jittery* (see "Jitteriness"). Newborns paralyzed with pancuronium to assist mechanical ventilation pose a special problem in seizure identification. In this circumstance physicians may be alerted to the possibility of seizures by the presence of rhythmic increases in systolic arterial blood pressure, heart rate, and oxygenation.

The term "subtle seizures" encompasses several different patterns in which tonic or clonic movements of the limbs are lacking. EEG monitoring has consistently failed to show that such movements are associated with epileptiform activity

<table>
<tr><td colspan="2">**Table 1–1 ◆** Movements That Resemble Neonatal Seizures</td></tr>
</table>

1. Benign nocturnal myoclonus
2. Jitteriness
3. Nonconvulsive apnea
4. Normal movement
5. Opisthotonos
6. Pathologic myoclonus

Table 1–2 ◆ Seizure Patterns in Newborns

1. Apnea with tonic stiffening of body
2. Focal clonic movements of one limb or both limbs on one side
3. Multifocal clonic limb movements
4. Myoclonic jerking
5. Paroxysmal laughing
6. Tonic deviation of the eyes, upward or to one side
7. Tonic stiffening of the body

(Mizrahi and Kellaway, 1987). One exception is tonic deviation of the eyes, which is almost always a seizure manifestation.

The definitive diagnosis of neonatal seizures requires EEG monitoring. This is best accomplished with split-screen, 16-channel video-EEG, but an ambulatory EEG cassette capable of marking the time of events can also be used. Epileptiform activity in newborns is usually widespread and can be detected even when the newborn is clinically asymptomatic (Figure 1–1).

Focal Clonic Seizures

Clinical Features. Focal clonic seizures are characterized by repeated, irregular jerking move-ments affecting one limb or both limbs on one side. The movements are rarely sustained for long periods, and they do not "march" as if spreading along the motor cortex. Focal clonic seizures in a full-term newborn who is otherwise alert and responsive suggest a cerebral infarction or intracerebral hemorrhage. In newborns with states of decreased consciousness, focal clonic seizures may indicate a focal infarction superimposed on a generalized encephalopathy (Clancy et al, 1985).

Diagnosis. During the seizure the EEG may show a unilateral focus of high-amplitude sharp waves adjacent to the Rolandic fissure. The discharge can spread to involve contiguous areas in the same hemisphere and can be associated with unilateral seizures of the limbs and adversive

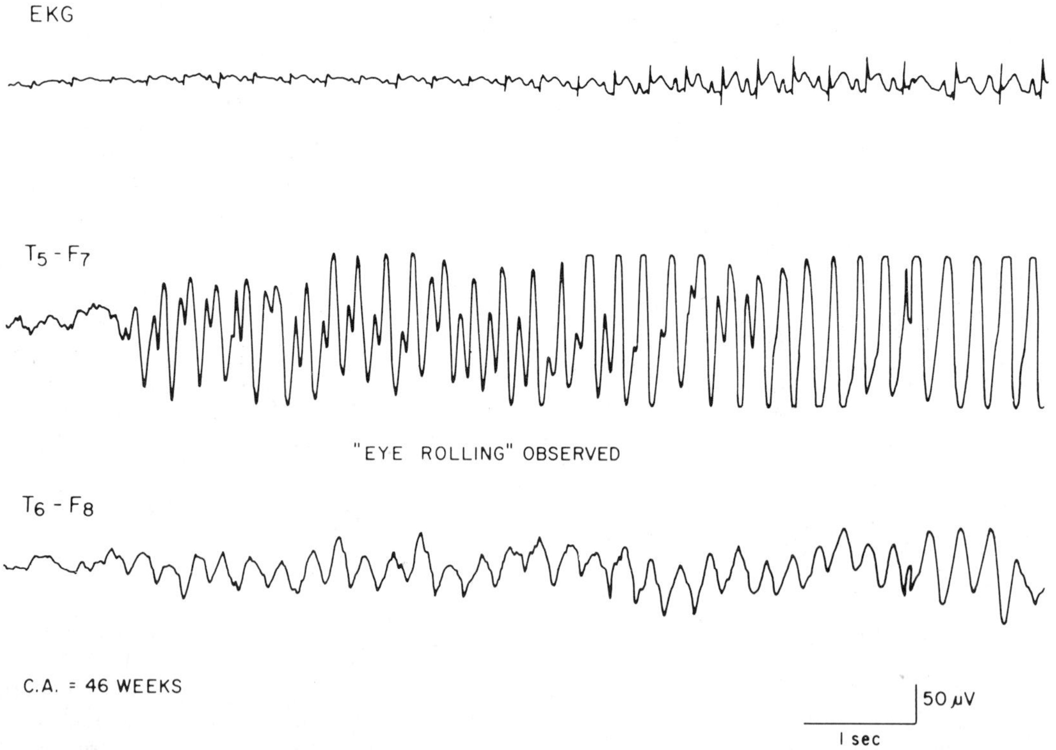

EKG

$T_5 - F_7$

"EYE ROLLING" OBSERVED

$T_6 - F_8$

C.A. = 46 WEEKS

50 µV

I sec

Figure 1–1   EEG tracing (A/EEG—ambulatory EEG). Electroconvulsive discharge from the left hemi-sphere (T_5-F_7) is associated with rolling back of the eyes.

movements of the head and eyes. In the interictal period the EEG usually demonstrates focal slowing or amplitude attenuation.

Newborns with focal clonic seizures should be evaluated by non-contrast-enhanced computed tomography (CT) or ultrasound to determine the presence of intracerebral hemorrhage. If the findings are normal but the affected limbs seem paretic after the seizure has subsided, CT should be performed a week later to look for cerebral infarction. Ultrasound is not useful in detecting small cerebral infarctions.

Multifocal Clonic Seizures

Clinical Features. In multifocal clonic seizures, migratory jerking movements are noted in first one limb and then another; face muscles may be involved as well. The migration appears random and does not follow expected patterns of epileptic spread. Movements in one limb are sometimes prolonged, suggesting a focal rather than a multifocal seizure. The multifocal nature is detected later, when nursing notes are found to be contradictory concerning the side or the limb affected. Multifocal clonic seizures are a neonatal equivalent of generalized tonic-clonic seizures. They are ordinarily associated with severe, generalized cerebral disturbances such as hypoxic-ischemic encephalopathy.

Diagnosis. Multifocal epileptiform activity can usually be detected on a standard EEG. If epileptiform activity is not observed, a 24-hour monitor is recommended.

Myoclonic Seizures

Clinical Features. Myoclonic seizures are characterized by brief, repeated extension and flexion movements of the arms, the legs, or all limbs. They constitute an uncommon seizure pattern in the newborn, but their presence suggests severe, diffuse brain damage.

Diagnosis. No specific EEG pattern is associated with myoclonic seizures in the newborn. Myoclonic jerks are often seen in babies born to drug-addicted mothers. Whether these movements are seizures, jitteriness, or myoclonus (discussed later) is not certain.

Tonic Seizures

Clinical Features. Tonic seizures are characterized by extension and stiffening of the body, usually associated with apnea and upward deviation of the eyes. Tonic posturing without the other features is rarely a seizure manifestation. Tonic sei-

zures are more common in premature neonates than in full-term newborns and usually indicate structural brain damage rather than a metabolic disturbance.

Diagnosis. Tonic seizures in premature newborns are often a symptom of intraventricular hemorrhage and are an indication for ultrasound study. Tonic posturing also occurs in newborns with forebrain damage, not as a seizure manifestation but as a disinhibition of brainstem reflexes. Prolonged disinhibition results in *decerebrate posturing*, an extension of the body and limbs associated with internal rotation of the arms, dilation of the pupils, and downward deviation of the eyes. Decerebrate posturing is often encountered as a terminal sign in premature infants with intraventricular hemorrhage caused by pressure on the upper brainstem (see Chapter 4).

Tonic seizures and decerebrate posturing must also be distinguished from *opisthotonos*, a prolonged arching of the back not necessarily associated with eye movements. Opisthotonos is probably caused by meningeal irritation and is seen in kernicterus, infantile Gaucher disease, and some aminoacidurias.

Apnea

Clinical Features. An irregular respiratory pattern with intermittent pauses of 3 to 6 seconds, often followed by 10 to 15 seconds of hyperpnea, is regularly observed in premature infants. The pauses are not associated with significant alterations in heart rate, blood pressure, body temperature, or skin color. This respiratory pattern, termed *periodic breathing*, is caused by immaturity of the brainstem respiratory centers. The incidence of periodic breathing correlates directly with the degree of prematurity. The rate of apnea is highest in active sleep and lowest in quiet sleep.

Apneic spells of 10 to 15 seconds are detectable at some time in almost all premature and some full-term newborns. Apneic spells of 10 to 20 seconds are usually associated with a 20% reduction in heart rate. Longer episodes of apnea are almost invariably associated with a 40% or greater reduction in heart rate. The frequency of these apneic spells correlates with brainstem myelination. At 40 weeks' conceptional age, premature infants continue to have a higher incidence of apnea than do full-term newborns (Albani et al, 1985). The incidence of apnea sharply decreases in all infants at 52 weeks' conceptional age.

Diagnosis. Apneic spells in otherwise normal-appearing newborns should be considered a sign of brainstem immaturity and not a pathologic condition. The brainstem auditory evoked response is

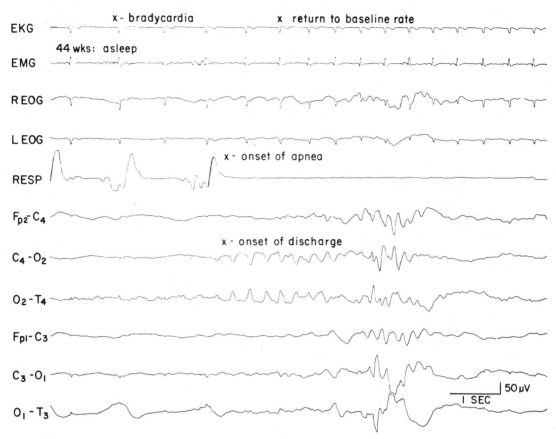

Figure 1–2   Convulsive apnea. The onset of apnea is concurrent with a theta discharge at the O_2 electrode. The duration of apnea exceeds the duration of discharge. (From Fenichel GM: Neonatal Neurology, 3rd edition. Churchill Livingstone, New York, 1990. By permission.)

useful in this regard. The interpeak latency between waves V and I is longer in premature infants with apnea than in those without apnea at the same conceptional age. Apnea is common when the interpeak latency is greater than 6 ms and decreases in frequency as latencies less than 5.6 ms are attained (Henderson-Smart et al, 1983).

The sudden onset of apnea and states of decreased consciousness, especially in a premature newborn, suggests an intracranial hemorrhage with brainstem compression. Immediate ultrasound examination is indicated.

Apneic spells are never a seizure manifestation unless they are associated with tonic deviation of the eyes, tonic stiffening of the body, or characteristic limb movements. The absence of bradycardia in association with prolonged apnea suggests the possibility of seizures (Figure 1–2).

Benign Nocturnal Myoclonus

Clinical Features.   Sudden jerking movements of the limbs during sleep occur in normal people of all ages (see Chapter 14). They appear primarily during the early stages of sleep as repeated flexion movements of the fingers, wrists, and elbows. When prolonged, they may be misdiagnosed as focal clonic or myoclonic seizures.

Diagnosis.   Nocturnal myoclonus can be distinguished from seizures and jitteriness because it occurs solely during sleep, it is not activated by a stimulus, and the EEG results are normal.

Treatment.   Treatment is not required.

Jitteriness

Clinical Features.   Jitteriness or tremulousness is an excessive response to stimulation. Touch, noise, and especially motion produce low-frequency, high-amplitude shaking of the limbs and jaw. Jitteriness is commonly associated with a low threshold for the Moro reflex, but it can occur in the absence of any apparent stimulation and be confused with myoclonic seizures.

Diagnosis.   Jitteriness usually occurs in newborns with perinatal asphyxia, some of whom have seizures as well. It can be distinguished from seizures by EEG monitoring, by the absence of eye movements or alteration in respiratory pattern, and by the presence of stimulus activation. Jitteriness is also encountered in newborns of addicted mothers and in newborns with metabolic disorders.

Treatment. Reduced stimulation decreases jitteriness. However, newborns of addicted mothers require sedation to facilitate feeding and to decrease energy expenditure.

DIFFERENTIAL DIAGNOSIS OF SEIZURES

Virtually any disorder of the brain in a newborn may result in a seizure. The time of onset of the first seizure is helpful in determining the cause (Table 1–3). Seizures occurring during the first 24 hours, and especially the first 12 hours, are usually due to hypoxic-ischemic encephalopathy. Sepsis, meningitis, and subarachnoid hemorrhage are next in frequency, followed by intrauterine infection and trauma. Direct drug effects, intraventricular hemorrhage at term, and pyridoxine dependency are relatively rare causes of seizures.

During the period from 24 to 72 hours after birth, seizures are most commonly caused by intraventricular hemorrhage in premature infants, by subarachnoid hemorrhage and cerebral contusion in large, full-term newborns, and by sepsis and meningitis at all gestational ages. Focal clonic seizures in full-term newborns suggest a cerebral infarction or an intracerebral hemorrhage. Cerebral dysgenesis may produce seizures at this time and remains an important cause of seizures throughout infancy. All other conditions are relatively rare. Newborns with metabolic disorders are usually lethargic and feed poorly before the onset of seizures.

After 72 hours, inborn errors of metabolism, especially aminoacidurias, become a more important consideration because protein and glucose feedings have been initiated. A battery of screening tests for metabolic disorders is outlined in Table 1–4. Herpes simplex infection is transmitted during delivery and does not become symptomatic until the second half of the first week. Among the conditions that cause early seizures and can also cause late seizures are cerebral dysgenesis, cerebral infarction, and intracerebral hemorrhage. In addition, familial neonatal seizures and those from kernicterus and neonatal adrenoleukodystrophy usually have their onset more than 72 hours after delivery.

Hypoxic-Ischemic Encephalopathy

Asphyxia at term is almost always an intrauterine event, and hypoxia and ischemia occur to-

---

Table 1–3 ◆ Differential Diagnosis of Neonatal Seizures by Peak Time of Onset

24 Hours
1. Bacterial meningitis and sepsis (see Chapter 4)
2. Direct drug effect
3. Hypoxic-ischemic encephalopathy
4. Intrauterine infection (see Chapter 5)
5. Intraventricular hemorrhage at term (see Chapter 4)
6. Laceration of tentorium or falx
7. Pyridoxine dependency
8. Subarachnoid hemorrhage

24 to 72 Hours
1. Bacterial meningitis and sepsis (see Chapter 4)
2. Cerebral contusion with subdural hemorrhage
3. Cerebral dysgenesis (see Chapter 18)
4. Cerebral infarction (see Chapter 11)
5. Drug withdrawal
6. Glycine encephalopathy
7. Glycogen synthase deficiency
8. Hypoparathyroidism-hypocalcemia
9. Incontinentia pigmenti
10. Intracerebral hemorrhage (see Chapter 11)
11. Intraventricular hemorrhage in premature newborns (see Chapter 4)
12. Pyridoxine dependency
13. Subarachnoid hemorrhage
14. Tuberous sclerosis
15. Urea cycle disturbances

72 Hours to 1 Week
1. Familial neonatal seizures
2. Cerebral dysgenesis (see Chapter 18)
3. Cerebral infarction (see Chapter 11)
4. Hypoparathyroidism
5. Intracerebral hemorrhage (see Chapter 11)
6. Kernicterus
7. Methylmalonic acidemia
8. Nutritional hypocalcemia
9. Propionic acidemia
10. Tuberous sclerosis
11. Urea cycle disturbances

1 Week to 4 Weeks
1. Adrenoleukodystrophy, neonatal (see Chapter 6)
2. Cerebral dysgenesis (see Chapter 18)
3. Fructose dysmetabolism
4. Gaucher disease type 2 (see Chapter 5)
5. Gm$_1$ gangliosidosis type 1 (see Chapter 5)
6. Herpes simplex encephalitis
7. Ketotic hyperglycinemias
8. Maple syrup urine disease, neonatal
9. Tuberous sclerosis
10. Urea cycle disturbances

Table 1–4 ◆ Screening for Inborn Errors of Metabolism That Cause Neonatal Seizures

Blood Glucose Low 1. Fructose-1,6,-diphosphatase deficiency 2. Glycogen storage disease, type 1 3. Maple syrup urine disease	**Metabolic Acidosis** 1. Fructose-1,6,-diphosphatase deficiency 2. Glycogen storage disease, type 1 3. Maple syrup urine disease 4. Methylmalonic acidemia 5. Multiple carboxylase deficiency 6. Propionic acidemia
Blood Calcium Low 1. Hypoparathyroidism 2. Maternal hyperparathyroidism	**Urine Ferric Chloride or Dinitrophenylhydrazine** 1. Maple syrup urine disease
Blood Ammonia High 1. Argininosuccinic acidemia 2. Carbamylphosphate synthetase deficiency 3. Citrullinemia 4. Methylmalonic acidemia (may be normal) 5. Multiple carboxylase deficiency 6. Ornithine transcarbamylase deficiency 7. Propionic acidemia (may be normal)	**No Rapid Screening Test** 1. Adrenoleukodystrophy, neonatal form 2. Glycine encephalopathy 3. Glycogen synthase deficiency 4. Infantile Gm₁ gangliosidosis, type 1
Blood Lactate High 1. Fructose-1,6, -diphosphatase deficiency 2. Glycogen storage disease, type 1 3. Mitochondrial disorders 4. Multiple carboxylase deficiency	

gether; the result is hypoxic-ischemic encephalopathy (HIE). Acute total asphyxia usually leads to death from circulatory collapse. Affected fetuses are stillborn or die in the perinatal period. Occasional survivors are born comatose and have evidence of cranial nerve dysfunction. The usual mechanism of HIE in surviving full-term newborns is partial, prolonged asphyxia. The fetal circulation accommodates to reductions in arterial oxygen by maximizing blood flow to the brain, and to a lesser extent the heart, at the expense of other organs.

Clinical experience indicates that the fetus may be subjected to considerable hypoxia without brain damage developing. The incidence of cerebral palsy among full-term newborns with a 5-minute Apgar score of 0 to 3 is only 1% if the 10-minute score is 4 or higher (Nelson and Ellenberg, 1981). Any episode of hypoxia sufficiently severe to cause brain damage also causes derangements in other organs. Newborns with mild to moderate HIE always have a history of irregular heart rate and usually pass meconium. Those with moderate to severe HIE may have lactic acidosis, elevated serum concentrations of hepatic enzymes, enterocolitis, renal failure, and fatal myocardial damage. HIE can be divided into three grades of severity by clinical symptoms: mild, moderate, and severe.

Clinical Features. Mild HIE is relatively common. Lethargy, without significant loss of consciousness, is noted immediately after birth. The characteristic features are jitteriness and sympathetic overactivity (tachycardia, dilation of pupils, and decreased bronchial and salivary secretions).

Muscle tone is normal at rest, tendon reflexes are normoreactive or hyperactive, and ankle clonus is usually elicited. The Moro reflex is complete, and repetitive extension and flexion movements are generated by a single stimulus. Seizures are not an expected feature, and their occurrence suggests concurrent hypoglycemia or the presence of a second condition.

Symptoms diminish and disappear during the first few days, although some degree of overresponsiveness may persist. Newborns with mild HIE probably recover completely; no evidence of a cause-and-effect relationship with epilepsy or learning disabilities has been found (Nelson and Broman, 1977).

Newborns with moderate HIE are lethargic or obtunded for at least the first 12 hours after delivery and are jittery when aroused. The resting posture indicates hypotonia, and spontaneous movement of the limbs is lacking. Proximal weakness is present and affects the shoulder more than the pelvic girdle. This weakness may be due in part to hypoxic-ischemic injury to the spinal cord, as well as the brain (Clancy et al, 1989). Between 48 and 72 hours after birth, some children with moderate HIE begin to improve and to resemble newborns with mild HIE.

In some newborns with moderate HIE, obtundation continues or progressive stupor and coma develop. Seizures are an ominous sign and indicate a worsening prognosis. An estimated 20% to 40% of newborns with moderate encephalopathy have permanent neurological sequelae (Hill and Volpe, 1989).

Newborns with severe HIE are stuporous or co-matose immediately after birth, and respiratory effort is usually periodic and insufficient to sustain life. Seizures begin within the first 12 hours. Hypotonia is severe, and tendon reflexes, the Moro reflex, and the tonic neck reflex are absent. Sucking and swallowing are depressed or absent, but the pupillary and oculovestibular reflexes are present.

Some newborns with severe HIE have a transitory improvement in state of consciousness between 12 and 24 hours post partum, but most remain comatose and have frequent seizures that progress to status epilepticus. The response to anticonvulsant drugs is usually incomplete. Generalized increased intracranial pressure develops between 24 and 72 hours of age. This is characterized by coma, bulging of the fontanelles, loss of pupillary and oculovestibular reflexes, and respiratory arrest.

The infant may die at this time or may remain stuporous for several weeks. The encephalopathy subsides after the third day, and survivors experience a decreasing frequency of seizures. Jitteri-ness is common as the child becomes arousable. Tone increases, and the infant becomes hypertonic in succeeding weeks.

The prognosis for newborns with severe HIE is poor. Neurologic sequelae can be expected in newborns with severe HIE who remain comatose for more than a week.

Diagnosis. EEG and CT are helpful in determining the severity and prognosis of HIE. In mild HIE the EEG background rhythms are normal or may be lacking in variability. In moderate to severe HIE the background is always abnormal and demonstrates suppression of background amplitude. The degree of suppression correlates well with the severity of HIE. The worst case is a flat EEG or one with a burst-suppression pattern (Figure 1–3). A bad outcome is invariable if the amplitude remains suppressed for 2 weeks or a burst-suppression pattern is present at any time (Grigg-Damberger et al, 1989). Epileptiform activity may also be present but is less predictive of outcome than is background suppression.

Between the second and fourth days following

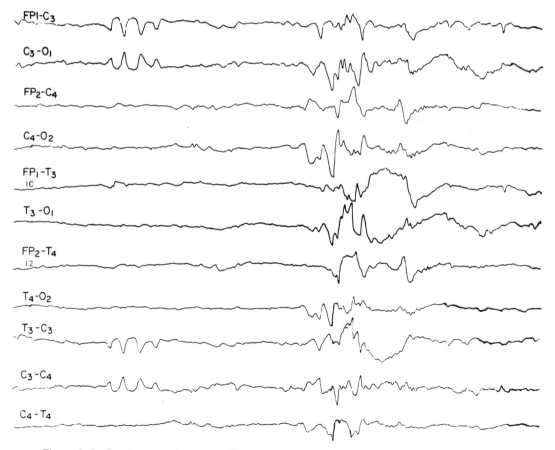

Figure 1–3 Burst-suppression pattern. Ten-second intervals of suppression are interrupted by bursts of slow and sharp waves in a full-term newborn with hypoxic-ischemic encephalopathy.

injury, CT shows the cerebral edema of severe HIE as a diffuse decrease in tissue attenuation (Lupton et al, 1988). Follow-up CT studies after 1 month show the full extent of injury.

Treatment.   The management of HIE in newborns requires immediate attention to derangements in several organs and correction of acidosis. No therapeutic regimen has proved effective in treating the encephalopathy (Vannucci, 1990). Nevertheless, clinical experience and some studies indicate that control of seizures, maintenance of adequate ventilation and perfusion, and prevention of fluid overload increase the chance of a favorable outcome.

The use of phenobarbital to treat seizures in newborns is detailed in a separate section. If phenobarbital proves ineffective, trying other drugs is probably unwise and often nonproductive. Seizures usually cease spontaneously during the second week, and anticonvulsants should be stopped after a further 2 weeks of control. The incidence of epilepsy among infants who had neonatal seizures caused by HIE is 30% to 40%. There is no evidence that continued therapy prevents the subsequent development of epilepsy.

Intracranial pressure may be lessened by the simple procedure of elevating the head to 30 degrees and reducing fluids by 10%.

Trauma and Intracranial Hemorrhage

Neonatal head trauma occurs most often in large, full-term newborns of primiparous mothers. Usually labor was prolonged and extraction was difficult because of fetal malposition or a precipitous delivery before the maternal cervix was sufficiently dilated. Intracranial hemorrhage may be subarachnoid, subdural, or intraventricular. Intraventricular hemorrhage is discussed in Chapter 4.

Primary Subarachnoid Hemorrhage

Clinical Features.   Blood in the subarachnoid space probably originates from tearing of the superficial veins by shearing forces during a prolonged delivery with the head engaged. Mild HIE is often associated with subarachnoid hemorrhage, but the newborn is usually well when an unexpected seizure occurs on the first or second day of life. Lumbar puncture is performed because of suspected sepsis, and blood is found in the cerebrospinal fluid. Most newborns with subarachnoid hemorrhage are neurologically normal later.

Diagnosis.   CT is useful to document the extent of hemorrhage. Blood is present in the interhemispheric fissure and the supratentorial and in-

fratentorial recesses. Routine ultrasound does not reliably demonstrate subarachnoid hemorrhage. Epileptiform activity may be seen on the EEG, but the background is not suppressed. This indicates that seizures are not due to HIE and that the prognosis is more favorable. Clotting studies should be performed to exclude the possibility of a coagulopathy.

Treatment.   Seizures usually respond to phenobarbital. Specific therapy is not available for the hemorrhage, and posthemorrhagic hydrocephalus is uncommon.

Subdural Hemorrhage

Clinical Features.   Subdural hemorrhage is usually the consequence of a tear in the tentorium near its junction with the falx. The lesion results from excessive vertical molding of the head in a vertex presentation, anteroposterior elongation of the head in face and brow presentations, or prolonged delivery of the aftercoming head in a breech presentation. Blood collects in the posterior fossa and may produce brainstem compression. The initial features are those of mild to moderate HIE. Clinical evidence of brainstem compression is delayed for 12 hours or longer and characterized by irregular respiration, abnormal cry, declining consciousness, hypotonia, seizures, and a tense fontanelle. Intracerebellar hemorrhage is sometimes present (Serfontein et al, 1980). Mortality is high, and neurologic impairment among survivors is common.

Diagnosis.   Subdural hemorrhage is readily visualized by CT and ultrasound.

Treatment.   Small hemorrhages do not require treatment, but large collections should be evacuated surgically to relieve brainstem compression.

Hypoglycemia

A transitory, asymptomatic hypoglycemia can be detected in 11% of newborns during the first hours post partum and before oral feeding is initiated. Hypoglycemia is not associated with neurologic impairment later in life. Symptomatic hypoglycemia may result from cerebral stress or inborn errors of metabolism (Table 1–5).

Clinical Features.   The time of onset of symptoms depends on the underlying disorder. Early onset is generally associated with perinatal asphyxia or intracranial hemorrhage, and late onset with inborn errors of metabolism. The syndrome includes any of the following symptoms: apnea, cyanosis, tachypnea, jitteriness, high-pitched cry,

Table 1–5 ◆ Causes of Neonatal Hypoglycemia

Primary Transitional Hypoglycemia
1. Complicated labor and delivery
2. Intrauterine malnutrition
3. Maternal diabetes
4. Prematurity

Secondary Transitional Hypoglycemia
1. Asphyxia
2. Central nervous system disorders
3. Cold injuries
4. Sepsis

Persistent Hypoglycemia
1. Aminoacidurias
   a. Maple syrup urine disease
   b. Methylmalonic acidemia
   c. Propionic acidemia
   d. Tyrosinosis
2. Congenital hypopituitarism
3. Defects in carbohydrate metabolism
   a. Fructose-1,6-diphosphatase deficiency
   b. Fructose intolerance
   c. Galactosemia
   d. Glycogen storage disease, type 1
   e. Glycogen synthase deficiency
4. Hyperinsulinism

poor feeding, vomiting, apathy, hypotonia, seizures, and coma. Symptomatic hypoglycemia is often associated with later neurologic impairment.

Diagnosis. Neonatal hypoglycemia is defined as a whole blood glucose concentration of less than 20 mg/dl (1 mmol/L) in premature and low-birth-weight newborns, less than 30 mg/dl (1.5 mmol/L) in full-term newborns during the first 72 hours, and less than 40 mg/dl (2 mmol/L) in full-term newborns after 72 hours.

Treatment. Normal blood glucose concentrations can be restored by intravenous administration of glucose, but the underlying cause must be determined before definitive treatment can be provided.

Hypocalcemia

Hypocalcemia is defined as a blood calcium concentration less than 7 mg/dl (1.75 mmol/L). The onset of hypocalcemia in the first 72 hours after delivery is associated with low birth weight, asphyxia, maternal diabetes, transient neonatal hypoparathyroidism, maternal hyperparathyroidism, and the DiGeorge syndrome. Later-onset hypocalcemia is seen in children fed evaporated cow's milk and other improper formulas, in maternal hyperparathyroidism, and in the DiGeorge syndrome.

Hypoparathyroidism in the newborn may result from maternal hyperparathyroidism or be a transient phenomenon of unknown cause. Hypocalcemia occurs in less than 10% of stressed newborns and enhances the vulnerability to seizures, but it is rarely the primary cause.

DiGeorge Syndrome

Clinical Features. DiGeorge syndrome is a congenital hypoplasia of organs derived from the third and fourth pharyngeal pouches (thymus, parathyroid gland, and great vessels) (Muller et al, 1988). The cause is unknown. The major features are multiple minor facial anomalies, hypocalcemic seizures, lymphocytopenia, and congenital heart disease. The symptoms may be due to congenital heart disease, hypocalcemia, or both. Jitteriness and tetany usually begin in the first 48 hours post partum. The peak onset of seizures is on the third day but may be delayed as long as 2 weeks. Many affected newborns die of cardiac causes during the first month; survivors fail to thrive and have frequent infections because of the failure of cell-mediated immunity.

Diagnosis. In newborns who come to medical attention because of heart disease, hypocalcemia may be suspected when a prolonged QT interval is detected on the electrocardiogram (EKG). All newborns with symptoms of hypocalcemia should be examined for cardiac defects.

Treatment. Hypocalcemia generally responds to parathyroid hormone or to oral calcium and vitamin D.

Aminoacidopathies
Maple Syrup Urine Disease

The neonatal form of maple syrup urine disease (MSUD) is caused by almost complete absence (less than 5% of normal) of branched-chain ketoacid dehydrogenase. Leucine, isoleucine, and valine cannot be decarboxylated, and they accumulate in blood, urine, and tissues (Figure 1–4). Later-onset forms are described in Chapters 5 and 10. The defect is transmitted by autosomal recessive inheritance.

Clinical Features. Affected newborns appear healthy at birth, but lethargy, feeding difficulty, and hypotonia develop after ingestion of protein. Seizures begin in the second week and are associated with the development of cerebral edema (Riviello et al, 1991). Once seizures begin, they continue with increasing frequency and severity. Without therapy, cerebral edema becomes progressively worse and results in coma and death within 1 month.

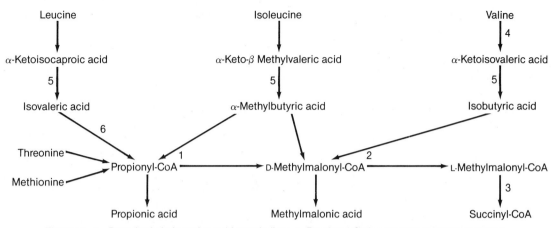

Figure 1–4   Branched-chain amino acid metabolism. *1,* Propionyl-CoA carboxylase (biotin cofactor). *2,* Methymalonyl-CoA racemase. *3,* Methymalonyl-CoA mutase (adenosylcobalamin). *4,* valine transaminase. *5,* Branched-chain ketoacid dehydrogenase. *6,* Isovaleryl-CoA dehydrogenase. (From Fenichel GM: Neonatal Neurology, 3rd edition. Churchill-Livingstone, New York, 1990. By permission.)

Diagnosis.   Rapid screening of urine for MSUD can be accomplished by the addition of ferric chloride, which colors urine deep blue, or with 2,4-dinitrophenylhydrazine, which causes a cloudy, yellow precipitate. Specific diagnosis requires the demonstration of increased plasma concentrations of the three branch-chained amino acids or enzyme deficiency in peripheral leukocytes. Heterozygotes can be detected by diminished levels of enzyme activity.

Treatment.   Exchange transfusions or peritoneal dialysis transiently lowers the plasma concentration of branch-chained amino acids and ketoacids. Administration of glucose and insulin provides a more prolonged reduction by promoting the uptake of amino acids into skeletal muscle.

A special diet, low in branched-chain amino acids (MSUD formula, Mead-Johnson), may prevent further encephalopathy and should be started immediately by nasogastric tube. Thiamine supplementation, 10 to 20 mg/kg/day, should be tried as well. Early diagnosis and treatment can result in normal intellectual outcome (Kaplan et al, 1991).

Glycine Encephalopathy

Glycine encephalopathy is due to a defect in the glycine cleaving system. It is inherited as an autosomal recessive trait.

Clinical Features.   Affected newborns are normal at birth but become irritable and refuse feeding during the first few days after delivery. Progressive lethargy, hypotonia, respiratory disturbances, and myoclonic seizures follow. Some newborns survive the acute illness, but their subsequent course is characterized by mental retardation, epilepsy, and spasticity (Trauner et al, 1983).

Diagnosis.   During the acute encephalopathy the EEG demonstrates a burst-suppression pattern, which evolves into hypsarrhythmia during infancy. Diagnosis is established by the demonstration of hyperglycinemia in the absence of hyperammonemia or organic acidemia.

Transitory hyperglycinemia, indistinguishable clinically and chemically from glycine encephalopathy, occurred in two newborns (Luder et al, 1989). One recovered in the second week and the other in the second month. The existence of such cases makes decisions concerning withdrawal of life support systems more difficult.

Treatment.   Exchange transfusion provides only temporary relief of the encephalopathy, and diet therapy has not proved successful in modifying the course. Diazepam, a competitor for glycine receptors, in combination with choline, folic acid, and sodium benzoate, may stop the seizures. Benzoate doses as high as 250 to 750 mg/kg are tolerated and should be tried (Nyhan, 1989).

Urea Cycle Disturbances

Carbamyl phosphate synthetase (CPS) deficiency, ornithine transcarbamylase (OTC) deficiency, citrullinemia, argininosuccinic acidemia, and *argininemia (arginase deficiency)* are the disorders caused by defects in the enzyme systems responsible for urea synthesis (Figure 1–5). Arginase deficiency does not produce symptoms in the newborn. OTC deficiency is an X-linked trait; all others are transmitted by autosomal recessive inheritance.

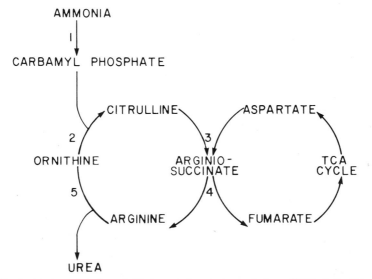

Figure 1–5 Ammonia metabolism. *1,* Carbamyl phosphate synthetase (CPS). *2,* Ornithine transcarbamylase (OTC). *3,* Argininosuccinate synthetase (AS). *4,* Argininosuccinate lyase (AL). *5,* Arginase. (From Fenichel GM: Neonatal Neurology. Churchill-Livingstone, 3rd edition, New York, 1990. By permission.)

Clinical Features. The clinical features of urea cycle disorders are due to ammonia intoxication (Table 1–6). Progressive lethargy, vomiting, and hypotonia may develop on the first postpartum day, even before the initiation of protein feeding, and are followed by progressive loss of consciousness and seizures on subsequent days. Vomiting and lethargy correlate well with plasma ammonia concentrations greater than 200 μg/dl (120 μmol/L); coma with concentrations greater than 300 μg/dl (180 μmol/L); and seizures with those greater than 500 μg/dl (300 μmol/L). Death follows quickly in untreated newborns.

Newborns with partial deficiency of CPS and female carriers of OTC deficiency may become symptomatic when given a large protein load.

Diagnosis. The diagnosis of a urea cycle disturbance should be suspected in every newborn with a compatible clinical syndrome and hyperammonemia without organic acidemia. Hyperammonemia can be life threatening, and diagnosis within 24 hours is essential (Bachmann, 1987). Blood ammonia concentration should be analyzed immediately, and plasma should be studied for acid-base status and concentrations of amino acids, creatinine, sodium, potassium, chloride, calcium, glucose, free and total carnitine, and lactate. A spot urine analysis should be performed for levels of amino acids, orotic acid, organic acids, and carnitine concentrations.

Definitive diagnosis requires identification of the specific enzyme defect in hepatic tissue or peripheral leuckocytes.

Treatment. Treatment cannot await specific diagnosis in newborns with symptomatic hyperammonemia caused by inborn errors of urea synthesis (Batshaw and Monahan, 1987). Nitrogen intake is limited to 1.2 to 2 g/kg/day, and a high percentage of the protein content should be essential amino acids. Arginine concentrations are low in all inborn errors of urea synthesis except for arginase deficiency and must be supplemented. Alternative pathways for nitrogen excretion must be provided. In addition to removal of ammonia by peritoneal dialysis or hemodialysis, waste nitrogen excretion through pathways other than urea synthesis can be promoted by sodium benzoate and phenylacetic acid. Nitrogen can be removed by

Table 1–6 ◆ Causes of Neonatal Hyperammonemia

Liver Failure

Primary Enzyme Defects in Urea Synthesis
1. Argininosuccinic acidemia
2. Carbamyl phosphate synthetase deficiency
3. Citrullinemia
4. Ornithine transcarbamylase deficiency

Other Disorders of Amino Acid Metabolism
1. Glycine encephalopathy
2. Isovaleric acidemia
3. Methylmalonic acidemia
4. Multiple carboxylase deficiency
5. Propionic acidemia

Transitory Hyperammonemia of Prematurity

peritoneal dialysis when blood ammonia concentrations become dangerously high.

Long-term management of disorders of urea synthesis requires a protein-restricted diet and arginine supplementation. Sodium benzoate and sodium phenylacetate (1.75 mmol/kg/day) should be continued as well. Even with optimal supervision, episodes of hyperammonemia may occur and may lead to coma and death (Brusilow et al, 1984). In such cases intravenous administration of sodium benzoate, sodium phenylacetate, and arginine, coupled with nitrogen-free alimentation, is indicated. Peritoneal dialysis or hemodialysis is indicated if the patient does not respond to drug therapy.

Organic Acid Disorders

Organic acid disorders are characterized by the accumulation of compounds, usually ketones or lactic acid, that cause acidosis in biologic fluids (Ozand and Gascon, 1991). More than 50 organic acid disorders have been described. They can be caused by abnormalities in vitamin metabolism, lipid metabolism, glycolysis, the citric acid cycle, oxidative metabolism, gluthathione metabolism, and 4-aminobutyric acid metabolism. The clinical presentations vary considerably and are described in several chapters.

Defects in the further metabolism of branched-chain amino acids are the organic acid disorders that most often cause neonatal seizures.

Isovaleric Acidemia

Isovaleric acid is a fatty acid derived from leucine. Its conversion to propionyl coenzyme A (CoA) is metabolized by the enzyme isovaleryl-CoA dehydrogenase (Figure 1–4). Isovaleric acidemia is transmitted by autosomal recessive inheritance, and the heterozygote state can be detected in cultured fibroblasts.

Clinical Features. Two phenotypes are associated with the same enzyme defect. One is an acute, overwhelming disorder of the newborn; the other is a chronic infantile form (Berry et al, 1988). Newborns are normal at birth but within a few days become lethargic, refuse to feed, and vomit. The clinical syndrome is similar to MSUD except that the urine is described as smelling like "sweaty feet" instead of maple syrup. Sixty percent of affected newborns die of ketoacidosis, pancytopenia, or intercurrent infection within 3 weeks. The survivors have a clinical syndrome identical to the chronic infantile phenotype.

Diagnosis. Isovaleric acidosis is detected by the excretion of isovaleryl-lysine in the urine. Isovaleryl-CoA dehydrogenase activity can be assayed in cultured fibroblasts. The clinical phenotype correlates not with the percentage of residual enzyme activity, but with the ability to detoxify isovaleryl-CoA with glycine.

Treatment. Dietary restriction of protein, especially leucine, decreases the occurrence of later psychomotor retardation. L-Carnitine, 50 mg/kg/day, is a beneficial supplement to the diet of some children with isovaleric acidemia. In acutely ill newborns, oral glycine, 250 to 500 mg/day, in addition to protein restriction and carnitine, lowers mortality.

Propionic Acidemia

Propionyl-CoA is formed as a catabolite of methionine, threonine, and the branched-chain amino acids. Its further carboxylation to D-methylmalonyl-CoA requires the enzyme propionyl-CoA carboxylase and the coenzyme biotin (Figure 1–4). Isolated deficiency of the enzyme causes propionic acidemia (Rosenberg and Fenton, 1989). The defect is transmitted as an autosomal recessive trait.

Clinical Features. Most affected children appear normal at birth; symptoms may begin as early as the first day post partum but can be delayed for months or years. In newborns the symptoms are nonspecific: feeding difficulty, lethargy, hypotonia, and dehydration. Recurrent attacks of profound metabolic acidosis often associated with hyperammonemia, which respond poorly to buffering, characterize the subsequent course. Untreated newborns rapidly become dehydrated, have generalized or myoclonic seizures, and become comatose.

Hepatomegaly caused by fatty infiltration occurs in 28% of patients. Neutropenia, thrombocytopenia, and occasionally pancytopenia may be present. A bleeding diathesis accounts for massive intracranial hemorrhage in some newborns.

Diagnosis. Propionic acidemia should be considered in any newborn with ketoacidosis but must also be considered in newborns with hyperammonemia and without ketoacidosis, since an erroneous diagnosis of carbamyl phosphate synthesis deficiency may be suggested. Propionic acidemia is the probable diagnosis when the plasma concentrations of glycine and propionate and the urinary concentrations of glycine, methylcitrate, and β-hydroxypropionate are increased. Although the urinary concentration of propionate may be normal, the plasma concentration is always elevated without a concurrent increase in the concentration of methylmalonate.

The definitive diagnosis of propionic acidemia requires the demonstration of deficiency enzyme activity in peripheral blood leukocytes or in skin fibroblasts. Prenatal diagnosis can be accomplished by the detection of methylcitrate, a unique metabolite of propionate, in the amniotic fluid, and by demonstration of deficient enzyme activity in amniotic fluid cells.

Treatment. The newborn in ketoacidosis requires dialysis to remove toxic metabolites, parenteral fluids to prevent dehydration, and protein-free nutrition. The frequency and severity of subsequent attacks are decreased by restricting protein intake to 0.5 to 1.5 g/kg/day. Oral administration of L-carnitine reduces the ketogenic response to fasting and may be useful as a daily supplement. Biotin supplementation is often used, although its benefit has not been established.

Methylmalonic Acidemia

D-Methylmalonyl-CoA is racemized to L-methylmalonyl-CoA by the enzyme D-methylmalonyl racemase and then isomerized to succinyl-CoA, which enters the tricarboxylic acid cycle. Isomerization is catalyzed by the enzyme D-methylmalonyl-CoA mutase, with the cobalamin (vitamin B_{12}) coenzyme adenosylcobalamin required as a cofactor. Several defects in this pathway are known; all are transmitted by autosomal recessive inheritance. Mutase deficiency is the most common abnormality (Rosenberg and Fenton, 1989). Propionyl-CoA, propionic acid, and methylmalonic acid accumulate and cause hyperglycinemia and hyperammonemia. Each of the enzyme defects responsible for methylmalonic acidemia is believed to be transmitted as an autosomal recessive trait.

Clinical Features. Affected children appear normal at birth. In 80% of those with complete mutase deficiency the symptoms appear during the first week post partum; those with defects in the synthesis of adenosylcobalamin generally show symptoms after 1 month. Symptoms include lethargy, failure to thrive, recurrent vomiting, dehydration, respiratory distress, and hypotonia after the initiation of protein feeding. Leukopenia, thrombocytopenia, and anemia are present in more than one half of patients. Intracranial hemorrhage may result from a bleeding diathesis. The outcome for newborns with complete mutase deficiency is usually poor. Most die within 2 months of diagnosis; survivors have recurrent acidosis, growth retardation, and mental retardation.

Diagnosis. The diagnosis should be suspected in any newborn with metabolic acidosis, especially if associated with ketosis, hyperammonemia, and hyperglycinemia. The diagnosis is confirmed by the demonstration of increased concentration of methylmalonate in the plasma and urine. The specific enzyme defect can be determined in fibroblasts. Techniques for prenatal detection are available.

Treatment. Treatment of newborns with mutase deficiency is confined to dietary therapy and management of metabolic disturbances as in propionic acidemia. Vitamin B_{12} supplementation is useful in some defects of adenosylcobalamin synthesis, and 1 mg of hydroxocobalamin should be administered while the definitive diagnosis is awaited. Treatment is then maintained with protein restriction (0.5 to 1.5 g/kg/day) and 1 mg hydroxocobalamin weekly. As in propionic acidemia, oral supplementation of L-carnitine reduces ketogenesis in response to fasting.

Herpes Simplex Encephalitis

Herpes genitalis (herpes simplex virus type 2, HSV-2) accounts for the majority of herpetic infections of the newborn. The newborn is most commonly infected during the second stage of labor by contact with maternal genital herpes. Symptomatic infections occur in 8% of newborns whose mothers have a history of recurrent genital HSV infection. The risk of fetal contamination at birth is highest (40%) when the mother acquires primary genital herpes during the pregnancy (Brown et al, 1987).

Clinical Features. The clinical spectrum of perinatal HSV infection is wide. Among symptomatic newborns, two thirds have disseminated disease and one third have localized involvement of the brain, eye, skin, or mouth. Whether disseminated or localized, approximately half of infections involve the central nervous system. The overall mortality rate is 62%, and 50% of survivors have permanent neurologic impairment.

Clinical manifestations may begin as early as the fifth day but usually appear in the second week. A vesicular rash is present in 30%, usually on the scalp after vertex presentation and on the buttocks after breech presentation. Conjunctivitis, jaundice, and a bleeding diathesis may be present. The first symptoms of encephalitis are irritability and seizures. Seizures may be focal or generalized and are frequently refractory to therapy. Neurologic deterioration is progressive and characterized by coma and quadriparesis.

Diagnosis. The EEG always shows abnormalities; a periodic pattern of slow waves or spike discharges. Examination of the cerebrospinal fluid reveals lymphocytic leukocytosis, red blood cells, and an elevated protein concentration.

A rising antibody titer in the newborn can be demonstrated by complement fixation. Because of the passive transfer of antibodies, a diagnosis of neonatal herpes infection requires the demonstration of specific IgM-HSV antibodies. Viral antigens may be demonstrated in cytologic smears from vesicles by immunofluorescence using monoclonal or polyclonal antibodies.

Treatment. The best treatment is prevention. Recurrent genital herpes in adults can be suppressed by administration of 800 mg of acyclovir as a single oral dose (Mostow et al, 1988). All women with genital herpes at term whose membranes are intact or ruptured for less than 4 hours should be delivered by cesarean section. Acyclovir, 10 mg/kg every 8 hours for 10 days, is recommended for therapy in the newborn, but the mortality rate remains 50% or greater in newborns with disseminated disease (Whitley et al, 1991).

Drug Withdrawal

Marijuana, alcohol, narcotic-analgesics, and hypnotic-sedatives are the drugs most commonly used during pregnancy. Marijuana and alcohol do not cause drug dependence in the fetus and are not associated with withdrawal symptoms. Hypnotic-sedatives, such as barbiturates, do not ordinarily produce withdrawal symptoms unless very large doses are ingested. Phenobarbital has a sufficiently long half-life in newborns that sudden withdrawal does not occur.

The prototype of narcotic withdrawal in the newborn is with heroin or methadone, but a similar syndrome occurs with codeine and propoxyphene.

Clinical Features. Symptoms of opiate withdrawal are more severe and tend to occur earlier in full-term (first 24 hours) than in premature (24 to 48 hours) newborns (Doberczak et al, 1991). The initial feature is a coarse tremor, present only during the waking state, that can shake an entire limb. This is followed by irritability; a shrill, high-pitched cry; and hyperactivity. The child seems hungry but has difficulty feeding and vomits afterward. Diarrhea and other symptoms of autonomic instability are common.

Myoclonic jerking is present in 10% to 25% of newborns undergoing withdrawal. Whether these movements are seizures or jitteriness is not clear. Definite seizures occur in less than 5%.

Maternal use of cocaine during pregnancy is associated with premature delivery, growth retardation, and microcephaly (Hadeed and Siegel, 1989). Newborns exposed to cocaine in utero or post partum through the breast milk often show features of cocaine intoxication, including tachycardia, tachypnea, hypertension, irritability, and tremulousness.

Diagnosis. Drug withdrawal should be suspected and anticipated in every newborn whose mother has a history of substance abuse. Even when such a history is not available, the combination of irritability, hyperactivity, and autonomic instability should provide a clue to diagnosis. Careful questioning of the mother concerning her use of prescription and nonprescription drugs is imperative. Specific drug identification is accomplished by blood and urine analyses.

Treatment. Symptoms remit spontaneously in 3 to 5 days, but appreciable mortality occurs among untreated newborns. Phenobarbital, 8 mg/kg/day, or chlorpromazine, 3 mg/kg/day, relieves symptoms and reduces mortality. Morphine, meperidine, opium, and methadone are not sufficiently secreted in breast milk to cause or relieve addiction in the newborn.

The occurrence of seizures does not in itself indicate a poor prognosis (Doberczak et al, 1988). Long-term outcome is closely related to the other risk factors associated with substance abuse in the mother.

Bilirubin Encephalopathy

Unconjugated bilirubin is bound to albumin in the blood. *Kernicterus*, a yellow discoloration of the brain especially severe in the basal ganglia and hippocampus, occurs when the serum unbound or free fraction becomes excessive. An excessive level of the free fraction in an otherwise healthy newborn is 20 mg/dl (340 μmol/L). Classic kernicterus was a complication of hemolytic disease, which is now uncommon. Other causes of hyperbilirubinemia in full-term newborns are generally managed without difficulty. The group now at greatest risk is critically ill premature infants with respiratory distress syndrome, acidosis, and sepsis. In such newborns a serum unbound level of 10 mg/dl (170 μmol/L) may be sufficient to cause bilirubin encephalopathy and even the albumin-bound fraction may pass the blood-brain barrier (Hansen and Bratlid, 1986).

Clinical Features. Three distinct clinical phases of bilirubin encephalopathy occur in full-term newborns with untreated hemolytic disease. Hypotonia, lethargy, and a poor sucking reflex are noted within 24 hours of delivery. Bilirubin staining of the brain is already evident in newborns who die during this first clinical phase. On the second or third day the newborn becomes febrile and shows increasing tone and opisthotonic posturing. Seizures are not a constant feature but may occur at this time. The third phase is characterized by apparent improvement with normalization of tone. This may cause second thoughts about the accuracy of the diagnosis, but the improvement is short lived. Evidence of neurologic dysfunction begins to appear toward the end of the second month and the symptoms become progressively worse throughout infancy.

In premature newborns the clinical presentation is more subtle and may lack the phases of increased tone and opisthotonos. The majority of affected premature infants are believed to die in the newborn period.

The typical clinical syndrome after the first year includes extrapyramidal dysfunction, usually athetosis, which occurs in virtually every case (see Chapter 14); disturbances of vertical gaze, upward more often than downward, in 90%; high-frequency hearing loss in 60%; and mental retardation in 25%.

Diagnosis.   In newborns with hemolytic disease a clinical diagnosis can be presumed on the basis of significant hyperbilirubinemia and a compatible evolution of symptoms. However, the diagnosis is difficult to establish in critically ill premature newborns, whose brain damage is more often caused by asphyxia and its consequences than by kernicterus.

The brainstem auditory evoked response (BAER) may be useful in assessing the severity of bilirubin encephalopathy and its response to treatment (Nakamura et al, 1985). The auditory nerve and pathways are especially susceptible to bilirubin encephalopathy. The generators of wave I and wave V of the BAER are the auditory nerve and the inferior colliculus, respectively. The latency of both waves increases in proportion to the concentration of free albumin and decreases after exchange transfusion.

Treatment.   Kernicterus can be prevented by maintaining serum bilirubin concentrations below the toxic range. Once kernicterus has occurred, further damage can be limited, but not reversed, by lowering serum bilirubin concentrations.

Pyridoxine Dependency

Pyridoxine dependency is a rare disorder transmitted as an autosomal recessive trait. It may be caused by impaired glutamic decarboxylase activity (Haenggeli et al, 1991).

Clinical Features.   Multifocal clonic seizures begin almost immediately after birth and progress rapidly to status epilepticus. However, a later onset, even after the first year, does not exclude the diagnosis. The seizures are refractory to standard anticonvulsants and respond only to pyridoxine. If pyridoxine supplementation is discontinued, seizures return within 3 weeks.

Diagnosis.   In most cases the diagnosis is suspected because a sibling was affected by the same syndrome and died. In the absence of a family history of the disorder the diagnosis need be considered only in newborns with continuous seizures. The infantile-onset variety may be characterized by intermittent myoclonic seizures, focal clonic seizures, or generalized tonic-clonic seizures. The EEG is continuously abnormal because of generalized or multifocal spike discharges. An intravenous injection of pyridoxine, 50 to 100 mg, stops the clinical seizure activity and often converts the EEG to normal in less than 10 minutes.

Pyridoxine-responsive seizures also occur in newborns of mothers treated with isoniazid. The onset of seizures is in the third week after delivery.

Treatment.   A lifelong dietary supplement of pyridoxine, which varies from 2 to 30 mg/kg/day, prevents further seizures. The higher dose is used during infancy and the smaller dose in childhood. Subsequent psychomotor development is best when treatment is initiated early, but this does not ensure a normal outcome.

Incontinentia Pigmenti (Bloch-Sulzberger Syndrome)

Incontinentia pigmenti is a rare neurocutaneous syndrome involving the skin, teeth, eyes, and central nervous system. It is probably transmitted as an X-linked trait lethal in the hemizygous male, but autosomal dominant transmission has not been excluded.

Clinical Features.   The female-to-male ratio is 20:1. An erythematous and vesicular rash resembling epidermolysis bullosa is present on the flexor surfaces of the limbs and lateral aspect of the trunk at birth or soon thereafter. Neurologic disturbances occur in less than half of cases. In newborns the prominent feature is the onset of seizures on the second or third day, often confined to one side of the body. The rash persists for the first few months and is replaced by a verrucous eruption that lasts weeks or months. Between 6 and 12 months of age, pigment is deposited in the previous area of rash in bizarre polymorphic arrangements. The pigmentation later regresses and may disappear.

Residual neurologic handicaps may include mental retardation, epilepsy, hemiparesis, and hydrocephalus. Two rare neurologic disturbances that may be associated with incontinentia pigmenti are (1) degeneration of anterior horn cells, producing clinical features similar to those of infantile spinal muscular atrophy (Larsen et al, 1987) (see Chapter 6), and (2) recurrent encephalomyelitis caused by transient loss of suppressor T cells (Brunquell, 1987).

Diagnosis. Information about the character and evolution of the rash is essential for diagnosis.

Treatment. Neonatal seizures caused by incontinentia pigmenti usually respond to standard anticonvulsant drugs.

Familial Neonatal Seizures

In some families several members experience neonatal seizures that generally remit with age. The trait is transmitted by autosomal dominant inheritance. Genetic heterogeneity is probable because the abnormal gene is localized to chromosome 20q in some but not all affected families (Ryan et al, 1991).

Clinical Features. Multifocal clonic seizures begin in a child who otherwise appears normal. The onset is usually in the first week but may be delayed as long as 4 weeks (Miles and Holmes, 1990). With or without treatment the seizures usually stop spontaneously within 3 weeks. Epilepsy develops later in life in 9% of affected newborns.

Diagnosis. The syndrome should be suspected when seizures develop without apparent cause in a healthy newborn. Laboratory tests, including the EEG, show no abnormalities. A family history of seizures is critical to diagnosis but may not be discovered until grandparents are interviewed; parents are frequently unaware that they had neonatal seizures.

A syndrome of clonic seizures, almost always on the fifth day, is also described in newborns lacking a family history of early seizures (Miles and Holmes, 1990). Whether this syndrome is a separate entity is not clear.

Treatment. Standard anticonvulsant therapy should be administered. After 4 weeks of complete seizure control the drug can be tapered and discontinued. If seizures return, a longer trial should be initiated.

TREATMENT OF NEONATAL SEIZURES

Animal studies have provided considerable evidence that continuous seizure activity, even in the normoxemic brain, may cause brain damage by inhibiting protein synthesis and breaking down polyribosomes. In human premature infants there is the additional concern that seizures increase cerebral blood flow and cause intraventricular hemorrhage.

Although seizure control is clearly in the child's best interest, anticonvulsant drugs are potentially harmful to the immature brain. Newborns with seizures that are difficult to control are presumably in this state because they already have brain damage. Toxic doses of multiple anticonvulsants are probably more harmful than the occasional seizure in a well-ventilated newborn and should be discouraged.

In premature infants, protein binding of anticonvulsant drugs may be impaired and the free fraction concentration may be toxic, whereas the measured protein-bound fraction appears therapeutic.

Phenobarbital

In newborns a unitary relationship exists between the intravenous dose of phenobarbital (measured in milligrams per kilogram of body weight) and the blood concentration (measured in milligrams per milliliter of blood or micromoles per liter). Approximately 40% of newborns with seizures respond to a phenobarbital blood concentration of 20 μg/ml (86 μmol/L) (Gilman et al, 1989). This level is achieved by a single intravenous loading dose of 20 mg/kg injected at a rate of 5 mg/min. Those who do not respond should be given additional boluses of 10 mg/kg to a total of 40 mg/kg. Phenobarbital monotherapy is effective in 70% to 85% of newborns with seizures when blood levels of 40 μg/ml are achieved. Either additional boluses of phenobarbital or a phenytoin load can be tried in refractory cases.

The half-life of phenobarbital in newborns varies from 50 to 200 hours, and additional doses should be administered only on the basis of current blood concentration information. After the tenth day the half-life shortens as the result of enzyme induction and a steady state is easier to achieve.

Phenytoin

Phenytoin should be administered to newborns only intravenously. Oral doses are poorly absorbed in newborns, and intramuscular doses are not absorbed at any age. A therapeutic blood concentration of 15 to 20 μg/ml (40 to 80 μmol/L) can be safely achieved by a single intravenous injection of 20 mg/kg at a rate of 0.5 mg/kg/min. The half-life is long during the first week, and further administration should be based on current knowledge of blood concentration. Most newborns require a maintenance dosage of 5 to 10 mg/kg/day.

Duration of Therapy

Seizures caused by an acute, self-limited encephalopathy, such as perinatal asphyxia, do not ordinarily require prolonged maintenance therapy. In most newborns seizures stop when the acute encephalopathy is over. No evidence suggests that continuous anticonvulsant therapy prevents the later development of epilepsy in newborns at risk. Therefore therapy should be discontinued after 2 weeks of complete seizure control. If seizures recur, anticonvulsant therapy can be reinitiated.

In contrast to newborns with seizures caused by acute encephalopathy, those with seizures caused by cerebral dysgenesis should be treated continuously. Eighty percent will be epileptic in childhood.

◆ Paroxysmal Disorders of Infancy

The pathophysiology of paroxysmal disorders is more varied in infants than in newborns

---

Table 1–7 ◆ Paroxysmal Disorders of Infancy

Apnea and Breathholding
1. Cyanotic
2. Pallid

Dystonia
1. Glutaric aciduria (see Chapter 14)
2. Transient paroxysmal dystonia of infancy

Migraine
1. Benign paroxysmal vertigo (see Chapter 10)
2. Cyclic vomiting
3. Paroxysmal torticollis (see Chapter 14)

Seizures
1. Febrile seizures
   a. Epilepsy triggered by fever
   b. Infection of the nervous system
   c. Simple febrile seizure
2. Nonfebrile seizures
   a. Generalized tonic-clonic seizures
   b. Partial seizures
      1. Benign
      2. Ictal laughter
3. Myoclonic seizures
   a. Infantile spasms
   b. Benign myoclonic epilepsy
   c. Severe myoclonic epilepsy
   d. Myoclonic status
   e. Lennox-Gastaut syndrome

(Table 1–7). Seizures, especially febrile seizures, remain the major cause of paroxysmal disorders, but apnea and syncope are relatively common as well. Infants with paroxysmal disorders are frequently referred for neurologic consultation because of the suspicion of seizures. The determination of which "spells" are seizures is often difficult and relies more on obtaining a complete description of the spell than on laboratory tests. The parents should be asked to provide a sequential history. If more than one spell occurred, they should first describe the one that was best observed or most recent. The following questions should be included: What was the child doing before the spell? Did anything provoke the spell? Did the child's color change? If so, when and what color? Did the eyes move in any direction? Was one part of the body affected more than another?

In addition to a home video of the spell, ambulatory EEG is useful to determine whether episodes of uncertain cause are seizures. Ambulatory EEG allows continuous recording at home and indicates whether the event in question is associated with epileptiform activity. In some children, prolonged split-screen video-EEG monitoring is the only way to identify the mechanism of paroxysmal activity.

APNEA AND SYNCOPE

Infant apnea is defined as cessation of breathing for 15 seconds or longer, or for less than 15 seconds if accompanied by bradycardia. Premature newborns with respiratory distress syndrome may continue to have apneic spells as infants, especially if they are neurologically abnormal. Persistent apnea is often thought to be a seizure manifestation, but EEG monitoring in children with this condition rarely demonstrates epileptiform activity in association with apneic spells or episodic tonic posturing.

Breathholding spells occur in almost 5% of children. They are a familial trait, probably transmitted by autosomal dominant inheritance with incomplete penetrance. Twenty-three percent of parents of affected children have a history of the condition. Cyanotic and pallid varieties, which occur with equal frequency, have been described. Most children experience only one or the other, but some have both.

Breathholding spells are involuntary responses to adverse stimuli. In approximately 80% of affected children the spells begin before 18 months of age, and in all cases spells start before 3 years of age. The last episode usually occurs by age 4 and no later than age 8.

Cyanotic Syncope

Clinical Features.   Cyanotic spells are usually provoked by anger, frustration, or fear. If the infant's sibling takes away a toy, the child cries and then stops breathing in expiration. Cyanosis develops rapidly, followed quickly by limpness and loss of consciousness. Occasionally cyanotic episodes are provoked by pain, and these may not be preceded by crying.

If the attack lasts only a few seconds, the infant may resume crying on awakening. Most spells, especially the ones referred for neurologic evaluation, are longer and are associated with tonic posturing of the body and clonic movements of the hands or arms. The eyes may roll upward. These movements are regarded as seizures by even experienced observers, but they are probably a brainstem release phenomenon not associated with abnormal electrical discharges.

After a short spell the child recovers rapidly and seems normal immediately; after a prolonged spell the child first arouses and then goes to sleep.

Once an infant begins having breathholding spells, the frequency increases for several months, then declines, and finally the spells cease.

Diagnosis.   The typical sequence of crying, cyanosis, and loss of consciousness is critical for diagnosis. Cyanotic syncope is often misdiagnosed as epilepsy because of lack of attention to the precipitating event. It is not sufficient to ask, "Did the child hold his breath?" The question conjures up the image of breathholding during inspiration. Instead, questioning should be focused on precipitating events, absence of breathing, facial color, and family history. The family may have a history of breathholding spells, febrile seizures, or both.

Between attacks the EEG shows no abnormalities. During an episode the EEG first shows diffuse slowing and then rhythmic slowing during the tonic-clonic activity.

Treatment.   No treatment is available to prevent future breathholding spells or to stop a spell in progress. The physician's major function is to identify the nature of the spell and explain that it is harmless. Children do not die during breathholding spells, and the episodes always cease spontaneously. (Does anyone know an adult who has breathholding spells?)

Pallid Syncope

Clinical Features.   Pallid syncope is a dramatic and frightening episode usually provoked by a sudden, unexpected, painful event such as a bump on the head. The child rarely cries but instead becomes white and limp and loses consciousness. Parents invariably believe the child is dead and begin mouth-to-mouth resuscitation. After the initial limpness the body may stiffen and clonic movements of the arms may occur. As in cyanotic syncope, these movements represent a brainstem release phenomenon and not seizure activity. The duration of the spell is difficult to determine. It is frightening to the observer, and seconds seem like hours. Afterward the child often falls asleep and is normal on awakening.

Diagnosis.   Pallid syncope is the result of reflex asystole. An attack sometimes can be provoked by pressure on the eyeballs to initiate a vagal reflex. I do not recommend provoking an attack as an office procedure, since the diagnosis can be made by history alone.

Treatment.   As with cyanotic spells, the major goal is to reassure the family that the child will not die during an attack. The physician must be very convincing.

SEIZURES
Febrile Seizures

An infant's first seizure often occurs at the time of fever. Three explanations are possible: (1) an infection of the nervous system; (2) an underlying seizure disorder in which the initial seizure is triggered by the stress of fever, although subsequent seizures may be afebrile; and (3) a *simple febrile seizure* (a genetic, age-limited epilepsy in which seizures are provoked only by fever). Infections of the nervous system are discussed in Chapters 2 and 4. The distinction between epilepsy and simple febrile seizures is often difficult and may require time rather than laboratory tests.

Clinical Features.   Febrile seizures, not caused by infection or other definable cause, occur in approximately 4% of children. Only 2% of children whose first seizure is associated with fever have nonfebrile seizures (epilepsy) by age 7. The most important predictor of subsequent epilepsy is an abnormal neurologic or developmental state. Complex seizures—defined as prolonged, focal, or multiple—slightly increase the probability of subsequent epilepsy.

A single, brief, generalized seizure occurring during the rise of fever is likely to be a simple febrile seizure. "Brief" and "fever" are difficult to define. Parents do not use a stopwatch, and when a child is having a seizure, seconds seem like minutes. Any child whose seizure is still in progress on arrival at the emergency room has had a prolonged seizure. Postictal sleep should not be counted as seizure time. Similarly, body temperature is not measured during a seizure and may be considerably different 30 minutes later.

Simple febrile seizures are familial and probably transmitted by autosomal dominant inheritance with incomplete penetrance. One third of infants who have a first simple febrile seizure will have a second at the time of a subsequent febrile illness, and half of these will have a third febrile seizure. The risk of recurrence is increased if the first febrile seizure occurs before 18 months of age or at a body temperature less than 40° C (El-Radhi and Banajeh, 1989). More than three episodes of simple febrile seizures are unusual and suggest that the child may later have nonfebrile seizures.

Diagnosis.   Any child who is thought to have an infection of the nervous system should undergo a lumbar puncture for examination of the cerebrospinal fluid. In approximately 15% of children with meningitis the initial manifestation is a febrile seizure, and infants may have no other signs of meningismus. However, a brief, generalized seizure from which the child recovers rapidly and completely is not caused by meningitis, especially if the fever subsides spontaneously or is otherwise explained.

Blood cell counts, measurements of glucose, calcium, and electrolytes, urinalysis, and EEG on a routine basis are not cost effective and should not be performed. The decision for laboratory testing can be individualized to the circumstances of the case. EEG should be performed on every infant who is neurologically abnormal or who has a family history of epilepsy. Magnetic resonance imaging (MRI) is indicated for infants with focal seizures or with focal deficits, even transitory, following a seizure.

Treatment.   Since only one third of children with an initial febrile seizure have a second seizure, treating every affected child is unreasonable. The low-risk group with a single, brief, generalized seizure should not be treated. No evidence has shown that a second seizure, even if prolonged, causes epilepsy or brain damage.

As a rule, I recommend anticonvulsant prophylaxis only if I believe the child has a condition other than simple febrile seizures. I follow these guidelines:

1. Infants with an abnormal neurologic state or a focal seizure should be considered candidates for prophylactic anticonvulsant therapy.
2. When the initial febrile seizure is multiple or prolonged but the child recovers rapidly and completely, treatment is not indicated unless the family has a history of nonfebrile seizures.
3. Infants who have had two prolonged or more than three brief febrile seizures are candidates for prophylactic anticonvulsant therapy.
4. A family history of simple febrile seizures is a relative contraindication to therapy in the situations just listed.

Rectal administration of diazepam, 0.5 mg/kg, at the time of febrile illness is a reasonable alternative to daily prophylaxis in children with frequent or prolonged simple febrile seizures. Phenobarbital prophylaxis, the usual treatment choice for infants with seizures other than the simple febrile type, is not significantly better than no treatment in reducing the recurrence rate of simple febrile seizures (McKinlay and Newton, 1989).

Nonfebrile Seizures

Disorders that produce nonfebrile tonic-clonic or partial seizures in infancy are not substantially different from those that cause nonfebrile seizures in childhood (see the section that follows). Major risk factors for the development of epilepsy in infancy and childhood are congenital malformations, neonatal seizures, and a family history of epilepsy.

A complex partial seizure syndrome that has its onset during infancy, sometimes in the newborn period, is ictal laughter associated with hypothalamic hamartoma (Berkovic et al, 1988). The attacks are brief, occur several times a day, and may be characterized by pleasant laughter or giggling. At first the laughter is thought to be normal, but then facial flushing and pupillary dilation are noted. With time the child begins to have drop attacks, generalized seizures, and personality change. Precocious puberty may be an associated condition.

A first partial motor seizure under the age of 2 is associated with a recurrence rate of 87%, whereas afterward the rate is 51% (Hirtz et al, 1984). The recurrence rate after a first nonfebrile, nonsymptomatic, generalized seizure is 60% to 70% at all ages (Elwes et al, 1985). The younger the age at onset of a nonfebrile seizure of any type, the more likely that the seizure is symptomatic rather than idiopathic.

Approximately 25% of children who have recurent seizures during the first year, excluding neonatal seizures and infantile spasms, are developmentally or neurologically abnormal at the time of the first seizure (Matsumoto et al, 1983). The initial EEG has prognostic significance; normal EEG results are associated with a favorable neurologic outcome.

Intractable seizures in children less than 2 years of age are often associated with later mental retardation (Huttenlocher and Hapke, 1990). The following relationship exists between the seizure type and probability of mental retardation: tonic-clonic 78%, myoclonic 94%, complex partial 60%, and simple partial 61%.

A benign complex partial epilepsy has been described in infants, with onset as early as 3 months (Watanabe et al, 1987). The seizures are characterized by motion arrest, decreased responsiveness, staring or blank eyes, and mild convulsive movements of the limbs. They are readily controlled with phenobarbital or carbamazepine and may disappear spontaneously within 2 to 4 years. The family generally has a history of benign early-onset seizures.

Infantile Spasms

Infantile spasms are age-dependent myoclonic seizures that occur with an incidence of 25 per 100,000 live births in the United States and Western Europe. An underlying cause can be determined in approximately 75% of patients; congenital malformations and perinatal asphyxia are common causes, and tuberous sclerosis accounts for 20% of cases in some series (Table 1–8). Despite considerable concern in the past, pertussis immunization is not a cause of infantile spasms (Institute of Medicine, 1991). The combination of infantile spasms, hypsarrhythmia, and mental retardation is sometimes referred to as *West syndrome*.

Clinical Features. The peak age of onset is between 4 and 7 months, and onset always occurs before 1 year of age. The spasm can be a flexor or an extensor movement; some children have both.

Spasms generally occur in clusters, shortly after the infant awakens from sleep, and are not activated by stimulation. A rapid flexor spasm involving the neck, trunk, and limbs is followed by a tonic contraction sustained for 2 to 10 seconds. Less severe flexor spasms are characterized only by dropping of the head and abduction of the arms or by flexion at the waist resembling colic. Extensor spasms resemble the second component of the Moro reflex: the head moves backward and the arms are suddenly spread. Whether flexor or extensor, the movement is almost always symmetric and brief.

When the cause of spasms is identifiable (symptomatic spasms), the infant is usually abnormal neurologically or developmentally when the spasms begin. Microcephaly is common in this group. Prognosis depends on the cause, but as a rule the symptomatic group does poorly: only 5% have normal development or only mild impairment (Glaze et al, 1988).

Idiopathic spasms characteristically occur in children who had been developing normally at the onset of spasms and have no history of prenatal or perinatal disorders. Neurologic findings, including head circumference, are normal. Approximately 40% of children with idiopathic spasms are neu-

---

Table 1–8 ◆ Neurocutaneous Disorders Causing Seizures in Infancy

Incontinentia Pigmenti
1. Seizure type
   a. Neonatal seizures
   b. Generalized tonic-clonic
2. Cutaneous manifestations
   a. Erythematous bullae (newborn)
   b. Pigmentary whorls (infancy)
   c. Depigmentated areas (childhood)

Linear Nevus Sebaceous Syndrome
1. Seizure type
   a. Infantile spasms
   b. Lennox-Gastaut syndrome
   c. Generalized tonic-clonic
2. Cutaneous manifestation
   a. Linear facial sebaceous nevus

Neurofibromatosis
1. Seizure type
   a. Generalized tonic-clonic
   b. Partial complex
   c. Partial simple motor
2. Cutaneous manifestations
   a. Café au lait spots
   b. Axillary freckles
   c. Neural tumors

Sturge-Weber Syndrome
1. Seizure type
   a. Epilepsia partialis continuans
   b. Partial simple motor
   c. Status epilepticus
2. Cutaneous manifestation
   a. Hemifacial hemangioma

Tuberous Sclerosis
1. Seizure type
   a. Neonatal seizures
   b. Infantile spasms
   c. Lennox-Gastaut syndrome
   d. Generalized tonic-clonic
   e. Partial simple motor
   f. Partial complex
2. Cutaneous manifestations
   a. Abnormal hair pigmentation
   b. Adenoma sebaceum
   c. Café au lait spots
   d. Depigmented areas
   e. Shagren patch

rologically normal or only mildly retarded subsequently.

Diagnosis. There is often considerable delay between spasm onset and diagnosis. Infantile spasms are so unlike the usual perception of seizures that even experienced pediatricians may be slow to realize the significance of the movements. Colic is often considered and treated for several weeks before seizures are suspected.

Infantile spasms must be differentiated from benign myoclonus of early infancy, benign myoclonic epilepsy of infants, severe myoclonic epilepsy of infancy, and the Lennox-Gastaut syndrome (Table 1–9). However, there is some reason to believe that infantile spasms, severe myoclonic encephalopathy, and the Lennox-Gestaut syndrome are a continuum of epileptic encephalopathies (Donat, 1992).

The EEG is the single most important test for diagnosis. However, EEG findings vary with duration of recording, sleep state, and underlying disorder (Hrachovy et al, 1984). Hypsarrhythmia is the usual pattern recorded during the early stages of infantile spasms. It is characterized by a chaotic and continuously abnormal background of very high-voltage and random slow waves and spikes. The spikes vary in location from moment to moment and at times become generalized, but they are never repetitive. Typical hypsarrhythmia is most often recorded during wakefulness or active sleep. During quiet sleep, greater interhemispheric synchrony occurs and the background may have a burst-suppression appearance.

The EEG may transiently become normal immediately on arousal, but when spasms occur, either an abrupt attenuation of the background or high-voltage slow waves appear.

Within a few weeks the original chaotic pattern of hypsarrhythmia is replaced by greater interhemispheric synchrony. The distribution of epileptiform discharges changes from multifocal to generalized, and the generalized discharges are followed by attenuation of the record.

Treatment. Hormonal therapy with adrenocorticotropic hormone (ACTH) or corticosteroids is effective in stopping infantile spasms, but it need not be used in every case (Aicardi, 1989). Hormonal therapy does not affect outcome in infants whose spasms are due to prenatal or perinatal brain abnormalities. In such infants clonazepam or nitrazepam should be tried first and usually proves effective, at least temporarily (Dreifuss et al, 1986). Valproate monotherapy controls spasms in 70% of infants when doses of 100 to 300 mg/kg are used (Prats et al, 1991). I prescribe valproate only as a last resort in this age group because of an unacceptable rate of fatal hepatotoxicity.

If clonazepam fails, hormonal therapy should be initiated. However, clonazepam should be continued in neurologically abnormal infants; ACTH or prednisone usually provides only temporary respite from seizures, and long-term anticonvulsant therapy is needed. The ideal dose and duration of ACTH or prednisone have not been established. Most reports favor smaller doses than previously recommended: ACTH gel, 20 IU/day by intramuscular injection, or oral prednisone, 2 mg/kg/day for 2 weeks and then a tapered dose and discontinuation in the following 2 weeks.

Some physicians believe that all infants with idiopathic infantile spasms who are neurologically and developmentally normal at the onset of spasms should be given ACTH as treatment of the underlying cause. However, no experimental data to support that notion have been presented, and some evidence to the contrary has been reported (Glaze et al, 1988).

The response to hormonal therapy is never graded; control is either complete or not at all. Even when the response is favorable, one third have relapses during or after the course of treatment. Failure to respond and relapse occur more often in symptomatic than idiopathic cases. A second course of treatment proves effective in 75% of cases in which the first course was successful, albeit at the price of increased adverse reactions.

High-dose pyridoxine should be considered in the treatment of infantile spasms when ACTH fails initially or relapses occur. Some cases of infantile spasms or other seizures of infancy may be atypical presentations of pyridoxine-dependent seizures (Goutieres and Aicardi, 1985). However, in most cases the anticonvulsant properties of pyridoxine and ACTH are unrelated to their physiologic func-

Table 1–9 ◆ Electroencephalographic (EEG) Appearance in Myoclonic Seizures of Infancy

Seizure Type	EEG Appearance
Infantile spasms	Hypsarrhythmia Slow spike and wave Burst-suppression
Benign myoclonus	Normal
Benign myoclonic epilepsy	Spike and wave (3 cps) Polyspike and wave (3 cps)
Severe myoclonic epilepsy	Polyspike and wave (>3 cps)
Lennox-Gastaut syndrome	Spike and wave (2-2.5 cps) Polyspike and wave (2-2.5 cps)

tions. The recommended dose of pyridoxine is 30 to 40 mg/kg/day.

Some children with idiopathic infantile spasms are shown by positron emission tomography to have unilateral foci of hypometabolism in the parietotemporooccipital region (Chugani et al, 1990). Surgical removal of the hypometabolic area, which usually proves to contain dysplastic tissue, provides seizure control.

Benign Myoclonus of Infancy

Clinical Features. Many series of patients with infantile spasms include a small number with normal EEG results. Such infants cannot be distinguished from others with infantile spasms by clinical features because the age at onset and the appearance of the movements are the same. The spasms occur in clusters, frequently at mealtime. Clusters increase in intensity and severity over weeks or months and then abate spontaneously. After 3 months the spasms usually stop altogether, and although occasional episodes may recur, no spasms occur after 2 years of age. Affected infants are normal neurologically and developmentally and remain so afterward. The term "benign myoclonus" is used because the spasms are believed to be an involuntary movement and not a seizure.

Diagnosis. A normal EEG result distinguishes this group from other causes of myoclonus in infancy. The CT findings are also normal.

Treatment. Infants who are neurologically normal and have normal EEGs should not be treated.

Benign Myoclonic Epilepsy

Clinical Features. Benign myoclonic epilepsy is a rare disorder of uncertain cause. A genetic basis is presumed because one third of patients have family members with epilepsy. Onset is between 4 months and 2 years of age. Affected infants are neurologically normal at onset of seizures and remain so afterward. The seizures are characterized by brief myoclonic attacks, which may be restricted to head nodding or may be so severe as to throw the infant to the floor. The head drops to the chest, eyes roll upward, arms are thrown upward and outward, and legs flex (Dravet et al, 1985a). Myoclonic seizures may be single or repetitive, but consciousness is not lost. No other seizure types are observed in infancy, but generalized tonic-clonic seizures may occur in adolescence.

Diagnosis. During a seizure the EEG demonstrates generalized 3 cps spike-wave or poly-spike-wave discharges. Sensory stimuli do not activate seizures. The pattern is consistent with primary, generalized epilepsy.

Treatment. Valproate produces complete seizure control. If left untreated, seizures may persist for years. The use of valproate is potentially dangerous in infants because of hepatotoxicity, but barbiturates and benzodiazepines are not effective.

Severe Myoclonic Epilepsy

Severe myoclonic epilepsy is an important but poorly understood disorder. A seemingly healthy infant has a seizure and then progressive neurologic deterioration that ends in a chronic brain damage syndrome. Because its nature is unknown, this disorder is blamed on any and all preceding events. It is often, but improperly, blamed on immunization.

Clinical Features. A family history of epilepsy is present in 25% of cases. The first seizures are frequently febrile, are usually prolonged, and can be generalized or focal clonic in type. Febrile and nonfebrile seizures recur, sometimes as status epilepticus (Dravet et al, 1985b). Generalized myoclonic seizures appear after 1 year of age. At first mild and difficult to recognize as a seizure manifestation, they later become frequent and repetitive and disturb function. Partial complex seizures with secondary generalization may also occur.

Coincident with the onset of myoclonic seizures are the slowing of development and the gradual appearance of ataxia and hyperreflexia.

Diagnosis. The initial differential diagnosis is febrile seizures. Because the febrile seizures are usually prolonged and sometimes focal, epilepsy should be suspected. A specific diagnosis is not possible until the appearance of myoclonic seizures in the second year.

Interictal EEG findings are normal at first. Paroxysmal abnormalities appear in the second year and are characterized by generalized spike-wave and polyspike-wave complexes with a frequency greater than 3 cps. Discharges are activated by photic stimulation, drowsiness, and quiet sleep.

Treatment. The seizures are resistant to therapy with anticonvulsant drugs. Valproate and benzodiazepines should be tried first. Carbamazepine may increase seizure frequency.

Lennox-Gastaut Syndrome

Lennox-Gastaut syndrome is characterized by the triad of seizures (atypical absence, atonic, and myoclonic), slow spike-wave complexes on EEG, and mental retardation. In most patients the seizures are secondary to underlying brain damage, but some are primary epilepsies. Some authorities reserve the term *myoclonic-astatic epilepsy* for Lennox-Gastaut syndrome that is due to primary epilepsy.

Clinical Features. The peak age at onset is 3 to 5 years; less than half of cases begin before 2 years of age. An underlying cause can be identified in approximately 60%; neurocutaneous disorders, perinatal disturbances, and postnatal brain injuries are most common. Twenty percent of children with the Lennox-Gastaut syndrome have a history of infantile spasms, sometimes with a seizure-free interval before development of the syndrome.

Although the syndrome can begin in a normal child, most children are identified as neurologically abnormal before its onset. The first seizures may be generalized tonic-clonic or focal clonic but are usually tonic. Tonic seizures are characterized by stiffening of the body, upward deviation of the eyes, dilation of the pupils, and alteration in the respiratory pattern. The seizures frequently occur during sleep, and enuresis may be an associated condition.

Atypical absence seizures occur in almost every patient. In addition to the stare, trembling of the eyelids and mouth occurs, followed by loss of facial tone so that the head leans forward and the mouth hangs open. Atonic seizures are characterized by sudden dropping of the head or body, at times throwing the child to the ground. More than 90% of patients are mentally retarded by 5 years of age.

Diagnosis. An EEG is essential for diagnosis. The characteristic feature during atypical absence or atonic seizures is a generalized burst of 2 to 2.5 cps spike-wave complexes. Tonic seizures are associated with 1 cps slow waves followed by generalized rapid discharges without postictal depression.

In addition to EEG, a thorough evaluation is needed to look for an underlying cause. Special attention should be given to skin manifestations suggesting a neurocutaneous syndrome (Table 1–8). MRI is useful for the diagnosis of congenital malformations, postnatal disorders, and neurocutaneous syndromes.

Treatment. Seizures are difficult to control. Valproate and clonazepam are the drugs most often effective. ACTH may provide transitory relief.

MIGRAINE

Clinical Features. Migraine attacks are uncommon in infancy, but when they occur, the clinical features are often "paroxysmal" and suggest the possibility of seizures. Cyclic vomiting is prob-

ably the most common manifestation. Attacks of vertigo (see Chapter 10) or torticollis (see Chapter 14) may be especially perplexing, and some infants have attacks in which they rock back and forth and appear uncomfortable.

Diagnosis. Migrainous vertigo *(benign paroxysmal vertigo)* is sufficiently stereotyped in presentation to be recognizable as a migraine variant. Other syndromes often remain undiagnosed until the episodes evolve into a typical migraine pattern. A history of migraine in one parent, usually the mother, is essential for diagnosis.

Treatment. Antimigraine drugs are generally not used in infants.

TRANSIENT PAROXYSMAL DYSTONIA OF INFANCY

Clinical Features. Transient paroxysmal dystonia of infancy is a nonfamilial disorder characterized by episodes of opisthotonos and symmetric or asymmetric dystonia of limbs, without alteration in consciousness. Onset is between 6 and 22 months of age (Angelini et al, 1988). At first the episodes usually last for several minutes but may last as long as 2 hours. Later the episodes increase in duration (up to 7 days) and frequency and are characterized by torsion dystonia of the neck and trunk. Eventually the episodes decrease in frequency and disappear. Afterward the child is neurologically and developmentally normal.

Diagnosis. The disorder must be differentiated from familial choreoathetosis and from glutaric aciduria (see Chapter 14). EEG findings during an episode is normal as are levels of serum electrolytes and organic acids.

Treatment. Treatment is not needed to ensure a favorable outcome, but centrally acting muscle relaxants may be useful during prolonged episodes.

◆ Paroxysmal Disorders of Childhood

Like infants, children with paroxysmal disorders are generally thought to have seizures until proven otherwise. Seizures are the most common paroxysmal disorder requiring medical consultation. Syncope, especially presyncope, is considerably more common but is generally diagnosed and managed at home unless associated symptoms suggest a seizure.

The prevalence of migraine in childhood is 10 times greater than epilepsy. Migraine syndromes that may suggest epilepsy are described in Chapters 2, 3, 10, 11, 14, and 15.

Sleep disorders often have a paroxysmal quality and may be confused with complex partial seizures. Adding to the confusion is the fact that complex partial seizures are often activated by sleep.

SYNDROMES SIMULATING SEIZURES
Syncope

Syncope is loss of consciousness because of a transitory decline in cerebral blood flow. This may be caused by an irregular cardiac rate or rhythm or by alterations of blood volume or distribution.

Clinical Features. Syncope is a common event in otherwise healthy children, especially in the second decade. The mechanism is a vasovagal reflex by which an emotional experience produces peripheral pooling of blood. The reflex may also be stimulated by overextension or sudden decompression of viscera, by the Valsalva maneuver, and by stretching with the neck hyperextended. Fainting in a hot, crowded church is especially common, when the worshiper rises to stand after prolonged kneeling.

Healthy children do not faint while lying down and rarely while seated. Fainting from anything but standing or arising suggests a cardiac arrhythmia and requires further investigation.

The child may first feel faint (described as "faint," "dizzy," or "lightheaded") or may lose consciousness without warning. Color drains from the face, and the skin becomes cold and clammy. With loss of consciousness the child falls to the floor. Consciousness may be regained rapidly, or stiffening of the body and clonic movements of the arms may occur. The latter is not a seizure. Afterward there may be a short period of confusion, but recovery is complete within minutes.

Diagnosis. The criteria for differentiating syncope from seizures are the precipitating factors and the child's appearance. Seizures do not produce pallor and cold, clammy skin. Laboratory investigations are not cost effective when syncope occurs in expected circumstances and the results of clinical examination are normal. Recurrent orthostatic syncope requires investigation of autonomic function, and any suspicion of cardiac abnormality deserves EKG monitoring.

Treatment. Infrequent syncopal episodes of obvious cause do not require treatment.

Hyperventilation Syndrome

Hyperventilation induces alkalosis by altering the proportion of blood gases. This is more readily accomplished in children than adults.

Clinical Features. During times of emotional upset, respiratory rate and depth may increase insidiously, first appearing like sighing and then as obvious hyperventilation. The occurrence of tingling of the fingers disturbs the patient further and may induce greater hyperventilation. Headache is an associated symptom. If hyperventilation is allowed to continue, the patient may lose consciousness.

Diagnosis. The observation of hyperventilation as a precipitating factor of syncope is essential to diagnosis. Often patients are unaware that they were hyperventilating, and probing questions are needed to elicit the history in the absence of a witness.

Treatment. An attack in progress can be aborted by having the patient breathe into a paper bag.

Narcolepsy-Cataplexy

Narcolepsy-cataplexy is a sleep disorder characterized by an abnormally short latency from sleep onset to rapid eye movement (REM) sleep. REM sleep is attained in less than 20 minutes instead of the usual 90 minutes. Normal REM sleep is characterized by dreaming and severe hypotonia. In narcolepsy-cataplexy these phenomena occur during wakefulness.

Clinical Features. Onset may occur at any time from early childhood to middle adulthood, but in 60% the syndrome begins before 20 years of age. (Kales et al, 1982). The syndrome has four components:

1. *Narcolepsy* refers to short sleep attacks. Three or four attacks occur each day, most often during monotonous activity, and are difficult to resist. Half of patients are easy to arouse from a sleep attack, and 60% feel refreshed afterward. Narcolepsy is usually a lifelong condition.
2. *Cataplexy* is a sudden loss of muscle tone induced by laughter, excitement, or startle. Almost all patients who have narcolepsy have cataplexy as well. The patient may collapse to the floor and then arise immediately. Partial paralysis, affecting just the face or hands, is more common than total paralysis. Two to four attacks occur daily, usually in the afternoon. They are embarrassing but do not cause physical harm.
3. *Sleep paralysis* occurs in the transition between sleep and wakefulness. The patient has generalized hypotonia and, although mentally awake, is unable to move any body part. Partial paralysis is less common. The attack may end spontaneously or when the

patient is touched. Two thirds of patients with narcolepsy-cataplexy also experience sleep paralysis once or twice each week. Occasional episodes of sleep paralysis may occur in people who do not have narcolepsy-cataplexy.

4. *Hypnagogic hallucinations* are vivid, usually frightening, visual and auditory perceptions occurring at the transition between sleep and wakefulness: a sensation of dreaming while awake. They are reported as an associated event by half of patients with narcolepsy-cataplexy. Episodes occur less than once a week.

Diagnosis. The syndrome should be recognizable by history. However, the symptoms are embarrassing or sound "crazy" to the patient and considerable prompting is often needed to elicit a full history.

Narcolepsy can be difficult to distinguish from other causes of excessive daytime sleepiness. The multiple sleep latency test is the standard for diagnosis. Patients with narcolepsy enter REM sleep within a few minutes of falling asleep.

Treatment. Symptoms of narcolepsy-cataplexy are distressing, and in many cases emotional problems develop. The realization that narcolepsy is not a mental disorder is comforting.

Amphetamine or methylphenidate is usually prescribed for narcolepsy but should be given with some caution because of potential abuse (Aldrich, 1990). Small doses should be used on schooldays or workdays and no medicine, if possible, on weekends and holidays. When not taking medicine, patients should be encouraged to schedule short naps.

Cataplexy can be treated with trihexyphenidyl, 2 mg three times a day, or imipramine, 50 mg three times a day.

Night Terrors

Night terrors are a partial arousal from non–rapid eye movement (non-REM) sleep.

Clinical Features. The onset usually occurs by 4 years of age and almost always by age 6. Two hours after falling asleep the child awakens in a terrified state, does not recognize people, and is inconsolable. An episode usually lasts for 5 to 15 minutes but can last an hour. During this time the child screams incoherently, may run if not restrained, and then goes back to sleep. Afterward the child has no memory of the event.

Most children with night terrors experience an average of one or more episodes each week. Night terrors stop by 8 years of age in one half of affected

children but continue into adolescence in one third (DiMario and Emery, 1986).

Diagnosis. Half of children with night terrors are also sleepwalkers, and many have a family history of either sleepwalking or night terrors. The diagnosis should be based on the history alone. A sleep laboratory evaluation may be helpful in unusual circumstances when the possibility of seizures cannot be excluded.

Treatment. Treatment is seldom needed, and regular bedtime sedation should be avoided except when spells are very frequent and intolerable to the family.

Startle Disease

Startle disease, also called *hyperekplexia*, is a rare disorder transmitted as an autosomal dominant trait (Andermann and Andermann, 1988).

Clinical Features. The onset is at birth or during infancy. When the onset is at birth, the newborn may appear hypotonic during sleep and develop generalized stiffening on awakening. Apnea and an exaggerated startle response may be associated signs. Hypertonia in the newborn is unusual and has a limited differential diagnosis (see Table 8–5). Rigidity diminishes but does not disappear during sleep. Tendon reflexes are brisk, and there is an increased spread of response.

The stiffness resolves spontaneously during infancy, and by 3 years of age the children are normal. However, episodes of stiffness may recur during adolescence or early adult life in response to startle, cold exposure, or pregnancy. A prominent startle response and nocturnal myoclonus are present throughout adult life.

Throughout life, affected individuals demonstrate a pathologically exaggerated startle response to visual, auditory, or tactile stimuli that would not startle normal individuals. In some the startle is associated with a transitory, generalized stiffness of the body that causes falling without protective reflexes, often leading to injury. The stiffening response is often confused with the stiff-man syndrome (see Chapter 8).

Diagnosis. A family history of startle disease is critical to the diagnosis but may be difficult to elicit because of partial expression or embarrassment. Epileptiform activity is not present on EEG, but an evoked response from the centroparietal region may be recorded at the time of startle.

Treatment. Valproate or clonazepam is useful in abolishing the falling attacks and reducing the startle. The natural history of the disease is variable; some children improve spontaneously, but others get worse.

Familial Paroxysmal Choreoathetosis

Familial paroxysmal choreoathetosis is transmitted by autosomal dominant inheritance. It is often regarded as a form of "reflex" epilepsy because the paroxysms are stimulus provoked and often responsive to prophylactic treatment with anticonvulsant drugs. However, the EEG does not demonstrate epileptiform activity, even during an attack (Lance, 1977).

Clinical Features. The age at onset varies from infancy to the third decade. The paroxysms, which are precipitated by sudden movement or startle, usually last less than 2 minutes but can continue for several hours. Each attack may include dystonia, choreoathetosis, or ballismus (see Chapter 14). One or both sides of the body can be affected. Some children have an "aura" described as tightness or tingling of the face or limbs. Attack frequency varies from once or twice each week to more than 100 each day. Consciousness is preserved during attacks. The disorder does not affect the life span.

In some families attacks are prolonged, not necessarily provoked by startle, and poorly responsive to anticonvulsants. Whether such families have a similar or different disease has not been determined.

Diagnosis. Approximately one fourth of cases are sporadic, some may be new mutations, and others are not genetic and may represent transient paroxysmal dystonia of infancy or idiopathic hypoparathyroidism (Barabas and Tucker, 1988). Serum calcium and phosphorus levels should be determined, and CT is useful to look for basal ganglia calcification.

Ictal and interictal EEGs show no abnormalities or demonstrate diffuse background slowing. Children with EEG evidence of epileptiform activity should be considered to have a seizure disorder and not familial paroxysmal choreoathetosis.

Treatment. Phenytoin or phenobarbital in ordinary anticonvulsant doses is effective in most cases.

MIGRAINE AND EPILEPSY

Migraine and epilepsy are thought to be linked because (1) they are both familial, paroxysmal, and associated with transitory neurologic disturbances, (2) there is an increased incidence of epilepsy in migraine sufferers and migraine in epileptics, (3) headache can be a seizure manifestation, and (4) abnormal EEGs occur in both disorders.

Clinical Features. In children who have epilepsy and migraine, both disorders may share a common aura and one may provoke the other. Basilar migraine (see Chapter 10) and benign occipital epilepsy best exemplify the fine line between epilepsy and migraine. Both are characterized by seizures, headache, and epileptiform activity.

Diagnosis. Asymptomatic central spikes are observed in 9% of children with migraine as compared with 1.9% of healthy children. Fourteen-and-six positive spikes, a normal adolescent pattern, is twice as common in children with migraine as in age-matched control subjects.

Treatment. Children who have both epilepsy and migraine must be treated for each condition separately.

STARING SPELLS

Daydreaming is a pleasant escape for people of all ages. Children feel the need for escape most acutely when in school, and they may stare vacantly out the window to the place they would rather be. Daydreams can be hard to break, and a child may not respond to verbal commands. Many dreamers are seen by neurologists, who may recommend EEG. Sometimes the EEG shows sleep-activated central spikes or another abnormality not related to staring, which may result in inappropriate anticonvulsant drug therapy.

Absence (petit mal) and complex partial seizures are characterized by staring. They have characteristic clinical and EEG features that establish the diagnosis. Precise diagnosis should be made in every case before treatment is initiated.

Absence Epilepsy

The term *petit mal* has been used generically for all small seizures in which consciousness is not lost. Such use of the term is not helpful and may lead to the wrong choice of anticonvulsant drug. "Absence" is the preferred term for generalized seizures characterized by staring. Absence epilepsy is a genetic disorder, transmitted as an autosomal dominant trait with age-dependent penetrance. The EEG is characteristic, and specific drug therapy is available.

Clinical Features. The peak age at onset is usually between 4 and 8 years with a range between 3 and 12 years. Absence never begins after 20 years of age but may persist from childhood into the seventh and eighth decades. Girls are affected more often than boys. Affected children are otherwise healthy.

The reported incidence of epilepsy in families of children with absence varies from 15% to 40%. Concurrence in monozygotic twins is 75% for seizures and 85% for the characteristic EEG abnormality.

Typical attacks last 5 to 10 seconds and occur up to 100 times each day. The child stops ongoing activity, stares vacantly, sometimes with rhythmic movements of the eyelids, and then resumes activity. There is never an aura or a period of postictal confusion. Longer seizures may last up to a minute and are indistinguishable by observation alone from complex partial seizures. Associated features may include myoclonus, increased or decreased postural tone, picking at clothes, turning of the head, and conjugate movements of the eyes. Occasional children and adults are brought to emergency rooms in a confusional state caused by absence status (see Chapter 2).

Approximately 50% of children with absence have at least one generalized tonic-clonic seizure. Some are actually brought for medical care because of a tonic-clonic seizure, even though absence attacks have occurred undiagnosed for months or years. The occurrence of a generalized tonic-clonic seizure does not change the diagnosis, prognosis, or treatment plan.

Diagnosis. The EEG is pathognomonic. Bilaterally synchronous and symmetric paroxysms of 3 cps spike-wave complexes appear concurrent with the clinical seizure (Figure 1–6). The amplitude of discharge is greatest in the frontocentral regions. Although the discharge begins with a frequency of 3 cps, it may slow to 2 cps as it ends. Hyperventilation almost always activates the discharge. The interictal EEG is usually normal. When it is abnormal, the typical features are focal or multifocal spike discharges or diffuse slowing. Children with interictal abnormalities are more likely to have mental retardation or developmental delay.

Although the EEG pattern of discharge is stereotyped, variations on the theme in the form of multiple spike and wave discharges are also acceptable. During sleep the discharges often lose their stereotype and become polymorphic in form and frequency, but remain generalized.

Once a correlation between clinical and EEG findings is made, looking for an underlying disease is unnecessary. Absence epilepsy is distinguished from two other primary generalized epilepsies in which absence occurs, *myoclonic absence* and *juvenile myoclonic epilepsy* (see "Myoclonic Seizures"), by the absence of myoclonic seizures (Berkovic et al, 1988).

Treatment. Ethosuximide and valproate are equally effective in the treatment of absence, with each providing complete relief of seizures in 80% of children. Ethosuximide is the treatment of choice because of its lower incidence of serious side effects. If neither drug alone provides seizure control, they should be used in combination at reduced dosages. The EEG becomes normal if treat-

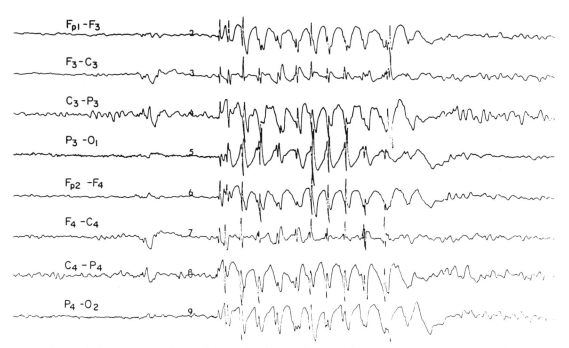

Figure 1–6 Absence epilepsy. A generalized burst of 3 cps spike-wave complexes appears during hyperventilation.

ment is successful, and repeating the EEG is useful to confirm the seizure-free state.

Children with only 3 cps spike-wave on EEG should first be treated with ethosuximide alone, even if a tonic-clonic seizure occurred before initiation of therapy. If tonic-clonic seizures recur after therapy is initiated, valproate should be substituted for ethosuximide. Other drugs that may be useful in the treatment of refractory absence include clonazepam, trimethadione, and methsuximide.

Complex Partial Seizures

Complex partial seizures arise in the cortex, most often the temporal lobe, but can originate from the frontal or parietal lobes as well.

Clinical Features. Complex partial seizures may occur spontaneously or be activated by sleep. Most last 1 to 2 minutes and rarely less than 30 seconds (Holmes and Mikati, 1991). An aura is reported in less than 30% of children. It is usually a nondescript, unpleasant feeling but might also be a stereotyped auditory hallucination or abdominal discomfort. The first manifestation of the seizure can be staring, automatic behavior, tonic extension of one or both arms, or loss of body tone. Staring is associated with a change in facial expression and is followed by automatic behavior. Automatisms vary from facial grimacing and fumbling movements of the fingers to walking, running, and resisting restraint. Automatic behavior in a given patient tends to be similar from seizure to seizure.

The seizure usually terminates with a period of postictal confusion, disorientation, or lethargy. Transitory aphasia is sometimes present. If the child is not treated or if treatment is abruptly withdrawn, secondary generalization is likely to occur.

Partial complex status epilepticus is a rare event manifested by impaired consciousness, staring alternating with wandering eye movements, and automatisms of the face and hands. Such children may arrive at the emergency room in a confused or delirious state (see Chapter 2).

Diagnosis. The etiology of complex partial seizures is heterogeneous, and a cause is often not determined. Brain tumor was thought to be an unusual cause in children, but contrast-enhanced MRI can demonstrate a low-grade glioma in many otherwise normal children with hard-to-control seizures and should be performed in all such cases. Focal dysplastic lesions, especially heterotopia, are another important cause of partial seizures that are identified on MRI (Palmini et al, 1991).

An EEG should be recorded in both the waking and sleeping states. Hyperventilation and photic stimulation are not useful as provocative measures. Results of a single EEG may be normal in the interictal period, but repeated EEGs usually reveal either a spike or slow-wave focus in the frontal or temporal lobe or multifocal abnormalities. During the seizure, repetitive focal spike discharges occur in the involved area of cortex, which change to spike-slow wave complexes and then slow waves with amplitude attenuation as the seizure ends.

Treatment. Carbamazepine, phenytoin, primidone, and phenobarbital are effective for seizure control, and the choice should be based on cost, side effects, and dosage schedule. Phenacemide, which had previously been discarded as an anticonvulsant because of adverse side effects, has been reappraised and found to be safe and useful in children with intractable complex partial seizures (Coker, 1986). My experience with phenacemide in similar cases has been positive.

Temporal lobectomy should be considered when seizures are refractory to anticonvulsant drugs (see "Surgical Approaches to Childhood Epilepsy").

MYOCLONIC SEIZURES

Myoclonus is a brief, involuntary muscle contraction (jerk) that may represent (1) a seizure manifestation, as in infantile spasms, (2) a physiologic response to startle or to falling asleep, or (3) an involuntary movement either alone or in combination with tonic-clonic seizures (see Table 14–8). Myoclonic seizures are often difficult to distinguish from myoclonus (the movement disorder) on clinical grounds alone. Essential myoclonus and other disorders in which myoclonus is clearly not a seizure manifestation are discussed in Chapter 14.

Myoclonic Absence

Myoclonic absence (also called *clonic absence*) is a rare epilepsy, probably distinct from absence epilepsy, in which 85% of patients are boys. It is not a homogeneous entity but may be genetic in some cases and symptomatic of an underlying brain disorder in others.

Clinical Features. Age at onset is between 2 and 12 years with the peak at 7. A family history of epilepsy is present in 25% of cases. Unlike absence epilepsy, 40% of affected children are mentally subnormal before the onset of seizures.

Seizures last 10 to 60 seconds and occur several times each day. They are characterized by a combination of absence and intense rhythmic, bilateral myoclonus affecting the muscles of the shoulders, arms, and legs. The child does not lose consciousness and may be aware of and disturbed by the jerking. Other seizure types seldom occur.

Myoclonic absence sometimes persists into adult life and other times ceases spontaneously. Some children, although intellectually normal before the onset of seizures, are retarded later.

Diagnosis. Myoclonic absence is thought to be intermediary between primary and secondary epilepsy, but an underlying cause has not been determined. The EEG demonstrates the same 3 cps spike-wave pattern associated with simple absence.

Treatment. The seizures are refractory to treatment. Occasional success may be achieved with a combination of valproate and ethosuximide.

Juvenile Myoclonic Epilepsy (Janz)

Juvenile myoclonic epilepsy (Janz) is a hereditary disorder, probably inherited as an autosomal recessive trait (Panayiotopoulos and Obeid, 1989), in which up to 40% of children have a family history of epilepsy. The responsible gene has been mapped to the short arm of chromosome 6 (Durner et al, 1991). Seizures in affected relatives may be tonic-clonic, myoclonic absence, or simple absence.

Clinical Features. The age at onset is between 12 and 18 years in 75% of cases. The characteristic feature is a brief, bilateral but not always symmetric, flexor jerk of the arms, which may be repetitive. The jerk sometimes affects the legs, causing the patient to fall. Consciousness is usually retained so that the patient is aware of the jerking movement. Seizures are precipitated by sleep deprivation, alcohol ingestion, and awakening from nocturnal or daytime sleep.

Most patients also have generalized tonic-clonic seizures, and one third experience absence but are otherwise normal neurologically. The potential for seizures of one type or another continues throughout adult life.

Diagnosis. Seizures are accompanied by generalized polyspike discharges followed by a slow wave. The polyspike discharge is concurrent with the clinical seizure, and the slow wave occurs afterward. Seizures are sometimes precipitated by photic stimulation or eye closure. The interictal record may be normal or may show 3.5 to 6 cps multispike-wave complexes (Figure 1–7).

Treatment. Valproate is the treatment of choice and provides complete relief of seizures in 75% of cases. Some children require a second drug for control of tonic-clonic seizures.

Progressive Myoclonus Epilepsies

The term "progressive myoclonus epilepsies" is used to cover several progressive disorders of the nervous system characterized by (1) myoclonus, (2) seizures that may be tonic-clonic, tonic, or myoclonic, (3) progressive mental deterioration, and (4) cerebellar ataxia, involuntary movements, or both (Berkovic et al, 1991). Some of these dis-

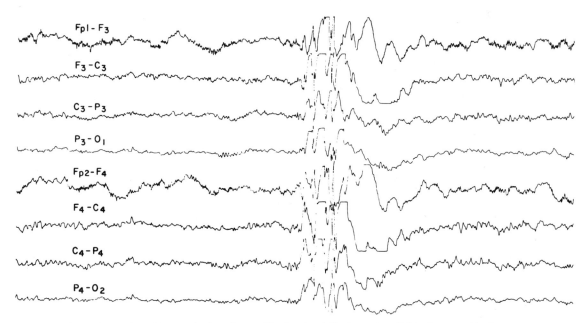

Figure 1–7 Juvenile myoclonic epilepsy. The interictal discharge is a 3.5 to 6 cps multispike-wave complex.

orders are due to specific lysosomal enzyme deficiencies, whereas others are probably mitochondrial disorders (Table 1–10).

Lafora Disease

Lafora disease is a rare hereditary disease probably transmitted by autosomal recessive inheritance.

Clinical Features.   Onset is between 11 and 18 years of age with the mean at age 14. Tonic-clonic or myoclonic seizures are the presenting symptoms in 80% of cases. Myoclonus becomes progressively worse, may be segmental or massive, and is increased by movement. Mental retardation begins early and is relentlessly progressive. Ataxia, spasticity, and involuntary movements occur late in the course. Death occurs 5 to 6 years from the onset of symptoms.

Diagnosis.   The EEG is normal at first and then shows the development of nonspecific generalized polyspike discharges that are not activated by sleep. The background becomes progressively disorganized and epileptiform activity more constant. Photosensitive discharges are a regular feature late in the course.

Antemortem diagnosis is accomplished by demonstrating periodic acid–Schiff (PAS)-positive inclusion bodies consisting of polyglucasan material in biopsy specimens from the liver or sweat glands.

Treatment.   The seizures become refractory to most anticonvulsant drugs, but the combination of valproate, clonazepam, and phenobarbital should be tried. Treatment of the underlying disease is not available.

Unverricht-Lundborg Syndrome

Unverricht-Lundborg syndrome is clinically similar to Lafora disease, except that inclusion bodies are not present. It is transmitted by autosomal recessive inheritance. The syndrome is most often reported in Finland and other Baltic countries

Table 1–10 ◆ Progressive Myoclonus Epilepsies

1. Ceroid lipofuscinosis, juvenile form
   (see Chapter 5)
2. Glucosylceramide lipidosis (Gaucher type 3)
   (see Chapter 5)
3. Lafora disease
4. Myoclonus epilepsy and ragged-red fibers
   (see Chapter 5)
5. Ramsay Hunt syndrome (see Chapter 10)
6. Sialidoses (see Chapter 5)
7. Unverricht-Lundborg syndrome

but has a worldwide distribution. Whether ethnic clusters are caused by distinct diseases is not known.

A combination of valproate, clonazepam, and phenobarbital is effective for seizure control.

PARTIAL SEIZURES

This section discusses several seizure types of focal cortical origin other than complex partial seizures. Such seizures may be purely motor or purely sensory or may affect higher cortical function. The most common partial seizure disorder is benign (Rolandic) epilepsy of childhood. Partial seizures are also secondary to underlying diseases, which can be focal, multifocal, or generalized.

Any seizure that originates in the cortex may discharge into the brainstem, causing a tonic-clonic seizure (secondary generalization). If the discharge remains focal for a few seconds, the patient experiences a focal seizure or an *aura* before losing consciousness. Often the secondary generalization occurs so rapidly that a tonic-clonic seizure is the initial symptom. In such cases, cortical origin of the seizure is detectable only on EEG. However, normal EEG findings are common during a simple partial seizure and do not exclude the diagnosis (Devinsky et al, 1988).

Benign Rolandic Epilepsy of Childhood

Benign Rolandic epilepsy of childhood is a genetic disorder thought to be transmitted as an autosomal dominant trait. Forty percent of close relatives have a history of febrile seizures or epilepsy. Absence and benign occipital epilepsy of childhood may be caused by the same genetic trait (Silvestri et al, 1989).

Clinical Features.   The age at onset is 18 months to 13 years, with the majority between 5 and 10 years of age (Loiseau et al, 1988). Seizures almost always stop spontaneously by 14 years of age. Even without drug therapy, 10% have only one seizure, 70% have infrequent seizures, and only 20% have frequent seizures. With drug therapy 20% have isolated seizures and 6% have frequent seizures. Seventy percent of children have only nocturnal seizures, 15% only when awake, and 15% both awake and asleep.

The typical seizure wakes the child from sleep. Paresthesias occur on one side of the mouth, followed by ipsilateral twitching of the face, mouth, and pharynx, resulting in speech arrest and drooling. Consciousness is preserved. The seizure lasts for 1 or 2 minutes. Daytime seizures do not generalize, but nocturnal seizures in children younger than 5 years old often spread to the arm or evolve into a generalized tonic-clonic seizure.

Diagnosis. Results of neurologic examination, CT, and MRI are normal. Interictal EEG demonstrates unilateral or bilateral spike discharges in the central or centrotemporal region. The spikes are typically of high voltage and are activated by drowsiness and sleep. The frequency of spike discharge does not correlate with the subsequent course.

Treatment. Treatment is not needed if seizures are infrequent and only nocturnal. A single bedtime dose of phenobarbital or phenytoin is usually satisfactory for seizure control. After 2 years of treatment, medication can be withdrawn and 80% remain seizure free. Those who resume having seizures should be treated until age 14. All children eventually stop having seizures whether they are treated or not.

Benign Occipital Epilepsy of Childhood

Benign occipital epilepsy of childhood is a genetic epilepsy, probably transmitted by autosomal dominant inheritance, that may be a phenotypic variation of benign Rolandic epilepsy.

Clinical Features. Age at onset is between 15 months and 17 years, generally between 4 and 8 years (Lerman and Kivity, 1991). One third of patients have a family history of epilepsy, frequently Rolandic epilepsy.

The initial seizure manifestation can consist of (1) visual hallucinations, usually flashing lights or spots, (2) blindness, hemianopia, or complete amaurosis, (3) visual illusions, such as micropsia, macropsia, or metamorphasia, or (4) loss of conciousness lasting up to 12 hours (Kivity and Lerman, 1992). More than one manifestation may occur simultaneously. The visual aura may be followed by unilateral clonic seizures, complex partial seizures, or generalized tonic-clonic seizures. Afterward the child may have migrainelike headaches and nausea. Attacks occur when the patient is awake or asleep, but the greatest frequency is at the transition from wake to sleep.

Diagnosis. Results of neurologic examination, CT, and MRI are normal. The interictal EEG demonstrates unilateral or bilateral, high-amplitude, occipital spike-wave discharges with a frequency of 1.5 to 2.5 cps. The discharges are inhibited by eye opening and enhanced by light sleep. During a seizure, rapid firing of spike discharges occurs in one or both occipital lobes.

Benign occipital epilepsy may be difficult to distinguish from basilar migraine (see Chapter 10). Reported cases of basilar migraine with occipital spikes are probably benign occipital epilepsy and not migraine. Such cases respond to anticonvulsant drugs and not antimigraine agents.

Treatment. Complete seizure control is accomplished with standard anticonvulsant drugs in the majority of children. Typical seizures do not persist beyond 12 years. However, not all children with occipital discharges have a benign epilepsy. The onset of seizures after 9 years of age suggests that epilepsy will continue in adult life.

Acquired Epileptiform Aphasia

Speech arrest and aphasia occur during some complex partial seizures and with absence status. In addition, acquired aphasia is associated with epileptiform activity on EEG in a disorder peculiar to children: the *Landau-Kleffner syndrome* (Deonna, 1991). The cases are probably not homogeneous, but a typical clinical profile has emerged.

Clinical Features. Age at onset ranges from 2 to 11 years with 75% beginning between 3 and 10 years (Lerman and Kivity, 1991). The first symptom may be aphasia or epilepsy. Aphasia is initially characterized by auditory verbal agnosia. The child has difficulty understanding what is said, spontaneous speech is reduced, and deafness or autism develops. Seizures, which may be partial or generalized, occur in 70% of children. Status epilepticus is sometimes the initial feature. Hyperactivity and personality change are noted in one half of affected children and may be caused by aphasia. Intelligence is not affected, and neurologic findings are otherwise normal.

Recovery of language is more likely to occur if the syndrome begins before 7 years of age. Seizures generally cease by age 10 and always by age 15.

Diagnosis. The Landau-Kleffner syndrome may be confused with autism, hearing loss, and psychotic behavior. The occurrence of seizures differentiates this syndrome from other possible disorders. The EEG demonstrates multifocal cortical spike discharges with a predilection for the temporal and parietal lobes. Involvement is bilateral in 88% of cases. An intravenous injection of diazepam may normalize the EEG and improve speech transiently, but this should not suggest that aphasia is caused by epileptiform activity. They both reflect an underlying cerebral disorder.

Treatment. Standard anticonvulsant drugs such as carbamazepine and phenytoin usually control the seizures but may not improve speech.

Epilepsia Partialis Continuans

Focal motor seizures that do not stop spontaneously are termed epilepsia partialis continuans. This is an ominous symptom and almost always indicates an underlying cerebral disorder. A seizure may last hours, days, or months.

Clinical Features. Focal jerking frequently begins in one body part, usually one side of the face or one hand, and then spreads to contiguous parts. Trunk muscles are rarely affected. The rate and intensity of the seizures vary at first, but then they become more regular and persist in sleep. The affected limbs become paretic and almost always remain so (see Chapter 11).

Diagnosis. Possible causes include infarction, hemorrhage, tumor, and inflammation. Epilepsia partialis continuans is the initial feature of a poorly defined entity of childhood called *Rasmussen encephalitis* (Honavar et al, 1992). Affected children have focal motor seizures that defy treatment and progress to affect first both limbs on one side of the body and then the limbs on the other side. Progressive hemiplegia and other neurologic deficits develop, and often they remain even after seizures have stopped. The syndrome is thought to be caused by a low-grade smoldering encephalitis, but evidence to support such a notion is lacking.

The EEG demonstrates continuous spike discharges originating in one portion of the cortex with spread to contiguous areas of the cortex and to a mirror focus on the other side. Secondary generalization may occur.

CT or MRI should be performed in every case, and arteriography is indicated if there is evidence of vascular disease.

Treatment. Every effort should be made to stop the seizures with intravenous anticonvulsant drugs (see "Treatment of Status Epilepticus"). Pentobarbital coma is often required, but seizures may return when the coma is lifted. Early hemispherectomy has been suggested as providing the best long-term results (see "Surgical Treatment of Epilepsy").

GENERALIZED TONIC-CLONIC SEIZURES

Generalized tonic-clonic seizures are the most common seizures of childhood. They are dramatic and frightening events that demand medical attention. Seizures that are prolonged or repeated without recovery are termed *status epilepticus*. The diagnostic considerations in a child who has had a generalized tonic-clonic seizure are summarized in Table 1–11.

Table 1–11 ◆ Diagnostic Considerations for a First Nonfebrile Tonic-Clonic Seizure After 2 Years of Age

1. Acute encephalopathy or encephalitis (see Chapter 2)
2. Isolated unexplained seizure
3. Partial seizure with secondary generalization
4. Primary generalized epilepsy
5. Progressive disorder of the nervous system (see Chapter 5)

Clinical Features. The onset may occur anytime after the neonatal period, but the onset of primary generalized epilepsy without absence is usually in the second decade. With absence, age at onset shifts to the first decade.

The initial feature is sudden loss of consciousness. The child falls to the floor and the body stiffens. This is followed by repetitive jerking (clonic) movements of the limbs; these movements at first are rapid and rhythmic and then become slower and more irregular as the seizure abates. The eyes roll backward in the orbits; breathing is rapid and deep, causing saliva to froth at the lips; and urinary and bowel incontinence may occur. Seizures are followed by a postictal sleep from which arousal is difficult. Afterward the child appears normal but may have sore limb muscles and a painful tongue, bitten during the seizure.

Diagnosis. A first, generalized tonic-clonic seizure requires laboratory evaluation. The extent of evaluation must be individualized. Important determining factors include body temperature, neurologic findings, family history, and known precipitating factors. An eyewitness report of focal features at the onset of the seizure, or the recollection of an aura, indicates a partial seizure with secondary generalization.

During the seizure the EEG demonstrates generalized repetitive spikes in the tonic phase and then periodic bursts of spikes in the clonic phase. The clonic portion is usually obscured by movement artifact. As the seizure ends, there is slowing of the background and amplitude attenuation.

Between seizures, brief generalized spike or spike-wave discharges that are polymorphic in appearance may occur. Discharge frequency is sometimes increased by drowsiness and light sleep. The presence of focal discharges indicates that the tonic-clonic seizure was secondarily generalized.

The cerebrospinal fluid is normal following a brief, tonic-clonic seizure caused by primary epilepsy. However, prolonged or repeated seizures may cause leukocytosis (up to 80 cells/mm³) with a polymorphonuclear predominance (Schmidley and Simon, 1981). Protein concentration can be mildly elevated, but the glucose concentration is normal.

Treatment. Phenobarbital, phenytoin, and carbamazepine are equally effective in preventing further seizures. Status epilepticus must be treated with intravenous drugs (see "Treatment of Status Epilepticus").

Pseudoseizures

"Hysterical" seizures are an effective method of seeking attention and secondary gain. They occur more often in adolescence than childhood and in females than males (3:1). There is often a history of sexual abuse. People with pseudoseizures may also have true seizures; the pseudoseizures begin when true seizures come under control and the secondary gain of epilepsy is lost.

Clinical Features. Pseudoseizures rarely simulate true seizures but sometimes may be difficult to distinguish by observation alone. They may be manifest as a rich variety of motor and behavioral phenomena, but three broad patterns are often observed (Gulick et al, 1982):

1. Unilateral or bilateral motor activity characterized by tonic posturing and tremulousness in which the patient's movements are thrashing or jerking rather than tonic-clonic; different movements may occur simultaneously
2. Behavioral or emotional changes in which distress or discomfort is expressed, followed by semipurposeless, but not stereotyped, behaviors such as fumbling with objects or walking
3. Periods of unresponsiveness

Attacks may be precipitated and ended by suggestion. Patients usually do not hurt themselves and are not incontinent.

Diagnosis. Pseudoseizures usually occur at home and are believed to be real. If the child has epilepsy, the seizures are reported by telephone to the physician and drug schedules are needlessly revised, often to the patient's detriment. The possibility of pseudoseizures must be considered when frequent seizures develop in children whose epilepsy has recently come under control.

Children who do not have epilepsy and in whom pseudoseizures develop are frequently brought to an emergency room and may be given anticonvulsant drugs before an investigation is initiated. It is then difficult to stop the medications and obtain a baseline EEG. Most pseudoseizures are diagnosed by observation alone. When doubt remains, video-EEG monitoring is the best method of diagnosis.

Treatment. The diagnosis of pseudoseizures should be presented in a positive and supportive manner (Shen et al, 1990). The diagnosis does not mean that the person is crazy or faking. The spells can be stopped but not with anticonvulsant drugs. Psychiatric referral is not always necessary. Pseudoseizures are managed best by determining the secondary gain provided by seizures and offering alternative methods of satisfaction. In 78% of children with pseudoseizures the attacks stop once the diagnosis is established (Wyllie et al, 1990).

◆ Anticonvulsant Drug Therapy

The goal of anticonvulsant therapy is to achieve the maximum normal function by balancing seizure control against drug toxicity.

INDICATIONS FOR STARTING THERAPY

Prophylactic therapy should be initiated whenever there is a reasonable expectation that seizures will recur. The risk of recurrence after a first unexplained and untreated tonic-clonic seizure in persons of all ages is 62% within 1 year and 72% within 2 years (Elwes et al, 1985). Among children younger than 7 years of age after a single unexplained nonfebrile seizure, 61% have a second seizure: 90% within 1 year and almost all within 2 years (Hirtz et al, 1984). After a second seizure 90% of children have a third seizure. When children of all ages and with partial or generalized nonfebrile seizures are considered together, the recurrence rate among untreated children is considerably lower (Shinnar et al, 1986). This can be explained by the relatively high prevalence of benign (Rolandic) epilepsy of childhood.

The majority of individuals who have a first nonfebrile seizure can be expected to have more seizures, but a significant minority have a single unexplained seizure that does not require therapy. Epileptiform activity on EEG, a family history of epilepsy, and an abnormal neurologic or developmental examination are factors that support initiating therapy after a single seizure.

In contrast to nonfebrile seizures, the risk of recurrence after a first febrile seizure is relatively small (see "Febrile Seizures").

DISCONTINUING THERAPY

Children who have an acute encephalopathy (e.g., anoxia, head trauma, encephalitis) and associated seizures should be treated with anticonvulsant drugs. When the acute encephalopathy is over and seizures have stopped, anticonvulsant therapy should be discontinued. Only a minority of children later have epilepsy, and they can be treated when seizures recur. There is no evidence that continuous anticonvulsant therapy prevents the development of epilepsy in such cases.

It has been the rule that children treated for epilepsy should be maintained seizure free for at least 2 years before attempts are made to discontinue therapy; this is certainly true in specific conditions such as the benign epilepsies of childhood. After a seizure-free period of 2 years and normalization of the EEG the recurrence rate is 25% (Arts et al, 1988). Three fourths of relapses occur in the withdrawal phase and in the 2 years thereafter. Contrary to popular belief, seizures are not caused by the rapid withdrawal of anticonvulsant drugs in a person who does not need them. Seizures occur in people with epilepsy when the blood concentration is no longer therapeutic, without regard to the rate of decline (Marks et al, 1991). Risk factors that predict a recurrence of seizures after therapy is discontinued include (1) an abnormal EEG at the time of discontinuing therapy, (2) seizures that were hard to control at onset, and (3) a child who is neurologically or developmentally abnormal.

PRINCIPLES OF THERAPY

Therapy should be started with a single drug. In approximately 75% of children with epilepsy the seizures can be fully controlled with monotherapy. Even patients whose seizures are never controlled are likely to do better on monotherapy than polytherapy. Polytherapy poses several problems: (1) drugs compete with each other for protein binding sites, (2) one drug can increase the rate and pathway of catabolism of a second drug, (3) drugs have cummulative toxicity, and (4) compliance is more difficult.

When more than one drug is needed, drugs that have different spectrums of activity or mechanisms of action should be chosen. Only one drug should be changed at a time. If several changes are made simultaneously, it is impossible to determine which drug is responsible for a beneficial or an adverse effect.

Anticonvulsant drugs should not be administered more often than three times each day. With many drugs an acceptable steady state can be attained using a twice-a-day regimen, and some can be administered once a day. Compliance usually falls when drugs are taken more than twice each day. Children often have problems taking medicine at school.

BLOOD CONCENTRATIONS

The development of techniques to measure blood concentrations of anticonvulsant drugs has been an important advance in the treatment of epilepsy. Measuring protein-bound fractions is customary even though the free fraction is responsible for efficacy and toxicity. While the ratio of free to bound fractions is relatively constant, some drugs, such as valproate, have a greater affinity for binding protein than other drugs and will displace them when used together. This raises the free concentration of the displaced drug and may have toxic effects even though the measured protein-bound fraction is "therapeutic."

Reference values of drug concentrations are guidelines. Some patients are seizure free with concentrations that are below the reference value, and others are unaffected by apparent toxic concentrations.

Most anticonvulsants follow first-order kinetics; that is, blood levels increase proportionately with increases in oral dose. The major exception is phenytoin, which follows zero-order kinetics. The drug is maximally metabolized until the responsible enzyme system is saturated, and then a small increment in oral dose produces large increments in blood concentration.

The half-lives of anticonvulsants listed in Table 1–12 are at steady state. Half-lives are generally longer when a patient is first exposed to a drug. Steady state is usually achieved after five half-lives. Similarly, five half-lives are required to eliminate a drug after administration has been discontinued. Drug half-lives vary from individual to individual and may be shortened or increased by the concurrent use of other anticonvulsants, antibiotics, and antipyretics. This is one reason that children with epilepsy may have a toxic response to drugs or increased seizures at the time of a febrile illness (Goulden et al, 1988).

Some anticonvulsants are metabolized to active metabolites that have anticonvulsant and toxic properties. With the exception of phenobarbital derived from primidone, these metabolites are not usually measured. Active metabolites may provide seizure control or have toxic effects when the blood concentration of the parent compound is low.

ADVERSE REACTIONS

Many anticonvulsant drugs irritate the gastric mucosa and produce nausea and vomiting. When this occurs, symptoms may be relieved by smaller doses at more frequent intervals, using enteric-

Table 1–12 ◆ Anticonvulsant Drugs For Children

Drug	Initial Dose (mg/kg/day)	Maintenance (mg/kg/day)	Blood Concentration (μg/ml)	Half-Life (hrs)
Acetazolamide	10	10-50	—*	24-72
Carbamazepine†	5	15-20	4-12	14-27
Clonazepam†	0.025	0.1-0.15	0.2-0.7*	20-40
Clorazepate	0.3	0.3-1	>1.2*	20-60
Ethosuximide	20	20-40	40-100	30-60
Methsuximide	20	20-40	—*	—*
Nitrazepam	0.2	0.5-1	—*	18-30
Phenacemide	20	40-50	50-75	24
Phenobarbital	3-5	3-5	10-40	37-73
Phenytoin	5-7	5-7	10-20	5-14
Primidone	2-5	10-15	8-12	5-11
Trimethadione	20	30-60	—*	16*
Valproate†	20	30-60	50-100	6-15

*Not clinically useful.
†May be administered rectally.

coated preparations, and administering the drug after meals.

Toxic adverse reactions are dose related. All anticonvulsant drugs cause sedation when blood concentrations are excessive. Subtle cognitive and behavioral disturbances, which are recognized only by the patient or family, often occur at low blood concentrations. The patient's observation of a toxic effect should not be discounted because the blood concentration is within the therapeutic range. As doses are increased, attention span, memory, and interpersonal relations become seriously impaired. This is especially common with barbiturates but can occur with any drug.

Idiosyncratic reactions are not dose related. They may occur on the basis of hypersensitivity (usually manifest as rash, fever, and lymphadenopathy) but may also be caused by the production of toxic metabolites. Idiosyncratic reactions are not always predictable, and the patient's observation should be respected, even when the reaction was not previously reported.

SELECTION OF AN ANTICONVULSANT DRUG

The use of generic drugs should be avoided whenever possible. Several different manufacturers provide generic versions of each drug; the bioavailability and half-life of these products vary considerably and maintaining a predictable blood concentration is impossible. The most common reasons for loss of seizure control in children who were previously seizure free are noncompliance and the use of generic drugs.

The drugs most often selected for the treatment of tonic-clonic and partial seizures are carbamazepine, phenobarbital, and phenytoin. Clonazepam, phenacemide, primidone, and valproate are used in refractory cases. Valproate is gaining in use as a primary drug in adults, but I believe that it has too many adverse effects in children to use it when other drugs are equally effective.

The initial drugs used to treat absence and myoclonic seizures are ethosuximide and valproate. Secondary drugs are benzodiazepines (clonazepam, clorazepate, and nitrazepam), methsuximide, and trimethadione. The ketogenic diet is an alternative to drug therapy.

Acetazolamide is used as an adjunct to therapy in children with refractory absence or myoclonic epilepsy and is sometimes administered the week before menses in women with catamenial epilepsy.

ACTH, prednisone, and pyridoxine provide transitory relief of intractable seizures in infants (see "Infantile Spasms") but are not ordinarily used in older children.

Acetazolamide (Diamox, Lederle)

Indications. Adjunct therapy for absence, myoclonic, and catamenial epilepsy.

Administration. The initial dose for children with absence or myoclonic seizures is 10 mg/kg/day. Increments of 10 mg/kg to a total of 50 mg/kg/day in two divided doses may be used. In woman with catamenial epilepsy, 250 mg/day is administered for the week preceding the expected time of menses.

Adverse Effects. Toxic reactions include tingling of the fingers and polyuria. Idiosyncratic reactions are rare.

Carbamazepine (Tegretol, Geigy)

Indications. Tonic-clonic and partial seizures. Atypical absence may be exacerbated (Snead and Hosey, 1985).

Administration. Absorption from the gastrointestinal tract is slow and variable. The rectal route may be used for maintenance if the dose is increased by one third. Approximately 85% of the drug is protein bound. Carbamazepine induces its own metabolism, and the initial dose should be 25% of the maintenance dose to prevent a toxic effect. The usual maintenance dose is 15 to 20 mg/kg/day to provide a blood concentration of 4 to 12 µg/ml (17 to 51 µmol/L). Half-life at steady state is 5 to 27 hours, and children usually require doses three times a day.

Concurrent use of erythromycin, propoxyphene, verapamil, and cimetidine interferes with carbamazepine metabolism and has a toxic effect.

Adverse Effects. A reduction in the number of peripheral leukocytes is expected but is rarely sufficient (absolute neutrophil count <1000) to warrant discontinuation of therapy. An initial white blood cell count should be performed 6 weeks after therapy is started. Repeating white blood cell counts each time the patient returns for a routine follow-up visit is not cost effective and does not allow the prediction of life-threatening events (Pellock and Willmore, 1991). The most informative time to repeat the white blood cell count is during a febrile illness.

Cognitive disturbances occur when doses are within the therapeutic range. Sedation, ataxia, and nystagmus occur at toxic blood concentrations.

Clonazepam (Klonopin, Roche)

Indications. Infantile spasms, myoclonic seizures, absence, and partial seizures. Tolerance to clonazepam often develops in children with severe myoclonic epilepsy such as those with infantile spasms and the Lennox-Gastaut syndrome (Specht et al, 1989). Once tolerance is established, discontinuation of the drug may actually improve seizure control.

Administration. The initial dosage is 0.025 mg/kg/day in two divided doses. Increments of 0.025 mg/kg are recommended every 3 to 5 days as needed and tolerated. The usual maintenance dosage is 0.1 mg/kg/day in three divided doses. Most children cannot tolerate more than 0.15 mg/kg/day. Therapeutic blood concentrations are 0.02 to 0.07 µg/ml; 47% is protein bound; and the half-life is 20 to 40 hours. The rectal route may be used for maintenance.

Adverse Effects. Toxic effects with doses within the therapeutic range include sedation, cognitive impairment, hyperactivity, and excessive salivation. Idiosyncratic reactions are unusual.

Clorazepate (Tranxene, Abbott)

Indications. Adjunct therapy for refractory myoclonic and partial seizures. Clorazepate should not be used as a primary anticonvulsant.

Administration. The smallest capsule, 3.75 mg, is given once each day and increased by one capsule every 3 days as needed and tolerated. Maintenance dosage is 1 to 3 mg/kg/day in three divided doses. The total dosage is limited by toxicity, and blood concentration measurements are not useful.

Adverse Effects. Sedation occurs within the therapeutic range and limits usefulness. Higher doses cause ataxia, diplopia, and impairment of cognitive function.

Ethosuximide (Zarontin, Parke-Davis)

Indications. Treatment of choice for absence, also useful for myoclonic absence.

Administration. The drug is absorbed rapidly, and peak blood concentrations appear within 4 hours. It is not bound to plasma proteins. The half-life is 30 hours in children and up to 60 hours in adults. The initial dosage is 20 mg/kg/day in three divided doses after meals to avoid gastric irritation. Increments of 10 mg/kg/day are administered as needed and tolerated to provide a blood concentration above 40 µg/ml (280 µmol/L).

Adverse Effects. Ethosuximide does not interact with other anticonvulsants because it is not protein bound. Idiosyncratic reactions include dystonia and a lupuslike syndrome. Aplastic anemia is a rare complication. Common toxic reactions include nausea, abdominal pain, headache, and sedation. Gastrointestinal symptoms occur within the therapeutic range and limit usefulness.

Methsuximide (Celontin, Parke-Davis)

Indications. A secondary drug for absence and myoclonic seizures if ethosuximide and valproate cannot be used. It may also be useful as a secondary drug for partial seizures.

Administration. Methsuximide is rapidly absorbed and reaches peak blood concentrations within 2 hours. However, active metabolites rather than the parent compound are probably responsible for efficacy and toxicity. Some of these accumulate for 30 to 40 hours. The initial dosage is 20 mg/kg/day in three divided doses. Increments of 10 mg/kg/day are administered as needed and tolerated. Measuring the blood concentration of the parent compound is not helpful.

Adverse Effects.   Drowsiness is the most common side effect, but gastric irritation and personality change may occur as well.

Nitrazepam (Mogadon, Roche)

Indications.   Infantile spasms and myoclonic seizures.

Administration.   Nitrazepam is not approved for use in the United States. The half-life is 18 to 30 hours. The initial dosage is 0.2 mg/kg/day in two divided doses. Biweekly increments of 0.3 mg/kg are administered as needed until a maintenance dosage of 0.5 to 1 mg/kg/day is achieved.

Adverse Effects.   Drowsiness, hypotonia, and increased secretions are the usual side effects.

Phenacemide (Phenurone, Abbott)

Indications.   Intractable complex partial seizures.

Administration.   Phenacemide has not been tested as initial monotherapy but can be effective when other drugs have failed. Therapy should be initiated at a dosage of 20 mg/kg/day in three divided doses and increased biweekly by 10 mg/kg/day. The usual maintenance dosage is 40 to 50 mg/kg/day to achieve a trough plasma level of 50 μg/dl (Coker et al, 1987).

Adverse Effects.   Phenacemide has an undeserved reputation for serious toxicity. Dose-related hepatotoxicity is the major concern. The actual incidence is lower than for valproate, and regular monitoring of hepatic enzymes should prevent irreversible liver damage. Aplastic anemia has also been attributed to phenacemide, but the evidence is not compelling.

Phenytoin (Dilantin, Parke-Davis)

Indications.   Tonic-clonic seizures, partial seizures, status epilepticus.

Administration.   Oral absorption is slow and unpredictable in newborns, erratic in infants, and probably not reliable until 3 to 5 years of age. Even in adults there is considerable individual variability. Once absorbed, phenytoin is 70% to 95% protein bound. A typical maintenance dosage is 7 mg/kg/day in newborns and 5 mg/kg/day in children. The half-life is up to 60 hours in full-term newborns, up to 140 hours in premature infants, 5 to 14 hours in children, and 10 to 34 hours in adults.

Capsules are usually taken in two divided doses, but tablets are more rapidly absorbed and may require three divided doses.

Rapid loading of phenytoin can be performed by giving three times the maintenance dose by either the oral or intravenous route (see "Treatment of Status Epilepticus"). Intramuscular injections are not absorbed and should not be used.

Blood concentrations less than 10 μg/ml (40 μmol/L) are metabolized by first-order kinetics, but higher concentrations are metabolized by zero-order kinetics. The usual therapeutic range is 10 to 20 μg/ml (40 to 80 μmol/L), and within that range, dosage increments must be small.

Adverse Reactions.   The major adverse reactions are hypersensitivity, gum hypertrophy, and hirsutism. Hypersensitivity reactions usually occur within 6 weeks of the initiation of therapy and are characterized by rash, fever, and lymphadenopathy. Once such a reaction has occurred, the drug should be discontinued. Concurrent use of antihistamines is not appropriate management. Continued use of the drug may produce a Stevens-Johnson syndrome or a lupuslike disorder.

Gum hypertrophy is caused by a combination of phenytoin metabolites and plaque on the teeth. Persons with good oral hygiene are less likely to have gum hypertrophy. The importance of good oral hygiene should be discussed at the onset of therapy.

Hirsutism is more a problem for girls than boys and is a valid reason for discontinuing therapy in favor of another drug.

Memory impairment, decreased attention span, and personality change may occur at therapeutic concentrations, but they occur less often and are less severe than with phenobarbital.

Phenobarbital

Indications.   Tonic-clonic and simple partial seizures.

Administration.   Oral absorption is slow, and daily doses are better given with the evening meal than at bedtime if seizures are hypnagogic. Since intramuscular absorption requires 1 to 2 hours, the intramuscular route should not be used for rapid loading (see "Treatment of Status Epilepticus"); 50% is protein bound, and 50% is free.

Initial and maintenance dosages are 3 to 5 mg/kg/day. The half-life is 46 to 136 hours in adults, 37 to 73 hours in children, and 61 to 173 hours in full-term newborns. Because of the very long half-life at all ages, once-a-day doses are usually satisfactory, and steady-state blood concentrations should be measured after 2 weeks of therapy. Therapeutic blood concentrations are 10 to 40 μg/ml (40 to 160 μmol/L).

Adverse Effects. Hyperactivity is the most common and limiting side effect in children. Adverse behavioral changes occur in one half of children between 2 and 10 years of age. Parents should be warned of this possibility at the onset of therapy. Behavioral changes are dose related, and other barbiturates that are converted to phenobarbital produce the same adverse effects at equivalent phenobarbital blood concentrations.

Drowsiness and cognitive dysfunction, rather than hyperactivity, are the usual adverse effects after 10 years of age. However, in one randomized trial of phenobarbital against carbamazepine, psychologic testing did not demonstrate any behavioral or cognitive difference between the two drugs (Mitchell and Chavez, 1987). Infants tolerate phenobarbital well, and it remains a drug of choice for oral use in newborns and infants. Idiosyncratic reactions are unusual.

Primidone (Mysoline, Ayerst)

Indications. Tonic-clonic and partial seizures.

Administration. Primidone is metabolized to at least two active metabolites, phenobarbital and phenyl-ethyl-malonamide (PEMA). Primidone half-life is 6 to 12 hours, and PEMA half-life is 20 hours. The usual maintenance dosage is 10 to 15 mg/kg/day, but the initial dose should be 25% of maintenance or intolerable sedation occurs. A therapeutic blood concentration of primidone is 8 to 12 μg/ml (36 to 52 μmol/L). The blood concentration of phenobarbital derived from primidone is generally four times greater, but this ratio is altered when other anticonvulsant drugs are administered concurrently.

Adverse Effects. The adverse effects are the same as for phenobarbital, except that the risk of intolerable sedation from the first tablet is great.

Trimethadione (Tridione, Abbott)

Indications. Simple absence, myoclonic absence, and myoclonic seizures. Trimethadione has been displaced by ethosuximide and valproate but should not be discarded. It may be effective in children whose seizures are refractory to other anticonvulsants.

Administration. Trimethadione is metabolized to the active metabolite 5,5-dimethyl-2,4-oxazolidindione (DMO). The half-life of trimethadione is 16 hours, and the half-life of DMO is 10 days. The initial dosage is 20 mg/kg in three divided doses; the dosage is increased incrementally as tolerated and needed to 60 mg/kg/day. The maintenance dose is usually limited by toxicity. Measuring blood concentrations of the parent compound is not as helpful as measuring blood concentrations of DOMA, which must be kept greater than 700 μg/ml.

Adverse Effects. The most common toxic effects are sedation and blurring of vision on exposure to bright light. The serious idiosyncratic complication is bone marrow suppression during the first 6 months of therapy, and monthly erythrocyte and leukocyte counts are mandatory during that time.

Valproate (Depakene, Abbott)

Indications. Myoclonic seizures, simple absence, myoclonic absence, myoclonus, and tonic-clonic seizures. Valproate is especially useful for mixed seizure disorders.

Administration. Oral absorption is rapid, and half-life is 6 to 15 hours. Doses three times a day are needed to achieve constant blood concentrations. An enteric-coated capsule (Depakote) slows absorption and allows twice-a-day doses in many children.

The initial dosage is 20 mg/kg/day. Increments of 10 mg/kg/day are administered to provide a blood concentration of 50 to 100 mg/ml (350 to 700 μmol/L). Blood concentrations of 80 to 120 μg/ml (560 to 840 μmol/L) are often required to achieve seizure control. Protein binding is 95% at blood concentrations of 50 μg/ml and 80% at 100 μg/ml. Therefore doubling the blood concentration increases the free fraction eightfold. Valproate has a strong affinity for plasma proteins and displaces other anticonvulsant drugs.

Valproate is absorbed when given rectally and can be administered by this route when oral administration is not possible. A peak concentration is attained 3 hours after rectal administration, and the serum concentration is approximately 75% of the oral dose (Holmes et al, 1989).

Adverse Effects. Valproate has dose-related and idiosyncratic hepatotoxicity. Dose-related hepatotoxicity is harmless and characterized by increased serum concentrations of transaminases. Important dose-related effects are a reduction in the platelet count, pancreatitis, and hyperammonemia. Thrombocytopenia may result in serious bleeding after trivial injury, while pancreatitis and hepatitis are both associated with nausea and vomiting. Hyperammonemia, caused by interference with the urea cycle, causes cognitive disturbances and nausea. These adverse reactions are reversible when the daily dose is reduced.

Plasma carnitine concentrations are reduced in children taking valproate, and some believe that carnitine supplementation helps relieve cognitive impairment.

The major idiosyncratic reaction is fatal liver necrosis caused by the production of an aberrant and toxic metabolite. The major risk (1:800) is in children younger than 2 years of age and receiving polytherapy (Dreifuss et al, 1989). Fatal hepatotoxicity has not been reported in children over 10 years of age treated with valproate alone.

The clinical manifestations of idiosyncratic hepatotoxicity are similar to those of Reye syndrome (see Chapter 2). It may begin after 1 day of therapy or not appear for 6 months. No reliable way exists to monitor patients for idiosyncratic hepatotoxicity or to predict its occurrence.

TREATMENT OF STATUS EPILEPTICUS
Immediate Management

Prolonged seizures or clusters of seizures in children with known epilepsy can sometimes be managed at home with rectal diazepam to prevent or abort status epilepticus (Kriel et al, 1991). A rectal preparation of diazepam is not available in the United States, but the intravenous preparation can be given rectally (0.3 to 0.5 mg/kg) through a lubricated syringe. If a single dose fails to stop seizures, the child should be brought to an emergency service.

Status epilepticus is a medical emergency requiring prompt attention. Initial assessment should be rapid and includes cardiorespiratory function, history leading up to the seizure, and neurologic examination. A controlled airway must be established immediately and mechanical ventilation made available. Venous access is established next. Blood is withdrawn for measurement of glucose, electrolyte, and anticonvulsant concentrations when applicable. Other tests (i.e., toxic screen) are performed as indicated. After blood is withdrawn, an intravenous infusion of saline solution is started for the administration of anticonvulsant drugs. An intravenous bolus of 50% glucose solution, 1 ml/kg, is then administered.

Drug Treatment

The ideal drug for treating status epilepticus is one that acts rapidly, has a long duration of action, and does not produce sedation. Diazepam is used widely for this purpose but is inadequate because the duration of action is brief. In addition, children who are given intravenous diazepam after a prior load of barbiturate often have respiratory depression. If diazepam is chosen as a first drug, the dose is 0.2 mg/kg, not to exceed 10 mg, at a rate of 1 mg/min. Lorazepam may be preferable to diazepam because of its longer action (Crawford et al, 1987). The usual dose in children 12 years or younger is 0.1 mg/kg. After age 12 it is 0.07 mg/kg.

My preference is intravenous phenytoin because of its long duration of action. A dose of 15 mg/kg is injected at a rate not to exceed 0.5 mg/kg/min. Infants generally require 20 mg/kg. The slow rate of administration is necessary to avoid causing cardiac arrhythmias.

Phenytoin is usually effective unless status epilepticus is caused by severe, acute encephalopathy. When phenytoin fails, several alternatives are available; my preference is pentobarbital coma.

The patient should have been transferred from the emergency room to an intensive care unit, intubated, and mechanically ventilated. After an arterial line is placed, the patient's blood pressure, cardiac rhythm, body temperature, and blood oxygen saturation are monitored.

With an EEG monitor recording continuously, 10 mg/kg boluses of pentobarbital are infused until a burst-suppression pattern appears on the EEG (Figure 1–8); a minimum of 30 mg/kg is generally required. Hypotension, when it occurs, is generally not observed until 40 to 60 mg/kg is administered. Barbiturates tend to accumulate, and the usual dose needed to maintain pentobarbital coma is 3 mg/kg/hr. The coma can be maintained safely for 3 days; longer periods may cause pulmonary edema. The EEG should be checked several times each day for the burst-suppression pattern. During barbiturate coma the patient has gastroparesis, and medications given through a nasogastric tube are not adequately absorbed but may remain in the stomach and then be rapidly absorbed when the coma is lifted. The coma can be lifted every 48 to 72 hours to see whether the seizures have stopped.

◆ Surgical Approaches to Childhood Epilepsy

Surgery is sometimes recommended for children with epilepsy that is intractable to optimal anticonvulsant therapy. Surgery is never a substitute for good medical therapy, and anticonvulsant drugs are often needed after surgery is performed. Three procedures are used: hemispherectomy, interhemispheric commissurotomy, and temporal lobectomy. None of these procedures is new, and all

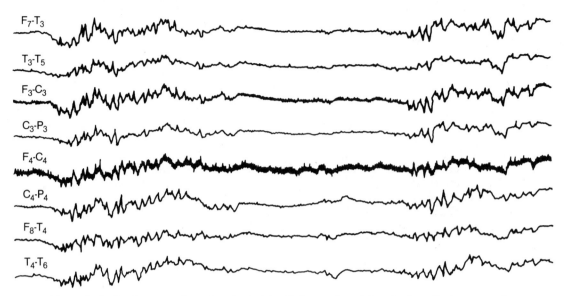

F_7-T_3

T_3-T_5

F_3-C_3

C_3-P_3

F_4-C_4

C_4-P_4

F_8-T_4

T_4-T_6

Figure 1–8   Burst-suppression pattern in pentobarbital coma. Long intervals of amplitude suppression are interrupted by bursts of mixed frequencies.

have gone through phases of greater or lesser popularity since being introduced.

HEMISPHERECTOMY

Hemispherectomy, or more correctly hemidecortication, has been used exclusively for children with intractable epilepsy and hemiplegia. It was first performed for that purpose in 1938 and became popular after 1950 (Goodman, 1986). The procedure consists of removing the cortex of one hemisphere along with a variable portion of the underlying basal ganglia. The extent of surgery depends partly on the underlying disease. The resulting cavity communicates with the third ventricle and becomes lined with a subdural membrane. The immediate results are good, with relief of seizures in about 80% of children. Improvements in behavior and spasticity, without deterioration of intellectual function, have been reported.

A postoperative mortality rate of 6.6% was considered acceptable, but the procedure fell from favor as late complication rates of 17% to 35% were reported. These complications, often fatal, included hemorrhage, hydrocephalus, and hemosiderosis. It is believed that the subdural membrane repeatedly tears, bleeding into the ventricular system and staining the ependymal lining and the pia arachnoid with iron.

Lindsay and associates (1987) have argued that optimal results and minimal complications are obtained by (1) selecting patients in whom the unaffected hemisphere is completely normal, (2) removing the cortex in a single piece, and (3) performing regular and careful follow-up of patients. Nevertheless, less radical alternatives are generally preferred. These alternatives are the Montreal-type hemispherectomy and interhemispheric commissurotomy.

The Montreal-type hemispherectomy is a modified procedure in which most of the damaged hemisphere is removed but portions of the frontal and occipital lobes are left in place, disconnected from the other hemisphere and brainstem. Only 20 such operations had been reported by 1988 (Tinuper et al, 1988). It appears that the percentage of patients who have become seizure free is less than with total hemispherectomy but that late complications are reduced.

INTERHEMISPHERIC COMMISSUROTOMY

Disconnecting the hemispheres from each other and from the brainstem is an alternative to hemispherectomy in children with intractable epilepsy and hemiplegia (Goodman et al, 1985). This operation is also used to decrease the occurrence of secondary generalized tonic-clonic seizures from partial or minor generalized seizures (Wyllie, 1988). The efficacy of commissurotomy and hemispherectomy in children with infantile hemiplegia is probably comparable, but the efficacy of commissurotomy in other forms of epilepsy has not been established.

Complete and partial commissurotomies have

been recommended. Complete commissurotomy entails division of the entire corpus callosum, anterior commissure, one fornix, and the hippocampal commissure. Complete commissurotomies may be performed in one stage or two. Partial commissurotomies vary from division of the corpus callosum and hippocampal commissure to division of only the anterior portion of the corpus callosum.

Two immediate, but transitory, postoperative complications may follow interhemispheric commissurotomy: (1) a syndrome of mutism, left arm and leg apraxia, and urinary incontinence and (2) hemiparesis. They are both more common after one-stage, complete commissurotomy than after two-stage procedures or partial commissurotomy and are probably caused by prolonged retraction of one hemisphere during surgery. Long-term complications may include stuttering and poorly coordinated movements of the hands.

TEMPORAL LOBECTOMY

Temporal lobectomy provided complete seizure relief in 50% and partial relief in 25% of selected children with intractable partial complex seizures of temporal lobe origin (Meyer et al, 1986). Only children who have a unilateral temporal focus are candidates for surgery. Positron emission tomography is proving valuable for identifying the epileptic focus (Chugani et al, 1988). The surgical procedure is a subpial resection of the superior temporal gyrus, hippocampus, and amygdala. The extent of resection is determined by intraoperative EEG. Benign tumors, gliomas and ganglioneuromas, are found in 12% of the specimens.

The most common complication is superior quadrantanopsia (40%), and the most serious complication is aphasia (10%), which is usually transitory.

References

Aicardi J: Current management of infantile spasms. Int Pediatr 4:188, 1989.

Albani M, Bentele KHP, Budde C, et al: Infant sleep apnea profile: Preterm vs. term infants. Eur J Pediatr 143:261, 1985.

Aldrich MS: Narcolepsy. N Engl J Med 323:389, 1990.

Andermann F, Andermann A: Startle disorders of man: Hyperekplexia, jumping, and startle epilepsy. Brain Dev 10:213, 1988.

Angelini L, Rumi V, Lamperti E, et al: Transient paroxysmal dystonia in infancy. Neuropediatrics 19:171, 1988.

Arts WFM, Vissar LH, Loonen MCB, et al: Follow-up of 146 children with epilepsy after withdrawal of antiepileptic therapy. Epilepsia 29:244, 1988.

Bachmann C: Diagnosis of urea cycle disorders. Enzyme 38:233-241, 1987.

Barabas G, Tucker SM: Idiopathic hypoparathyroidism and paroxysmal dystonic choreoathetosis. Arch Neurol 45:585, 1988.

Batshaw ML, Monahan PS: Treatment of urea cycle disorders. Enzyme 38:242-250, 1987.

Berkovic SF, Andermann F, Melanson D, et al: Hypothalamic hamartoma and ictal laughter: Evolution of a characteristic epileptic syndrome and diagnostic value of magnetic resonance imaging. Ann Neurol 23:429, 1988.

Berkovic SF, So NK, Andermann F: Progressive myoclonus epilepsies: Clinical and neurophysiological diagnosis. J Clin Neurophysiol 8:261, 1991.

Berry GT, Yudkoff M, Segal S: Isovaleric acidemia: Medical and neurodevelopmental effects of long-term therapy. J Pediatr 113:58, 1988.

Brown ZA, Vontner LA, Benedetti J, et al: Effects on infants of a first episode of genital herpes during pregnancy. N Engl J Med 317:1246-1251, 1987.

Brunquell PJ: Recurrent encephalomyelitis associated with incontinentia pigmenti. Pediatr Neurol 3:174, 1987.

Brusilow SW, Danney M, Waber LJ, et al: Treatment of episodic hyperammonemia in children with inborn errors of urea synthesis. N Engl J Med 310:1630, 1984.

Chugani HT, Shewmon DA, Peacock WJ, et al: Surgical treatment of intractable neonatal-onset seizures: The role of positron emission tomography. Neurology 38:1178, 1988.

Chugani HT, Shields WD, Shewmon A, et al: Infantile spasms. I. PET identifies focal cortical dysgenesis in cryptogenic cases for surgical treatment. Ann Neurol 27:406, 1990.

Clancy R, Legido A, Lewis D: Occult neonatal seizures. Epilepsia 29:256, 1988.

Clancy R, Malin S, Laraque D, et al: Focal motor seizures heralding stroke in full-term neonates. Am J Dis Child 139:601, 1985.

Clancy RR, Sladky JT, Rorke LB: Hypoxic-ischemic spinal cord injury following perinatal asphyxia. Ann Neurol 25:185-189, 1989.

Coker SB, Holmes EW, Egel RT: Phenacemide therapy of complex partial epilepsy in children: Determination of plasma drug concentrations. Neurology 37:1861, 1987.

Crawford TO, Mitchell WG, Snodgrass SR: Lorazepam in childhood status epilepticus and serial seizures: Effectiveness and tachyphylaxis. Neurology 37:190, 1987.

Danner R, Shewmon A, Sherman MP: Seizures in an atelencephalic infant: Is the cortex essential for neonatal seizures? Arch Neurol 42:1014, 1985.

Deonna TW: Acquired epileptiform aphasia in childhood (Landau-Kleffner syndrome). J Clin Neurophysiol 8:288, 1991.

Devinsky O, Kelley K, Porter RJ, et al: Clinical and electroencephalographic features of simple partial seizures. Neurology 38:1347, 1988.

DiMario FJ Jr, Emery ES: The natural history of night terrors. Ann Neurol 20:440, 1986.

Doberczak TM, Kandall SR, Wilets I: Neonatal opiate abstinence syndrome in term and preterm infants. J Pediatr 118:933, 1991.

Doberczak TM, Shanzer S, Cutler R, et al: One-year follow-up of infants with abstinence-associated seizures. Arch Neurol 45:649, 1988.

Donat J: The age-dependent epileptic encephalopathies. J Child Neurol 7:7, 1992.

Dravet C, Bureau M, Roger J: Benign myoclonic epilepsy in infants. In Roger J, Dravet C, Bureau M, et al, eds: Epileptic Syndromes in Infancy, Childhood and Adolescence. John Libbey Eurotext, London, 1985a, p 51.

Dravet C, Bureau M, Roger J: Severe myoclonic epilepsy in infants. In Roger J, Dravet C, Bureau M, et al, eds: Epileptic Syndromes in Infancy, Childhood and Adolescence. John Libbey Eurotext, London, 1985b, p 58.

Dreifuss FE, Langer DH, Moline KA, et al: Valproic acid hepatic fatalities. II. US experience since 1984. Neurology 39:201, 1989.

Durner M, Sander T, Greenberg DA, et al: Localization of idiopathic generalized epilepsy on chromosome 6p in families of juvenile myoclonic epilepsy patients. Neurology 41:1651, 1991.

El-Radhi AS, Banajeh S: Effect of fever on recurrence rate of febrile convulsions. Arch Dis Child 64:869, 1989.

Elwes RDC, Chesterman P, Reynolds EH: Prognosis after a first untreated tonic-clonic seizure. Lancet 2:752, 1985.

Gilman JT, Gal P, Duchowny MS, et al: Rapid sequence phenobarbital treatment of neonatal seizures. Pediatrics 83:674, 1989.

Glaze DG, Hrachovy RA, Frost JD Jr, et al: Prospective study of outcome of infants with infantile spasms treated during controlled studies of ACTH and prednisone. J Pediatr 112:389, 1988.

Goodman R: Hemispherectomy and its alternatives in the treatment of intractable epilepsy in patients with infantile hemiplegia. Dev Med Child Neurol 28:251, 1986.

Goodman RN, Williamson PD, Reeves AG, et al: Interhemispheric commissurotomy for congenital hemiplegics with intractable epilepsy. Neurology 35:1351, 1985.

Goulden KJ, Camfield PR, Camfield CS, et al: Changes in serum anticonvulsant levels with febrile illness in children with epilepsy. Can J Neurol Sci 15:281, 1988.

Goutieres F, Aicardi J: Atypical presentations of pyridoxine-dependent seizures: A treatable cause of intractable epilepsy in infants. Ann Neurol 17:117, 1985.

Gulick TA, Spinks IP, King DW: Pseudoseizures: Ictal phenomena. Neurology 32:24, 1982.

Hadeed AJ, Siegel SR: Maternal cocaine use during pregnancy: Effect on the newborn infant. Pediatrics 84:205, 1989.

Haenggeli C-A, Girardin E, Paunier L: Pyridoxine-dependent seizures, clinical and therapeutic aspects. Eur J Pediatr 150:452, 1991.

Hansen TWR, Bratlid D: Bilirubin and bilirubin toxicity. Acta Paediatr Scand 75:513, 1986.

Henderson-Smart DJ, Pettigrew AG, Campbell DJ: Clinical apnea and brainstem function in preterm infants. N Engl J Med 308:353, 1983.

Hill A, Volpe JJ: Perinatal asphyxia: Clinical aspects. Clin Perinatol 16:435, 1989.

Hirtz DG, Ellenberg JH, Nelson KB: The risk of recurrence of nonfebrile seizures in children. Neurology 34:637, 1984.

Holmes G, Mikati M: Temporal lobe epilepsy in children. Int Pediatr 6:201, 1991.

Holmes GB, Rosenfeld WE, Graves NM, et al: Absorption of valproate suppositories in human volunteers. Arch Neurol 46:906, 1989.

Honavar M, Janota I, Polkey CE: Rasmussen's encephalitis in surgery for epilepsy. Dev Med Child Neurol 34:3, 1992.

Hrachovy RA, Frost JD Jr, Kellaway P: Hypsarrhythmia: Variations on a theme. Epilepsia 25:317, 1984.

Huttenlocher PR, Hapke RJ: A follow-up study of intractable seizures in childhood. Ann Neurol 28:699, 1990.

Institute of Medicine: Adverse Effects of Pertussis and Rubella Vaccines. National Academy Press, Washington, DC, 1991.

Kales A, Cadieux RJ, Soldatos CR, et al: Narcolepsy-cataplexy. I. Clinical and electrophysiologic characteristics. Arch Neurol 39:164, 1982.

Kaplan P, Mazur A, Field M, et al: Intellectual outcome in children with maple syrup urine disease. J Pediatr 119:46, 1991.

Kivity S, Lerman P: Stormy onset with prolonged loss of conciousness in benign childhood epilepsy with occipital paroxysms. J Neurol Neurosurg Psychiat 55:45, 1992.

Kriel RL, Cloyd JC, Hadsall RS, et al: Home use of rectal diazepam for cluster and prolonged seizures: Efficacy, adverse reactions, quality of life, and cost analysis. Pediatr Neurol 7:13, 1991.

Lance JW: Familial paroxysmal dystonic choreoathetosis and its differentiation from related syndromes. Ann Neurol 2:285, 1977.

Larsen R, Ashwal S, Peckham N: Incontinentia pigmenti: Association with anterior horn cell degeneration. Neurology 37:446, 1987.

Lerman P, Kivity S: The benign nonrolandic epilepsies. J Clin Neurophysiol 8:275, 1991.

Lindsay J, Ounsted C, Richards P: Hemispherectomy for childhood epilepsy: A 36 year study. Dev Med Child Neurol 29:592, 1987.

Loiseau P, Duché B, Cordova S, et al: Prognosis of benign childhood epilepsy with centrotemporal spikes: A follow-up study of 168 patients. Epilepsia 29:229, 1988.

Luder AS, Davidson A, Goodman SI, et al: Transient nonketotic hyperglycinemia in neonates. J Pediatr 114:1013, 1989.

Lupton BA, Hill A, Roland EH, et al: Brain swelling in the asphyxiated term newborn: Pathogenesis and outcome. Pediatrics 82:139, 1988.

Marks DA, Katz A, Scheyer R, et al: Clinical and electrographic effects of acute anticonvulsant withdrawal in epileptic patients. Neurology 41:508, 1991.

Matsumoto A, Watanabe K, Sugiura M, et al: Prognostic factors of convulsive disorders in the first year of life. Brain Dev 5:469, 1983.

McKinlay I, Newton R: Intention to treat febrile convulsions with rectal diazepam, valproate or phenobarbitone. Dev Med Child Neurol 31:617, 1989.

Meyer FB, Marsh WR, Laws ER Jr, et al: Temporal lobectomy in children with epilepsy. J Neurosurg 64:371, 1986.

Miles DK, Holmes GL: Benign neonatal seizures. J Clin Neurophysiol 7:369, 1990.

Mitchell WG, Chavez JM: Carbamazepine versus phenobarbital for partial onset seizures in children. Epilepsia 28:56, 1987.

Mizrahi EM, Kellaway P: Characterization and classification of neonatal seizures. Neurology 37:1837, 1987.

Mostow SR, Mayfield JL, Marr JJ, et al: Suppression of recurrent genital herpes by single daily dosages of acyclovir. Am J Med 85(suppl 2A):30-33, 1988.

Muller W, Peter HH, Wilken M, et al: The DiGeorge syndrome. I. Clinical evaluation and course of partial and complete forms of the syndrome. Eur J Pediatr 147:496, 1988.

Nakamura H, Takeda S, Shimabuku R, et al: Auditory nerve and brainstem responses in newborns with hyperbilirubinemia. Pediatrics 75:703, 1985.

Nelson KB, Broman SH: Perinatal risk factors in children with serious motor and mental handicaps. Ann Neurol 2:371, 1977.

Nelson KB, Ellenberg JH: Apgar scores as predictors of chronic neurologic disability. Pediatrics 68:36, 1981.

Nyhan WL: Nonketotic hyperglycinemia. In Scriver CR, Beaudet AL, Sly WS, et al, eds: The Metabolic Basis of Inherited Disease, 6th edition. McGraw-Hill Information Services, New York, 1989, p 743.

Ozand PT, Gascon GG: Organic acidurias: A review. Part 1. J Child Neurol 6:196, 1991.

Palmini A, Andermann F, Olivier A, et al. Focal neuronal migration disorders and intractable partial epilepsy: a study of 30 patients. Ann Neurol 30:741, 1991.

Panayiotopoulos CP, Obeid T: Juvenile myoclonic epilepsy: An autosomal dominant disease. Ann Neurol 25:440, 1989.

Pellock JM, Willmore LJ: A rational guide to routine blood monitoring in patients receiving antiepileptic drugs. Neurology 41:961, 1991.

Piatt JH Jr, Hwang PA, Armstrong DC, et al: Chronic focal encephalitis (Rasmussen syndrome): Six cases. Epilepsia 29:268, 1988.

Prats JM, Garaizar C, Rua MJ, et al: Infantile spasms treated with high doses of sodium valproate: Initial response and follow-up. Dev Med Child Neurol 33:617, 1991.

Riviello JJ, Rezvani I, DeGeorge AM, et al: Cerebral edema causing death in children with maple syrup urine disease. J Pediatr 119:42, 1991.

Rosenberg LE, Fenton WA: Disorders of propionate and methylmalonate metabolism. In Scriver CR, Beaudet AL, Sly WS, et al, eds: The Metabolic Basis of Inherited Disease, 6th edition. McGraw-Hill Information Services, New York, 1989, p 821.

Ryan SG, Wiznitzer M, Hollman C, et al: Benign familial neonatal convulsions: Evidence for clinical and genetic heterogeneity. Ann Neurol 29:469, 1991.

Schmidley JW, Simon RP: Postictal pleocytosis. Ann Neurol 9:81, 1981.

Serfontein GL, Rom S, Stein S: Posterior fossa subdural hemorrhage in the newborn. Pediatrics 65:40, 1980.

Shen W, Bowman ES, Markand ON: Presenting the diagnosis of pseudoseizure. Neurology 40:756, 1990.

Shinnar S, Zeitlin-Gross L, Moshe SL, et al: The low risk of seizure recurrences following a first unprovoked seizure in children and adolescence: A prospective study. Ann Neurol 20:388, 1986.

Silvestri R, Ciliberto R, Domenico PD, et al: Paroxysmal electroencephalographic abnormalities genetically transmitted. Eur Neurol 29:216, 1989.

Snead OC, Hosey LC: Excerbation of seizures in children by carbamazepine. N Engl J Med 313:916, 1985.

Specht U, Boenigk HE, Wolf P: Discontinuation of clonazepam after long-term treatment. Epilepsia 30:458, 1989.

Tinuper P, Andermann F, Willemure J-G, et al: Functional hemispherectomy for treatment of epilepsy associated with hemiplegia: Rationale, indications, results, and comparison with callosotomy. Ann Neurol 24:27-34, 1988.

Trauner DA, Page T, Greco C, et al: Progressive neurodegenerative disorder in a patient with nonketotic hyperglycinemia. J Pediatr 98:272, 1983.

Vannucci RC: Current and potentially new management strategies for perinatal hypoxic-ischemic encephalopathy. Pediatrics 85:961, 1990.

Watanabe K, Yamamoto N, Negoro T, et al: Benign complex partial epilepsies in infancy. Pediatr Neurol 3:208, 1987.

Whitley R, Arvin A, Prober C, et al: A controlled trial comparing vidarabine with acyclovir in neonatal herpes simplex virus infection. N Engl J Med 324:444, 1991.

Wyllie E: Corpus callosotomy for intractable generalized epilepsy. J Pediatr 113:255, 1988.

Wyllie E, Friedman D, Rothner AD, et al: Psychogenic seizures in children and adolescents: Outcome after diagnosis by ictal video and electroencephalographic recording. Pediatrics 85:480, 1990.

Altered States of Consciousness

The terms used in this text to describe states of decreased consciousness are provided in Table 2–1. With the exception of "coma," these definitions are not standard. However, they are more precise and therefore more useful than such terms as "semicomatose" and "semistuporous." The term "encephalopathy" is used to describe a diffuse disorder of the brain in which at least two of the following symptoms are present: (1) altered states of consciousness, (2) altered cognition or personality, and (3) seizures. Encephalitis is an encephalopathy accompanied by cerebrospinal fluid pleocytosis.

Lack of responsiveness does not always equal lack of consciousness. For example, infants with botulism (see Chapter 6) may have such severe hypotonia and ptosis that they cannot move their limbs or eyelids in response to stimulation. They appear to be in coma or stupor but are actually alert. The locked-in syndrome (a brainstem disorder in which the individual can process information but cannot respond) and catatonia are other examples of diminished responsiveness in the alert state.

Freemon (1976) has described two "roads" to coma. The "high road" is characterized by increased neuronal excitability. The patient becomes restless, then confused; next tremor, hallucinations, and delirium (an agitated confusional state) develop. Myoclonic jerks may be noted. Seizures herald the end of delirium and are followed by stupor or coma. Table 2–2 summarizes the differential diagnosis of the "high road." Tumors and other mass lesions are not expected causes. Instead, the diagnosis is weighted in favor of metabolic, toxic, and inflammatory disorders.

The "low road" is characterized by decreased neuronal excitability and lacks an agitated stage. Instead the patient shows progressive deterioration from lethargy to obtundation, stupor, and coma. The differential diagnosis is considerably larger than that of the "high road" and includes mass lesions and other causes of increased intracranial pressure (Table 2–3). Conditions that may cause a recurrent encephalopathy are listed in Table 2–4.

A comparison of Tables 2–2 and 2–3 shows a considerable overlap between conditions whose first manifestations are agitation and confusion and those that begin with lethargy or coma. Therefore the disorders responsible for each are described together in the text to prevent repetition.

◆ Diagnostic Approach to Delirium

Any child with the acute behavioral changes of delirium (agitation, confusion, delusions, or hallucinations) should be assumed to have an organic encephalopathy until proven otherwise. Delirium is usually caused by a toxic or metabolic disorder diffusely affecting both cerebral hemispheres. Schizophrenia should not be a consideration in a prepubertal child with acute delirium. *Delusions* are fixed beliefs that cannot be altered by reason. The paranoid delusions of schizophrenia are logical

Table 2–1 ◆ States of Decreased Consciousness

Term	Definition
Lethargy	Difficulty in maintaining the aroused state
Obtundation	Responsive to stimulation other than pain*
Stupor	Responsive only to pain*
Coma	Unresponsive to pain

*Responsive indicates cerebral alerting and not just reflex withdrawal.

Table 2–2 ◆ Causes of Agitation and Confusion

Epileptic
1. Absence status (see Chapter 1)
2. Complex partial seizure (see Chapter 1)
 	
Infectious Disorders
1. Bacterial infections
  a. Cat scratch disease
  b. Meningitis (see Chapter 4)
2. Rickettsial infections
  a. Lyme disease
  b. Rocky Mountain spotted fever
3. Viral infections
  a. Aseptic meningitis
  b. Arboviruses
  c. Herpes simplex encephalitis
  d. Measles encephalitis
  e. Postinfectious encephalomyelitis
  f. Reye syndrome
 	
Metabolic and Systemic Disorders
1. Disorders of osmolality
  a. Hypoglycemia
  b. Hyponatremia
2. Endocrine disorders
  a. Adrenal insufficiency
  b. Hypoparathyroidism
  c. Thyroid disorders
3. Hepatic encephalopathy
4. Inborn errors of metabolism
  a. Disorders of pyruvate metabolism (see Chapter 5)
  b. Primary carnitine deficiency
  c. Urea cycle disorder, heterozygote (see Chapter 1).
5. Renal disease
  a. Hypertensive encephalopathy
  b. Uremic encephalopathy
	Migraine
	1. Acute confusional
	2. Aphasic
	3. Transient global amnesia
	
	Psychologic
	1. Panic disorder
	2. Schizophrenia
	
	Toxic
	1. Prescription drugs
	2. Substance abuse
	3. Toxins
	
	Vascular
	1. Congestive heart failure
	2. Embolism
	3. Hypertensive encephalopathy
	4. Lupus erythematosus
	5. Subarachnoid hemorrhage
	6. Vasculitis

to the patient and frequently part of an elaborate system of irrational thinking in which the patient feels menaced. Delusions associated with organic encephalopathy are less logical, are not systematized, and tend to be stereotyped.

A *hallucination* is the perception of sensory stimuli that are not present. Visual hallucinations are almost always caused by organic encephalopathy, and auditory hallucinations, especially if accusatory, usually indicate psychiatric illness. Stereotyped auditory hallucinations that represent a recurring memory are an exception and suggest temporal lobe seizures.

HISTORY AND PHYSICAL EXAMINATION

Delirious children, even with stable vital function, must be assessed rapidly because the potential for deterioration to a state of diminished consciousness is always present. Careful history must be obtained of (1) the events leading to the behavioral change, (2) drug or toxic exposure (prescription drugs are more often at fault than substances of abuse, and a medicine cabinet inspection should be ordered in every home the child has visited), (3) personal or family history of migraine or epilepsy, (4) recent or concurrent fever, infectious disease, or systemic illness, and (5) previous personal or family history of encephalopathy.

Examination of the eyes, in addition to determining the presence or absence of papilledema, provides other etiologic clues. Drug or toxic exposure is suggested by small or large pupils that respond poorly to light, nystagmus, or impaired eye movements. Fixed deviation of the eyes in one lateral direction may indicate that (1) the encephalopathy has focal features, (2) seizures are a cause

Table 2-3 ◆ Causes of Lethargy and Coma

Epilepsy
1. Postictal state (see Chapter 1)
2. Status epilepticus (see Chapter 1)

Hypoxia-Ischemia
1. Cardiac arrest
2. Cardiac arrhythmia
3. Congestive heart failure
4. Hypotension
   a. Autonomic dysfunction
   b. Dehydration
   c. Hemorrhage
   d. Pulmonary embolism
5. Near-drowning
6. Neonatal (see Chapter 1)

Increased Intracranial Pressure
1. Cerebral abscess (see Chapter 4)
2. Cerebral edema (see Chapter 4)
3. Cerebral tumor (see Chapters 4 and 10)
4. Herniation syndromes (see Chapter 4)
5. Hydrocephalus (see Chapters 4 and 18)
6. Intracranial hemorrhage
   a. Spontaneous (see Chapter 4)
   b. Traumatic

Infectious Disorders
1. Bacterial infections
   a. Cat scratch disease
   b. Gram-negative sepsis
   c. Hyperpyrexia (hemorrhagic shock) and en-
      cephalopathy syndrome
   d. Meningitis (see Chapter 4)
   e. Toxic shock syndrome
2. Rickettsial infections
   a. Lyme disease
   b. Rocky Mountain spotted fever
3. Viral infections
   a. Aseptic meningitis
   b. Arboviruses
   c. Herpes simplex encephalitis
   d. Measles encephalitis
   e. Postinfectious encephalomyelitis
   f. Reye syndrome
4. Postimmunization encephalopathy

Metabolic and Systemic Disorders
1. Disorders of osmolality
   a. Diabetic ketoacidosis (hyperglycemia)
   b. Hypoglycemia
   c. Hypernatremia
   d. Hyponatremia
2. Endocrine disorders
   a. Adrenal insufficiency
   b. Hypoparathyroidism
   c. Thyroid disorders
3. Hepatic encephalopathy
4. Inborn errors of metabolism
   a. Disorders of pyruvate metabolism (see Chap-
      ter 5)
   b. Glycogen storage disorders (see Chapter 1)
   c. Neonatal presentation (see Chapter 1)
   d. Primary carnitine deficiency
   e. Urea cycle disorder, heterozygote (see Chap-
      ter 1)
5. Renal disorders
   a. Acute uremic encephalopathy
   b. Chronic uremic encephalopathy
   c. Dialysis encephalopathy
   d. Hypertensive encephalopathy
6. Other metabolic disorders
   a. Burn encephalopathy
   b. Hypomagnesemia
   c. Parenteral hyperalimentation
   d. Vitamin B complex deficiency

Migraine Coma

Toxic
1. Prescription drugs
2. Substance abuse
3. Toxins

Trauma
1. Concussion
2. Contusion
3. Intracranial hemorrhage
   a. Epidural hematoma
   b. Subdural hematoma
   c. Intracerebral hemorrhage
4. Neonatal (see Chapter 1)

Vascular
1. Hypertensive encephalopathy
2. Intracranial hemorrhage—nontraumatic (see
   Chapter 4)
3. Lupus erythematosus (see Chapter 11)
4. Vasculitis (see Chapter 11)

of the confusional state, or (3) seizures are a part of the encephalopathy.

The general and neurologic examinations should specifically include a search for evidence of trauma, needle marks on the limbs, meningismus, and cardiac disease.

LABORATORY INVESTIGATIONS

Laboratory evaluation should be individualized; not every test is essential for each clinical situation. The first step is to obtain blood and urine. Studies of potential interest include culture, complete blood

Table 2–4 ◆ Causes of Recurrent Encephalopathy

1. Burn encephalopahty
2. Epilepsy
3. Hashimoto thyroiditis
4. Hypoglycemia
5. Increased intracranial pressure (recurrent)
6. Mental disorders
7. Migraine
8. Mitochondrial disorders
9. Primary carnitine deficiency
10. Pyruvate metabolism disorders
11. Substance abuse
12. Urea cycle disorder

cell count, sedimentation rate, toxicity screen, concentrations of glucose, electrolytes, calcium and phosphorus, urea nitrogen, ammonia, and thyroid-stimulating hormone, and liver function tests. If possible, a computed tomography (CT) of the head should be performed while these results are pending. If sedation is required to perform the study, a short-acting benzodiazepine is preferred. Nondiagnostic blood studies and normal CT results are an indication for lumbar puncture looking for infection, hemorrhage, and increased intracranial pressure. A manometer should always be available

to measure the pressure of the cerebrospinal fluid.

An electroencephalogram (EEG) can be useful in the evaluation of delirious patients and should be obtained at an opportune time. Findings are almost always abnormal in acute organic encephalopathies and normal in psychiatric illnesses. The minimal EEG finding in encephalopathy is slowing of the posterior rhythm; more severe encephalopathies are characterized by diffuse theta and delta activity, absence of faster frequencies, and intermittent rhythmic delta activity (Fig. 2–1). Specific abnormalities may include epileptiform activity consistent with absence or complex partial status, triphasic waves indicating hepatic or uremic encephalopathy (Fig. 2–2), and periodic lateralizing epileptiform discharges in one temporal lobe, suggesting herpes encephalitis.

◆ Diagnostic Approach to Lethargy and Coma

The diagnostic approach to states of diminished consciousness in children is similar to that suggested for delirium, except for greater urgency. Progressive decline in state of consciousness can

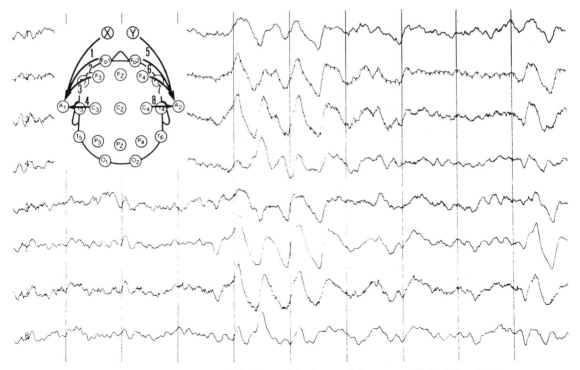

Figure 2–1 Frontal intermittent rhythmic delta activity. Bursts of slow waves with frontal predominance are a nonspecific abnormality in early encephalopathy. (From Epstein C, Andriola M: Introduction to EEG and Evoked Potentials. Lippincott, Philadelphia, 1983.)

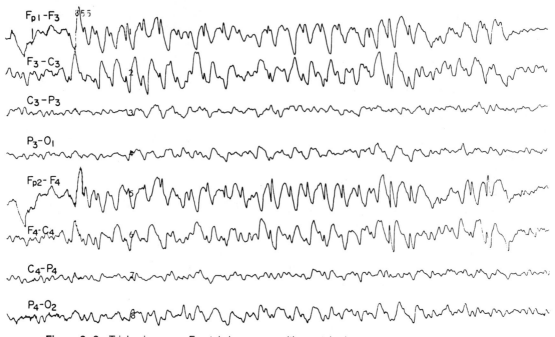

Figure 2-2 Triphasic waves. Frontal slow waves with a notched appearance are a feature of uremic and hepatic encephalopathy. (From Epstein C, Andriola M: Introduction to EEG and Evoked Potentials. Lippincott, Philadelphia, 1983.)

be caused by diffuse or multifocal disturbances of the cerebral hemispheres or by focal injury to the brainstem. The anatomic site of abnormality can often be determined by physical examination.

HISTORY AND PHYSICAL EXAMINATION

The historical data to be obtained are the same as for delirium, except that mass lesions are an important consideration. Further inquiry must be made concerning trauma or preceding symptoms of increasing intracranial pressure.

Physical examination is directed at determining both the anatomic site of disturbed cerebral function and its cause. The important variables in locating the site of abnormality are state of consciousness, pattern of breathing, pupillary size and reactivity, eye movements, and motor responses (Plum and Posner, 1980). Lethargy and obtundation are generally caused by mild depression of hemispheric function. Stupor and coma are characteristic of much more extensive disturbance of hemispheric function or involvement of the diencephalon and upper brainstem. Derangements of the dominant hemisphere may have a greater effect on consciousness than derangements of the non-dominant hemisphere.

Cheyne-Stokes respiration, in which periods of hyperpnea alternate with periods of apnea, results from an extensive, usually bilateral diencephalic disturbance with the brainstem intact. Hypothalamic and midbrain damage causes a sustained, rapid, deep hyperventilation (central neurogenic hyperventilation). Abnormalities within the medulla and pons affect the respiratory centers and cause several different patterns of respiratory control: (1) *apneustic breathing,* a pause at full inspiration; (2) *ataxic breathing,* haphazard breaths and pauses without a predictable pattern; or (3) *Ondine's curse,* failure of automatic breathing when asleep.

The pupillary light reflex is usually retained in metabolic disturbances, and its absence in a comatose patient indicates a structural abnormality. The major exception is drugs: a fixed dilated pupil in an alert patient is caused by topical administration of mydriatics. In comatose patients, hypothalamic damage causes unilateral pupillary constriction and a Horner syndrome; midbrain lesions cause midposition fixed pupils; pontine lesions cause small but reactive pupils; and lateral medullary lesions cause a Horner syndrome.

Tonic lateral deviation of both eyes indicates a seizure originating in the hemisphere opposite the direction of gaze or a destructive lesion in the hemisphere in the direction of gaze. Ocular motility in comatose patients can be assessed by instilling ice water sequentially 15 minutes apart in each ear to chill the tympanic membrane. Ice water in the right ear causes both eyes to deviate rapidly to the right and then slowly return to the midline. The rapid movement to the right is a brainstem reflex, and its presence indicates that much of the brainstem is intact. Abduction of the right eye with failure of left eye adduction demonstrates a lesion in the medial longitudinal fasciculus (see Chapter 15). The slow movement that returns the eye to the left requires a corticopontine pathway originating in the right hemisphere and terminating in the left pontine lateral gaze center. Its presence demonstrates unilateral hemispheric function.

Trunk and limb position at rest, spontaneous movements, and response to noxious stimuli must be carefully observed. Spontaneous movement of all limbs generally indicates a mild depression of hemispheric function without structural disturbance. Monoplegia or hemiplegia, except in the postictal state, suggests a structural disturbance of the contralateral hemisphere. An extensor response of the trunk and limbs to a noxious stimulus is termed *decerebrate rigidity*. The most severe form is called *opisthotonos:* the neck is hyperextended and the teeth are clenched; the arms adducted, hyperextended, and hyperpronated; and the legs extended with the feet plantar flexed. Decerebrate rigidity indicates brainstem compression and should be considered an ominous sign whether present at rest or in response to noxious stimuli. Flexion of the arms and extension of the legs is termed *decorticate rigidity*. It is uncommon in children except following head injury and indicates hemispheric dysfunction with brainstem integrity.

LABORATORY INVESTIGATIONS

Laboratory investigations are similar to those described for the evaluation of delirium. Head CT with contrast enhancement should be performed promptly to exclude the possibility of a mass lesion and herniation. It is a great error to send a child whose condition is uncertain for CT without a physician in attendance who knows how to monitor deterioration and intervene appropriately.

◆ Hypoxia and Ischemia

Hypoxia and ischemia usually occur together. Prolonged hypoxia causes personality change first and then loss of consciousness; acute anoxia results in immediate loss of consciousness.

PROLONGED HYPOXIA

Clinical Features. Prolonged hypoxia can result from severe anemia (oxygen-carrying capacity reduced by at least half), congestive heart failure, chronic lung disease, and neuromuscular disorders.

The best studied model of prolonged, mild hypoxia is ascent to high altitudes. Mild hypoxia causes impaired memory and judgment, confusion, and decreased motor performance. Greater degrees of hypoxia result in obtundation, multifocal myoclonus, and sometimes focal neurologic signs such as monoplegia and hemiplegia. Children with chronic cardiopulmonary disease may have an insidious alteration in behavioral state as arterial oxygen concentration slowly declines.

Neuromuscular disorders that weaken respiratory muscles, such as muscular dystrophy, often produce nocturnal hypoventilation as a first symptom of respiratory insufficiency. This is characterized by frequent awakenings and fear of sleeping (see Chapter 7).

Diagnosis. Hypoxia should be considered in children with chronic cardiopulmonary disorders who become depressed or undergo personality change. Arterial Po_2 values below 40 mm Hg are regularly associated with obvious neurologic disturbances, but minor mental disturbances may occur at a Pao_2 of 60 mm Hg, especially when hypoxia is chronic.

Treatment. Encephalopathy usually reverses when Pao_2 is increased, but persistent cerebral dysfunction may occur in mountain climbers after returning to sea level (West, 1986), and permanent cerebral dysfunction may develop in children with chronic hypoxia (O'Dougherty et al, 1985). As a group, children with chronic hypoxia from congenital heart disease have a lower IQ than nonhypoxic children. The severity of mental decline is related to the duration of hypoxia.

Children with neuromuscular disorders who have symptoms during sleep can be treated overnight with intermittent positive-pressure ventilation applied by mouth (see Chapter 7).

ACUTE ANOXIA AND ISCHEMIA

The usual circumstance in which acute anoxia and ischemia occur is cardiac arrest or sudden hypotension. Anoxia without ischemia occurs with suffocation (near-drowning, choking). Prolonged anoxia leads to bradycardia and cardiac arrest. In adults hippocampal and Purkinje cells begin to die after 4 minutes of total anoxia and ischemia and the outside limit of brain viability is believed to be 10 minutes. Exact timing may be difficult in clinical situations when ill-defined intervals of anoxia and hypoxia occur. Remarkable survivals are sometimes associated with near-drowning in water cold enough to lower cerebral temperature and metabolism.

The pattern of hypoxic-ischemic brain injury in newborns is different and depends largely on brain maturity (see Chapter 1).

Clinical Features. Consciousness is lost within 8 seconds of cerebral circulatory failure, but the loss may take longer when anoxia occurs without ischemia. Presyncopal symptoms of lightheadedness and visual disturbances sometimes precede loss of consciousness. Seizures and extensor rigidity follow.

Considerable effort has been made to identify predicters of outcome after hypoxic-ischemic events. Only 13% of adults who have had a cardiac arrest regain independent function in the first year after arrest (Levy et al, 1985). Outcome in children is somewhat better because the incidence of preexisting cardiopulmonary disease is lower. Absence of pupillary responses on initial examination is an ominous sign; such patients do not recover independent function. Twenty-four hours after arrest, patients with poor prognoses are identified by lack of motor responses in the limbs and eyes. In contrast, a favorable outcome can be predicted for patients who rapidly recover roving or conjugate eye movements and limb withdrawal from pain.

Two delayed syndromes of neurologic deterioration follow anoxia. The first is *delayed postanoxic encephalopathy*, the appearance of apathy or confusion 1 to 2 weeks after apparent recovery. This is followed by motor symptoms, usually rigidity or spasticity, and may progress to coma or death. Demyclination is the suggested mechanism. The other syndrome is *postanoxic action myoclonus*. This usually follows a severe episode of anoxia and ischemia caused by cardiac arrest. All voluntary activity initiates disabling myoclonus (see Chapter 14). Symptoms of cerebellar dysfunction are also present.

Diagnosis. Cerebral edema is prominent during the first 72 hours following severe hypoxia. CT at that time demonstrates decreased density with loss of the differentiation between gray and white matter. Severe, generalized loss of density on CT correlates with a poor outcome.

An EEG that shows a burst-suppression pattern or absence of activity is associated with poor neurologic outcome or death; lesser abnormalities are not useful in predicting prognosis.

Treatment. The principles of treating patients who have sustained hypoxic-ischemic encephalopathy do not differ substantially from the principles of caring for other comatose patients. Oxygenation, circulation, and blood glucose concentration must be maintained. Intracranial pressure must be lowered sufficiently to allow satisfactory cerebral perfusion (see Chapter 4). Seizures are managed with anticonvulsant drugs (see Chapter 1). Anoxia is invariably associated with lactic acidosis, and acid-base balance must be restored.

Barbiturate coma is frequently used to slow cerebral metabolism, but neither clinical nor experimental evidence indicates a beneficial effect following cardiac arrest (Dearden, 1985) or near-drowning (Nussbaum and Maggi, 1988). Hypothermia prevents brain damage during the time of hypoxia and ischemia but has questionable value after the event. Corticosteroids do not improve neurologic recovery in patients with global ischemia following cardiac arrest (Jastremski et al, 1989).

Postanoxic action myoclonus can be treated effectively with valproate.

PERSISTENT VEGETATIVE STATE

The terms "persistent vegetative state" and "neocortical death" are used interchangeably to describe patients who, after recovery from coma, return to a state of wakefulness without cognition. A persistent vegetative state is "a form of eyes-open permanent unconsciousness in which the patient has periods of wakefulness and physiological sleep/wake cycles, but at no time is the patient aware of him- or herself or the environment" (American Academy of Neurology, 1989). Brainstem functions such as respiration and circulation are intact, and with good nursing care survival is indefinite. A persistent vegetative state occurs in 12% of adults who survive nontraumatic coma but is probably less common in children. The usual causes in order of frequency are anoxia and ischemia, metabolic or encephalitic coma, and head trauma. Recovery is rare when the vegetative state has persisted for 1 month in adults. The prognosis may be better in children, but little reason for hope remains after 3 months.

The American Academy of Neurology (1989) has adopted the policy that all medical treatment, including the provision of nutrition and hydration, may be ethically discontinued when a patient's condition has been diagnosed as a persistent vegetative state, it is clear that the patient would not want to be maintained in this state, and family agrees to discontinue therapy.

BRAIN DEATH

Various standards for the diagnosis of brain death have been proposed, but guidelines established by a presidential commission have been endorsed by major specialty societies and are now generally accepted (President's Commission, 1981). The important features of the report are summarized in Table 2–5. The commission urged caution in applying the criteria to children younger than 5 years, but subsequent experience supports the validity of the standards in the newborn and through childhood (Alvarez et al, 1988; Ashwal and Schneider, 1989; Fackler et al, 1988). Absence of cerebral blood flow is the earliest and most definitive proof of brain death. EEG activity may still be present 24 hours after cessation of cerebral blood flow but subsequently becomes isoelectric.

◆ Infectious Disorders
BACTERIAL INFECTIONS
Cat Scratch Disease

Cat scratch disease is caused by a gram-negative bacillus inoculated by a cat scratch (English et al, 1988). Three thousand cases were diagnosed in the United States between 1959 and 1987. Most cases are probably undiagnosed. The age range is 1 to 65 years, and males and females are equally affected. Eighty-two percent of cases occur in children less than 12 years of age (Carithers and Margileth, 1991).

Clinical Features. The major feature is lymphadenopathy proximal to the site of scratch. Fever is present in only 60% of cases. The disease is usually benign and self-limited. Unusual sys-temic manifestations are oculoglandular disease, erythema nodosum, osteolytic lesions, and thrombocytopenic purpura. The most common neurologic manifestation is encephalopathy. Rare cases of transverse myelitis and cerebral arteritis have been reported.

Encephalitis occurs in less than 1% of patients with cat scratch disease. The mechanism is unknown, but it may be caused by direct infection or vasculitis. The male-to-female ratio is 2:1. Only 17% occur in children less than 12 years, and 15% in children 12 to 18 years. The frequency of fever and the site of scratch are no different in patients with cat scratch disease encephalitis than in those who have the disease without encephalitis. The initial and most prominent manifestation is a decreased state of consciousness, ranging from lethargy to coma. Seizures occur in 46% and combative behavior in 40%. Focal findings are rare.

Diagnosis. The diagnosis requires local lymphadenopathy, history of contact with a cat, an identifiable site of inoculation, and a positive skin test or recovery of the organism. The cerebrospinal fluid is normal in 70% of cases. The cat scratch disease skin test, not yet commercially available, is positive for the disease in 4% to 8% of the general population, 18% of relatives of patients with cat scratch disease, and 23% of animal workers. The test becomes positive 24 to 48 hours after inoculation. The organism is identified from lymph nodes or from the inoculation site when a Warthin-Starry stain is used.

Lymphocytosis in the cerebrospinal fluid, when present, does not exceed 30 cells/mm^3. The EEG shows diffuse slowing. MRI and CT of the head show no abnormalities.

Treatment. All affected children recover completely, 50% within 4 weeks. Intravenous gentamicin, 5 to 7 mg/kg/day, may speed recovery.

GRAM-NEGATIVE SEPSIS

Clinical Features. The onset of symptoms of gram-negative sepsis may be explosive and is characterized by fever or hypothermia, chills, hyperventilation, hemodynamic instability, and mental changes (irritability, delirium, or coma). Multiple organ failure follows (1) renal shutdown caused by hypotension, (2) hypoprothrombinemia caused by vitamin K deficiency, (3) thrombocytopenia caused by nonspecific binding of immunoglobulin, (4) disseminated intravascular coagulation with infarction or hemorrhage in several organs, and (5) progressive respiratory failure (Karakusis, 1986).

Diagnosis. Sepsis must always be considered in the differential diagnosis of shock, and blood cultures must be obtained. When shock is the initial

---

Table 2–5 ◆ Diagnosis of Brain Death

An experienced physician must determine that:
I. Cessation of all brain function has occurred
  A. Cerebral functions are absent (coma)
  B. Brainstem reflexes are absent
    1. Pupillary light reflex
    2. Corneal reflex
    3. Oculocephalic reflex
    4. Oculovestibular reflex
    5. Oropharyngeal reflex
    6. Respiratory reflexes
II. Cessation of brain function is irreversible
  A. Sufficient cause is established
  B. Possibility of recovery is excluded
III. Period of observation is appropriate
  A. With confirmatory test,* minimum period is 6 hours
  B. Without confirmatory test
    1. If cause is not anoxia, minimum period is 12 hours
    2. If cause is anoxia, minimum period is 24 hours

*Confirmatory tests include cerebral angiography, radioisotope cerebral blood flow study, and EEG.

manifestation, gram-negative sepsis is likely. In *Staphylococcus aureus* infection, shock is more likely to occur during the course of the infection and not as an initial symptom.

Treatment. Septic shock is a medical emergency. Antibiotic therapy should be initiated promptly at maximal doses. Hypotension must be treated by restoration of intravascular volume, and each factor contributing to coagulopathy must be addressed. Mortality is high even with optimal treatment.

HYPERPYREXIA (HEMORRHAGIC SHOCK) AND ENCEPHALOPATHY SYNDROME

Hyperpyrexia and encephalopathy syndrome is presumed to be caused by bacterial sepsis, but this has not been proved (Chaves-Carballo et al, 1990).

Clinical Features. Most affected children are younger than 1 year of age, but cases are described up to 26 months. One half of children have mild prodromal symptoms of a viral gastroenteritis or respiratory illness. In the rest the onset is explosive; a previously well child is found unresponsive and having seizures. Fever of 38° C or higher is a constant feature. Marked hypotension with poor peripheral perfusion is followed by profuse watery or bloody diarrhea with metabolic acidosis and compensatory respiratory alkalosis. Disseminated intravascular coagulopathy develops, and bleeding is noted from every venipuncture site.

The mortality rate is 50%; the survivors have mental and motor impairment.

Diagnosis. The syndrome resembles toxic shock syndrome, gram-negative sepsis, heatstroke, and Reye syndrome. Abnormal renal function occurs in every case, but serum ammonia concentrations remain normal, hypoglycemia is unusual, and blood cultures yield no growth.

Cerebrospinal fluid is normal except for increased pressure. CT demonstrates small ventricles and loss of sulcal marking caused by cerebral edema. The EEG background rhythms are diffusely slow.

Treatment. Affected children require intensive care with ventilatory support, volume replacement, correction of acid-base and coagulation disturbances, anticonvulsant therapy, and control of cerebral edema.

TOXIC SHOCK SYNDROME

Toxic shock syndrome is a potentially lethal illness caused by infection or colonization with some strains of *S. aureus* (Chesney et al, 1982).

Clinical Features. The onset is abrupt and characterized by high fever, hypotension, vomiting, diarrhea, myalgia, headache, and a desquamating rash. Multiple organ failure may occur during desquamation. Serious complications include cardiac arrhythmia, pulmonary edema, and oliguric renal failure. Initial encephalopathic features are agitation and confusion. These may be followed by lethargy, obtundation, and generalized tonic-clonic seizures.

The majority of pediatric cases have occurred in menstruating girls who use tampons, but this syndrome is also a complication of influenza and influenza-like illness in children with staphylococcal colonization of the respiratory tract (MacDonald et al, 1987).

Diagnosis. No diagnostic laboratory test is available. The diagnosis is based on the typical clinical and laboratory findings. Over half of patients have sterile pyuria, immature granulocytic leukocytes, coagulation abnormalities, hypocalcemia, low serum albumin and total protein concentrations, and elevated concentrations of blood urea nitrogen, transaminase, bilirubin, and creatine kinase. Cultures of specimens from infected sites yield *S. aureus*.

Treatment. Hypotension usually responds to volume restoration with physiologic saline solution. Some patients require vasopressors or fresh-frozen plasma. Antibiotic therapy should be initiated promptly with an agent effective against *S. aureus*.

RICKETTSIAL INFECTIONS
Lyme Disease

Lyme disease, caused by a spirochete *(Borrelia burgdorferi)* and transmitted by tick bite, is now the most common vector-borne infection in the United States (Steere, 1989). Six northeastern states account for 80% of cases.

Clinical Features. Three stages of disease are described, but their sequence is variable. The first symptom (stage 1) in 60% to 80% of patients is a skin lesion of the thigh, groin, or axilla (erythema chronicum migrans), which may be associated with fever and regional lymphadenopathy. The rash fades within 3 to 4 weeks but may recur. Neurologic manifestations develop weeks or months after the skin lesion and are indicative of systemic infection (stage 2). Most patients have only aseptic meningitis, which clears completely within 6 weeks, but some have encephalitis, which may cause persistent neurologic impairment. The aseptic meningitis is characterized by recurrent attacks of severe headache, mild stiffness of the neck, nausea, and vomiting. Fever may not occur. Other neurologic syndromes that may occur in combination with aseptic meningitis or alone include Bell palsy, multiple cranial neuropathies, radiculopathy, and polyneuropathy. Transitory cardiac involvement (myopericarditis and atrioventricular block) may occur in stage 2. A year or more of continual migratory arthritis begins weeks to years after the onset of neurologic manifestations (stage 3). Only one joint, often the knee, or a few large joints are affected. During stage 3 the patient feels ill. Fatigue may be the most prominent symptom, but chronic encephalopathy and polyneuropathy are also reported (Logigian et al, 1990).

Diagnosis. The spirochete can be grown on cultures from the skin rash during stage 1 of the disease. At the time of meningitis the cerebrospinal fluid may be normal at first but then shows a lymphocytic pleocytosis (about 100 cells/mm^3), an elevated protein concentration, and a normal glucose concentration. The diagnosis of neuroborreliosis is established by showing the production of specific intrathecal IgA, IgG, and IgM (Hansen and Lebach, 1991). Antibody production begins 2 weeks after infection, and IgG is always detectable at 6 weeks.

Treatment. Intravenous therapy for 2 weeks with either ceftriaxone, 2 g/day as a single dose, or penicillin G, 20 million U/day in six divided doses, is used for children with neurologic manifestations. However, oral amoxicillin, 250 mg three times a day, or tetracycline, 250 mg three times a day, can be used if Bell palsy is the only manifestation.

ROCKY MOUNTAIN SPOTTED FEVER

Rocky Mountain spotted fever is an acute, tickborne disorder caused by *Rickettsia rickettsii* (Kirk et al, 1990). Its geographic name is now a misnomer; the disease occurs in much of the United States with a special predilection for southwestern and southeastern states.

Cinical Features. Fever, myalgia, and rash are constant symptoms. The rash appears within 14 days of onset (average 4 days) and may be maculopapular, petechial, or both. Headache is present in 66% of patients; meningismus in 33%, focal neurologic signs in 14%, and seizures in 6%.

Diagnosis. The diagnosis is confirmed by a fourfold rise in the Weil-Felix agglutination reaction or by the presence of complement-fixing or immunofluorescent antibody. The cerebrospinal fluid shows a mild pleocytosis.

VIRAL INFECTIONS

Since encephalitis usually affects the meninges as well as the brain, the term "meningoencephalitis" may be more accurate. However, distinguishing encephalitis from aseptic meningitis is useful for viral diagnosis because most viruses cause primarily one or the other, but not both. An annual incidence of 7.4:100,000 for encephalitis and 10.9:100,000 for aseptic meningitis remained relatively constant in one Minnesota county over a 30-year period (Beghi et al, 1984). Both conditions were more common in the summer, in childhood, and in males.

Routine childhood immunization has reduced the number of pathogenic viruses circulating in the community. Enteroviruses and herpes simplex virus are now the most common viral causes of meningitis and encephalitis in children. However, specific viral identification is established in only 15% to 20% of cases (Beghi et al, 1984; Kennard and Swash, 1981).

The classification of viruses undergoes frequent change, but a constant first step is the separation of viruses with a DNA nucleic acid core from those with an RNA core. The only DNA virus that produces acute, postnatal encephalitis in immunocompetent hosts is herpes simplex. RNA viruses causing encephalitis are myxoviruses (influenza and measles encephalitis), arboviruses (St. Louis encephalitis, eastern equine encephalitis, western equine encephalitis, and LaCrosse-California encephalitis), retroviruses (acquired immune deficiency syndrome [AIDS] encephalitis), and rhabdoviruses (rabies). RNA viruses (especially enteroviruses and mumps) are responsible for aseptic meningitis.

In addition to viruses that directly infect the brain and meninges, encephalopathies may also follow systemic viral infections. These are thought to result from demyelination caused by immune-mediated responses of the brain to infection.

Aseptic Meningitis

The term "aseptic meningitis" is used to define a syndrome of meningismus and cerebrospinal fluid leukocytosis without bacterial or fungal infection. Aseptic meningitis is a benign, self-limited disease from which 95% of children recover completely.

Clinical Features. Twenty percent of children have a history of antecedent respiratory infection or gastrointestinal illness. The onset of symptoms is abrupt and characterized by fever, headache, and stiff neck. Irritability, lethargy, and vomiting are also common. "Encephalitic" symptoms are not part of the syndrome, but febrile seizures may occur in predisposed infants. Systemic illness is uncommon, but its presence may suggest specific viral disorders (parotitis suggestive of mumps, myalgia of coxsackie virus infection, rash of echovirus infection and Lyme disease, diarrhea of enterovirus infection).

The actue illness usually lasts less than 1 week, but malaise and headache may continue for several weeks. Communicating hydrocephalus is an unusual long-term sequela.

Diagnosis. In most cases of aseptic meningitis the cerebrospinal fluid contains 10 to 200 leukocytes/mm^3, but counts of 1000 cells/mm^3 or greater may occur with lymphocytic choriomeningitis. The response is primarily lymphocytic, but polymorphonuclear leukocytes may predominate early in the course. Protein concentration is generally between 50 and 100 mg/dl (0.5 and 1 g/L), and glucose concentration is normal, although it may be slightly reduced in mumps and lymphocytic choriomeningitis.

Aseptic meningitis usually occurs in the spring or summer, and enteroviruses are responsible for most cases in children. The mumps and poliomyelitis viruses remain important causative agents in countries where immunization is not mandatory. Nonviral causes of aseptic meningitis are rare but must be considered; these include Lyme disease, Kawasaki disease, leukemia, systemic lupus erythematosus, migraine, and irritation of the meninges from blood, drugs, and contrast materials.

Patients with a personal or family history of migraine may have attacks of severe headache associated with stiff neck and focal neurologic disturbances such as hemiparesis and aphasia (Bartleson et al, 1981; Brattstrom et al, 1984). Cerebrospinal fluid examination reveals a pleocytosis (5 to 300 cells/mm^3) that is mainly lymphocytes and a protein concentration of 50 to 100 mg/dl (0.5 to 1 g/L). Whether the attacks are migraine provoked by intercurrent aseptic meningitis or represent a "meningitic" form of migraine is not known. The recurrence of attacks in some patients suggests that the mechanism is wholly migrainous.

Bacterial meningitis is the major concern when a child has meningismus. Although cerebrospinal fluid examination provides several clues that differentiate bacterial from viral meningitis, antibiotic therapy should be initiated for every child with a clinical syndrome of aseptic meningitis until a cerebrospinal fluid culture is negative for bacteria (see Chapter 4). This is especially true for children who received antibiotic therapy before examination of the cerebrospinal fluid.

Treatment. Children with viral meningitis or encephalitis are now routinely treated for herpes encephalitis until that diagnosis can be excluded; treatment with acyclovir is harmless. Treatment of viral aseptic meningitis is directed at the symptoms. Bed rest in a quiet environment and mild analgesics provide satisfactory relief of symptoms in most children.

Arboviral (Arthropod-Borne) Encephalitis

Arboviruses are classified on the basis of ecology rather than structure. Ticks and mosquitoes are the usual vectors, and epidemics occur in the spring and summer. Each encephalitis has a defined geographic area. Japanese encephalitis is the most widespread, occurring worldwide. Arboviruses account for 10% of encephalitis cases reported in the United States.

California-LaCrosse Encephalitis

LaCrosse virus is the most common cause of encephalitis by California serogroup viruses in the United States.

Clinical Features. Before 1984 most cases were reported from Wisconsin and Minnesota. Recent epidemics have occurred in Indiana, and sporadic cases have been reported throughout the Midwest and western New York. Small woodland mammals serve as a reservoir and mosquitoes as the vector.

Most cases of encephalitis occur in children, and asymptomatic infection is common in adults. The initial feature is a flulike syndrome that lasts 2 or 3 days. Encephalitis is heralded by headache followed by seizures and rapid progression to coma (Chun et al, 1968). Focal neurologic disturbances are present in 20% of cases. Symptoms begin to resolve 3 to 5 days after onset, and most children recover without neurologic sequelae. Death is uncommon and occurs mainly in infants.

Diagnosis. Examination of cerebrospinal fluid reveals a mixed pleocytosis with lymphocytes predominating. The count is usually 50 to 200 cells/mm^3 but may range from zero to 600. The virus is difficult to grow on culture, and diagnosis depends on the demonstration of a fourfold or greater increase in hemagglutination inhibition and neutralizing antibody titers between acute and convalescent sera.

Treatment. Treatment is supportive. No effective antiviral agent is available.

Eastern Equine Encephalitis

Clinical Features. Eastern equine encephalitis is a perennial infection of horses from New York to Florida. Human cases do not exceed five each year, and they follow epidemics in horses (Eastern equine encephalitis, 1991). The mortality rate is 30%. Wild birds serve as a reservior and mosquitoes as a vector. Consequently, almost all cases occur during the summer months.

Onset is usually abrupt and characterized by high fever, headache, and vomiting, followed by drowsiness, coma, and seizures (Przelomski et al, 1988). The longer the duration of nonneurologic prodromal symptoms, the better the outcome. In infants seizures and coma are often the first manifestations. Signs of meningismus are usually present in older children. Children usually survive the acute encephalitis, but mental impairment, seizures, and disturbed motor function can be expected in survivors.

Diagnosis. The cerebrospinal fluid pressure is usually elevated, and examination reveals 200 to 2000 leukocytes/mm^3, of which half are polymorphonuclear leukocytes. Diagnosis relies on the demonstration of a fourfold or greater rise in complement fixation and neutralizing antibody titers between acute and convalescent sera.

Treatment. Treatment is supportive. No effective antiviral agent is available.

Japanese B Encephalitis

Japanese B encephalitis is a major form of encephalitis in Asia and is an important health hazard to nonimmunized travelers during summmer months.

Clinical Features. The initial features are malaise, fever, and headache or irritability lasting 2 to 3 days. These are followed by meningismus, confusion, and delirium. During the second or third week, photophobia and generalized hypotonia develop. Seizures may occur at any time. Finally, rigidity, a masklike facies, and brainstem dysfunction ensue. Mortality rates are high among indigenous populations and lower among Western travelers, probably because of a difference in the age of the exposed populations.

Diagnosis. Examination of the cerebrospinal fluid shows pleocytosis (20 to 500 cells/mm^3). The cells are initially mixed, but later lymphocytes predominate. Protein concentration is usually between 50 and 100 mg/dl (0.5 and 1 mg/L), and glucose concentration is normal. Diagnosis depends on demonstrating a fourfold or greater elevation in the level of complement-fixing antibodies between acute and convalescent sera.

Treatment. Treatment is supportive. No effective antiviral agent is available, but two immunizations with an inactivated vaccine protects against encephalitis in more than 90% of individuals (Hoke et al, 1988).

St. Louis Encephalitis

Clinical Features. St. Louis encephalitis is endemic in the western United States and epidemic in the Mississippi valley and Atlantic states. It is the most common type of epidemic viral encephalitis in the United States (St. Louis encephalitis outbreak, 1991). The vector is a mosquito, and birds are the major reservior.

Most infections are asymptomatic. The spectrum of neurologic illness varies from aseptic meningitis to severe encephalitis leading to death within days. The mortality rate is low. Headache, vomiting, and states of decreased consciousness are typical features. Stiff neck and seizures are less common, and focal neurologic disturbances are rare. The usual duration of illness is 1 to 2 weeks. Children usually recover completely, but adults may be left with mental or motor impairment.

Diagnosis. Cerebrospinal fluid examination reveals a lymphocytic pleocytosis (50 to 500 cells/mm^3) and a protein concentration between 50 and 100 mg/dl (0.5 and 1 g/L). Glucose concentration is normal.

The virus is difficult to grow on culture, and diagnosis requires a fourfold or greater increase in complement fixation and hemagglutination inhibition antibody titers between acute and convalescent sera.

Treatment. Treatment is supportive. No effective antiviral agent is available.

Western Equine Encephalitis

Clinical Features. Western equine encephalitis is a rare disorder. Wild birds serve as the reservoir and mosquitoes as the vector. All recent cases have been reported from North Dakota, South Dakota, and Canada. Between 20% and 30% of cases occur in infants.

In infants the infection is characterized by irritability, fever, meningismus, bulging of the fontanelles, seizures, and coma. Older children may have a flulike syndrome before symptoms of meningoencephalitis develop. The initial symptom is usually behavioral change, including delirium, which is followed by drowsiness and coma. The EEG shows focal abnormalities lateralizing to one temporal lobe that suggest herpes encephalitis.

Symptoms last 1 to 2 weeks, and although the overall mortality rate is 10%, most fatalities are infants. Fifty percent of surviving infants have permanent mental impairment and seizures.

Diagnosis. Cerebrospinal fluid pleocytosis is first a mixture of polymorphonuclear leukocytes and lymphocytes and then lymphocytes alone. Protein concentration is between 50 and 100 mg/dl

(0.5 and 1 g/L). Diagnosis relies on demonstrating a fourfold or greater rise in complement-fixing or neutralizing antibodies between acute and convalescent sera.

Western equine encephalitis may be difficult to distinguish from herpes encephalitis without brain biopsy.

Treatment. Treatment is supportive. The child should be treated for herpes encephalitis until a definitive diagnosis is made. No effective antiviral agent is available for western equine encephalitis.

Herpes Simplex Encephalitis

Two similar strains of herpes simplex virus (HSV) are pathogenic to humans. HSV-1 is associated with orofacial infections and HSV-2 with genital infections. Both have worldwide distribution (Corey and Spear, 1986). Forty percent of children have antibodies to HSV-1, but antibodies to HSV-2 are not routinely detected until puberty. HSV-1 is the important causative agent of acute postnatal herpes simplex encephalitis, and HSV-2 of encephalitis in the newborn (see Chapter 1).

Initial orofacial infection with HSV-1 may be asymptomatic. The virus replicates in the skin, infecting nerve fiber endings and then the trigeminal ganglia. Further replication occurs within the ganglia before the virus enters a latent stage during which it cannot be recovered from the ganglia. Reactivation occurs during time of stress, especially intercurrent febrile illness. The reactivated virus ordinarily retraces its neural migration to the facial skin but occasionally spreads proximally to the brain, causing encephalitis. The host's immunocompetence maintains the virus in a latent state. An immunocompromised state results in frequent reactivation and severe, widespread infection.

Herpes simplex is the single most common cause of nonepidemic encephalitis and accounts for 10% to 20% of cases. The annual incidence is estimated at 2.3 cases per million population. Thirty-one percent of cases occur in children (Whitley et al, 1982).

Clinical Features. Primary infection is often the cause of encephalitis in children. Only 22% of patients give a history of recurrent labial herpes infection. Typically the patient has an acute onset of fever, headache, lethargy, nausea, and vomiting. Eighty percent of patients show focal neurologic disturbances (hemiparesis, cranial nerve deficits, visual field loss, aphasia, and focal seizures), and the remainder show behavioral changes or generalized seizures without clinical evidence of focal neurologic deficits. However, both groups have fo-

cal abnormalities on neuroradiographic studies or EEG. The acute stage of encephalitis lasts approximately a week. Recovery takes several weeks and is often incomplete.

Herpes meningitis (Corey and Spear, 1986) is usually associated with genital lesions and caused by HSV-2. The clinical features are similar to those of aseptic meningitis caused by other viruses.

Diagnosis. Prompt diagnosis of herpes simplex encephalitis is important because treatment is available. Cerebrospinal fluid pleocytosis is present in 97% of cases. The median count is 130 leukocytes/mm^3 (range zero to 1000). Up to 500 red blood cells/mm^3 may be present as well. Median protein concentration is 80 mg/dl (0.8 g/L), but 20% of patients have normal protein concentrations and 40% have concentrations exceeding 100 mg/dl (1 g/L). The glucose concentration in cerebrospinal fluid is usually normal, but in 7% of cases it is less than half of the blood glucose concentration (Whitley et al, 1982).

In the past the demonstration of periodic lateralizing epileptiform discharges on EEG was considered presumptive evidence of herpes encephalitis. However, MRI has proved to be a more sensitive early indicator of herpes encephalitis (Schroth et al, 1987). T$_2$-weighted studies reveal increased signal intensity in one or both temporal lobes (Fig. 2–3).

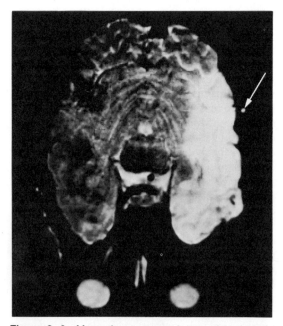

Figure 2–3 Magnetic resonance image of herpes encephalitis. T$_2$-weighted images show increased signal intensity in both temporal lobes.

Brain biopsy with virus isolation by tissue culture is the only method for definitive diagnosis but is not a standard of practice. Herpes infection may be patchy, and biopsy may remove an unaffected portion of the temporal lobe. Most physicians begin treatment on the basis of a compatible clinical history and an EEG or MRI that supports the clinical impression.

Treatment. Acyclovir has replaced vidarabine as the treatment of choice (Whitley et al, 1986). The dosage is 10 mg/kg every 8 hours, infused in 100 ml of standard intravenous fluid over a 1-hour period. The mortality rate is 28% and is highest in patients who are already in coma when treatment is initiated. In 38% of patients function returns to normal. The prognosis is best for noncomatose children younger than 10 years of age.

Measles (Rubeola) Encephalitis

Compulsory immunization had almost eliminated natural measles infection in the United States, but the incidence began climbing again in 1990 because of reduced immunization rates. The risk of encephalitis from natural disease is 1:1000. During the first 20 years of the measles vaccine program an estimated 52 million cases of measles, 5200 deaths, and 17,400 cases of mental retardation were prevented (Bloch et al, 1985). The mechanism of measles encephalitis has been contested, but evidence for both direct viral infection and allergic demyelination has been presented (Johnson et al, 1984). A chronic form of measles encephalitis (subacute sclerosing panencephalitis) is described in Chapter 5.

Clinical Features. Measles is a neurotropic virus, and EEG abnormalities are often present even without clinical symptoms of encephalopathy. Symptoms of encephalitis usually begin 1 to 8 days after the appearance of rash but can be delayed for 3 weeks. The onset is usually abrupt and is characterized by lethargy or obtundation that may rapidly progress to coma. Generalized seizures occur in half of patients. The spectrum of neurologic disturbances includes hemiplegia, ataxia, and involuntary movement disorders. Acute transverse myelitis may be present as well (see Chapter 12). The incidence of neurologic morbidity (mental retardation, epilepsy, and paralysis) is high but does not correlate with the severity of acute encephalitis.

Measles encephalitis may occur as a consequence of measles immunization. Fever and rash develop 7 to 12 days after immunization and are quickly followed by lethargy and irritability (Peltola and Heinonen, 1986). Generalized seizures may occur. The systemic features and the enceph-

alopathy have their onset during the second week following immunization; symptoms that occur earlier are not related to immunization. Recovery is complete. Although clearly an increased risk of febrile seizures follows measles immunization, no evidence of permanent neurologic disturbances has been found (Centers for Disease Control, 1984; Pollock and Morris, 1983).

Diagnosis. Examination of cerebrospinal fluid reveals a lymphocytic pleocytosis. The number of lymphocytes is usually highest in the first few days but rarely exceeds 100 cells/mm³. Protein concentrations are generally between 50 and 100 mg/dl (0.5 and 1 g/L), and glucose concentration is normal.

Treatment. Treatment is supportive. Anticonvulsant drugs usually provide satisfactory seizure control.

Postinfectious Encephalomyelitis

Demyelinating disorders that occur during or after systemic viral illnesses are called postinfectious and are presumed to be immune mediated. The nervous system is not thought to be infected. Either central or peripheral myelin may be affected, but whether both can be affected simultaneously has not been determined. Examples of postinfectious disorders appear in several chapters of the text and include the Guillain-Barré syndrome (see Chapter 7), acute cerebellar ataxia (see Chapter 10), transverse myelitis (see Chapter 12), brachial neuritis (see Chapter 13), optic neuritis (see Chapter 16), and Bell palsy (see Chapter 17). The incidence of some postinfectious disorders is increased in immunocompromised populations, which provides further support for the immune hypothesis.

The cause-and-effect relationship between viral infection and many of these syndromes is virtually impossible to establish if the latency period between viral infection and onset of neurologic dysfunction is 30 days. The average school-aged child has four to six "viral illnesses" each year, so that 33% to 50% of children have a viral illness 30 days before any life event. A greater than 50% incidence of viral illness, 30 days before onset, is not reported for any postinfectious disorder listed previously.

Clinical Features. MRI has expanded the spectrum of clinical features associated with postinfectious encephalopathy by allowing the demonstration of small demyelinating lesions. Lethargy and weakness are at one end of the spectrum, and coma is at the other.

The encephalopathy is often preceded by lethargy, headache, and vomiting. Whether these "systemic features" are symptoms of a viral illness or of early encephalopathy is not clear. The onset of neurologic symptoms is abrupt and characterized by declining consciousness and seizures. In some cases the generalized encephalopathy is preceded by optic neuritis, transverse myelitis, or both (see "Devic Syndrome," Chapter 12). Some children never have focal neurologic signs, whereas others have hemiplegia, quadriplegia, ataxia, and cranial nerve dysfunction (Sriram and Steinman, 1984).

Mortality is highest in the first week. Although recovery among survivors is variable, the degree of recovery may be astonishing.

Diagnosis.   Diagnosis is based on T_2-weighted MRI that reveals a marked increase in signal intensity throughout the white matter (Fig. 2–4). The lesions resolve in the weeks that follow, and no new lesions develop (Kesselring et al, 1990). Adrenoleukodystrophy must be excluded in boys.

The cerebrospinal fluid is frequently normal. Occasional abnormalities are a mild lymphocyte pleocytosis and elevation of protein concentration.

Treatment.   Most children with severe demyelinating encephalopathies are treated with corticosteroids, despite the absence of conclusive evidence that such treatment is beneficial.

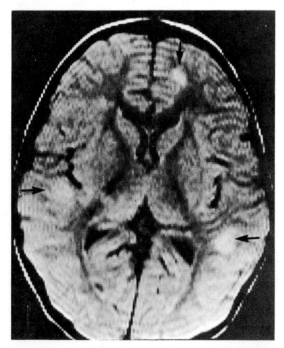

Figure 2–4   Postinfectious demyelination of the cerebral hemispheres. Areas of increased signal intensity are seen in both hemispheres *(arrows).*

Reye Syndrome

Reye syndrome is a systemic disorder of mitochondrial function that occurs during or following viral infection. The disorder occurs more often when salicylates are administered during viral illness for relief of symptoms (Hurwitz et al, 1987). Recognition of this relationship has led to decreased use of salicylates in children and a marked decline in the incidence of Reye syndrome.

Clinical Features.   In the United States sporadic cases are generally associated with varicella (chickenpox) or nonspecific respiratory infections; small epidemics are associated with influenza B infection. When varicella is the precipitating infection, the initial stage of Reye syndrome occurs 3 to 6 days after the appearance of rash.

The clinical course is relatively predictable and has been divided into five stages:

Stage 0—vomiting but no symptoms of brain dysfunction
Stage I—vomiting, confusion, and lethargy
Stage II—agitation, delirium, decorticate posturing, and hyperventilation
Stage III—coma and decerebrate posturing
Stage IV—flaccidity, apnea, dilated fixed pupils

The progression from stage I to stage IV may be explosive, evolving in less than 24 hours. More commonly the period of recurrent vomiting and lethargy lasts for a day or longer. In most children with vomiting and laboratory evidence of hepatic dysfunction following varicella or respiratory infection, liver biopsy reveals features of Reye syndrome (Lichtenstein et al, 1983) despite normal cerebral function. This has been designated Reye stage 0. Stages I and II represent increasing degrees of encephalopathy with metabolic dysfunction and edema. Stages III and IV indicate generalized increased intracranial pressure and herniation.

Focal neurologic disturbances and meningismus are not part of the syndrome. Fever is not a prominent feature, and hepatomegaly occurs in one half of patients late in the course.

Outcome is variable, but as a rule infants do worse than older children. Progression to stages III and IV at all ages is associated with a high death rate and impaired neurologic function in survivors.

Diagnosis.   Typical blood abnormalities are hypoglycemia, hyperammonemia, and increased concentration of hepatic enzymes. Serum bilirubin concentration remains normal, and jaundice does not occur. Acute pancreatitis sometimes develops and can be identified by increased concentrations of serum amylase.

The cerebrospinal fluid is normal except for increased pressure. The EEG shows abnormalities consistent with a diffuse encephalopathy.

Liver biopsy is definitive. Light microscopy reveals panlobular accumulation of small intracellular lipid droplets and depletion of succinic acid dehydrogenase in the absence of other abnormalities. Electron microscopic changes include characteristic mitochondrial abnormalities, peroxisomal proliferation and swelling, proliferation of smooth endoplasmic reticulum, and glycogen depletion.

Conditions that mimic Reye syndrome are primary carnitine deficiency, ornithine transcarbamylase deficiency, and valproate hepatotoxicity. Inborn errors of metabolism should be assumed and sought in any child with recurrent Reye syndrome or a family history of similar illness. Metabolic products of valproate are mitochondrial poisons that have been used to produce an experimental model of Reye syndrome.

Treatment. Children with stage I or II disease should be watched closely in a pediatric intensive care unit and treated with intravenous hypertonic (10% to 15%) glucose solution at normal maintenance volumes. Stages III and IV require treatment of increased intracranial pressure (see Chapter 4) by elevation of the head, controlled mechanical ventilation, and mannitol (Shaywitz et al, 1986; Trauner, 1986). Corticosteroids are of limited benefit and should not be used routinely. Some authorities continue to advocate intracranial pressure monitors and pentobarbital coma, although they have never been demonstrated to affect outcome. Fortunately, this once common and deadly disease has almost disappeared with discontinuation of salicylate therapy for children.

POSTIMMUNIZATION ENCEPHALOPATHY

Three types of vaccines are in general use in the United States: live-attenuated viruses, whole or fractionated killed organisms, and toxoids.

Live-attenuated virus vaccines (measles, mumps, rubella, varicella, and oral poliomyelitis) are intended to produce a mild and harmless infection with subsequent immunity. However, even under ideal circumstances of vaccine preparation and host resistance, symptoms of the natural disease and its known neurologic complications may develop in vaccine recipients. Measles is the only live-attenuated virus vaccine that has the potential of causing encephalitis (see "Measles Encephalitis").

Whole killed organisms (pertussis, influenza, rabies, and parenteral poliomyelitis) do not reproduce their natural disease but are alleged to injure the nervous system by a toxic or allergic mechanism. Pertussis vaccine can cause seizures, but no evidence exists that it causes any chronic brain damage syndrome (Institute of Medicine, 1991). Rabies vaccine had been an important cause of encephalomyelitis in the past, but the present vaccine, prepared from virus grown on human diploid cells, has been only rarely implicated as a cause of polyneuropathy (Bernard et al, 1982). Several case reports have suggested that influenza immunization may cause encephalopathy, but considering the millions of doses administered, the number of cases reported is less than might be expected by chance alone. None of the other whole-killed organism vaccines causes encephalopathy.

Toxoids are produced by the inactivation of toxins produced by bacteria. Diphtheria and tetanus toxoids are the only such vaccines now in use, and neither is associated with encephalopathy.

◆ Metabolic and Systemic Disorders
DISORDERS OF OSMOLALITY

The osmolality of a solution is determined by the number of particles in the solution. Sodium salts, glucose, and urea are the primary osmoles of the extracellular space, potassium salts of the intracellular space, and plasma proteins of the intravascular space. Because cell membranes are permeable to water and osmotic equilibrium must be maintained, the volume of intracellular fluid is determined by the osmolality of the extracellular space.

Hypernatremia and hyperglycemia are the major causes of serum hyperosmolality, and hyponatremia is the main cause of serum hypoosmolality.

Diabetic Ketoacidosis

The major cause of symptomatic hyperglycemia in children is diabetic ketoacidosis. Nonketotic, hyperglycemic coma, associated with mild or non-insulin-requiring diabetes, is unusual in children.

Clinical Features. Diabetic ketoacidosis develops rapidly in children who have neglected to take prescribed doses of insulin or who have a superimposed infection. Initial features are polydipsia, polyuria, and fatigue. The child hyperventilates to compensate for the metabolic acidosis. Lethargy rapidly progresses to coma. Ketoacidosis is the leading cause of death in children with diabetes, and mortality rates are still as high as 10%.

Cerebral edema is an early and almost constant feature of diabetic ketoacidosis. It may not be part of the natural progression of disease but can be caused instead by the administration of large volumes of hypotonic fluid (Duck and Wyatt, 1988). The severity of cerebral edema correlates with changes in level of consciousness. Edema may contribute to death in some cases. Other, less common neurologic complications of diabetic ketoacidosis are venous sinus thrombosis and intracerebral hemorrhage (Atluru, 1986). Both are associated with focal or generalized seizures.

Diagnosis. The diagnosis is based on the combination of a blood glucose level greater than 400 mg/dl (22 mmol/L), the presence of serum and urinary ketones, an arterial pH less than 7.25, and a serum bicarbonate concentration less than 15 mmol/L.

Treatment. In children with moderate to severe diabetic ketoacidosis, the rapid administration of hypotonic fluids at a time of high serum osmolality should be avoided (Harris et al, 1988). Fluid deficits should be replaced evenly over 48 hours. The sodium deficit should be reduced by half in the first 12 hours and the remainder eliminated over the next 36 hours. Bicarbonate ion should be given in physiologic proportions.

Hypoglycemia

Symptomatic hypoglycemia after the neonatal period is usually associated with insulin use in the treatment of diabetes mellitus. Sepsis and inborn errors of metabolism account for only a minority of cases.

Clinical Features. Clinical features are not precisely predictable from blood glucose concentration (Malouf and Brust, 1985). Hypoglycemia does not usually become symptomatic until blood concentrations are less than 50 mg/dl (2.8 mmol/L). The rate of fall may be important in determining the clinical manifestations. Dizziness and tremor may occur at blood concentrations less than 60 mg/dl (3.1 mmol/L) and serve as a warning of insulin overdose. Greater declines in blood glucose concentration result in confusion, delirium, and loss of consciousness. Sudden hemiplegia, usually transitory and sometimes shifting between the two sides, is a rare feature of hypoglycemia. The mechanism is unknown, and CT shows no evidence of infarction.

Diagnosis. Hypoglycemia should be suspected in diabetic children with an altered mental status or decreased consciousness. Blood glucose concentration should be measured promptly.

Treatment. Diabetic children should be encouraged to carry a source of sugar for use at the first symptom of hypoglycemia. Children who are comatose from hypoglycemia should receive immediate intravenous glucose replacement. Complete recovery is the rule.

Hypernatremia

Hypernatremia is usually caused by dehydration in which water loss exceeds sodium loss and by overhydration with hypertonic saline solution. It is a medical emergency and, if not corrected promptly, may lead to permanent brain damage and death.

Clinical Features. Hypernatremic dehydration may be a consequence of vomiting or diarrhea, especially if water intake is restricted. Iatrogenic hypernatremia is usually caused by overzealous correction of hyponatremia. Rapid alterations in sodium concentration are much more likely to cause encephalopathy than are equivalent concentrations attained slowly. The symptoms of hypernatremia are referable to the nervous system and include irritability, lethargy progressing to coma, and seizures. The presence of focal neurologic deficits suggests cerebral venous sinus thrombosis.

Diagnosis. Symptomatic hypernatremia develops at sodium concentrations greater than 160 mEq/L (160 mmol/L). The EEG demonstrates the nonspecific slowing associated with metabolic encephalopathies. Focal slowing on the EEG or focal abnormalities on examination warrant CT to look for venous sinus thrombosis.

Chronic or recurrent episodes of hypernatremia may result from hypodipsia (lack of thirst), a rare condition encountered in children with congenital or acquired brain disorders (Hammond et al, 1986). The syndrome is usually associated with a defect in secretion of antidiuretic hormone.

Treatment. Rapid water replacement can lead to cerebral edema. The recommended approach is to correct abnormalities of intravascular volume before correcting the water deficit.

Hyponatremia

Hyponatremia may result from water retention, sodium loss, or both. Water retention is often caused by the syndrome of inappropriate antidiuretic hormone secretion (SIADH), and sodium loss results from renal disease, vomiting, and diarrhea. Permanent brain damage from hyponatremia is uncommon but may occur if the serium sodium concentration is allowed to remain less than 115 mEq/L for several hours (Arieff, 1986).

Syndrome of Inappropriate Antidiuretic Hormone Secretion

SIADH occurs in association with a variety of neurologic disorders, including head trauma, infections, and intracranial hemorrhage.

Clinical Features.   Most patients with SIADH have a preexisting loss of consciousness from their underlying neurologic disorder. In such patients hyponatremia is the only feature of SIADH. In those who are alert, lethargy develops from the hyponatremia but rarely progresses to coma or seizures.

Diagnosis.   Those who provide care for children with acute intracranial disorders must be vigilant for SIADH; repeated determinations of serum sodium concentration are required. Once hyponatremia is documented, urinary sodium concentration must be measured. The urinary sodium concentration is usually greater than 20 mEq/L (20 mmol/L) and parallels intake. Definitive diagnosis requires the demonstration of inappropriately high plasma concentrations of arginine vasopressin in the presence of hyponatremia.

Treatment.   All signs of SIADH respond to fluid restriction. A daily intake of 50% to 75% of fluid maintenance is generally satisfactory.

Sodium Loss

Clinical Features.   Hyponatremic encephalopathy is caused by the movement of water into the brain. Nausea, vomiting, muscular twitching, and lethargy appear when the serum sodium concentration falls below 125 mEq/L (125 mmol/L). A further decline to less than 115 mEq/L (115 mmol/L) is associated with seizures and coma.

Diagnosis.   Hyponatremia should be recognized as a potential problem in children with vomiting or diarrhea or with renal disease. Serum and urinary sodium concentrations are both decreased.

Treatment.   The treatment of acute symptomatic hyponatremia remains controversial. Rapid correction of the sodium concentration is important, but only to mildly hypotonic concentrations (Ayus et al, 1985). Sudden corrections of greater than 20 mEq/L (20 mmol/L) are associated with seizures, hypernatremic encephalopathy, and the possibility of central pontine myelinolysis (Norenberg, 1983). Half-normal saline solution should be administered at a rate that requires at least 24 hours for complete correction.

ENDOCRINE DISORDERS
Adrenal Disorders

Adrenal hypersecretion causes agitation or depression but does not produce coma. Adrenal failure may result from sepsis, abrupt withdrawal of corticosteroid therapy, or adrenal hemorrhage. Initial symptoms are nausea, vomiting, abdominal pain, and fever. Lethargy progresses to coma and is associated with hypovolemic shock. Prompt intravenous infusion of fluids, glucose, and corticosteroids is lifesaving.

Parathyroid Disorders

The neurologic features of hyperparathyroidism are related to hypercalcemia. Weakness and myopathy are relatively common. Alterations in mental status occur in 50% of patients and include apathy, delirium, paranoia, and dementia. Apathy and delirium occur at serum calcium concentrations greater than 11 mg/dl (2.75 mmol/L), and psychosis and dementia develop at concentrations of 16 mg/dl (4 mmol/L) or greater.

Seizures are the major manifestation of hypoparathyroidism and hypocalcemia. They may be generalized or focal and are often preceded by tetany. Hypocalcemic seizures do not respond to anticonvulsant drugs and must be treated with calcium replacement.

Thyroid Disorders

Hyperthyroidism produces exhilaration bordering on mania and may be associated with seizures and chorea (see Chapter 14). Thyroid storm (crisis) is a life-threatening event characterized by restlessness, cardiac arrhythmia, vomiting, and diarrhea. Delirium is an early feature and may progress to coma.

Acquired hypothyroidism affects both the central and the peripheral nervous system. Peripheral effects include neuropathy and myopathy. Central effects are cranial nerve abnormalities, ataxia, psychoses, dementia, seizures, and coma. Delusions and hallucinations occur in more than half of patients with long-standing disease. Myxedema coma, a rare manifestation of long-standing hypothyroidism in adults, is even more uncommon in children. It is characterized by profound hypothermia without shivering.

Hashimoto Encephalopathy

Hashimoto thyroiditis is an immune-mediated disease associated with high titers of antithyroid antibodies (Shaw et al, 1991).

Clinical Features.   The progression of symptoms is variable but usually begins with headache and confusion that progress to stupor. Focal or generalized seizures and transitory neurologic deficits (strokelike episodes) may be an initial or a late feature. Tremulousness and myoclonus commonly occur during some stage in the illness. The encephalopathy lasts several days and then gradually disappears. Recurrent episodes are the rule and lead to permanent neurologic sequelae.

Diagnosis. Hashimoto thyroiditis should be suspected in every case of recurrent encephalopathy. The cerebrospinal fluid protein concentration is elevated, sometimes above 100 mg/dl (1 g/L), but the pressure and cell count are normal. Affected individuals are usually euthyroid. The diagnosis depends on the demonstration of antithyroid antibodies. Antibodies against thyroglobulin and the microsomal fraction are most common, but antibodies against other thyroid elements and other organs may be present as well.

Treatment. Corticosteroids and other immunosuppressive agents are beneficial in ending an attack and preventing further episodes.

HEPATIC ENCEPHALOPATHY

Fulminant hepatic failure in children is caused by viral hepatitis, drugs, toxins, and Reye syndrome. The encephalopathy that accompanies hepatic failure cannot be explained by abnormalities of any single factor, such as ammonia concentration, but is due to multifactorial metabolic derangements. Severe viral hepatitis with marked elevation of the unconjugated bilirubin concentration may even lead to kernicterus in older children (Ho et al, 1980).

In children with chronic cholestatic liver disease, demyelination of the posterior columns and peripheral nerves may develop as a result of vitamin E deficiency. The major features are ataxia, areflexia, and gaze paresis, without evidence of encephalopathy (see Chapter 10).

Clinical Features. Malaise and fatigue are early symptoms that accompany features of hepatic failure: jaundice, dark urine, and abnormal results of liver function tests. Nausea and vomiting occur when hepatic failure is fulminant. The onset of coma may be spontaneous or induced by gastrointestinal bleeding, infection, high protein intake, and excessive use of tranquilizers or diuretics. The first features are disturbed sleep and a change in affect. These are followed by drowsiness, hyperventilation, and asterixis, a flapping tremor at the wrist when the arms are extended and the wrists flexed. Hallucinations sometimes occur during early stages, but a continuous progression to coma is more common. Seizures and decerebrate rigidity develop as the patient becomes comatose.

Diagnosis. In hepatic coma the EEG pattern is not specific but is always abnormal and suggests a metabolic encephalopathy: loss of posterior rhythm, generalized slowing of background, and frontal triphasic waves (Fig. 2–2).

Biochemical markers of liver failure include a sharp rise in transaminase activity (serum glutamic oxaloacetic transaminase [SGOT] and serum glutamic pyruvate transaminase [SGOT]), increased prothrombin time, mixed hyperbilirubinemia, and a decline in serum albumin concentration.

Treatment. The goal of treatment is to maintain cerebral, renal, and cardiopulmonary function until liver regeneration or transplantation can occur. Cerebral function is impaired, not only by abnormal concentrations of metabolites but also by cerebral edema.

INBORN ERRORS OF METABOLISM

Inborn errors of metabolism that produce states of decreased consciousness are associated with hyperammonemia, hypoglycemia, or organic aciduria. Neonatal seizures are an early feature in most of these conditions (see Chapter 1), but some may not cause symptoms until infancy or childhood. Inborn errors with a delayed onset of encephalopathy include disorders of pyruvate metabolism and respiratory chain disorders (see Chapters 5, 6, 8, and 10); hemizygotes for ornithine carbamylase deficiency and heterozygotes for carbamyl phosphate synthetase deficiency (see Chapter 1); glycogen storage diseases (see Chapter 1); and primary carnitine deficiency.

Primary Carnitine Deficiency

L-Carnitine is essential for the transfer of long-chain fatty acids across the inner mitochondrial membrane, the facilitation of branched chain alpha-ketoacid oxidation, the shuttle of acyl-coenzyme A (CoA) products of peroxisomal beta-oxidation to the mitochondrial matrix in the liver, the modulation of the acyl-CoA/CoA ratio, and the esterification of potentially toxic acyl-CoA metabolites. The transfer of fatty acids across the mitochondrial membrane requires the conversion of acyl-CoA to acylcarnitine. If the carnitine concentration is deficient, toxic levels of acyl-CoA accumulate and impair the citric acid cycle, gluconeogenesis, the urea cycle, and fatty acid oxidation (De Vivo and Tein, 1990).

Primary carnitine deficiency is a genetic disorder of carnitine metabolism caused by deficiency of medium-chain acyl-CoA dehydrogenase (MCAD). It is transmitted by autosomal recessive inheritance. A systemic and a myopathic form are recognized. Both are considered variant phenotypes of MCAD deficiency. Similar clinical phenotypes are caused by deficiencies of long-chain and short-chain acyl-CoA dehydrogenase (Tein et al, 1991).

Clinical Features. Primary systemic carnitine deficiency is a disease of infancy and early childhood. It is characterized by attacks of vomiting, confusion, lethargy, and coma provoked by intercurrent illness or fasting. Recurrent attacks are the rule, and the mortality rate is high in the absence of prompt treatment. Between attacks the child may appear normal. In some families the deficiency causes cardiomyopathy, whereas in others it causes only mild to moderate proximal weakness (see Chapters 6 and 7).

Diagnosis. The acute attacks resemble Reye syndrome in both clinical and laboratory findings: hypoglycemia, hypoprothrombinemia, hyperammonemia, elevated concentrations of liver enzymes, and fatty deposition in hepatocytes are present.

The deficiency is diagnosed by demonstration of low carnitine concentrations in blood or tissues. Insufficient serum or tissue carnitine concentrations may also result from other inborn errors of metabolism and from acquired systemic and iatrogenic disorders (Table 2–6).

Blood carnitine concentrations in patients with primary carnitine deficiency are less than 20 μmol/mg noncollagen protein. Those with secondary deficiency have higher, but less than normal, concentrations.

Table 2–6 ◆ Differential Diagnosis of Carnitine Deficiency

Primary Genetic Carnitine Deficiency

Secondary to Other Metabolic Errors
1. Aminoacidurias
   a. Glutaric aciduria
   b. Isovaleric acidemia
   c. Methylmalonic acidemia
   d. Propionic acidemia
2. Disorders of pyruvate metabolism
   a. Multiple carboxylase deficiency
   b. Pyruvate carboxylase deficiency
   c. Pyruvate dehydrogenase deficiency
3. Disorders of the respiratory chain
4. Phosphoglucomutase deficiency

Secondary to Acquired Conditions
1. Hemodialysis
2. Malnutrition
3. Pregnancy
4. Reye syndrome
5. Total parenteral nutrition
6. Valproate hepatotoxicity

Treatment. Dietary supplementation with L-carnitine is recommended. The initial dosage is 50 mg/kg/day, which is increased as tolerated (up to 800 mg/kg/day) until the desired blood concentration is attained. Adverse effects of carnitine include nausea, vomiting, diarrhea, and abdominal cramps. During an acute attack a diet rich in medium-chain triglycerides and low in long-chain triglycerides should be provided in addition to carnitine. General supportive care is required for hypoglycemia and hypoprothrombinemia.

RENAL DISORDERS

Children with chronic renal failure are at risk for acute or chronic uremic encephalopathy, dialysis encephalopathy, hypertensive encephalopathy, and neurologic complications of the immunocompromised state.

Acute Uremic Encephalopathy

Clinical Features. In children with acute renal failure, symptoms of cerebral dysfunction develop over several days. Asterixis is often the initial feature. This is followed by periods of confusion and headache, sometimes progressing to delirium and then to lethargy. Weakness, tremulousness, and muscle cramps develop. Myoclonic jerks and tetany may be present. If uremia continues, decreasing consciousness and seizures follow.

Transitory or permanent hemiparesis may occur in children with *hemolytic-uremic syndrome.* Encephalopathy is the usual initial feature, but hemiparesis and aphasia caused by thrombotic stroke can occur in the absence of seizures or altered states of consciousness (Trevathan and Dooling, 1987).

Diagnosis. The mechanism is multifactorial and does not correlate with concentrations of blood urea nitrogen alone. Hyperammonemia and disturbed equilibrium of ions between the intracellular and extracellular spaces are probably important factors.

Late in the course, acute uremic encephalopathy may be confused with hypertensive encephalopathy. A distinguishing feature is that increased intracranial pressure is an early feature of hypertensive encephalopathy but not acute uremic encephalopathy. Early in the course the EEG demonstrates slowing of the background rhythms and periodic triphasic waves.

Treatment. Hemodialysis reverses the encephalopathy and should be performed as quickly as possible after diagnosis.

Chronic Uremic Encephalopathy

Clinical Features.   Chronic uremic encephalopathy is usually caused by congenital renal hypoplasia. Renal failure begins during the first year, and encephalopathy occurs between 1 and 9 years of age (Foley et al, 1981; Rotundo et al, 1982). Growth failure precedes the onset of encephalopathy. Three stages are described.

Stage 1 consists of delayed motor development, dysmetria and tremor, or ataxia. Examination during this stage reveals hyperreflexia, mild hypotonia, and extensor plantar responses. Within 6 to 12 months the disease progresses to stage 2.

Stage 2 is characterized by myoclonus of the face and limbs, partial motor seizures, dementia, and then generalized seizures. Facial myoclonus and lingual apraxia make speech and feeding difficult, and limb myoclonus interferes with ambulation. The duration of stage 2 is variable and may be months to years.

In stage 3 there are progressive bulbar failure, a vegetative state, and death.

Diagnosis.   The diagnosis is based on clinical findings. Initially the EEG reveals progressive slowing and then the development of superimposed epileptiform activity. CT demonstrates progressive cerebral atrophy. The disorder may be difficult to distinguish from dialysis encephalopathy; they may be the same disease.

Hyperparathyroidism with hypercalcemia has been noted in some children with chronic uremic encephalopathy, but parathyroidectomy does not reverse the process (Geary et al, 1980). A suggested cause is aluminum toxicity from antacids administered as phosphate binders (Sedman et al, 1984). Plasma concentrations of aluminum should be determined during stage 1, and if they are elevated, aluminum ingestion should be discontinued.

Treatment.   Hemodialysis and renal transplantation have not altered the course in most patients.

Dialysis Encephalopathy

Long-term dialysis may be associated with acute, transitory neurologic disturbances attributed to the rapid shift of fluids and electrolytes between intracellular and extracellular spaces. Most common are vascular headaches and seizures. Seizures usually occur toward the end of dialysis or up to 24 hours later and may be preceded by lethargy and delirium.

In contrast, progressive encephalopathies associated with dialysis are often fatal. Two important causes exist: (1) encephalitis resulting from immunosuppression and (2) the dialysis dementia syndrome. Opportunistic infections in the immunodeficient host are usually due to cytomegalovirus, toxoplasmosis, and mycoses.

Dialysis Dementia Syndrome

Clinical Features.   The mean interval between commencement of dialysis and onset of symptoms is 4 years (range 1 to 7 years), and subsequent progression of symptoms varies from weeks to years (O'Hare et al, 1983). Patients have a characteristic speech disturbance either as an initial feature or later in the course. It begins as intermittent hesitancy of speech (stuttering and slurring) and may progress to aphasia. Agraphia and apraxia may be present as well. Subtle personality changes suggestive of depression occur early in the course. A phase of hallucinations and agitation may occur, and then progressive dementia develops.

Myoclonic jerking of the limbs is often present before the onset of dementia. First noted during dialysis, it soon becomes continuous and interferes with normal activity. Generalized tonic-clonic seizures develop in most patients and become more frequent and severe as the encephalopathy progresses. Complex partial seizures may be observed, but focal motor seizures are unusual.

Neurologic examination reveals the triad of speech arrest, myoclonus, and dementia. In addition, many patients show symmetric proximal weakness (myopathy) or distal weakness and sensory loss (neuropathy) with loss of tendon reflexes.

Diagnosis.   EEG changes correlate with disease progress. A characteristic early feature is the appearance of paroxysmal high-amplitude delta activity in the frontal areas, despite a normal posterior rhythm. Eventually the background becomes generally slow and frontal triphasic waves are noted. Epileptiform activity develops in all patients with dialysis dementia and is the EEG feature that differentiates dialysis dementia from uremic encephalopathy. The activity consists of sharp, spike, or polyspike discharges that may have a periodic quality.

Treatment.   Evidence suggests that aluminum toxicity is an important contributory cause, but no single factor has been established as etiologic. Excessive aluminum may be derived from orally administered aluminum gels or from the dialysate. Removal of aluminum from dialysate prevents the appearance of new cases and progression in some established cases, even if oral gels are still administered.

Renal transplantation prevents development of

the syndrome but does not always provide relief in established cases.

Benzodiazepines are useful in treating myoclonus and seizures and may improve the speech disturbance.

Hypertensive Encephalopathy

Hypertensive encephalopathy occurs when increases in systemic blood pressure exceed the limits of cerebral autoregulation. The result is damage to small arterioles, which leads to patchy areas of ischemia and edema. Therefore focal neurologic deficits are relatively common.

Clinical Features. The initial features are transient attacks of cerebral ischemia and headache. Such symptoms may be dismissed as part of uremic encephalopathy, despite the warning signs of focal neurologic deficits. Headache persists and is accompanied by visual disturbances and vomiting. Seizures and diminished consciousness follow. The seizures are frequently focal at onset and then generalized. Examination reveals papilledema and retinal hemorrhages.

Diagnosis. Because the syndrome occurs in children receiving long-term renal dialysis while awaiting transplantation, the differential diagnosis includes disorders of osmolality, uremic encephalopathy, and dialysis encephalopathy. The EEG shows nonspecific abnormalities, including generalized slowing of the background rhythms and sometimes paroxysmal discharges and periodic complexes.

Hypertensive encephalopathy can be distinguished from other encephalopathies associated with renal disease by the greater elevation of blood pressure and the presence of focal neurologic disturbances.

Treatment. Hypertensive encephalopathy is a medical emergency. Treatment consists of anticonvulsant therapy and aggressive efforts to reduce hypertension. Measures to reduce cerebral edema are required in some patients.

OTHER METABOLIC ENCEPHALOPATHIES

Several less common causes of metabolic encephalopathy are listed in Table 2–3. Some are attributable to derangements of a single substance, but most are multifactorial.

In 5% of children with burns covering 30% of the body surface, an encephalopathy that may be intermittent develops *(burn encephalopathy)*. The onset may be days to weeks after the burn. Altered mental states (delirium or coma) and seizures (generalized or focal) are the major features. Multiple metabolic alterations are present, and the encephalopathy usually cannot be attributed to a single factor (Mohnot et al, 1982).

Encephalopathies that occur during total parenteral hyperalimentation are generally due to hyperammonemia caused by excessive loads of amino acids (Grazer et al, 1984).

Hypomagnesemia in infancy may be caused by prematurity, maternal deficiency, maternal or infant hypoparathyroidism, high-phosphorus diets, exchange transfusion, intestinal disorders, and specific defects in magnesium absorption. These conditions are often associated with hypocalcemia. Excessive use of diuretics causes hypomagnesemia in older children. Symptoms develop when plasma magnesium concentrations are less than 1.2 mg/dl (0.5 mmol/L) and include jitteriness, hyperirritability, and seizures. Further decline in serum magnesium concentration leads to obtundation and coma.

Deficiency of one or more B vitamins may be associated with lethargy or delirium, but only thiamine deficiency causes coma. Thiamine deficiency is relatively common in alcoholic adults and produces Wernicke encephalopathy but is uncommon in children. Subacute necrotizing encephalopathy is a thiamine deficiency–like state in children (see Chapters 5 and 10).

◆ Migraine

Migraine produces a large variety of neurologic syndromes and is discussed in several chapters. Among its less common manifestations are a confusional state, an amnestic state, and coma.

ACUTE CONFUSIONAL MIGRAINE

Clinical Features. A confused and agitated state resembling toxic-metabolic psychosis occurs as a migraine variant in children between the ages of 5 and 16. Most affected children are 10 years or older. The symptoms develop rapidly. The child becomes delirious and appears to be in pain but does not complain of headache. Impaired awareness of environment, retarded responses to painful stimuli, hyperactivity, restlessness, and combative behavior are evident. The duration of an attack is usually 3 to 5 hours but may be as long as 20 hours. The child eventually falls into a deep sleep, appears normal on awakening, and has no memory of the episode. Confusional attacks tend to recur over a period of days or months and then evolve into typical migraine episodes (Ehyai and Fenichel, 1978).

Diagnosis.   Migraine is always a clinical diagnosis and should be arrived at only after other possibilities are excluded. The diagnosis relies heavily on a family history of migraine, but not necessarily of confusional migraine. During or shortly after a confusional attack the EEG demonstrates unilateral temporal or occipital slowing.

Treatment.   The acute attack can be treated with intramuscular chlorpromazine, 1 mg/kg. Propranolol provides prophylaxis (see Chapter 3).

MIGRAINE COMA

Migraine coma is a rare but extreme form of migraine that can be fatal (Fitzsimon and Wolfenden, 1985).

Clinical Features.   The major features of migraine coma are (1) recurrent episodes of coma precipitated by trivial head injury and (2) apparent meningitis associated with life-threatening cerebral edema. Migraine coma has been reported in a kindred with *familial hemiplegic migraine* (see Chapter 11), but a similar syndrome may occur in sporadic cases. Coma develops following trivial head injury and is associated with fever. Intracranial pressure is increased because of cerebral edema, which can be localized to one hemisphere and cause sufficient midline shift to produce herniation. States of decreased consciousness may last several days. Recovery is then complete.

Diagnosis.   Coma following even trivial head injury causes concern for intracranial hemorrhage. The initial CT scan may not show abnormalities, especially if obtained early in the course. Scans obtained between 24 and 72 hours show generalized or focal edema.

Examination of the cerebrospinal fluid reveals increased pressure and pleocytosis (up to 100 cells/mm^3). The combination of fever, coma, and cerebrospinal fluid pleocytosis suggests viral encephalitis, and herpes is a possibility if edema is localized to one temporal lobe.

Treatment.   Patients who have experienced migraine coma should be treated afterward with a prophylactic agent to prevent further attacks (see Chapter 3). The major treatment goal during the attack is to decrease intracranial pressure by reducing cerebral edema (see Chapter 4).

TRANSIENT GLOBAL AMNESIA

Transient global amnesia usually occurs in adults and is characterized by sudden inability to form new memories and repetitive questioning about events, but no other neurologic symptoms or signs. Migraine is the probable cause when such attacks occur in children or in more than one family member (Dupuis et al, 1987).

Clinical Features.   Attacks last from 20 minutes to several hours, and retrograde amnesia is present on recovery. Many adults with transient global amnesia have a history of migraine, and a similar syndrome may be seen in children with migraine following trivial head injury (Haas and Ross, 1986). The attacks are similar to acute confusional migraine except that the patient has less delirium and greater isolated memory deficiency.

Diagnosis.   A personal or family history of migraine is essential for diagnosis. The CT scan shows no abnormalities, but the EEG may demonstrate slowing of the background rhythm in one temporal lobe.

Treatment.   Management is the same as for classic migraine (see Chapter 3).

◆ Psychologic Disorders

Panic disorders and schizophrenia may have an acute onset of symptoms suggesting delirium or confusion and must be distinguished from acute organic encephalopathies.

PANIC DISORDER

Clinical Features.   Panic attacks were thought to be confined to adults but now are recognized to occur in adolescents and school-aged children (Herskowitz, 1986). A panic attack is an agitated state caused by anxiety. Principal features are paroxysmal dizziness, headache, and dyspnea. Hyperventilation often occurs and results in further dizziness, paresthesias, and lightheadedness. Attacks may be provoked by phobias, such as fear of going to school. They can last for minutes to hours and recur daily.

Diagnosis.   Panic attacks simulate cardiac or neurologic disease, and many children undergo extensive and unnecessary medical evaluation before the correct diagnosis is reached. Panic disorder should be suspected in children with recurrent attacks of hyperventilation, dizziness, or dyspnea.

Treatment.   Antidepressant drugs have varying degrees of efficacy. Imipramine has the best success rate. Initial dosages are less than those used for depression (0.25 mg/kg/day), but higher dosages may be needed if concurrent depression must be treated.

SCHIZOPHRENIA

Clinical Features.   Schizophrenia is a disorder of adolescence or early adult life and should not be suspected in prepubertal children. Schizophrenic individuals have no antecedent history of an affective disorder. An initial feature is often declining work performance simulating dementia. Intermittent depersonalization (not knowing where or who one is) may occur early in the course and suggests complex partial seizures.

Thoughts move with loose association from one idea to another until they become incoherent. Delusions and hallucinations are common and usually have paranoid features. Motor activity can be either lacking, with the patient remaining stationary, or excessive and purposeless. This combination of symptoms in an adolescent may be difficult to distinguish clinically from drug encephalopathy.

Diagnosis. The diagnosis is established by careful evaluation of mental status. The family may have a history of schizophrenia. Neurologic and laboratory findings are normal. A normal EEG in an awake child with the clinical symptoms of acute encephalopathy points to psychologic disturbances, including schizophrenia.

Treatment. Schizophrenia is generally considered a chemical disorder of the brain. It is incurable, but many of the symptoms are alleviated by antipsychotic drugs. Phenothiazines and haloperidol are most often used.

◆ Toxic Encephalopathies

Accidental poisoning with drugs and chemicals left carelessly within reach is relatively common in children from ages 1 to 4. Between ages 4 and 10 there is a trough in the frequency of poisoning, which is followed by an increasing frequency of intentional poisoning with substances of abuse and prescription drugs.

PRESCRIPTION DRUG OVERDOSES

Most intentional overdoses are with prescription drugs, since they are readily available. Delirium or coma may be due to toxic effects of psychoactive drugs (anticonvulsants, antidepressants, antipsychotics, and tranquilizers), hypoglycemia (insulin and oral hypoglycemic agents), and acid-base disturbances (salicylates).

The encephalopathies that occur when drugs cause disorders of osmolality or organ failure are described in the section on metabolic encephalopathies.

Clinical Features. Psychoactive drugs are present in many households and are a frequent cause of poisoning. As a rule, toxic doses produce lethargy, nystagmus or ophthalmoplegia, and loss of coordination. Higher concentrations result in coma and seizures. Involuntary movements may occur as an idiosyncratic or dose-related effect.

Diazepam is remarkably safe when taken alone, and no instances of coma or death from overdose have been reported. Other benzodiazepines are also reasonably safe.

Tricyclic antidepressants are the most widely prescribed drugs in the United States and account for 25% of serious overdoses (Braden et al, 1986). The major features of overdose are coma, hypotension, and anticholinergic effects (flushing, dry skin, dilated pupils, tachycardia, decreased gastrointestinal motility, and urinary retention). Seizures and myocardial depression may be present as well.

The onset of symptoms following phenothiazine or haloperidol administration may be delayed for 6 to 24 hours, and symptoms may be intermittent (Knight and Roberts, 1986). Extrapyramidal disturbances (see Chapter 14), and symptoms of anticholinergic poisoning are prominent features. Fatalities are uncommon and probably caused by cardiac arrhythmia.

Diagnosis. Most drugs can be identified by the laboratory within 2 hours. A drug screen of the urine should be performed in all cases of unidentified coma or delirium. If an unidentifiable product is found in the urine, further identification may be possible in the plasma. Blood concentration should be determined when the identity of a drug is known.

Treatment. The degree of supportive care needed depends on the severity of the poisoning. Every child needs an intravenous line and careful monitoring of cardiorespiratory status. A continuous electrocardiogram (EKG) is often required because of concern for arrhythmia. Unabsorbed drug must be removed from the stomach by lavage and repeated doses of activated charcoal (30 mg every 6 hours) administered to prevent absorption and increase drug clearance. Extrapyramidal symptoms are treated with intravenous diphenhydramine, 2 mg/kg.

POISONING

Most accidental poisonings occur in small children who ingest common household products. The ingestion is usually discovered quickly because the child becomes sick and vomits. Insecticides, herbicides, and products containing hydrocarbons or alcohol are frequently implicated. Clinical features vary depending on the agent ingested. Optimal management requires identification of constituent poisons, estimation of amount ingested, interval since exposure, cleansing of the gastrointestinal tract, specific antidotes when available, and supportive measures.

SUBSTANCE ABUSE

Alcohol remains the most common substance of abuse in the United States. More than 90% of high school seniors have used alcohol one or more times, and 6% are daily drinkers (Kulberg, 1986). Approximately 6% of high school seniors use marijuana daily, but less than 0.1% are regular users of hallucinogens or opiates. The use of cocaine, stimulants, and sedatives has been increasing in recent years. Daily use of stimulants is reported by up to 1% of high school seniors.

Clinical Features.   The American Psychiatric Association defines the diagnostic criteria for substance abuse as (1) a pattern of pathologic use with inability to stop or reduce use, (2) impairment of social or occupational functioning, which includes school performance in children, and (3) persistence of the problem for 1 month or longer.

The clinical features of acute intoxication vary with the substance used. Almost all disturb judgment, intellectual function, and coordination. Alcohol and sedatives lead to drowsiness, sleep, and obtundation. In contrast, hallucinogens cause bizarre behavior, which includes hallucinations, delusions, and muscle rigidity. Such drugs as phencyclidine (angel dust) and lysergic acid diethylamide (LSD) produce a clinical picture that simulates schizophrenia.

The usual symptoms of marijuana intoxication are euphoria and a sense of relaxation at low doses and a dreamlike state with slow response time at higher doses. Very high blood concentrations produce depersonalization, disorientation, and sensory disturbances. Hallucinations and delusions are unusual with marijuana and suggest mixed drug use.

Amphetamine abuse should be considered when an agitated state is coupled with peripheral evidence of adrenergic toxicity: mydriasis, flushing, diaphoresis, and reflex bradycardia caused by peripheral vasoconstriction.

Cocaine affects the brain and heart. Early symptoms include euphoria, mydriasis, headache, and tachycardia. Higher doses produce emotional lability, nausea and vomiting, flushing, and a syndrome that simulates paranoid schizophrenia. Life-threatening complications are hyperthermia, seizures, cardiac arrhythmia, and stroke. Associated stroke syndromes include transient ischemic attacks in the distribution of the middle cerebral artery, lateral medullary infarction, and anterior spinal artery infarction (Mody et al, 1988).

Diagnosis.   The major challenge is to differentiate acute substance intoxication from schizophrenia. Important clues are a history of substance abuse obtained from family or friends, associated autonomic and cardiac disturbances, and alterations in vital signs. Urine and plasma screening generally detects the substance or its metabolites.

Treatment.   Management of acute substance abuse depends on the substance used and the amount ingested. Physicians must be alert to the possibility of multiple drug or substance exposure. An attempt should be made to empty the gastrointestinal tract of substances taken orally. Support of cardiorespiratory function and correction of metabolic disturbances are generally required. Intravenous diazepam reduces the hallucinations and seizures produced by stimulants and hallucinogens. Standard cardiac drugs are used to combat arrhythmias.

The most vexing problem with substance abuse is generally not the acute management of intoxication, but rather breaking the habit. This requires the patient's motivation and long-term inpatient and outpatient treatment.

◆ Trauma

Trivial head injuries, without loss of consciousness, are commonplace in children, and are an almost constant occurrence in toddlers. Migraine should be suspected whenever transitory neurologic disturbances (e.g., amnesia, ataxia, blindness, coma, confusion, hemiplegia) follow trivial head injuries. Important causes of significant head injuries are child abuse in infants, sports and play injuries in children, and motor vehicle accidents in adolescents.

Neonatal head injuries generally cause seizures (see Chapter 1). Loss of consciousness is the major feature of head injuries beyond the neonatal period. Mild head injuries are characterized by temporary loss of consciousness without evidence of focal neurologic disturbances. Such events are usually termed concussion. Severe head injuries are characterized by prolonged intervals of coma associated with brain swelling and intracranial hemorrhage.

MILD HEAD INJURIES

Clinical Features.   Mild closed head injuries are associated with temporary loss of consciousness and the absence of localizing neurologic signs. The child may be stunned without definite loss of consciousness or may be obtunded for several hours but is not in coma. Once consciousness is restored, the child is invariably tired and sleeps long and soundly if left undisturbed. As a rule recovery is complete, but the child may not remember the event or the period before and after it. The length of the amnestic interval correlates with the severity of injury.

Many children complain of headache and dizziness for several days or weeks following concussion. They may be irritable and have memory disturbances. The severity and duration of these symptoms usually correlate with the severity of injury but sometimes seem disproportionate.

Focal or generalized seizures, and sometimes status epilepticus, may occur 1 or 2 hours after mild head injury (Snoek et al, 1984). Seizures may even occur in children who did not lose consciousness. Such seizures rarely portend later epilepsy.

Diagnosis. A CT scan of the head is usually obtained when a child is brought to an emergency room with a mild head injury. This is probably cost effective, since it reduces the number of hospital admissions. EEG should be performed if there is any suspicion that the head injury occurred during a seizure or if neurologic disturbances are disproportionate to the severity of injury.

Treatment. Mild head injuries do not require treatment, and in the absence of skull fracture a child whose neurologic findings are normal does not require hospitalization (Rosenthal and Bergman, 1989). If the child does not need hospitalization, asking the parents to awaken the child at regular intervals and assess neurologic status is unreasonable. Normal children are difficult to arouse from sleep, and a child who has had a head injury and spent several hours in an emergency room will sleep all the sounder. A child who does not need hospital observation does not need home observation.

SEVERE HEAD INJURIES

The outcome following severe head injuries is usually better for children than for adults, but it is not clear that younger children do better than older children (Kriel et al, 1989; Luerssen et al, 1988).

Shaking Injuries

Clinical Features. Shaking is a common method of child abuse in infants. An unconscious infant is brought to the emergency room with bulging fontanelles. Seizures may have precipitated the hospital visit. The history is fragmentary and inconsistent among informants. Typically the child has been left in the care of a babysitter or the mother's boyfriend.

The child shows no external evidence of head injury, but ophthalmoscopic examination reveals retinal and optic nerve sheath hemorrhages (Lambert et al, 1986). Many of the hemorrhages may

be old, suggesting repeated shaking injuries. On the thorax or back the examiner may note bruises that conform to hand prints where the child was held during the shaking. Healing fractures of the posterior rib cage indicate child abuse.

Death may result from uncontrollable increased intracranial pressure or contusion of the cervicomedullary junction (Hadley et al, 1989).

Diagnosis. The CT scan reveals a swollen brain but may not show subdural collections of blood if bleeding is recent. A subdural tap should be performed whether or not subdural blood is observed on the CT scan. It is both diagnostic and therapeutic.

Treatment. Bilateral subdural taps should be performed immediately with the intention of removing as much blood as possible. The amount available for drainage through a subdural tap is only a small percentage of the total volume in the subdural space. The goal of the subdural tap is not to remove all subdural blood, but rather to remove a sufficient quantity to relieve increased intracranial pressure and to aid reabsorptive mechanisms. Taps are repeated daily until the removable volume begins to decline; then an every-other-day schedule of subdural taps allows continued reduction of the accumulated fluid. A subdural-peritoneal shunt may be required if permanent effusion develops.

Transfusion may be needed if the peripheral hematocrit value is low and falling.

Protective service must be sought to prevent further injuries. Overall, the neurologic and visual outcome among victims of shaking is poor. Most are left with a considerable handicap.

Closed Head Injuries

Supratentorial subdural hematomas are venous in origin, are frequently bilateral, and usually occur without associated skull fracture. Supratentorial epidural hematomas are usually associated with skull fracture and are described in the section on open head injuries. Epidural and subdural hematomas are almost impossible to distinguish on clinical grounds alone. Progressive loss of consciousness is a feature of both types, and both may be associated with a lucid interval between time of injury and neurologic deterioration.

Posterior fossa epidural and subdural hemorrhages occur most often in newborns (see Chapter 1) and older children with posterior skull fractures.

Clinical Features. Loss of consciousness is not always immediate; a lucid period of several minutes may intervene between injury and onset of neurologic deterioration (Snoek et al, 1984). The Glasgow Coma Scale is used widely to quantify the degree of responsiveness following head injuries (Table 2–7). Scores of 8 or less correlate well with severe injury.

Acute brain swelling and intracranial hemorrhage account for the clinical manifestations. Increased intracranial pressure is always present and may lead to herniation if uncontrolled. Focal neurologic deficits suggest intracerebral hemorrhage.

Mortality rates in children with severe head injury are usually between 10% and 15% and have not changed substantially in the past decade (Kalff et al, 1989). Low mortality rates are sometimes associated with higher percentages of survivors in chronic vegetative states. Duration of coma is the best guide to long-term morbidity (Filley et al, 1987). Permanent neurologic impairment is produced when coma persists for 1 month or longer.

Diagnosis.   A head CT should be performed as rapidly as possible after closed head injuries. Brain swelling and subarachnoid hemorrhage with blood collecting along the falx are typical findings. Intracranial hemorrhage may also be detected. Immediately after injury some subdural hematomas are briefly isodense and may not be observed. Later the hematoma appears as a region of increased density, convex toward the skull and concave toward the brain. With time the density decreases.

Intracerebral hemorrhage is usually superficial but may extend deep into the brain. Frontal or temporal lobe contusion is common. Discrete deep hemorrhages without a superficial extension are not usually caused by trauma.

Children with head injuries must be kept with the neck immobilized until radiographic examination for fracture-dislocation of the cervical spine is done, since the force of a blow to the skull is frequently propagated to the neck. The child must be examined for limb and organ injury when head injury occurs in a motor vehicle accident.

Treatment.   Severe head injuries should be managed in an intensive care unit. Essential support includes controlled ventilation, prevention of hypotension, and sufficient reduction in brain swelling to maintain cerebral perfusion. Methods to reduce cerebral edema are reviewed in Chapter 4. Barbiturate coma does not affect outcome (Ward et al, 1985).

Acute expanding intracranial hematomas warrant immediate surgery. Small subdural collections that do not produce a mass effect can be left in place until the patient's condition is stabilized and the options are considered.

Phenytoin is routinely administered intravenously to prevent posttraumatic epilepsy. It decreases seizure frequency during the first week but is ineffective in preventing subsequent epilepsy (Temkin et al, 1990).

Open Head Injuries

The clinical features, diagnosis, and management of open head injuries are much the same as described for closed injuries. The major differences are the greater risk of epidural hematoma and infection and the possibility of damage to the brain surface from depression of the bone.

Supratentorial epidural hematomas are usually temporal or temporoparietal in location. The origin of the blood may be arterial (tearing of the middle meningeal artery), venous, or both. Skull fracture is present in 75% of cases. Epidural hematoma has a characteristic lens-shaped appearance (Fig. 2–5). Infratentorial epidural hematoma is venous in origin and produces signs of brainstem compression.

Skull fractures, other than linear fractures, are associated with an increased risk of infection. A fracture is referred to as depressed if the inner table fragment is displaced by at least the thickness of the skull. Depressed fractures are termed compound if the scalp is lacerated and penetrating if the dura is torn. Infants with penetrating injuries may develop growing skull fractures (Scarfo et al, 1989). The rapid growth of the brain causes the fracture line to spread further in order to accommodate the increasing intracranial volume.

Depressed fractures of the skull vault may injure the underlying brain and tear venous sinuses. The result is hemorrhage into the brain and subdural space. Treatment includes elevation of depressed

Table 2–7 ◆ Glasgow Coma Scale*

Eye Opening (E)

Spontaneous	4
To speech	3
To pain	2
None	1

Best Motor Response (M)

Obeys	6
Localizes	5
Withdraws	4
Abnormal flexion	3
Abnormal extension	2
None	1

Verbal Response (V)

Oriented	5
Confused conversation	4
Inappropriate words	3
Incomprehensible sounds	2
None	1

*Coma Score = E + M + V.

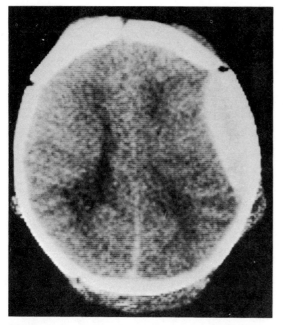

Figure 2–5 Epidural hematoma. The hematoma appears as a lens-shaped density just below the skull.

fragments, debridement and closure of the scalp laceration, and systemic penicillin.

Basal skull fractures with dural tear may result in leakage of cerebrospinal fluid from nose or ear and meningitis. Such leaks usually develop within 3 days of injury. The timing and need for dural repair are somewhat controversial, but the need for intravenous antibiotic coverage has been established.

Posttraumatic Epilepsy

Posttraumatic epilepsy develops in 53% of patients with penetrating head injuries (Salazar et al, 1985). Half continue to have seizures as long as 15 years after injury. Two thirds have seizure onset during the first year after the injury, and 90% by 5 years, but onset is delayed by 10 to 15 years in 7%. Patients with focal neurologic deficits and large cerebral lesions immediately after injury have the greatest risk for posttraumatic epilepsy. Initial seizures are generalized in 70% to 80% of cases.

Posttraumatic epilepsy is much less common with closed head injuries (Annegers et al, 1980). The 5-year incidence is 11.5% after severe head trauma (brain contusion, intracranial hemorrhage, or 24 hours of unconsciousness or amnesia) and 1.6% after moderate head trauma (skull fracture or 30 minutes to 24 hours of unconsciousness or amnesia). Mild head injuries (less than 30 minutes of

unconsciousness or amnesia) are not associated with an increased incidence of posttraumatic epilepsy.

References

Alvarez LA, Moshe SL, Belman AL, et al: EEG and brain death determination in children. Neurology 38:227, 1988.

American Academy of Neurology: Position of the American Academy of Neurology on certain aspects of the care and management of the persistent vegetative state patient. Neurology 39:125, 1989.

Annegers JF, Grabow JD, Groover RV, et al: Seizures after head trauma: A population study. Neurology 30:683, 1980.

Arieff AI: Hyponatremia, convulsions, respiratory arrest, and permanent brain damage after elective surgery in healthy women. N Engl J Med 314:1529, 1986.

Ashwal S, Schneider S: Brain death in the newborn. Pediatrics 84:429, 1989.

Atluru VL: Spontaneous intracerebral hematomas in juvenile diabetic ketoacidosis. Pediatr Neurol 2:167, 1986.

Ayus JC, Krothapalli RK, Arieff AI, et al: Changing concepts in treatment of severe symptomatic hyponatremia: Rapid correction and possible relation to central pontine myelinolysis. Am J Med 78:897, 1985.

Bartleson JD, Swanson JW, Whisnat JP: A migrainous syndrome with cerebrospinal fluid pleocytosis. Neurology 31:1257, 1981.

Beghi E, Nicolosi A, Kurland LT, et al: Encephalitis and aseptic meningitis, Olmsted county, Minnesota, 1950–1981. I. Epidemiology. Ann Neurol 16:283, 1984.

Bernard KW, Smith PW, Kader EJ, et al: Neuroparalytic illness and human diploid cell rabies vaccine. JAMA 248:3136, 1982.

Bloch AB, Orenstein WA, Stetler HC, et al: Health impact of measles vaccination in the United States. Pediatrics 76:524, 1985.

Braden NJ, Jackson JE, Walson PD: Tricyclic antidepressant overdose. Pediatr Clin North Am 33:287, 1986.

Brattstrom L, Hindfelt B, Nilsson O: Transient neurological symptoms associated with mononuclear pleocytosis of the cerebrospinal fluid. Acta Neurol Scand 70:104, 1984.

Carithers HA, Margileth AM: Cat-scratch disease: Acute encephalopathy and other neurologic manifestations. AJDC 145:98, 1991.

Centers for Disease Control: Adverse Events Following Immunization. Surveillance Report No. 2, 1982–1984. Issued December 1986.

Chaves-Carbello E, Montes JE, Nelson B, et al: Hemorrhagic shock and encephalopathy: Clinical definition of a catastrophic syndrome in infants. AJDC 144:1079, 1990.

Chesney PJ, Crass BA, Polyak MB, et al: Toxic shock syndrome: Management and long-term sequelae. Ann Intern Med 96:847, 1982.

Chun RWM, Thompson WH, Grabow JD, et al: California arbovirus encephalitis in children. Neurology 18:369, 1968.

Corey L, Spear PG: Infections with herpes simplex viruses (parts 1 and 2). N Engl J Med 314:686, 749, 1986.

De Vivo DC, Tein I: Primary and secondary disorders of carnitine metabolism. Int Pediatr 5:134, 1990.

Dearden NM: Ischaemic brain. Lancet 2:255, 1985.

Duck SC, Wyatt D: Factors associated with brain herniation in the treatment of diabetic ketoacidosis. J Pediatr 113:10, 1988.

Dupuis MJM, Pierre Ph, Gonsette RE: Transient global amnesia and migraine in twin sisters [letter]. J Neurol Neurosurg Psychiatry 50:816, 1987.

Eastern equine encephalitis—Florida, Eastern United States. MMWR 40:533, 1991.

Ehyai A, Fenichel GM: The natural history of acute confusional migraine. Arch Neurol 35:368, 1978.

English CK, Wear DJ, Margileth AM, et al: Cat scratch disease: Isolation and culture of the bacterial agent. JAMA 259:1347, 1988.

Fackler JC, Troncosco JC, Gioia FR: Age-specific characteristics of brain death in children. AJDC 142:999, 1988.

Filley CM, Cranberg LD, Alexander MP, et al: Neurobehavioral outcome after closed head injury in childhood and adolescence. Arch Neurol 44:194, 1987.

Fitzsimon RB, Wolfenden WH: Migraine coma: Meningitic migraine with cerebral oedema associated with a new form of autosomal dominant cerebellar ataxia. Brain 108:555, 1985.

Foley CM, Polinsky MS, Gruskin AB, et al: Encephalopathy in infants and children with chronic renal disease. Arch Neurol 38:656, 1981.

Freemon FR: Two roads to coma: The Scottish hypothesis. Med Hypotheses 2:82, 1976.

Geary DF, Fennell RS, Andriola M, et al: Encephalopathy in children with chronic renal failure. J Pediatr 96:41, 1980.

Grazer RE, Sutton JM, Friedstrom S, et al: Hyperammonemic encephalopathy due to essential amino acid hyperalimentation. Arch Intern Med 144:2278, 1984.

Haas DC, Ross GS: Transient global amnesia triggered by mild head trauma. Brain 109:251, 1986.

Hadley MN, Sonntag VKH, Rekate HL, et al: The infant whiplash-shake injury syndrome: A clinical and pathological study. Neurosurgery 24:536, 1989.

Hammond DN, Moll GW, Robertson GL, et al: Hypodipsic hypernatremia with normal osmoregulation of vasopressin. N Engl J Med 315:433, 1986.

Hansen K, Lebach A-M: Lyme neuroborreliosis: A new sensitive diagnostic assay for intrathecal synthesis of *Borrelia burgdorferi*—specific immunoglobulin G, A, and M. Ann Neurol 30:197, 1991.

Harris GD, Fiordalisi I, Finberg L, et al: Safe management of diabetic ketoacidosis. J Pediatr 113:65-68, 1988.

Herskowitz J: Neurologic presentations of panic disorder in childhood and adolescence. Dev Med Child Neurol 28:617, 1986.

Ho K-C, Hodach R, Varma R, et al: Kernicterus and central pontine myelinolysis in a 14-year-old boy with viral hepatitis. Ann Neurol 8:633, 1980.

Hoke CH, Nisalak A, Sangawhipa N, et al: Protection against Japanese encephalitis by inactivated vaccines. N Engl J Med 319:608, 1988.

Hurwitz ES, Barrett MJ, Bregman D, et al: Public Health Service study of Reye's syndrome and medications. JAMA 257:1905, 1987.

Institute of Medicine: Adverse Effects of Pertussis and Rubella Vaccines. National Academy Press, Washington, DC, 1991.

Jastremski M, Sutton-Tyrrell K, Vaagenes P, et al: Glucocorticoid treatment does not improve neurological recovery following cardiac arrest. JAMA 262:3427, 1989.

Johnson RT, Griffin DE, Hirsch RL, et al: Measles encephalomyelitis—clinical and immunologic studies. N Engl J Med 310:137, 1984.

Kalff R, Kocks W, Pospiech J, et al: Clinical outcome after head injury in children. Child Nerv Syst 5:156, 1989.

Karakusis PH: Considerations in the treatment of septic shock. Med Clin North Am 70:933, 1986.

Kennard C, Swash M: Acute viral encephalitis: Its diagnosis and outcome. Brain 104:129, 1981.

Kesselring J, Miller DH, Robb SA, et al: Acute disseminated encephalomyelitis: MRI findings and the distinction from multiple sclerosis. Brain 113:291, 1990.

Kirk JL, Fine DP, Sexron DJ, et al: Rocky Mountain spotted fever: A clinical review based on 48 confirmed cases, 1943–1986. Medicine 69:35, 1990.

Knight ME, Roberts RJ: Phenothiazine and butyrophone intoxication in children. Pediatr Clin North Am 33:299, 1986.

Kriel RL, Krach LE, Panser LA: Closed head injury: Comparison of children younger and older than 6 years of age. Pediatr Neurol 5:296, 1989.

Kulberg A: Substance abuse: Clinical identification and management. Pediatr Clin North Am 33:325, 1986.

Lambert SR, Johnson TE, Hoyt CS: Optic nerve and retinal hemorrhages associated with the shaken baby syndrome. Arch Ophthalmol 104:1509, 1986.

Levy DE, Caronna JJ, Singer BH, et al: Predicting outcome from hypoxic-ischemic coma. JAMA 253:1420, 1985.

Lichtenstein PK, Heubi JE, Daugherty CC, et al: Grade I Reye's syndrome: A frequent cause of vomiting and liver dysfunction after varicella and upper-respiratory-infection. N Engl J Med 309:133, 1983.

Logigian EL, Kaplan RF, Steere AC: Chronic neurologic manifestations of Lyme disease. N Engl J Med 323:1438, 1990.

Luerssen TG, Klauber MR, Marshall LF: Outcome from head injury related to patient's age: A longitudinal prospective study of adult and pediatric head injury. J Neurosurg 68:409, 1988.

MacDonald KL, Osterholm MT, Hedberg CW, et al: Toxic shock syndrome: A newly recognized complication of influenza and influenzalike illness. JAMA 257:1053, 1987.

Malouf R, Brust JCM: Hypoglycemia: Causes, neurological manifestations, and outcome. Ann Neurol 17:421, 1985.

Mody CK, Miller BL, McIntyre HB, et al: Neurologic complications of cocaine abuse. Neurology 38:1189, 1988.

Mohnot D, Snead OC, Benton JW Jr: Burn encephalopathy in children. Ann Neurol 12:42, 1982.

Norenberg MD: A hypothesis of osmotic endothelial injury: A pathogenetic mechanism in central pontine myelinolysis. Arch Neurol 40:66, 1983.

Nussbaum E, Maggi JC: Pentobarbital therapy does not improve neurologic outcome in nearly drowned flaccid-comatose children. Pediatrics 81:630, 1988.

O'Dougherty M, Wright FS, Loewenson RB, et al: Cerebral dysfunction after chronic hypoxia in children. Neurology 35:42, 1985.

O'Hare JA, Callaghan NM, Murnaghan DJ: Dialysis encephalopathy: Clinical, electroencephalographic and interventional aspects. Medicine 62:129, ,1983.

Peltola H, Heinonen OP: Frequency of the true adverse reactions to measles-mumps-rubella vaccine: A double-blind-controlled trial in twins. Lancet 1:939, 1986.

Plum F, Posner JB: The Diagnosis of Stupor and Coma, 3rd edition. FA Davis, Philadelphia, 1980, p 19.

President's Commission: Guidelines for the determination of death. JAMA 246:2184, 1981.

Przelomski MM, O'Rourke E, Grady GF, et al: Eastern equine encephalitis in Massachusetts: A report of 16 cases, 1970–1984. Neurology 38:736, 1988.

Rosenthal BW, Bergman I: Intracranial injury after moderate head trauma in children. J Pediatr 115:346, 1989.

Rotundo A, Nevins TE, Lipton M, et al: Progressive encephalopathy in children with chronic renal disease. Kidney Int 21:486, 1982.

St. Louis encephalitis outbreak—Arkansas, 1991. MMWR 40:605, 1991.

Salazar AM, Jabbari B, Vance SC, et al: Epilepsy after penetrating head injury. I. Clinical correlates: A report of the Vietnam Head Injury Study. Neurology 35:1406, 1985.

Scarfo GB, Mariottini A, Tomaccini D, et al: Growing skull fractures: Progressive evolution of brain damage and effectiveness of surgical treatment. Child Nerv Syst 5:163, 1989.

Schroth G, Gawehn J, Thron A, et al: Early diagnosis of herpes simplex encephalitis by MRI. Neurology 37:179, 1987.

Sedman AB, Wilkening GN, Warady BA, et al: Encephalopathy in childhood secondary to aluminum toxicity. J Pediatr 105:836, 1984.

Shaw PJ, Walls TJ, Newman MB, et al: Hashimoto's encephalopathy: A steroid-responsive disorder associated with high anti-thyroid antibody titers—report of 5 cases. Neurology 41:228, 1991.

Shaywitz BA, Lister G, Duncan CC: What is the best treatment for Reye's syndrome? Arch Neurol 43:730, 1986.

Snoek JW, Minderhould JM, Wilmink JT: Delayed deterioration following mild head injury in children. Brain 107:15, 1984.

Sriram S, Steinman L: Postinfectious and postvaccinial encephalomyelitis. Neurol Clin North Am 2:341, 1984.

Steere AC: Lyme disease. N Engl J Med 321:586, 1989.

Tein I, De Vivo DC, Hale DE, et al: Short-chain L-3-hydroxy-acyl-CoA dehydrogenase deficiency in muscle: A new cause for recurrent myoglobinuria and encephalopathy. Ann Neurol 30:415, 1991.

Temkin NR, Dikmen SS, Wilensky AJ, et al: A randomized double-blind study of phenytoin for the prevention of post-traumatic seizures. N Engl J Med 323:497, 1990.

Trauner DA: What is the best treatment for Reye's syndrome? Arch Neurol 43:729, 1986.

Trevathan E, Dooling EC: Large thrombotic strokes in hemolytic-uremic syndrome. J Pediatr 111:863, 1987.

Ward JD, Becker DP, Miller JD, et al: Failure of prophylactic barbiturate coma in the treatment of severe head injury. J Neurosurg 62:383, 1985.

West JB: Do climbs to extreme altitude cause brain damage? Lancet 2:387, 1986.

Whitley RJ, Alford CA, Hirsch MS, et al: Vidarabine versus acyclovir therapy in herpes simplex encephalitis. N Engl J Med 314:144, 1986.

Whitley RJ, Soong S-J, Linneman C Jr, et al: Herpes simplex encephalitis: Clinical assessment. JAMA 247:317, 1982.

Headache

◆ Approach to Headache

An epidemiologic study of headache in one Maryland county showed that 12% of adolescents missed a day of school in the preceding month because of headache (Linet et al, 1989). Headache had caused 13% of males and 20% of females to consult a physician. Among those seeking medical opinion, 7.7% of the boys and 2.2% of the girls had seen a neurologist. To some, this last statistic will suggest a bias against women, but I believe that neurologic consultation is sought more often for boys than girls because they have a higher incidence of head injuries.

Parents seek medical attention for a child with headache, not so much looking for relief of pain as seeking assurance that the headache is not a sign of intracranial disease such as brain tumor. If this is the understood purpose of consultation, identifying the cause of headache may not be necessary in all cases. The paramount goal is to provide assurance that headache is not a sign of serious illness. In some circumstances, this assurance is the only possible achievement. Not every headache can be explained, and the term "psychogenic" should not be used as a synonym for idiopathic. It is usually possible, often by history and physical examination alone but sometimes with the aid of diagnostic studies, to distinguish headaches that are only painful from those that are harmful. This distinction is usually made by identifying the structure or structures that are generating pain and is almost always insured by imaging the brain.

SOURCES OF PAIN

Pain-sensitive structures of the head and neck are summarized in Table 3–1. The major pain-sensitive structures inside the skull are blood vessels. Mechanisms that stimulate pain from blood vessels are vasodilation, inflammation, and traction-displacement. Increased intracranial pressure causes pain mainly by the traction and displacement of intracranial arteries (see Chapter 4). The brain parenchyma, its ependymal lining, and the meninges are insensitive to pain.

Pain from supratentorial intracranial vessels is transmitted by the trigeminal nerve, whereas pain from infratentorial intracranial vessels is transmitted by the first three cervical nerves. Arteries in the superficial portion of the dura are innervated by the ophthalmic division of the trigeminal nerve and refer pain to the eye and forehead. The middle meningeal artery is innervated by the second and third divisions of the trigeminal nerve and refers pain to the temple. Cerebral arteries are innervated by all three divisions of the trigeminal nerve and refer pain to the eye, forehead, and temple. In contrast, pain from all structures in the posterior fossa is referred to the occiput and neck.

Several extracranial structures are pain sensitive. Major scalp arteries are present around the eye, forehead, and temple and produce pain when dilated or stretched. Cranial bones are insensitive, but periosteum, especially in the sinuses and near the teeth, is painful when inflamed. The inflamed periosteum is usually tender to palpation or other forms of physical stimulation. Muscles attached to the skull are a possible source of pain. The largest groups of such muscles are the neck extensors, which attach to the occipital ridge, the masseter muscles, and the frontalis muscle. The mechanism of muscle pain is not fully understood but probably involves prolonged contraction. The extraocular muscles are a source of muscle contraction pain in patients with heterophoria. When an imbalance exists, especially in convergence, long periods of close work cause difficulty in maintaining conjugate gaze and pain is felt in the orbit.

Pain from the cervical roots and cranial nerves

Table 3–1 ◆ Sources of Headache Pain

Intracranial
1. Cerebral and dural arteries
2. Large veins and venous sinuses

Extracranial
1. Cervical roots
2. Cranial nerves
3. Extracranial arteries
4. Muscles attached to skull
5. Periosteum/sinuses

is generally due to mechanical traction from injury or malformation. Pain follows this nerve distribution: the neck and back of the head up to the vertex for the cranial roots, and the face for the cranial nerves.

DESCRIPTIONS OF PAIN

History is everything in the attempt to diagnose the cause of headache. Yet children, especially very young ones, are incapable of describing this pain. A child asked to describe the quality of pain usually responds with sullen silence and looks imploringly at his or her mother to answer the foolish question. Encouraging remarks from the mother do not stimulate a response. To children, the only quality of pain is that it hurts and this should be self-evident. The physician tries to help the child with a litany of words that can be used to describe pain, such as throbbing, pulsating, tight, and sharp, and the child seeks approval by confessing to all.

Asking a child younger than 10 years of age how often headaches occur or how long they last is rarely productive. Young children have no sense of time, but parents are usually quite helpful in this regard. The exception is the parent who replies, either through conviction or to impress the physician with the severity of the situation, that the child who is sitting comfortably in the examining room has had a headache every day for the past 6 months or 1 year. Two questions should be asked in response. The first is, "How many days of school have been missed?" The answer provides a sense of frequency, severity, and disability. The second is, "How many different kinds of headache do you have?" The usual response is that the child has two kinds of headache: the bad headache, of which the child complains spontaneously, and the mild headache, of which the child complains when asked, "Are you having a headache?" When such history is obtained, the physician should direct further inquiry to the bad headache and give short shrift to the other. Another explanation for the complaint

of daily headaches of a year's duration is that the child has a flurry of headaches over a period of a week or two, then after a prolonged headache-free interval experiences another flurry of daily headaches. This pattern is identified by asking, "What is the longest period of time that you have been headache free?"

Helpful responses to traditional questions concerning the history of headache can be obtained from children aged 10 or older (Table 3–2). Several typical headache patterns, when present, allow recognition of either the source or the mechanism of pain. Temporal pain is usually vascular in origin; steady, tight pain, especially in the occipital region or in a band around the head, is likely to be muscular in origin. Periosteal pain, especially inflammation of the sinuses, is localized and tender to palpation. Cervical root and cranial nerve pain has a radiating or shooting quality. Confusion arises when several mechanisms of pain are experienced concurrently. Individuals with migraine commonly also have a tension headache.

Sinusitis is overdiagnosed as a cause of headache. Computed tomography (CT) evidence of sinusitis is commonplace in children. In my experience "sinusitis" is the most frequent radiologic finding in children evaluated for dementia. The physician should no sooner conclude that CT evidence of sinusitis is causally related to headache than that it is related to dementia.

A continuous, low-intensity, chronic headache, in the absence of associated symptoms or signs, is not likely to indicate intracranial disease. Intermittent headaches, especially those associated with nausea, from which the child recovers completely and is normal between attacks, are likely to be migraine. The recent onset of a severe headache, unlike anything previously experienced, from which the child never returns to a normal baseline is probably due to significant intracranial disease.

Most headaches are bilateral. Unilateral headache suggests migraine or intracranial mass lesions that are displacing local vessels without producing generalized increased intracranial pressure. Time of onset may indicate a stressful period for a child, such as school or visitation by a separated parent.

Table 3–2 ◆ Diagnostic Features of Headache

1. Associated features
2. Factors that precipitate
3. Factors that relieve
4. Frequency and duration
5. Length of illness
6. Location
7. Time of day

EVALUATION

Children referred to a pediatric neurologist for headache commonly arrive with a CT scan or at least a report of a normal CT scan. The only question asked by the primary physician was, "Does this child have a brain tumor?" Unfortunately, a normal CT scan neither explained nor cured the headache. A routine brain imaging study on every child with chronic headache is not a substitute for adequate history and physical examination.

◆ Migraine

Migraine accounts for 75% of headache in young children referred for neurologic consultation (Chu and Shinnar, 1992). It is a hereditary disorder transmitted by autosomal dominant inheritance. A history of migraine in at least one parent is reported in 90% of cases if both parents are interviewed by the physician and in 80% if only one parent is interviewed (Bille, 1962). The prevalence of migraine is 2.5% under the age of 7 (both sexes equally affected), 5% from age 7 to puberty (female-to-male ratio of 3:2), 5% in postpubertal boys, and 10% in postpubertal girls (Deubner, 1982; Sillanpaa, 1983). The prevalence in preschool children is probably higher than the recorded figure because migraine symptoms in preschool children tend to be atypical and are rarely identified as migraine at the time. The higher incidence of migraine in pubertal girls than in boys is probably related to the triggering effect of the menstrual cycle on migraine attacks.

TRIGGERING FACTORS

Among persons with a predisposition to migraine, individual attacks are usually provoked by an idiosyncratic triggering factor. Common triggering factors are stress, exercise, head trauma, and the premenstrual decline in circulating estrogen. An allergic basis for migraine has been considered but has not been substantiated.

Stress and Exercise

Migraine symptoms may first occur during stress or exercise or during the period of relaxation that follows. Therefore stress rarely provokes attacks upon awakening but is likely to contribute when attacks occur during school or shortly after returning home. No personality type of migrainous children has been established.

Head Trauma

The mechanism by which blows to the head and whiplash head movements provoke migraine attacks is unknown. Trivial blows to the head during competitive sports are significant triggering factors because they occur on a background of vigorous exercise and stress. A severe migraine attack—headache, vomiting, transitory neurologic deficits—following a head injury suggests the possibility of intracranial hemorrhage. The number of diagnostic tests can be reduced if the cause-and-effect relationship between head trauma and migraine is appreciated and the diagnosis of migraine established.

Transient cerebral blindness, as well as other transitory neurologic deficits, sometimes occurs after head trauma in children with migraine (see Chapter 16).

Menstrual Cycle

The higher rate of migraine among postpubertal girls as compared either with prepubertal children of both sexes or with postpubertal boys supports the observation that hormonal changes in the normal female cycle trigger attacks of migraine. The widespread use of oral contraceptives has provided some insight into the relationship between the female hormonal cycle and migraine. Oral contraceptives increase the frequency and intensity of migraine attacks in women with a history of migraine and may precipitate the initial attack in genetically predisposed women who have previously been migraine free. Among women taking oral contraceptives the greatest increase in frequency of migraine occurs at midcycle. The decline in concentration of circulating estrogens is probably the critical factor in precipitating an attack (Silberstein and Merriam, 1991).

CLINICAL SYNDROMES

Three major headache syndromes are associated with migraine: classic migraine, common migraine, and cluster headache. Classic and common migraine are probably a variable expression of the same genetic defect; different members of a family may have symptoms of classic or common migraine. Cluster headache is probably a distinct genetic entity with relatively uniform symptoms within the same family.

In addition to the headache syndromes of migraine, there are migraine equivalents in which the cardinal features are transitory disturbances in neurologic function. Headache is a minor feature or not present. Migraine equivalent syndromes are discussed in several other chapters (Table 3–3). The syndromes are variants of classic and common migraine, never of cluster headache.

Classic Migraine

Classic migraine is a biphasic event. In the initial phase a wave of excitation followed by depression of cortical function spreads over both hemispheres from back to front. This is associated with decreased regional cerebral blood flow and transitory neurologic disturbances. These disturbances are caused primarily by neuronal depression rather than ischemia. The second phase is usually, but not necessarily, associated with increased blood flow in both the internal and external carotid circulation. Headache, nausea, and sometimes vomiting occur in the second phase. The mechanism of headache and nausea remains uncertain but is not explained by increased cerebral blood flow.

During an individual attack the major clinical symptoms may be related only to the first phase (migraine equivalents), only to the second phase (headache and vomiting), or both. The most common symptoms of the initial phase are visual aberrations: the perception of sparkling lights or colored lines, blind spots, blurred vision, hemianopia, transitory blindness, micropsia, and visual hallucinations. With proper interviewing techniques, visual symptoms can be identified in 41% of children with migraine (Hachinski et al, 1973). The visual symptoms tend to be stereotypes for each child and may be perceived in one eye, in one field, or without localization.

Visual hallucinations and other visual distortions may be associated with impairment of time sense and body image. This symptom complex in migraine has been referred to as the *Alice-in-Wonderland syndrome* (Golden, 1979). More extreme disturbances in mental state—amnesia, confusion, and psychosis—are discussed in the sections on confusional migraine and transient global amnesia (see Chapter 2).

After visual aberrations, dysesthesias of the

Table 3–3 ◆ Migraine Equivalents

1. Acute confusional migraine (see Chapter 2)
2. Basilar migraine (see Chapter 10)
3. Benign paroxysmal vertigo (see Chapter 10)
4. Cyclic vomiting
5. Hemiplegic migraine (see Chapter 11)
6. Ophthalmoplegic migraine (see Chapter 15)
7. Paroxysmal torticollis (see Chapter 14)
8. Transient global amnesia (see Chapter 2)

limbs and perioral region are the next most common sensory symptoms in classic migraine. The occurrence of focal motor deficit, usually hemiplegia or ophthalmoplegia, is referred to as *complicated migraine*. Such deficits, although alarming, are transitory; normal function usually returns within 24 hours and always within 72 hours.

A migraine attack may terminate at the end of the initial phase, without headache. Alternatively, the initial phase may be brief or asymptomatic and headache the major symptom. Frequently, the pain is dull at first and then becomes throbbing, pulsating, or pounding. Severe headache that is maximal at onset is not migraine. Pain is unilateral in approximately two thirds of patients and bilateral in the rest. It is most intense in the region of the eye, forehead, and temple. Eventually the pain becomes constant and diffuse. The headache lasts 2 to 6 hours and is associated with nausea and sometimes vomiting. Anorexia and photophobia are concomitant symptoms. The child appears ill and needs to lie down. Vomiting frequently heralds the end of the attack. As discomfort diminishes, the fatigued child falls into a deep sleep. Normal function resumes when the child awakens.

Most patients have one to four attacks a month. However, the child may be symptom free for long intervals and have attacks more than once a week during other periods. Those with frequent headaches are probably experiencing stress.

Common Migraine

Common migraine differs from classic migraine because the symptoms are more variable and do not regularly evolve in a biphasic mode of neurologic aura and headache. Consequently the attacks are less readily identified as migrainous. A preheadache phase is not prominent. Visual disturbances, such as those described for classic migraine, may occur, but the more typical symptoms are personality change, malaise, dizziness, and nausea. Recurrent vomiting may be the only manifestation of common migraine in preschool children.

The headache may be unilateral and pounding, but more often the child has difficulty localizing the pain and describing its quality. When the headache is prolonged, the pain is not of uniform intensity; instead, intermittent severe headaches are superimposed on a background of chronic discomfort in the neck and other pericranial muscles (Olesen, 1978). Common migraine may be difficult to differentiate from other headache syndromes. The important clue is that the child appears sick, wants to lie down, and is sensitive to light and sound.

Nausea and vomiting may occur repeatedly, do not herald the termination of the attack, and can be more prominent than the headache.

Cluster Headache

Cluster headache is uncommon in children. Its prevalence in the United States is 0.4% for men and 0.08% for women (Kudrow, 1980). The onset occurs almost exclusively after age 10 but may occur in children as young as age 3 (Kudrow, 1980). Eighty percent of patients have clusters of headaches over periods of weeks or months separated by intervals of 1 to 2 years. The other 20% have chronic headache; because of associated features, such headaches are considered to be the cluster type despite the lack of "clustering" (Pearce, 1980).

Headache is the initial symptom; pain is unilateral and the same side of the head is affected in each attack. It begins behind and around one eye, then spreads to the entire hemicranium. During an attack the child cannot lie still but typically walks the floor in anguish; this is an important distinguishing feature from migraine, in which the child wants to go to bed. Pain is intense and may be described as throbbing or constant. The scalp may seem edematous and tender. One third of individuals with cluster experience sudden intense jabs of pain, suggesting tic douloureux. Nausea and vomiting do not occur, but symptoms of hemicranial autonomic dysfunction—injection of the conjunctiva, tearing of the eye, Horner syndrome, sweating, flushing of the face, and stuffiness of the nose—develop ipsilateral to the headache. The attack may be as brief as 10 minutes or as long as 4 hours, but 30 minutes to 2 hours is typical. As a rule, only one attack occurs each day, but several attacks within 24 hours are not unusual. A cluster of daily attacks lasting 4 to 8 weeks may occur once or twice a year, often in the autumn or spring. Patients are headache free in the interim.

Alcohol ingestion is a common trigger of cluster headaches, but only during the period of susceptibility.

DIAGNOSIS

The diagnosis of migraine is based on clinical observation; migraine is one of the few remaining disorders in which the physician cannot stumble on the diagnosis by imaging the brain. Salient features are a family history of migraine and some combination of recurrent headache, nausea, or neurologic disturbances, especially if the symptoms are relieved by sleep. The physician should be reluctant to make the diagnosis if questioning of both parents does not elicit a family history of migraine. Motion sickness is present in 45% of children with migraine (Barabas et al, 1983). Whether this is a significant association is uncertain; the incidence of motion sickness in the general population can approach 100% depending on the amount of motion experienced.

Diagnostic tests have no value in migraine, but every child with chronic headache probably should have one brain imaging study to exclude the possibility of an underlying disorder that is increasing intracranial pressure.

The most common electroencephalographic (EEG) abnormality during a classic migraine attack is a slow wave focus in the temporal lobe of one hemisphere. Asymptomatic central spikes are observed in 9% of children with migraine as compared with 1.9% of healthy children, suggesting a link between Rolandic epilepsy (see Chapter 1) and migraine (Kinast et al, 1982). Fourteen-and-six positive spikes, a normal adolescent pattern, occurs twice as commonly in children with migraine as in age-matched control subjects (Jay, 1982); the significance of this increased prevalence in children with migraine is uncertain.

TREATMENT

The essential caveat for the treatment of migraine in children is that irrespective of treatment, about half of patients have more than a 50% reduction in headache frequency in the 6 months following the initial visit to a neurologist (Prensky and Sommer, 1979). Once the child's parents are convinced that headache is due to migraine and not brain tumor, they are less anxious, the child is more relaxed, and headaches either decrease in frequency or are discussed less often. The therapeutic efficacy of neurologic consultation has the dual effect of making drug evaluation difficult and at the same time reinforcing the neurologist's belief that the drug regimen selected is useful.

There are two approaches to migraine therapy: treatment of the acute attack and prophylaxis. Whichever approach is selected, the patient and family must be taught "how to live with migraine":

1. Avoid, when possible, activities that are known to trigger attacks.
2. When attacks occur, give in and go to bed.
3. Use as little pain medication as possible because repeated dosages only lead to further gastrointestinal upset.
4. Do not use narcotics or other addictive drugs to treat severe attacks.

5. Any medication that puts the child to sleep will abort the attack.

Treating the Acute Attack

Over-the-counter analgesics may relieve pain in children who have only mild headaches. Ergotamine is the drug most often prescribed for the acute treatment of migraine. The response is variable and should never be used for the purpose of diagnosis. Oral ergotamine is not more effective than placebo in double-blind controlled studies (Waters, 1970).

The best treatment for migraine is to have the child go to sleep. I generally prescribe promethazine, 25 to 50 mg, as either a tablet or a suppository. It relieves nausea and causes drowsiness. Intramuscular chlorpromazine, 1 mg/kg, is a safe and effective alternative for severe attacks. In one report 96% of adult migraineurs treated at an emergency room were relieved of pain and nausea within 1 hour of injection (Iserson, 1983). The only adverse reaction is orthostatic hypotension, but this is less likely to occur in children than in adults.

Sumatriptan, a selective agonist of 5-hydroxytryptamine−like receptors, has recently proved effective in the management of acute attacks (Subcutaneous Sumatriptan International Study Group, 1991). A subcutaneous injection of 6 mg decreases the severity of the attack within 60 minutes in 72% of adults. The dose in children is not established.

Migraine Prophylaxis

An extraordinary number of agents with diverse pharmacologic properties have been administered daily to prevent migraine attacks. Among these agents are hormones, serotonin agonists and antagonists, tranquilizers, antidepressants, antihistamines, anticonvulsants, calcium channel blocking agents, vasoconstrictors, and vasodilators. In double-blind controlled trials in adults many of these agents have significantly reduced the frequency of migraine as compared with placebo. Unfortunately, success in the treated group rarely exceeds 50% and statistical significance is achieved because patients given placebo have done worse than might be expected.

Propranolol is the only agent that consistently demonstrates efficacy greater than a placebo's and has been the drug of choice in migraine prophylaxis. Calcium channel blocking agents have undergone recent trials in children and adults, but evidence of definite efficacy is still insufficient.

Propranolol

Propranolol is a beta-adrenergic blocking agent that was serendipitously found useful in preventing migraine attacks in patients being treated for cardiovascular disease. This observation led to several control trials in which propranolol was found effective in 55% to 84% of patients (Rosen, 1983). There is no reason to believe that its mechanism of action in preventing migraine is by beta-adrenergic blockade. The mechanism is more likely a central action. Propranolol must have central action because it causes depression. Other beta-adrenergic blocking agents have not been studied in migraine and should not be used.

The dosage in children is 2 mg/kg in three divided doses (Ludvigsson, 1974). Because depression is a dose-related reaction and because lower doses may be effective, treatment should be initiated at 1 mg/kg/day. Depression is the most common reason to discontinue therapy, and parents should be warned of this reaction when the drug is started. The drug should not be used in children with asthma because it may provoke an attack. Hypotension and pulse rate reduction do not occur in children with normal cardiovascular systems. Once a maintenance dose is established, the sustained release tablet can be used by increasing the daily dose by one third. Plasma levels of propranolol are not useful in determining the effective dose for migraine (Cortelli et al, 1985).

Patients who respond to propranolol do not develop tolerance. However, if the drug is abruptly stopped after 6 to 12 months of therapy, some patients have rebound headaches of increased frequency. Others continue to demonstrate the benefits achieved during therapy.

Calcium Channel Blocking Agents

Calcium channel blocking agents have vasodilators that prevent the influx of calcium into vascular smooth muscle. They have been used extensively for coronary artery disease and are effective dilators of the cerebral vasculature. Specific agents that have been tested in migraine are listed in Table 3−4. Cyproheptadine and nifedipine have been studied in children, and a dosage in milligrams per kilogram is available. Nimodipine, flunarizine, and verapamil have not been tested in children with migraine, and the dosages provided in Table 3−4 are for adults. Calcium channel blocking agents as a group have little or no toxicity in children with normal cardiovascular systems.

Cyproheptadine should be an especially potent prophylactic agent for migraine. It is not only a

Table 3–4 ◆ Calcium Channel Blocking Agents

Drug	Dosage
Cyproheptadine	0.2-0.4 mg/kg
Flunarizine	5 mg b.i.d.
Nifedipine	1 mg/kg
Nimodipine	40 mg t.i.d.
Verapamil	80 mg t.i.d.

calcium blocking agent but also an antihistamine with mild to moderate antiserotonin activity. However, in large clinical trials less than 50% of patients reported improvement (Lance et al, 1970). In contrast, 80% improvement rates are reported for flunarizine (Louis, 1981), verapamil (Markley, 1991; Solomon et al, 1983), and nifedipine (Meyer and Hardenberg, 1983). However, these reports are based on very small numbers of patients. A 2- to 3-week delay is expected between the onset of treatment and the result.

Treating Cluster Headache

The treatment of cluster headache is usually directed at suppressing recurrent headaches rather than treating a headache in progress. Lithium is becoming the prophylactic agent of choice. The inhalation of 100% oxygen at a rate of 8 to 10 L/min relieves an acute attack in 82% of patients (Fogan, 1985).

Methysergide Maleate

Methysergide maleate, a serotonin agonist, was popularized as a prophylactic agent for migraine and for cluster headache in 1964 (Graham, 1964). Methysergide prevents attacks in more than 50% of migraineurs. The dose in adults is 2 mg three times a day, after meals to avoid gastric upset. A dosage in milligrams per kilogram has not been established for children. Unfortunately, retroperitoneal fibrosis, as well as other fibrotic syndromes, occurs in patients taking the medication regularly for periods greater than 1 year. The fibrosis is ordinarily reversible when medication is stopped. Methysergide maleate can be used safely for periods of less than 6 months and is particularly useful for short-term therapy in patients with cluster headache.

Prednisone

Prednisone suppresses bouts of cluster headache in three fourths of patients who are unresponsive to methysergide (Kudrow, 1980). An initial dosage of 1 mg/kg is administered for the first 5 days and then tapered over the following 2 weeks. If headaches reappear during the tapering process, the dose is increased and maintained at a level sufficient to keep the patient headache free. If the bout of cluster headache is prolonged, the prednisone dosage should be tapered before the appearance of adverse side effects.

Lithium Carbonate

Lithium is used in patients with the chronic form of cluster in which headache never ceases. Increasing doses are used to achieve a blood concentration of 1.2 mEq/L (1.2 mmol/L). Most patients have at least a partial response to lithium, but only 50% are relieved completely. The beneficial effect of lithium is enhanced by the addition of daily oral ergotamine (Stagliano and Gallagher, 1983).

◆ Nonmigrainous Vascular Headaches

Other than migraine, vascular headache may be caused by traction or displacement of intracranial vessels, vasodilation of intracranial or extracranial vessels, and vasculitis. Traction-displacement of intracranial vessels is the primary mechanism of headache in patients with increased intracranial pressure and is discussed in Chapter 4.

VASCULITIS

Headaches caused by vasculitis, especially temporal arteritis, are important in the differential diagnosis of vascular headaches in adults. Cerebral vasculitis is uncommon in childhood and usually occurs as part of a collagen vascular disease, as the result of a hypersensitivity reaction, or as part of an infection of the nervous system.

Connective Tissue Disorders

Headache is a relatively common feature of systemic lupus erythematosus and mixed connective tissue disease (Bronshvag et al, 1978). In patients with connective tissue disease, it is not clear that neurologic symptoms, including headache, are caused by vasculitis of the cerebral arteries.

Clinical Features. Headache is not an early symptom of lupus in children. The common early symptoms are fever, arthritis, and skin rash. Symptoms referable to the nervous system—seizures and mental changes—are the initial manifestation in less than 5% of affected children. Hepatosplenomegaly and lymphadenopathy are present in approximately 70% of children, a rate twice as great as in adults.

Mixed connective disease is a syndrome with features of lupus erythematosus, scleroderma, and polymyositis. It usually has a more benign course than lupus. Thirty-five percent of patients with mixed connective disease report vascular headaches. The headaches are moderate and generally do not interfere with activities of daily living. Headaches may be unilateral or bilateral but are generally throbbing. More than half of patients report a visual aura, and some have nausea and vomiting. Headaches with visual aura and vascular headaches may be classified as migraine, but it is statistically unlikely that such a high percentage of patients with mixed connective disease also have migraine.

Diagnosis.　The diagnosis of connective tissue disease depends on the combination of a compatible clinical syndrome and the demonstration of antinuclear antibodies in the blood. The presence of antinuclear antibodies in a child with headache who has no systemic symptoms of connective tissue disease should suggest the possibility of a hypersensitivity reaction.

Treatment.　Children with connective tissue disease are ordinarily treated with corticosteroids. In many cases headaches develop while the child is already taking corticosteroids, and this should not be an indication to increase the dose. Headache is not a disabling symptom, it does not indicate a generalized encephalopathy, and it should be treated with analgesics.

Hypersensitivity Vasculitis

The important causes of hypersensitivity vasculitis in children are serum sickness, Henoch-Schonlein purpura (see Chapter 11), amphetamine abuse (Matick et al, 1983), and cocaine abuse. Patients with serum sickness and Henoch-Schonlein purpura have systemic symptoms that precede the headache. In contrast, amphetamine abusers may have only cerebral vasculitis and their symptoms are headache, encephalopathy, focal neurologic deficits, and subarachnoid hemorrhage.

VASODILATIVE HEADACHES

Table 3–5 lists several conditions that cause vasodilation in the internal carotid circulation, the external carotid circulation, or both, and result in headache. The list is not intended to be exhaustive but focuses on headaches that are likely to be encountered in childhood and adolescence. Vasodi-

Table 3–5 ◆ Nonmigrainous Vasodilative Headaches

1. Drugs and toxins
   a. Alcohol
   b. Caffeine withdrawal
   c. Food additives
   d. Marijuana
2. Effort headache
3. Fever
4. Hypertension
5. Posttraumatic headache

lative headaches are generally bitemporal or diffuse and are described as pounding, throbbing, or pulsating. The pain is made worse by sudden jarring or movement of the head. Differentiating migrainous from nonmigrainous vascular headaches may be difficult on the basis of the description of pain. Furthermore, many factors that trigger vascular headache in nonmigrainous individuals also trigger migraine in migraineurs. Severe vascular headache of any cause is often compounded by tension headache.

Benign Exertional Headache

Exertion, especially during competitive sports, is a known trigger for migraine in predisposed individuals (see "Migraine" earlier in this chapter). Others, who do not have migraine, may be subject to vascular headaches only during exertion. Headache during sexual intercourse is probably a form of benign exertional headache, and affected individuals often experience the same headache during exercise (Silbert et al, 1991).

Clinical Features.　Physical exertion is more likely to produce headache when effort is prolonged and sufficient to sustain the pulse at twice its resting rate for 10 minutes or longer (Diamond and Dalessio, 1982). Pain begins during or just after exercise and may last as long as 4 hours. It is throbbing and bitemporal. Benign exertional headache may also occur during prolonged sexual arousal.

More than one kind of headache is associated with sexual intercourse. A dull headache, primarily occipital but also in a band distribution, may be experienced as sexual excitement increases (Lance, 1982). It is not incapacitating and does not disrupt sexual activity. A more severe and dangerous headache is one that occurs just before and at the moment of orgasm. This headache, caused by sudden increase in blood pressure, is similar to the headache associated with pheochromocytoma. Blood pressure elevation during orgasm is considerable and can be associated with subarachnoid hemorrhage in adolescents with arteriovenous malformations.

Diagnosis. The association between exertion and headache is easily recognized. Medical consultation is seldom requested unless the patient is a serious athlete whose performance is impaired.

Treatment. Exertional headache can sometimes be prevented by taking indomethacin before activities known to induce benign exertional headache. The prophylactic use of indomethacin, 25 mg three times a day, or propranolol, 1 to 2/mg/kg/day, is reported to reduce the incidence of attacks (Diamond and Dalessio, 1982; Johns, 1986).

Drugs and Toxins

Many psychotropic drugs, analgesics, and cardiovascular agents have vasodilating properties. Cocaine use produces a migrainelike headache in individuals who do not have migraine at other times (Dhuna et al, 1991). Drug-induced headache should be suspected in a child who has vascular headache following the administration of any drug.

Alcohol Headache

Ethyl alcohol produces vasodilation and may precipitate migraine or cluster headache in a predisposed individual. Hangover headache is probably due to vasodilation as well, but the mechanism is not fully understood. Acetaldehyde, an oxidation product of alcohol, is an established cause of vascular headache and may be responsible for the hangover.

Most hangover headaches are not treated. Concurrent gastritis prevents the use of oral medication.

Caffeine Withdrawal

Clinical Features. Many children, especially adolescents, drink large volumes of carbonated beverages containing caffeine each day. Caffeine has vasoconstricting properties and does not in itself cause headache. However, rebound vasodilation occurs when blood caffeine concentrations fall. Individuals who regularly drink large amounts of caffeine-containing beverages often notice a dull frontotemporal headache an hour or more after last use. More caffeine is taken to relieve the headache, and caffeine addiction is initiated (Greden et al, 1980). Withdrawal symptoms eventually become severe and include throbbing headache, anxiety, and malaise.

Diagnosis. Most people associate caffeine with coffee and are unaware of the caffeine content of soft drinks. Adolescent girls frequently use diet colas as a substitute for food and become caffeine dependent.

Treatment. Caffeine addiction, like other addictions, is hard to break. Some patients can be weaned from caffeine, but most require abrupt cessation and experience withdrawal symptoms. Hospitalization and sedation are sometimes necessary to help patients through withdrawal.

Food Additives

Clinical Features. Chemicals are added to food to preserve it and enhance its appearance. Ordinarily the concentration is low and adverse effects occur only in individuals who are genetically sensitive. Nitrites are powerful vasodilators used to enhance the appearance of cured meats such as hot dogs, salami, bacon, and ham. Diffuse, throbbing headaches may occur just after ingestion.

Monosodium glutamate (MSG) is used primarily in Chinese cooking and may produce generalized vasodilation. A syndrome described in sensitive individuals includes both a throbbing bitemporal headache and a band headache, sometimes associated with pressure and tightness of the face and a burning sensation over the body (Schaumberg et al, 1969). Symptoms occur 20 minutes after MSG ingestion.

Diagnosis. The association between ingestion of a specific food and vascular headache quickly becomes evident to the patient.

Treatment. Headache can be prevented only by avoidance of the offending chemical. This may not be easy, since determining which additives prepared foods contain is often difficult.

Marijuana

Marijuana is a peripheral vasodilator and produces a sensation of warmth, injection of the conjunctivae, and sometimes frontal headache. The headache is mild and ordinarily experienced only during marijuana use. However, marijuana metabolites remain in the blood for several days and prolonged vasodilative headaches may occur in children who are regular users.

Fever

Clinical Features. Fever is the most common cause of vascular headache. The degree of vasodilation parallels the rise of body temperature. Vasodilation is both intracranial and extracranial. Headache is bitemporal or diffuse in location and throbbing in quality.

Diagnosis. The association between fever and headache is ordinarily self-evident and does not lead to diagnostic studies unless infection of the nervous system or subarachnoid hemorrhage is suspected. Suspicion is raised when headache or personality change is disproportionate to the degree of fever and when meningismus is present.

Treatment. Aspirin or acetaminophen combats both fever and headache, but aspirin is contraindicated in children because of the possibility of Reye syndrome (see Chapter 2).

Hypertension

An acute rise in systemic blood pressure causes the explosive throbbing headache associated with orgasm and pheochromocytoma. Several authorities have suggested that individuals with chronic hypertension may have low-grade occipital headache on awakening that diminishes as they get up and begin activity. However, there is no convincing evidence that chronic hypertension is a cause of headache and usually hypertension is a silent disease. The development of chronic headache in children with renal disease should not be ascribed to hypertension (see Chapter 2). Instead, alternative causes must be pursued. Headaches are common in patients undergoing dialysis and may be due to psychologic tension, the precipitation of migraine attacks, and dialysis itself (Bana et al, 1972). Dialysis headache begins a few hours after the procedure is terminated and is characterized by mild bifrontal throbbing headache, which may be associated with nausea and vomiting.

Posttraumatic Headache

Several different kinds of headache may be associated with head trauma. Vascular headache is experienced by 40% patients in the first day or two after head injury. It is a diffuse pounding headache made worse by movement of the head or by coughing and straining. Dizziness may be an associated feature. Posttraumatic vascular headaches subside spontaneously. Prolonged posttraumatic headaches are not fully understood; they may be psychogenic but are not vascular in origin (see Chapter 2).

◆ Chronic Mixed Headache

I am using the term "chronic mixed headache" to describe chronic headache that is of uncertain origin and lacks any identifiable cause. *"Tension headache"* is an alternative term, but it is not always clear that the child is experiencing stress.

When a stressful situation is identified (e.g., divorce of the parents, unsuitable school placement, physical or sexual abuse), the headache cannot be managed without resolution of the stress. When adults with chronic tension headache are asked about the onset of their symptoms, almost 50% date the onset before age 20 and 15% before age 10 (Lance et al, 1965). Females are affected three times more frequently than males.

Clinical Features. Individuals with chronic headache of any cause may have depression and anxiety. Pain is almost always bilateral and diffuse, and the site of most intense pain may shift during the course of the day. Much of the time, headache is dull and aching; sometimes it has a pounding vascular quality and is more intense. Headache is generally present on awakening and may continue all day. Most children describe an undulating course characterized by long periods in which headache occurs almost every day and shorter intervals when they are headache-free.

Chronic mixed headache is not associated with nausea, vomiting, or transitory neurologic disturbances. When these features are present, they usually occur only a few times a month and suggest that the patient has both intermittent migraine and chronic mixed headache. Neurologic findings should be normal.

Diagnosis. The diagnosis of chronic tension headache is to some extent a diagnosis of exclusion. The physician must be certain that chronic headache is not caused by migraine or increased intracranial pressure, conditions requiring specific treatment. Brain imaging should be performed on every child with chronic headache. No matter how convinced the physician is, on the basis of history and physical examination, that the child does not have increased intracranial pressure, parents are rarely convinced by anything less than an imaging study. The cause of chronic tension headache is easier to investigate when the specter of brain tumor has been laid to rest. EEG is indicated when the intermittent nature of the headache or associated features suggest the possibility of epilepsy.

All children with chronic headache must be asked, "Do you have more than one kind of headache?" This is important to separate concurrent headache syndromes such as migraine and chronic mixed headache. Once the diagnosis of chronic mixed headache is established, the severity of depression must be analyzed to determine whether psychiatric consultation is indicated.

Treatment. Chronic mixed headache is by definition difficult to treat or it would not be a chronic headache. Most children have tried and received no benefit from several over-the-counter analgesics before coming to a physician. The use of more powerful analgesics or analgesic-muscle relaxant combinations also has limited value. Long-term use of analgesics usually adds an upset stomach to the child's distress.

Amitriptyline is probably the most useful drug for chronic mixed headache. It has analgesic properties beyond its effect as an antidepressant. I always start with a small bedtime dose (approximately 0.25 to 0.5 mg/kg) and slowly increase the dose as tolerated (Lance, 1982).

Many children with chronic mixed headache benefit from relaxation exercises or biofeedback. I routinely refer children for such therapy when the response to amitriptyline is unsatisfactory.

Benzodiazepines may be useful when anxiety is a significant concurrent symptom. Diazepam has been the one most often administered, but longer acting benzodiazepines such as alprazolam are becoming more popular. A small dose is first given at bedtime and then during daytime as well; sedation is the limiting factor.

◆ Other Pain Syndromes

ACUTE TENSION HEADACHE

Clinical Features.   Acute tension headache is common in people of all ages and both sexes. It is generally brought on by fatigue, exertion, and temporary life stress. The mechanism is prolonged contraction of muscles attached to the skull. The pain is described as constant, aching, and tight. It is localized mainly to the back of the head and neck, sometimes becomes diffuse, and may be described as a constricting band around the head. Vascular headache and acute tension headache may be concurrent. Nausea, vomiting, and other symptoms are not present.

Diagnosis.   Acute tension headache should be differentiated from chronic mixed headache, which has similar clinical features but persists for weeks, months, and years. Acute tension headache is self-diagnosed, and the individual rarely seeks medical attention.

Treatment.   Pain is relieved by rest or relaxation and also responds to aspirin or acetaminophen.

EYESTRAIN

Clinical Features.   Prolonged ocular near-fixation in a child with a latent disturbance in convergence may cause dull aching pain behind the eyes that is quickly relieved when the eyes are closed. The pain is of muscular origin and caused by the continuous effort to maintain conjugate gaze. If work is continued despite ocular pain, acute tension headache may develop.

Diagnosis.   Children who complain of eyestrain are often thought to have refractive errors, and eyeglasses are fitted. However, refractive errors do not cause eyestrain in children as presbyopia does in adults.

Treatment.   Eyestrain is relieved by resting the eyes.

SINUSITIS

In giving a family history of migraine, parents often identify their own episodic headache, preceded by scintillating scotoma and followed by nausea and vomiting, as sinusitis. This diagnosis is favored by physicians and patients to describe chronic or episodic headaches and is usually wrong.

Clinical Features.   Children with sinusitis are usually sick. They are febrile, feel stuffy, and have difficulty maintaining a clear airway. Localized tenderness is present over the infected frontal or maxillary sinuses, and inflammation of the ethmoidal or sphenoidal sinuses causes deep midline pain behind the nose. Pain is exaggerated by blowing the nose or by quick movements of the head, especially bending forward. Vascular headache caused by fever may be concurrent.

Diagnosis.   Radiographs reveal clouding of the sinuses and sometimes a fluid level. CT of the skull is exceptionally accurate in identifying sinusitis but is usually an unnecessary expense. It is impressive how often CT of the head, performed for reasons other than headache, demonstrates radiographic evidence of asymptomatic sinusitis. Clearly, radiographic evidence of sinusitis does not necessarily explain a patient's headache.

Treatment.   The primary objective of treatment is to allow the sinus to drain. This is usually accomplished with decongestants, but sometimes surgery is required. Antibiotics have limited usefulness if drainage is not established.

TEMPOROMANDIBULAR JOINT SYNDROME

Any discussion of temporomandibular joint (TMJ) syndrome must begin with the caveat that the association between TMJ disease and headache is not clearly understood.

The TMJ syndrome has been described in children 8 years of age and older (Katzberg et al, 1985). The duration of symptoms before diagnosis may be as long as 5 years and averages 21 months.

TMJ syndrome is not generally recognized as a disease of childhood. The primary disturbance is an arthritis of the joint that produces localized pain in the lower face and crepitus in the joint. Because of pain on one side, chewing is performed on the opposite side. Unfortunately, this has the unwanted effect of overuse of the affected side. The overused masseter muscle becomes tender; a muscle contraction headache ensues and is felt on the side of the face and at the vertex. The cause of arthritis is generally attributed to dental malocclusion, but a prior injury of the jaw is reported in one third of children with TMJ syndrome.

Diagnosis. Radiographs of the TMJ demonstrate some internal derangement in 94% of affected children and degenerative arthritis in 39% (Katzberg et al, 1985). Magnetic resonance imaging (MRI) using surface coils is said to be the most effective technique of demonstrating disturbed joint architecture (Katzberg et al, 1986).

Treatment. Treatment for TMJ syndrome has not been established based on controlled experiments. Placebos provide considerable benefit, and extensive oral surgery is not indicated. Nonsteroidal antiinflammatory agents, application of heat to the tense muscles, and dental splints may prove useful.

WHIPLASH AND OTHER NECK INJURIES

Whiplash and other neck injuries produce pain by rupture of cervical disks, damage to soft tissue, injury to occipital nerves, and excessive muscle contraction. The muscle contraction is an effort to splint the area of injury and thereby reduce further tissue damage. Constant contraction of the neck extensors produces a dull aching pain not only in the neck but also in the shoulders and upper arms. The head is generally kept in a fixed position. Nausea and vomiting are not associated symptoms.

Diagnosis. Following any neck or head injury, radiographs of the cervical spine are needed to determine the presence of fracture or dislocation. Shooting pains that radiate either to the occiput or down the arm and into the fingers suggest the possibility of disk herniation and require further study with myelography or CT.

Treatment. Muscle contraction headache following cervical spine injuries is relieved by lying or sitting with the head supported, by superficial application of heat to the painful muscles, by muscle relaxants, and by simple analgesics.

◆ Seizure Headache

Diffuse headache caused by vasodilation of cerebral arteries is a frequent postictal symptom following a generalized tonic-clonic convulsion. In patients who have both epilepsy and migraine, one can trigger the other, so that concurrent headache and seizure occur frequently. Approximately 1% of epileptic patients report headache as a seizure manifestation (Young and Blume, 1983). This phenomenon has been termed seizure headache (Swaiman and Frank, 1978). Most patients with seizure headaches are known epileptics, but in some children headache is the only manifestation of their seizure disorder. The association of migraine and epilepsy is discussed in Chapters 1 and 10.

Clinical Features. Headache is a manifestation of several epilepsy syndromes. In some children the sequence suggests migraine. Headaches are paroxysmal, generally bifrontal, frequently accompanied by nausea and vomiting, and followed by lethargy and sleep (Swaiman and Frank, 1978). However, a family history of migraine is lacking and no triggering factor for attacks can be identified. Attacks may occur during sleep or anytime during the day and last for several hours. The EEG shows spike and wave discharges. Regular administration of anticonvulsant drugs prevents further attacks.

I have seen one eloquent adolescent who complained of paroxysmal "head pain that is not like other headaches" that was associated with EEG evidence of generalized epileptiform activity. The head pain was relieved by anticonvulsants.

Headache may also occur as a seizure manifestation in patients known to have a seizure disorder. Such individuals usually have a long history of partial or generalized seizures before headache becomes part of the syndrome. Associated ictal events depend on the site of the cortical focus and may include auditory hallucinations, visual disturbances, vertigo, déjà vu, and focal motor seizures. Headache is usually the initial manifestation of the seizure but can follow other partial seizure manifestations, such as déjà vu and vertigo. The headache may be described as throbbing, sharp, or without an identified quality. Complex partial seizures, simple partial seizures, or generalized tonic-clonic seizures follow the headache phase. Spike foci in patients with seizure headaches may arise in any region of the brain but occur predominantly in the temporal lobe.

Two children with seizure headaches were studied with depth electrodes before surgery (Laplante et al, 1983). Both were found to have seizure activity confined to the right hippocampus and amygdala during seizure headaches. In one, pain was localized to the vertex and associated with shortness of breath and lightheadedness. At times the seizure progressed to aphasia, but consciousness was preserved. The other child had frequent attacks of dizziness and tinnitus associated with the sudden onset of pain in the temporal region; the pain lasted 30 to 60 seconds. Temporal lobe surgery provided complete relief of seizure activity in both patients.

Diagnosis. Most seizure headaches in children are diagnosed by the demonstration of interictal spike discharges on the EEG. The presence of interictal spike discharges, especially Rolandic spikes, in a child with headache does not necessarily mean that the headaches are a seizure manifestation. For example, children with migraine have a 9% incidence of Rolandic spikes. A child who has a clinical syndrome of migraine and a family history of migraine, and who has never had a clinical seizure, should be considered to have migraine and not epilepsy despite the presence of interictal spike discharges.

EEG is indicated for children with chronic paroxysmal headache who do not have a family history of migraine. If interictal spike discharges are demonstrated, an effort should be made to record a seizure headache with an ambulatory EEG monitor. The demonstration of continuous epileptiform activity during a headache provides reassurance that headache is a seizure manifestation and that anticonvulsant drugs are indicated. However, the site of the seizure focus does not necessarily match the location of the headache.

Treatment. The response to anticonvulsant therapy is usually considered diagnostic as well as therapeutic. Since the seizure focus is usually cortical and most often in the temporal lobe, carbamazepine or phenytoin is recommended.

References

Bana DS, Yap AU, Graham JR: Headache during hemodialysis. Headache 12:1, 1972.

Barabas G, Matthews WS, Ferrari M: Childhood migraine and motion sickness. Pediatrics 72:188, 1983.

Bille B: Migraine in school children. Acta Paediatr 51:13, 1962.

Bronshvag MM, Prystowsky SD, Traviesa DC: Vascular headaches in mixed connective tissue disease. Headache 18:154, 1978.

Chu ML, Shinnar S: Headache in children younger than 7 years of age. Arch Neurol 49:79, 1992.

Cortelli P, Sacquengna T, Albani F, et al: Propranolol plasma levels and relief of migraine: Relationship between plasma propranolol and 4-hydroxypropranolol concentrations and clinical effects. Arch Neurol 42:46, 1985.

Deubner DC: An epidemiologic study of migraine and headache in 10-20 year olds. Headache 22:268, 1982.

Dhuna A, Pascuel-Leone A, Belgrade M: Cocaine-related vascular headaches. J Neurol Neurosurg Psychiatry 54:803, 1991.

Diamond S, Dalessio DJ: The Practicing Physician's Approach to Headache, 3rd edition. Williams & Wilkins, Baltimore, 1982, p 72.

Fogan L: Treatment of cluster headache: A double-blind comparison of oxygen vs. air inhalation. Arch Neurol 42:362, 1985.

Golden GS: The Alice in Wonderland syndrome in juvenile migraine. Pediatrics 63:517, 1979.

Graham JR: Methysergide for prevention of headache: Experience in 500 patients over three years. N Engl J Med 270:67, 1964.

Greden JF, Victor BS, Fontaine P, et al: Caffeine-withdrawal headache: A clinical profile. Psychosomatics 21:411, 1980.

Hachinski VC, Prochawka J, Steele JC: Visual symptoms in the migraine syndrome. Neurology 23:570, 1973.

Iserson KV: Parenteral chlorpromazine treatment of migraine. Ann Emerg Med 12:756, 1983.

Jay GW: Epilepsy, migraine, and EEG abnormalities in children: A review and hypothesis. Headache 22:110, 1982.

Johns DR: Benign sexual headache within a family. Arch Neurol 43:1158, 1986.

Katzberg RW, Bessette RW, Tallents RH, et al: Normal and abnormal temporomandibular joint: MR imaging with surface coil. Radiology 158:183, 1986.

Katzberg RW, Tallents RH, Hayakawa K, et al: Internal derangement in the temporomandibular joint: Findings in the pediatric age group. Radiology 154:125, 1985.

Kinast M, Leuders H, Rother AD, et al: Benign focal epileptiform discharges in childhood migraine (BFEDC). Neurology 32:1309, 1982.

Kudrow L: Cluster Headache: Mechanisms and Management. Oxford University Press, Oxford, Eng, 1980.

Lance JW: Mechanism and Management of Headache, 4th edition. Butterworths, London, 1982, p 78.

Lance JW, Anthony M, Somerville B: Comparative trial of serotonin antagonists in the management of migraine. Br Med J 2:327, 1970.

Lance JW, Curran DA, Anthony M: Investigators into the mechanisms and treatment of chronic headache. Med J Aust 2:909, 1965.

Laplante P, Saint-Hilaire JM, Bouvier G: Headache as an epileptic manifestation. Neurology 33:1493, 1983.

Linet MS, Stewart WF, Celentano DD, et al: An epidemiologic study of headache among adolescents and young adults. JAMA 261:2211, 1989.

Louis P: A double-blind placebo-controlled prophylactic study of flunarizine (sibelium) in migraine. Headache 21:235, 1981.

Ludvigsson J: Propranolol used in prophylaxis of migraine in children. Acta Neurol Scand 50:109, 1974.

Markley HG: Verapamil and migraine prophylaxis: Mechanisms and efficacy. Am J Med 90(suppl 5A):49, 1991.

Matick H, Anderson D, Brumlik J: Cerebral vasculitis associated with oral amphetamine overdose. Arch Neurol 40:253, 1983.

Meyer JS, Hardenberg J: Clinical effectiveness of calcium entry blockers in prophylactic treatment of migraine and cluster headaches. Headache 23:266, 1983.

Olesen J: Some clinical features of the acute migraine attack: An analysis of 750 patients. Headache 18:268, 1978.

Pearce JMS: Chronic migrainous neuralgia: A variant of cluster headache. Brain 103:149, 1980.

Prensky AL, Sommer D: Diagnosis and treatment of migraine in children. Neurology 29:506, 1979.

Rosen JA: Observations on the efficacy of propranolol for the prophylaxis of migraine. Ann Neurol 13:92, 1983.

Schaumberg HH, Byck R, Gerstl R, et al: Monosodium L-glutamate: Its pharmacology and role in the Chinese restaurant syndrome. Science 163:826, 1969.

Silberstein SD, Merriam GR: Estrogens, progestins, and headache. Neurology 41:786, 1991.

Silbert PL et al: Benign vascular sexual headache and exertional headache. Br Med J 54:417, 1991.

Sillanpaa M: Changes in the prevalence of migraine and other headaches during the first seven school years. Headache 23:15, 1983.

Solomon GD, Steel JG, Spaccavento LJ: Verapamil prophylaxis of migraine: A double-blind, placebo-controlled study. JAMA 250:2500, 1983.

Stagliano RA, Gallagher RM: Combination ergotamine tartrate and lithium carbonate therapy in the chronic cluster headache patient. Headache 23:147, 1983.

Subcutaneous Sumatriptan International Study Group: Treatment of migraine attacks with sumatriptan. N Engl J Med 325:316, 1991.

Swaiman KF, Frank Y: Seizure headaches in children. Dev Med Child Neurol 20:580, 1978.

Waters WE: Controlled clinical trial of ergotamine tartrate. Br Med J 2:325, 1970.

Young GB, Blume WT: Painful epileptic seizures. Brain 106:537, 1983.

Increased Intracranial Pressure

Patients do not come to a physician complaining of increased intracranial pressure (Table 4–1). Most often it is brought to attention because of headache, vomiting, personality change, and alterations in states of consciousness. Less frequently the initial complaint is diplopia or the observation that one or both eyes are turning in. Some children are referred for neurologic consultation because a primary physician believes the child has papilledema. Conditions causing increased intracranial pressure are described elsewhere in the book, especially in chapters on altered states of consciousness, headache, ataxia, and disorders of ocular motility. This chapter is restricted to conditions in which symptoms of increased intracranial pressure are initial and prominent features.

◆ Pathophysiology

Once the cranial bones fuse during childhood, the contents of the skull are enveloped by a rigid box. Intracranial pressure is then the sum of the individual pressures exerted by the brain, blood, and cerebrospinal fluid. An increase in the size of any of these three compartments must be accommodated by an equivalent decrease in size of one or both of the other compartments, if intracranial pressure is to remain constant. Because cerebral blood flow must be kept relatively constant to provide oxygen and nutrients, the major adaptive mechanisms available to relieve pressure are the compressibility of the brain and the rapid reabsorption of cerebrospinal fluid by arachnoid villi. Infants and young children, in whom the cranial bones are still unfused, have the additional adaptive mechanism of spreading the cranial bones apart to increase volume.

CEREBROSPINAL FLUID

The choroid plexus accounts for at least 70% of cerebrospinal fluid production, and the transependymal movement of fluid from the brain to the ventricular system accounts for the remainder. The average volumes of cerebrospinal fluid are 90 ml in children from 4 to 13 years of age and 150 ml in adults. The rate of formation is approximately 0.35 ml/min, or 500 ml/day (Cutler and Spertell, 1982). Therefore approximately 14% of total volume turns over every hour. The rate at which cerebrospinal fluid is formed remains relatively constant and declines only slightly as cerebrospinal fluid pressure increases. In contrast, the rate of absorption increases linearly as cerebrospinal fluid pressure exceeds 70 mm H_2O. At a pressure of 200 mm H_2O the rate of absorption is three times the rate of formation.

Therefore impaired absorption, not increased formation, is the usual mechanism of progressive hydrocephalus. Choroid plexus papilloma is the only pathologic process in which formation can sometimes overwhelm absorption. When absorption is impaired, efforts to decrease the formation of cerebrospinal fluid are not likely to have a significant effect on volume.

CEREBRAL BLOOD FLOW

Systemic arterial pressure is the primary determinant of cerebral blood flow. Normal cerebral blood flow remains remarkably constant from newborn to adult life and is generally 50 to 60 ml/min/100 g brain weight. Blood vessels on the surface and at the base of the brain are more richly innervated by autonomic nerve fibers than are vessels of any other organ. These nerve fibers allow

**Table 4–1 ◆ Manifestations of Increased
Intracranial Pressure**

In Infants
1. Bulging fontanelle
2. Failure to thrive
3. Large head (see Chapter 18)
4. Setting sun sign
5. Shrill cry

In Children
1. Diplopia (see Chapter 15)
2. Headache (see Chapter 3)
3. Mental changes
4. Nausea and vomiting
5. Papilledema

the autoregulation of cerebral blood flow. Autoregulation refers to a buffering effect by which cerebral blood flow remains constant despite changes in systemic arterial perfusion pressure. Alterations in the arterial blood concentration of carbon dioxide have an important effect on total cerebral blood flow. Hypercarbia dilates cerebral blood vessels and increases blood flow, whereas hypocarbia constricts cerebral blood vessels and decreases flow. Alterations in blood oxygen content have the reverse effect, but are less potent stimuli for vasoconstriction or vasodilation than are alterations in blood carbon dioxide concentration.

Cerebral perfusion pressure is the difference between mean systemic arterial pressure and intracranial pressure. It can be reduced to dangerous levels either by reducing systemic arterial pressure or by increasing intracranial pressure. The autoregulation of the cerebral vessels is lost when cerebral perfusion pressure falls below 50 cm H_2O or severe acidosis is present. Increased intracranial blood volume can be caused by arterial vasodilation or by obstruction of cerebral veins and venous sinuses. Increased intracranial blood volume, like increased cerebrospinal fluid volume, results in increased intracranial pressure.

CEREBRAL EDEMA

Cerebral edema is an increase in the brain's volume caused by an increase in its water and sodium content. Edema may be localized or generalized; when generalized, it increases intracranial pressure. Cerebral edema is generally categorized as *vasogenic, cytotoxic,* or *interstitial.*

Vasogenic edema is caused by increased capillary permeability and is encountered with brain tumor, abscess, trauma, and hemorrhage. The fluid is located primarily in the white matter and re-

sponds to treatment with corticosteroids. Osmotic agents have no effect on vasogenic edema, but they can decrease the volume of normal brain tissue and in that way reduce total intracranial pressure.

Cytotoxic edema is caused by swelling of neurons, glia, and endothelial cells. It is usually due to hypoxia, ischemia, or infection of the nervous system. Increased fluid is located in both gray and white matter. Corticosteroids do not decrease edema, but osmotic agents may relieve intracranial pressure by reducing brain volume.

Interstitial edema is due to transependymal movement of fluid from the ventricular system to the brain. This occurs when cerebrospinal fluid absorption is blocked and the ventricles are enlarged. The fluid collects chiefly in the periventricular white matter. Agents intended to reduce cerebrospinal fluid production, such as acetazolamide and furosemide, may be useful. Corticosteroids and osmotic agents are not effective (Fishman, 1980).

MASS LESIONS

Mass lesions (e.g., tumor, abscess, hematoma, arteriovenous malformation) increase intracranial pressure by occupying space at the expense of other intracranial compartments, provoking cerebral edema, blocking the circulation and absorption of cerebrospinal fluid, increasing blood flow, and obstructing venous return.

◆ Symptoms and Signs

The clinical features of increased intracranial pressure depend on the child's age and the rate at which pressure increases. Newborns and infants present a special case because increased pressure can be partially vented by expanding the volume of the skull. The rate of intracranial pressure increase is important at all ages. Intracranial structures accommodate slowly increasing pressure remarkably well, but sudden changes are intolerable and result in some combination of headache, personality change, and states of decreasing consciousness.

INCREASED INTRACRANIAL PRESSURE IN INFANCY

Measurement of head circumference and palpation of the anterior fontanelle are readily available methods to assess intracranial volume and pressure rapidly. Head circumference is measured by determining its greatest anteroposterior circumference. Normal standards are different for premature and full-term newborns. Normal head growth in a full-term newborn is 2 cm/month for the first 3 months, 1 cm/month for the second 3 months, and 0.5 cm/month for the next 6 months. Excessive head growth is a major feature of increased intracranial pressure throughout the first year and even up to 3 years of age. However, normal head growth does not preclude the presence of increased intracranial pressure. In posthemorrhagic hydrocephalus, considerable ventricular dilation precedes any measurable change in head circumference by compressing the brain parenchyma.

The palpable tension of the anterior fontanelle is an excellent measure of intracranial pressure. In a quiet child a fontanelle that bulges above the level of the bone edges and is sufficiently tense to cause difficulty in determining where bone ends and fontanelle begins is abnormal and indicates increased intracranial pressure. A full fontanelle, which is clearly distinguishable from the surrounding bone edges, may indicate increased intracranial pressure but can also be caused by crying, edema of the scalp, subgaleal hemorrhage, and extravasation of intravenous fluids. The normal fontanelle is clearly demarcated from bone edges, falls below the surface, and pulsates under the examining finger.

Although the size of the anterior fontanelle and its rate of closure are variable, increased intracranial pressure should be suspected when the metopic and coronal sutures are sufficiently separated to admit a fingertip.

When the separation of cranial sutures is no longer sufficient to decompress increased intracranial pressure, the infant experiences lethargy and vomiting and fails to thrive. Palsies of the sixth cranial nerve, impaired upward gaze (setting sun sign), and disturbances of blood pressure and pulse may ensue. Papilledema is uncommon.

INCREASED INTRACRANIAL PRESSURE IN CHILDREN
Headache

Headache is one of the more common symptoms of increased intracranial pressure at all ages. Traction and displacement of intracranial arteries are the major cause of headache from increased intracranial pressure (see Chapter 3). As a rule, pain fibers from supratentorial intracranial vessels are innervated by the trigeminal nerve and pain is referred to the eye, forehead, and temple. In contrast, infratentorial intracranial vessels are innervated by cervical nerves and pain is referred to the occiput and neck.

When increased intracranial pressure is gener-alized, as may occur from cerebral edema or obstruction of the ventricular system, headache is generalized and more often prominent in the morning on awakening and rising to a standing position. Pain is constant but may vary in intensity. Coughing, sneezing, straining, and other maneuvers that transiently increase intracranial pressure exaggerate the headache. The quality of pain is often difficult to describe. Vomiting in the absence of nausea, especially on arising in the morning, is often a concurrent feature.

In the absence of generalized increased intracranial pressure, localized, or at least unilateral, headache can occur if a mass causes traction on contiguous vessels.

In children younger than 10 years, symptoms of increased intracranial pressure can be temporarily relieved by the separation of sutures. Such children may have a symptom-free interval of several weeks following weeks or months of chronic headache and vomiting. The relief of pressure is temporary, and symptoms return with their prior intensity. An intermittent course of symptoms should not direct attention away from the possibility of increased intracranial pressure.

An individual who was previously well and then experiences an acute, intense headache described as "the worst headache I ever had in my life" has surely suffered a subarachnoid hemorrhage. A small hemorrhage may not cause loss of consciousness but still produces sufficient meningeal irritation to cause intense headache and some stiffness of the neck. Fever may be present.

Diplopia and Strabismus

Paralysis of one or both abducens nerves is a relatively common feature of generalized increased intracranial pressure and may be a more prominent feature than headache in children with pseudotumor cerebri (see Chapter 15).

Papilledema

Papilledema is passive swelling of the optic disk caused by increased intracranial pressure (Table 4–2). The mechanism of swelling is uncertain but generally is believed to be the obstruction of venous return from the retina and nerve head. The edema is usually bilateral and, when unilateral, suggests a mass lesion behind the affected eye. Early papilledema is asymptomatic, and only when it is advanced does the patient experience transitory obscuration of vision. Preservation of visual acuity differentiates papilledema from primary optic nerve disturbances such as optic neuritis, in which

Table 4–2 ◆ Differential Diagnosis of Swollen Disk

1. Congenital disk elevation
2. Increased intracranial pressure
3. Ischemic neuropathy
4. Juvenile diabetes
5. Optic glioma
6. Papillitis
7. Retinitis
8. Retrobulbar mass
9. Uveitis

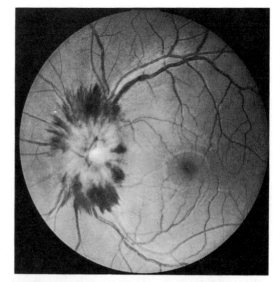

Figure 4–1 Acute papilledema. The optic disk is swollen with peripapillary nerve fiber layer hemorrhages.

visual acuity is always profoundly impaired early in the course (see Chapter 16).

The observation of papilledema in a child with headache or diplopia confirms the diagnosis of increased intracranial pressure. However, the diagnosis of papilledema is not always easy, and congenital variations of disk appearance may confuse the issue. The earliest sign of papilledema is loss of spontaneous venous pulsations in the vessels around the disk margin. Spontaneous venous pulsations are said to occur in approximately 80% of normal eyes, but this is closer to 100% in children. Spontaneous venous pulsations cease when intracranial pressure exceeds 200 mm H_2O. Therefore papilledema is not present if spontaneous venous pulsations are present, no matter how obscure the disk margin may appear. Conversely, when spontaneous venous pulsations are lacking in children, papilledema should be suspected even though the disk margin is flat and well visualized.

As edema progresses, the disk swells and is raised above the plane of the retina, causing obscuration of the disk margin and tortuosity of the veins (Figure 4–1). Associated features include small flame-shaped hemorrhages and nerve fiber infarcts known as "cotton-wool" (Figure 4–2). If the process continues, the retina surrounding the disk becomes edematous so that the disk appears greatly enlarged and retinal exudates radiate from the fovea. Eventually the hemorrhages and exudates clear, but optic atrophy ensues and blindness may be permanent. Even if increased intracranial pressure is relieved during the early stages of disk edema, 4 to 6 weeks is required before the retina appears normal again.

Congenitally elevated disks that give the false impression of papilledema are usually caused by hyaline bodies (drusen) within the nerve head. The actual drusen are not observable during the first decade, and therefore only the elevated nerve head is apparent. Drusen continue to grow and can be seen in older children and their parents (Figure 4–3). Drusen are inherited as an autosomal dominant trait and occur more often in whites than other racial groups. Anomalous nerve head elevations can be easily distinguished from papilledema because spontaneous venous pulsations are present.

HERNIATION SYNDROMES

Increased intracranial pressure may cause portions of the brain to shift from their normal location into other compartments, compressing structures already occupying that space. Such shifts may oc-

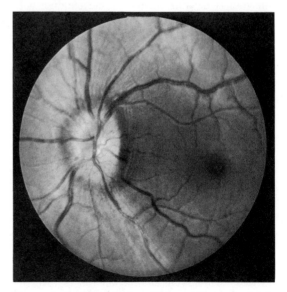

Figure 4–2 Established papilledema. The optic disk is elevated with opacification of the nerve fiber layer around the disk margin and retinal folds (Paton lines) temporally.

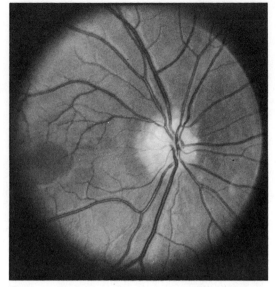

Figure 4–3   Drusen. The disk margin is indistinct, the physiologic cup is absent, and yellowish, globular bodies are present on the surface.

cur under the falx cerebri, through the tentorial notch, and through the foramen magnum (Table 4–3).

Lumbar puncture is generally contraindicated in patients with increased intracranial pressure because of the fear that a change in fluid dynamics will cause herniation. It is especially hazardous when pressure between cranial compartments is unequal. This prohibition is relative, and early lumbar puncture is the rule in infants and children with suspected infections of the nervous system despite the presence of increased intracranial pressure. In other situations lumbar puncture is rarely essential for diagnosis, but it is usually accomplished safely in the absence of papilledema. Patients at increased risk for herniation following lumbar puncture can be defined by the following computed tomography (CT) criteria: lateral shift of midline structures, loss of the suprachiasmatic and basilar cisterns, obliteration of the fourth ventricle, or obliteration of the superior cerebellar and quadrigeminal plate cisterns (Gower et al, 1987).

Falx Herniation

Herniation of one cingulate gyrus under the falx cerebri is common when one hemisphere is enlarged. The major feature is compression of the internal cerebral vein and the anterior cerebral artery, resulting in still greater increased intracranial pressure because of reduced venous outflow and arterial infarction.

Unilateral (Uncal) Transtentorial Herniation

The tentorial notch allows structures to pass from the posterior to the middle fossa. Normally it is filled with the brainstem, the posterior cerebral artery, and the third nerve. Unilateral transtentorial herniation characteristically occurs when enlargement of one temporal lobe causes the uncus or hippocampus to bulge into the tentorial notch. Falx herniation is usually an associated feature. Because intracranial pressure must be considerable to cause such a shift, consciousness is decreased even before the herniation and continues to decline as the brainstem is compressed. Direct pressure on the oculomotor nerve causes ipsilateral dilation of the pupil; sometimes the contralateral pupil is dilated because the displaced brainstem compresses the opposite oculomotor nerve against the incisura of the tentorium. Contralateral homonymous hemianopia occurs (but is impossible to test in an unconscious patient) because of compression of the ipsilateral posterior cerebral artery. With further pressure on the midbrain, both pupils become dilated and fixed, respirations become irregular, decerebrate posturing is noted, and death results from cardiorespiratory collapse.

Bilateral (Central) Transtentorial Herniation

Central herniation is usually associated with generalized cerebral edema. Both hemispheres are displaced downward, and the diencephalon and midbrain are pushed caudad through the tentorial

Table 4–3 ◆ Herniation Syndromes

Unilateral (Uncal) Transtentorial Herniation
1. Declining consciousness
2. Respiratory irregularity
3. Dilated and fixed pupil
4. Homonymous hemianopia
5. Increased blood pressure, slow pulse
6. Decerebrate rigidity

Bilateral (Central) Transtentorial Herniation
1. Declining consciousness
2. Pupillary constriction or dilation
3. Impaired upward gaze
4. Irregular respiration
5. Decerebrate or decorticate rigidity

Cerebellar (Downward) Herniation
1. Neck stiffness or head tilt
2. Declining consciousness
3. Impaired upward gaze
4. Irregular respirations
5. Lower cranial nerve palsies

notch. The diencephalon becomes edematous, and the pituitary stalk may be avulsed. The clinical features are states of decreasing consciousness, pupillary constriction and then dilation, impaired upward gaze, irregular respiration, disturbed control of body temperature, decerebrate or decorticate posturing, and death.

Cerebellar Herniation

Increased pressure in the posterior fossa may cause upward herniation of the cerebellum through the tentorial notch or downward displacement of one or both cerebellar tonsils through the tentorial notch. Upward displacement causes compression of the midbrain, resulting in impairment of upward gaze, dilated or fixed pupils, and respiratory irregularity. Downward cerebellar herniation causes compression of the medulla, resulting in states of decreasing consciousness, impaired upward gaze, and lower cranial nerve palsies. One of the earliest features of cerebellar herniation into the foramen magnum is neck stiffness or head tilt as an effort is made to relieve the pressure by enlarging the surface area of the foramen magnum.

◆ Medical Treatment

Several measures to lower increased intracranial pressure are available, even in circumstances where surgical intervention is required (Table 4–4).

MONITORING INTRACRANIAL PRESSURE

The enthusiasm for continuous monitoring of intracranial pressure in children is declining. Despite advances in technology, the effect of pressure monitoring on outcome is questionable. It has no value in children with hypoxic-ischemic encephalopathies and has marginal value in children with other kinds of encephalopathies (Le Roux et al, 1991). The symptoms and prognosis of increased

Table 4–4 ◆ Medical Measures to Decrease Intracranial Pressure

1. Elevation of head
2. Hyperventilation
3. Osmotic diuretics
   a. Mannitol
   b. Glycerol
4. Corticosteroids
5. Hypothermia
6. Pentobarbital coma

intracranial pressure depends at least as much on its cause as on the level of pressure attained.

HEAD ELEVATION

Elevating the head of the bed 30 to 45 degrees above horizontal decreases intracranial pressure by improving jugular venous drainage. Systemic blood pressure is not affected, so that the overall result is increased cerebral perfusion. A continuous wave Doppler technique has been used to measure the effect of head elevation on intracranial pressure in normal and asphyxiated newborns (Emery and Peabody, 1983). Pressure is higher in the dependent position and lower in the elevated position in both groups, but the effect is greater in asphyxiated newborns.

HYPERVENTILATION

Intracranial pressure is reduced within seconds of the initiation of hyperventilation. The mechanism is vasoconstriction resulting from hypercarbia. The goal is to lower the arterial pressure of carbon dioxide to 25 cm H_2O from 40 cm H_2O. Further reduction may cause ischemia and is contraindicated. Vasoconstriction is not maintained so long as hyperventilation is continued. However, as the vessels redilate and blood flow returns to normal, "rebound," is which blood flow increases above baseline, does not occur.

OSMOTIC DIURETICS

Mannitol and glycerol are the two osmotic diuretics most widely used in the United States. Mannitol, 0.5 g/kg, is given intravenously as a 20% solution. Much larger doses were previously recommended, but the lower dose is equally effective and produces less rebound. Mannitol does not cross the blood-brain barrier. It remains in the plasma and creates an osmotic gradient that draws water from the brain into capillaries. Onset of action is within 30 minutes, and the peak effect is generally 1 to 2 hours after administration. The effect is short lasting, and infusions must be given three to six times each day to keep serum osmolality below 320 mOsm/L (320 nmol/L). Because repeated infusions of mannitol produce dehydration, as well as fluid and electrolyte imbalance, it is generally used for only 2 to 3 days. Rebound may occur when mannitol is discontinued.

Glycerol, 1 g/kg, is given intravenously as a 10% solution three or four times a day. The onset of action is within 30 minutes, and the effect usually lasts 24 hours or longer. As with mannitol, dehydration and electrolyte disturbances may follow repeated administration. Rebound is less prominent than with mannitol.

CORTICOSTERIODS

Corticosteroids such as dexamethasone are effective in the treatment of vasogenic edema. The intravenous dose is 0.1 to 0.2 mg/kg every 6 hours. Onset of action is 12 to 24 hours, and peak action may be delayed even longer. The mechanism is uncertain. Cerebral blood flow is not affected. Corticosteroids are most useful for reducing edema surrounding mass lesions.

HYPOTHERMIA

Hypothermia decreases cerebral blood flow and is frequently used concurrently with pentobarbital coma. Body temperature is generally kept between 27° and 31° C. It is not clear how much is gained by hypothermia in addition to other measures that decrease cerebral blood flow, such as head elevation, hyperventilation, and pentobarbital coma.

PENTOBARBITAL COMA

Barbiturates reduce cerebral blood flow, decrease edema formation, and lower the brain's metabolic rate (Steer, 1982). These effects do not occur at anticonvulsant plasma concentrations but require brain concentrations sufficient to produce a burst-suppression pattern on the electroencephalogram (EEG). Barbiturate coma is particularly useful in patients with increased intracranial pressure resulting from disorders of mitochondrial function such as Reye syndrome. Pentobarbital is preferred to phenobarbital (see Chapter 1).

◆ Hydrocephalus

Hydrocephalus is a condition marked by an excessive volume of intracranial cerebrospinal fluid. It is termed *communicating* or *noncommunicating* depending on whether there is communication of cerebrospinal fluid between the ventricular system and subarachnoid space. Congenital hydrocephalus occurs in approximately one birth per thousand. It is generally associated with other congenital malformations and may be caused by genetic disturbances or intrauterine disorders such as infection and hemorrhage. Often no cause can be determined. Congenital hydrocephalus is discussed in Chapter 18 because its initial manifestation is almost always macrocephaly.

Acquired hydrocephalus may be caused by brain tumor, intracranial hemorrhage, or infection. Solid brain tumors generally produce hydrocephalus by obstructing the ventricular system, whereas nonsolid tumors such as leukemia impair the reabsorptive mechanism in the subarachnoid space.

Intracranial hemorrhage and infection may produce communicating and noncommunicating hydrocephalus and also may increase intracranial pressure through the mechanisms of cerebral edema and impaired venous return. Because several factors contribute to increased intracranial pressure, the discussion of acquired hydrocephalus is categorized by cause in the sections that follow.

◆ Brain Tumor

Primary tumors of the posterior fossa and middle fossa are discussed in Chapters 10, 15, and 16 (Table 4–5). This section deals with tumors of the cerebral hemispheres. Supratentorial tumors occur

Table 4–5 ◆ Brain Tumors in Children

Hemispheric Tumors
1. Choroid plexus papilloma
2. Neuroepithelial tumors
   a. Astrocytoma
   b. Ependymoma
   c. Oligodendroglioma
   d. Primitive neuroectodermal tumors
3. Pineal region tumors
   a. Pineal-parenchymal tumors
      (1) Pineoblastoma
      (2) Pineocytoma
   b. Germ cell tumors
      (1) Embryonal cell carcinoma
      (2) Germinoma
      (3) Teratoma
   c. Glial tumors
      (1) Astrocytoma
      (2) Ganglioglioma
4. Other tumors
   a. Angiomas
   b. Dysplasia
   c. Meningioma
   d. Metastatic tumors

Middle Fossa Tumors
1. Optic glioma (see Chapter 16)
2. Sellar and parasellar tumors (see Chapter 16)

Posterior Fossa Tumors
1. Astrocytoma (see Chapter 10)
2. Brainstem glioma (see Chapter 15)
3. Ependymoma (see Chapter 10)
4. Hemangioblastoma (see Chapter 10)
5. Medulloblastoma (see Chapter 10)

more commonly in children less than 2 years old and again in adolescents.

Tumors of glial origin make up approximately 40% of supratentorial tumors in infancy and childhood. The common glial tumors of childhood in order of frequency are astrocytoma, ependymoma, and oligodendroglioma. A mixture of two or more cell types is the rule. Oligodendroglioma occurs exclusively in the cerebral hemispheres, whereas astrocytoma and ependymoma may be found in either a supratentorial or an infratentorial location.

Oligodendroglioma is rare in childhood and generally not encountered until adolescence. These tumors grow slowly and tend to calcify. The initial symptom is usually a seizure rather than increased intracranial pressure.

CHOROID PLEXUS PAPILLOMA

Choroid plexus papilloma is an unusual tumor, representing between 1% and 4% of childhood brain tumors. It generally occurs during infancy and may be present at birth.

Clinical Features. Choroid plexus tumors are usually located in one lateral ventricle (Ellenbogen et al, 1989). They are manifest as symptoms and signs of increased intracranial pressure resulting from hydrocephalus. Communicating hydrocephalus may be caused by excessive production of cerebrospinal fluid by the tumor, but noncommunicating hydrocephalus caused by obstruction of the ventricular foramen is more common. If the tumor is pedunculated, its movement may cause intermittent ventricular obstruction by a ball-valve mechanism. The usual course is one of rapid progression with only a few weeks from first symptoms to diagnosis.

Infants with choroid plexus tumors usually have macrocephaly and are thought to have congenital hydrocephalus. Older children have nausea, vomiting, diplopia, headaches, and weakness. Papilledema is the rule.

Diagnosis. Because affected children show clear evidence of increased intracranial pressure, CT is usually the first test performed. The tumor is visualized within one ventricle as a mass of increased density with marked contrast enhancement. Hydrocephalus of one or both lateral ventricles is visualized as well. Because choroid plexus papillomas are highly vascular, angiography should be performed before surgery. Many tumors bleed spontaneously, and the spinal fluid may be xanthochromic or grossly bloody. The concentration of protein in the cerebrospinal fluid is usually elevated.

Treatment. Complete surgical extirpation is the treatment of choice. The 5-year survival rate is 50% with most deaths occurring within 7 months of surgery. Operative mortality may be high because the tumor has a tendency to hemorrhage. If the tumor is removed completely, hydrocephalus is relieved without the need of a shunt and recurrences are unusual.

ASTROCYTOMA

Hemispheric astrocytomas are graded by histologic appearance into three classes: low-grade, anaplastic, and glioblastoma multiforme. Anaplastic tumors and glioblastoma multiforme are referred to as high-grade tumors. Glioblastoma multiforme accounts for fewer than 10% of childhood supratentorial astrocytomas and is more likely to occur in adolescence than in infancy. High-grade tumors may evolve from low-grade tumors (Dropcho et al, 1987).

Clinical Features. The initial manifestations of glial tumors in children depend on location and may include seizures, hemiparesis, and movement disorders affecting one side of the body. Seizures are the most common initial manifestation of low-grade gliomas. Tumors infiltrating the basal ganglia and internal capsule are less likely to cause seizures than those closer to cortical structures. A mass effect may not be present early in the course because slow-growing, infiltrating tumors can be accommodated by surrounding neural structures. Such tumors may cause only seizures for several years before causing weakness of the contralateral limbs.

Headache is a relatively common complaint and may be focal if the tumor is producing localized displacement of vessels without increasing intracranial pressure. A persistent focal headache usually correlates well with tumor location.

Symptoms of increased intracranial pressure— generalized headache, nausea, and vomiting—are initial manifestations of hemispheric astrocytoma in only 37% of children but are features at time of diagnosis in 79%. Intracranial pressure is likely to increase when rapidly growing tumors provoke edema of the hemisphere. A mass effect is produced that causes collapse of one ventricle, shift of midline structures, and pressure on the aqueduct. When herniation occurs, or when the lateral ventricles are dilated because of pressure on the aqueduct, the early features of headache, nausea, vomiting, and diplopia are followed by generalized weakness or fatigability, lethargy, and declining consciousness.

Papilledema occurs in children with generalized increased intracranial pressure except those under

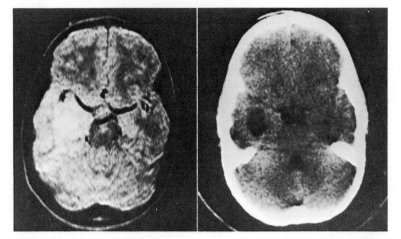

Figure 4–4   Low-grade glioma. MRI *(left)* reveals an area of increased signal intensity in right temporal lobe, which appears as a cystic lesion on CT *(right)*.

2 years of age, in whom macrocephaly may develop instead. When papilledema is present, abducens palsy is usually associated. Other neurologic findings depend on the site of the tumor and may include hemiparesis, hemisensory loss, or homonymous hemianopia.

Diagnosis.   High-grade hemispheric astrocytomas are readily identified by contrast-enhanced CT, but low-grade tumors are much better visualized with magnetic resonance imaging (MRI). MRI rather than CT should be used when tumor is suspected as the cause of seizures. Low-grade gliomas appear as low-density or cystic areas that are enhanced when contrast material is injected (Figure 4–4). Cerebral edema is identified as a low-density area surrounding the tumor that does not demonstrate contrast enhancement.

High-grade gliomas have patchy areas of low and high density, sometimes evidence of hemorrhage, and cystic degeneration. Marked contrast enhancement is noted, often in a ring pattern. When a mass effect is present, CT shows a shift of midline structures, deformity of the ipsilateral ventricle, and swelling of the affected hemisphere with obliteration of sulcal markings (Figure 4–5). A mass effect is identified in 50% of low-grade astrocytomas, 90% of anaplastic tumors, and 100% of glioblastoma multiforme (Weisberg, 1980).

Treatment.   All children with increased intracranial pressure caused by hemispheric astrocytoma should be treated with dexamethasone to reduce vasogenic cerebral edema. Headache and nausea are frequently relieved within 24 hours, and neurologic deficits are often improved as well. Surgical resection of the tumor is the next step in treatment. Complete removal is rarely possible, except with cystic cerebral astrocytoma, which re-

sembles cerebellar astrocytomas in having a mural nodule within the cyst. With these tumors the 5-year survival rate following surgery alone is 90% (Palma et al, 1983).

Postoperative radiation is recommended for anaplastic astrocytomas, but its value in the treatment of low-grade astrocytomas remains controversial (Cairncross and Laperriere, 1990; Shaw, 1990).

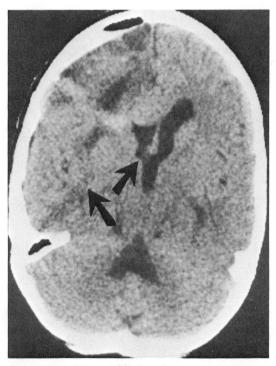

Figure 4–5   Mass effect. Invasive tumor of left hemisphere *(arrow)* compresses the lateral ventricle on that side *(arrow)* and causes herniation under the falx.

Children with anaplastic astrocytomas have less than a 30% 5-year survival rate even with radiation, and those with glioblastoma multiforme have less than a 3% 5-year survival (Duffner et al, 1986).

Because the 5-year survival rate is poor with high-grade astrocytomas, several chemotherapy protocols have been tried. Although this approach does provide some short-term benefits, long-term survival is not affected substantially.

EPENDYMOMA

Ependymomas are tumors derived from cells that line the ventricular system, and they may be found in either a supratentorial or an infratentorial location. Infratentorial ependymoma is discussed in Chapter 10 because the initial symptom is often ataxia. However, symptoms of increased intracranial pressure are the first manifestation in 90% of children with posterior fossa ependymoma, and papilledema is present in 75% at the time of initial examination. Approximately 60% of children with ependymoma are younger than 5 years at the time of diagnosis, and only 4% are older than 15 (Dohrmann et al, 1976). As a rule, children with infratentorial ependymoma are younger than children with supratentorial ependymoma.

The expected location of supratentorial ependymoma is in relation to the third and lateral ventricles. However, ependymal tumors may arise within the hemispheres at a site distant from the ventricular system. Such tumors are thought to be derived from ependymal cell rests.

Clinical Features.   Symptoms of increased intracranial pressure are less prominent with supratentorial tumors than infratentorial tumors. Common manifestations are focal weakness, seizures, and visual disturbances. Papilledema is a common physical finding in patients with ependymoma. Hemiparesis, hyperreflexia, and hemianopia are typical features, but some children demonstrate only ataxia. The duration of symptoms before diagnosis averages 7 months but can be as little as 1 month for malignant tumors and as long as several years for low-grade tumors.

Diagnosis.   Tumor density on CT is usually greater than brain density, and contrast enhancement is present. Small cysts within the tumor are relatively common. Approximately one third of supratentorial ependymomas contain calcium.

Tumors within the third ventricle cause marked dilation of the lateral ventricles with edema of the hemispheres and obliteration of sulcal markings. High-grade tumors are likely to seed the subarachnoid space, producing metastases in the spinal cord and throughout the ventricular system. In such cases tumor cells may line the lateral ventricles and produce a "cast" of contrast enhancement around the ventricles.

Treatment.   Surgical resection is the first step in management but is not curative. Low-grade supratentorial ependymomas are associated with a low risk of metastases and should be treated with local irradiation. Children with high-grade supratentorial tumors should receive at least whole brain irradiation, and complete craniospinal irradiation should be considered as well (Cohen and Duffner, 1984). Several studies of chemotherapy are in progress. No significant increase in long-term survival has been demonstrated. Overall, the 5-year survival rate in children with ependymoma is only 28% (Duffner et al, 1986). Children with tumors that are supratentorial or of low-grade malignancy have a better prognosis than do children in whom the tumors are infratentorial or anaplastic.

PRIMITIVE NEUROECTODERMAL TUMORS

Primitive neuroectodermal tumors (PNETs) are tumors of childhood consisting of small, undifferentiated, darkly staining cells that have neuronal, glial, and mesenchymal elements. These tumors resemble medulloblastoma; some classifications include medulloblastoma as a PNET, whereas others reserve the term for tumors in the cerebral hemispheres (Schut et al, 1989).

Clinical Features.   Age at onset may be anytime during childhood but is usually in the first decade. Males and females are affected equally. Because these tumors are highly malignant, the progression of symptoms is rapid and time to diagnosis is usually less than 3 months. Approximately half of children show features of increased intracranial pressure. Other manifestations are determined by tumor site. Two thirds of tumors are in the frontal or parietal lobe. Seizures, monoparesis, hemiplegia, and ophthalmoplegia are initial manifestations in approximately 10% of patients. Hydrocephalus or head enlargement is unusual early in the course.

Diagnosis.   CT and MRI are effective techniques for determining tumor location and size. On CT, PNETs appear as poorly defined, infiltrating and lobular masses, sometimes containing multiple cysts and hemorrhage. The tumor mass is surrounded by cerebral edema, and midline structures are frequently shifted under the falx.

Treatment.   Cerebral edema may be relieved by the use of dexamethasone. Complete tumor resection is attempted but rarely accomplished. Postoperative craniospinal irradiation is believed to prolong survival. Several chemotherapeutic trials are ongoing.

Unfortunately, the mean survival of all patients is only 26 months. The best results are attributed to complete surgical resection, postoperative radiotherapy, and aggressive chemotherapy (Tomita et al, 1988). However, the tumor metastasizes throughout the subarachnoid space of brain and spinal cord, so recurrence is possible even when the primary tumor is believed to be fully resected.

PINEAL REGION TUMORS

Tumors in the pineal region may be derived from several histologic types. Germ cell tumors are the most common, then tumors of the pineal parenchyma, and finally other histologic types. The incidence of pineal region tumors is 10 times higher in Japan than in the United States or Western Europe. Pineal region tumors are more common in boys than girls and generally become symptomatic during the second decade.

Clinical Features.   Because pineal region tumors are in a midline location, where they can invade or compress the third ventricle or aqueduct, symptoms of increased intracranial pressure are common. The first pressure symptoms may be acute and accompanied by midbrain dysfunction (Packer et al, 1984). Midbrain dysfunction resulting from pressure by pineal region tumors on the periaqueductal gray matter is usually referred to as *Parinaud syndrome*: loss of pupillary light reflex, supranuclear palsy of upward gaze with preservation of downward gaze, and retraction-convergence nystagmus when upward gaze is attempted. Eventually paralysis of both upward and downward gaze and loss of accommodation may occur.

Tumors growing into or compressing the anterior hypothalamus produce loss of vision, diabetes insipidus, precocious puberty, and emaciation. Precocious puberty occurs almost exclusively in males. Extension of tumor into the posterior fossa produces multiple cranial neuropathies and ataxia, and lateral extension causes hemiparesis.

Diagnosis.   CT and MRI accurately image tumor location and the presence of secondary hydrocephalus but cannot distinguish histologic types. As a rule, germinomas are isodense and noncalcified and have irregular margins. Contrast enhancement is not homogeneous. Teratomas appear lobulated and have both hyperdense and multicystic areas. Calcification may be present, and contrast enhancement is not uniform. Tumors that spread into the ventricular system and have intense contrast enhancement are likely to be malignant. Tumors that contain abundant amounts of calcium are likely to be benign.

Asymptomatic nonneoplastic pineal cysts are sometimes identified by CT or MRI in children who are being imaged for other reasons. These are developmental variants of the pineal gland that may contain calcium. Only rarely do they grow to sufficient size to obstruct the aqueduct or cause a Parinaud syndrome.

Treatment.   Stereotactic biopsy is essential to establish histologic type and plan therapy. Ventricular drainage may be needed to relieve hydrocephalus. Germinomas are highly radiosensitive, and 5-year survival rates of 50% to 80% are reported. Other tumors of the pineal region are less radiosensitive. Complete surgical removal of pineal region tumors has been discouraged in the past because mortality and morbidity rates have been prohibitive. Improved surgical techniques are now allowing successful removal in many cases (Schulte et al, 1987).

OTHER TUMORS

Cerebral metastatic disease is unusual in childhood. Tumors with the highest frequency of producing cerebral metastases are osteogenic sarcoma and rhabdomyosarcoma in patients younger than 15 years and testicular germ cell tumors after age 15 (Graus et al, 1983). The cerebral hemispheres are affected more often than posterior fossa structures. Pulmonary involvement always precedes cerebral metastasis. Brain metastasis is rarely present at the time of initial cancer diagnosis.

The symptoms of different hemispheric tumors are similar and are generally some combination of increased intracranial pressure, seizures, and hemiparesis. CT is useful in each case to identify the presence of tumor. Complete surgical excision is the treatment of choice when possible; if not, partial resection or biopsy is performed to relieve tumor burden and establish tissue diagnosis. Radiation is administered following partial resection and especially when there is evidence of malignancy.

◆ Intracranial Arachnoid Cysts

Primary arachnoid cysts are cavities that are within the arachnoid and are filled with cerebrospinal fluid. The cause of cyst formation is uncertain, but cysts are generally considered a minor disturbance in arachnoid formation and not a pathologic process (Naidich et al, 1986). Arachnoid cysts are identified in 0.5% of postmortem examinations: two thirds are supratentorial and one third infratentorial.

Clinical Features.   Most cysts are asymptomatic structures identified by CT or MRI. Deciding whether the cyst is the cause of the symptom for which the imaging study was ordered is sometimes a problem. Subarachnoid cysts are usually present from infancy, but may develop, or at least enlarge enough to be detected, during adolescence.

Large cysts can produce symptoms by compressing adjacent structures or by increasing intracranial pressure. Focal neurologic disturbances vary with location but are most often hemiparesis or seizures when the cyst is supratentorial and ataxia when infratentorial. Compression of the parietal lobe from early infancy may result in undergrowth of contralateral limbs.

Increased intracranial pressure can be caused by mass effect or hydrocephalus and is associated with cysts in all locations. Manifestations include macrocephaly, headache, and behavioral change.

Diagnosis. It has become commonplace for children with headache, learning or behavioral disorders, and suspected seizures to undergo imaging studies of the brain. Many have incidental arachnoid cysts. A cause-and-effect relationship should be considered only if the cyst is large and if it clearly explains the symptoms.

Treatment. Simple drainage of the cyst often results in reaccumulation of fluid and recurrence of symptoms. The definitive procedure is to shunt the cyst into the peritoneal space (Harsh et al, 1986).

◆ Intracranial Hemorrhage

HEAD TRAUMA

Head trauma is a major cause of intracranial hemorrhage from the newborn period through childhood and adolescence. It is associated with intracerebral hemorrhage, subarachnoid hemorrhage, subdural hematoma, and epidural hema-

toma. Increased intracranial pressure is a constant feature of intracranial hemorrhage and also occurs from cerebral edema following concussion without hemorrhage. Intracranial hemorrhage from head trauma is discussed in Chapter 2.

INTRAVENTRICULAR HEMORRHAGE OF THE NEWBORN

Intraventricular hemorrhage is primarily a disorder of liveborn premature newborns with respiratory distress syndrome. The autoregulation of cerebral blood flow, which meets local tissue needs by altering cerebrovascular resistance, is impaired in premature newborns with respiratory distress syndrome. During episodes of systemic hypotension, cerebral blood flow is decreased and the potential for cerebral infarction exists. Such infarctions usually occur symmetrically in the white matter adjacent to the lateral ventricles and are termed *periventricular leukomalacia*. Low-density lesions in the periventricular white matter can be identified on CT at 40 weeks' conceptional age in 89% of newborns with a birth weight less than 1500 g (McCarton-Daum et al, 1983).

During episodes of systemic hypertension, cerebral blood flow increases. Hemorrhage occurs first in the subependymal germinal matrix and then bursts through the ependymal lining into the lateral ventricle. Such hemorrhages are called *periventricular-intraventricular hemorrhage*. The predilection of the germinal matrix for hemorrhage during episodes of increased cerebral blood flow has not been fully explained. The likely explanation is prior ischemic injury that weakens the capillary walls and their supporting structures, making them vulnerable to rupture during episodes of increased cerebral blood flow (Figure 4–6). Echo-dense lesions consistent with periventricular leukomalacia

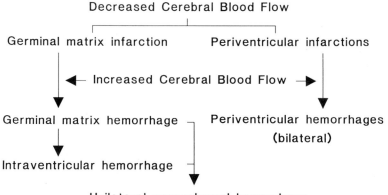

Figure 4–6   Pathophysiology of periventricular-intraventricular hemorrhage. (From Fenichel GM: Neonatal Neurology, 3rd edition. Churchill Livingstone, New York, 1990. By permission.)

can be detected by ultrasound in 36% of premature newborns with intraventricular hemorrhage (McMenamin et al, 1984).

Intraventricular hemorrhage also occurs in full-term newborns, but the mechanism of hemorrhage at term is different from that before term.

Periventricular-Intraventricular Hemorrhage of Premature Newborns

The incidence of periventricular-intraventricular hemorrhage (PIVH) in premature newborns whose birth weight is less than 2000 g has fallen in recent years from 40% to 25% (Philip et al, 1989). The reason for the decline has not been fully explained. PIVH is still identified in 62% of very small premature newborns (birth weights between 500 and 700 g) and is associated with a high mortality rate. In newborns weighing less than 1500 g the incidence is approximately 40%. A grading system has been developed to quantify the severity of hemorrhage:

I. Isolated subependymal hemorrhage
II. Intraventricular hemorrhage without ventricular dilation
III. Intraventricular hemorrhage with ventricular dilation
IV. Intraventricular hemorrhage with ventricular dilation and hemorrhage into the parenchyma of the brain

Hemorrhage into the parenchyma of the brain (grade IV) is a coexistent process caused by hemorrhagic infarction *(periventricular hemorrhagic infarction)* and is not an extension of intraventricular hemorrhage.

Clinical Features. Routine ultrasound examinations are now the standard of care for all newborns whose birth weight is 1800 g or less. Ultrasound often shows PIVH in newborns for whom there was no clinical suspicion of hemorrhage. Among this group some have blood in the cerebrospinal fluid and others have clear cerebrospinal fluid. Only 54% of newborns with PIVH have clinical signs and symptoms, and these are generally the ones with grade III or IV hemorrhage (Lazzara et al, 1980).

In some premature newborns, PIVH produces rapid neurologic deterioration characterized by decreasing states of consciousness, severe hypotonia, and respiratory insufficiency. Within minutes to hours the infant shows obvious evidence of increased intracranial pressure: bulging fontanelle, decerebrate posturing, loss of pupillary reflexes, and respiratory arrest. Hypothermia, bradycardia, hypotension, and a 10% fall in the hematocrit value may be associated findings.

More commonly the hemorrhage is manifested subacutely with stepwise progression of symptoms over hours or even days. The initial symptoms are subtle and include a change in behavior, diminished spontaneous movement, and either an increase or a decrease in appendicular tone. The fontanelles remain soft, and vital signs are stable. These first symptoms may correspond to grade I hemorrhage. Some newborns then become stable and have no further difficulty. Others undergo clinical deterioration characterized by hypotonia and declining consciousness. This deterioration probably corresponds to the presence of blood in the ventricles. The child becomes lethargic or obtunded and then may stabilize. If continued bleeding causes acute ventricular dilation, apnea and coma follow. Seizures occur when blood dissects into the cerebral parenchyma.

Newborns with intraventricular hemorrhage are at risk for progressive hydrocephalus. The likelihood is much greater among children with grade III or IV hemorrhage. Initial ventricular dilation is probably due to plugging of the arachnoid villi and impaired reabsorption of cerebrospinal fluid (Hill et al, 1982). The ventricles can enlarge by compressing the brain without causing a measurable change in head circumference. Therefore weekly ultrasound studies are imperative to follow the progression of hydrocephalus.

Progressive hydrocephalus develops in 10% to 15% of preterm newborns with PIVH (Dykes et al, 1989). The hydrocephalus ultimately arrests or regresses in two thirds of these children and progresses to severe hydrocephalus in the remainder.

Diagnosis. Ultrasound is the standard for the diagnosis of intraventricular hemorrhage in the newborn. CT is equally effective, but ultrasound is preferred because it can be performed in the intensive care nursery, study time is briefer, and no radiation is involved.

Prevention. Prevention is the best treatment for PIVH. This could be accomplished, to a great extent, by preventing prematurity and by delivering preterm newborns at specialized perinatal centers. A premature newborn transported to an intensive care nursery has a far greater chance of hemorrhage than a fetus transported to the delivery room in utero. Normal tensions of carbon dioxide and oxygen, normal osmolality and viscosity, normal perfusion pressure without episodic hypertension from undue stimulation, and good ventilatory control in the early hours post partum can best be maintained in a specialized neonatal unit (Volpe, 1989).

Several promising medical interventions for preventing PIVH have been introduced (Table 4–6); none of the drug treatments has gained wide ac-

Table 4–6 ◆ Prevention of Periventricular-
Intraventricular Hemorrhage

Antenatal
1. Prevention of prematurity
2. Delivery in specialized center
3. Treatment of mothers with
   a. Phenobarbital
   b. Vitamin K supplementation

Postnatal
1. Avoidance of rapid volume expansion
2. Maintenance of stable systemic blood pressure
3. Muscle paralysis of ventilated premature
4. Correction of coagulation abnormalities
5. Potential pharmacologic agents
   a. Ethamsylate
   b. Indomethacin
   c. Phenobarbital
   d. Vitamin E

ceptance (Vannucci, 1990). Even more vexing is the management of progressive posthemorrhagic hydrocephalus, for which no medical therapy has seemed promising.

Treatment. Once intraventricular hemorrhage has occurred, treatment is directed at preventing or stabilizing progressive posthemorrhagic hydrocephalus. The efficacy of treatment for posthemorrhagic hydrocephalus is difficult to assess because ventricular dilation's role in causing chronic neurologic impairment has not been established. Newborns with progressive posthemorrhagic hydrocephalus have also experienced asphyxial encephalopathy, germinal matrix hemorrhage, and periventricular leukomalacia. Neurologic morbidity correlates better with the degree of parenchymal damage than with ventricular size (Dykes et al, 1989).

Children with progressive posthemorrhagic hydrocephalus require a ventriculoperitoneal shunt. However, early shunt placement, while the ventricles still contain blood, has a high incidence of shunt failure and infection. Several methods of preventing posthemorrhagic hydrocephalus have been tried to either delay the time of shunt surgery or obviate the need for it.

The procedure that has undergone the greatest scrutiny is serial lumbar punctures. A major problem is the technical difficulty of performing repeated lumbar punctures on a small premature newborn. Different groups have reported contradictory results on the efficacy of serial lumbar punctures. Although its value is not established, the method is recommended for at least temporary amelioration of posthemorrhagic hydrocephalus if, in response to the procedure, a decrease in ventric-

ular size is shown by ultrasound (Kreusser et al, 1985).

An alternative to serial lumbar punctures is external ventricular reservoir drainage (Marro et al, 1991). This method is technically easier than serial lumbar punctures but may cause ventriculitis.

A final approach is the use of chemical agents such as acetazolamide and furosemide, which are presumed to reduce the production of spinal fluid (Shinnar et al, 1985). Acetazolamide is started at a dosage of 25 mg/kg/day for 1 day and then increased by 25 mg/kg/day each day to a maximum of 100 mg/kg/day. Metabolic acidosis may occur at the maintenance dosage of 100 mg/kg/day. Base replacement with a systemic alkalizing agent must be initiated simultaneously to maintain a serum bicarbonate level greater than 18 mEq/L (18 mmol/L). Furosemide is started at a dosage of 1 mg/kg/day in three divided doses and may be increased to 3 mg/kg/day. The results with this protocol are encouraging, but the number of treated infants reported is not large enough to support a definite conclusion.

The neurologic outcome for newborns following PIVH is linked to the grade of hemorrhage. Following grade II hemorrhage up to 75% of children may have normal intellectual and motor development, whereas virtually all children with grade IV hemorrhage have some neurologic morbidity. However, some newborns who have only grade I hemorrhage may be neurologically impaired while others with grade III hemorrhage are normal (Williamson et al, 1983). Neurologic outcome is determined by multiple factors of which asphyxia and periventricular infarction probably play an important role.

Intraventricular Hemorrhage at Term

Unlike intraventricular hemorrhage in premature newborns, which originates almost exclusively from the germinal matrix, intraventricular hemorrhage at term may originate from the veins of the choroid plexus, from the germinal matrix, or both.

Clinical Features. Full-term newborns with intraventricular hemorrhage may be divided into two groups. More than half are delivered with difficulty, frequently in the breech position, and have had some degree of intrauterine asphyxia (Fenichel et al, 1984). These babies are usually bruised and require resuscitation. At first they appear to be improving, and then multifocal seizures occur on the second day post partum. The fontanelle is tense, and the cerebrospinal fluid is bloody.

The other half have experienced neither trauma nor asphyxia and appear normal at birth. During the first hours post partum, however, apnea, cyanosis, and a tense fontanelle develop. The mechanism of hemorrhage is not understood.

Posthemorrhagic hydrocephalus is common in both groups, and 35% require shunt placement (Scher et al, 1982).

Diagnosis.   Ultrasound is as useful for diagnosis of intraventricular hemorrhage in full-term newborns as in premature newborns.

Treatment.   Full-term newborns with intraventricular hemorrhage are treated in the same manner as premature newborns with intraventricular hemorrhage.

ARTERIAL ANEURYSMS

Arterial aneurysms are vestiges of the embryonic circulation and are present in a rudimentary form before birth. Only rarely do they rupture during infancy. More often they become symptomatic after age 10 and usually after age 20. Symptomatic arterial aneurysms in childhood may be associated with coarctation of the aorta or polycystic kidney disease. Aneurysms tend to be located at the bifurcation of major arteries at the base of the brain.

Clinical Features.   The first manifestation is usually subarachnoid hemorrhage. The presentation may be catastrophic: sudden loss of consciousness, tachycardia, hypotension, and evidence of increased intracranial pressure. However, in most patients the first bleeding from an aneurysm is not catastrophic but is a "warning leak" that may go unrecognized. The warning leak is characterized by severe headache, stiff neck, and low-grade fever. Occasionally aneurysms produce neurologic signs by exerting pressure on adjacent cranial nerves. The oculomotor nerve is most frequently affected, resulting in disturbances of gaze and pupillary function.

Physical activity is not related to time of rupture. Aneurysmal size is the only predictor of rupture; those smaller than 1 cm in diameter have a low probability of rupture (Weibers et al, 1981).

The patient's state of consciousness is the most important predictor of survival (Kassell and Torner, 1984). Approximately 50% of patients die during the first hospitalization, some from the initial hemorrhage during the first 14 days. Untreated, another 30% die from recurrent hemorrhage in the next 10 years.

Diagnosis.   On the day of aneurysmal rupture, CT demonstrates intracranial hemorrhage in 96% of patients. However, the blood is rapidly reabsorbed and can be demonstrated in only 64% of patients on the fifth day after rupture. Most aneurysms can be visualized by standard MRI or MRI angiography.

Lumbar puncture is often performed because the stiff neck, headache, and fever suggest bacterial meningitis. The fluid is usually grossly bloody and therefore indicative of subarachnoid hemorrhage. Unfortunately, blood in the cerebrospinal fluid is often attributed to a traumatic tap when time is not taken to centrifuge the fluid and examine it for xanthochromia. Once a diagnosis of subarachnoid hemorrhage is established, either by imaging studies or by lumbar puncture, four-vessel cerebral arteriography is essential. All vessels must be visualized to determine the aneurysmal site and the presence of multiple aneurysms.

Treatment.   The initial goals of therapy are to prevent early rebleeding and cerebral ischemia from arterial spasm. Nimodipine, a calcium channel blocking agent, reduces the incidence of spasm and should be administered as soon as possible (Allen et al, 1983).

The definitive treatment is surgical clipping and excision of the aneurysm. Early surgery is recommended in conscious patients to prevent rebleeding. The 6-month survival rate in patients who are conscious at time of admission is approximately 86%. In contrast, only 20% of patients who are comatose on admission are alive 6 months later.

ARTERIOVENOUS MALFORMATIONS

Arteriovenous malformations account for almost 9% of subarachnoid hemorrhage at all ages but make up a considerably larger share of subarachnoid hemorrhage in childhood. Approximately 0.1% to 0.2% of the population has an arteriovenous malformation. No familial occurrence has been documented. Two types of malformations are described. The first arises from an abnormal communication between primitive choroidal arteries and veins. Such malformations are in the midline and give rise to the vein of Galen malformation, malformations involving the choroid plexus, and shunts between cerebellar arteries and the straight sinus. The other type arises between superficial arteries and veins and results in an arteriovenous malformation within the parenchyma of the cerebral hemisphere. The vessels of the scalp, skull, and dura are interconnected, causing anastomotic channels between the extracranial and intracranial circulations to remain patent. Approximately 90% of arteriovenous malformations are supratentorial and 10% are infratentorial.

Deep Midline Malformations

Large deep midline malformations, especially those involving the great vein of Galen, produce hydrocephalus and cardiac failure during infancy. These are discussed in Chapter 18.

Clinical Features. Small, deep midline malformations become manifest because of spontaneous bleeding. The peak onset is after age 20, but symptoms may appear as early as age 5. Small malformations are more likely than large ones to bleed. The hemorrhage is into the parenchyma of the brain in two thirds of cases and into the subarachnoid space in one third. Because bleeding is often from the venous rather than the arterial side of the malformation, the first symptoms are not as catastrophic as with arterial aneurysms. Symptoms may evolve over several hours, and no characteristic clinical syndrome has been described. Most patients describe sudden severe headache, neck stiffness, and vomiting. Fever is frequently an associated symptom. Focal neurologic deficits depend on the location of the malformation and may include hemiparesis, sensory disturbances, and oculomotor palsies. Many patients recover completely from the first hemorrhage; the risk of recurrent hemorrhage is 6% in the first year and 2% each year afterward (Graf et al, 1983).

Diagnosis. Most arteriovenous malformations are easily visualized on MRI or CT with contrast enhancement. The degree of ventricular enlargement is shown by either study. However, the development of a therapeutic plan requires four-vessel arteriography to demonstrate fully all arterial and venous channels.

Treatment. Deep midline malformations are usually managed by a combination of embolization and surgical ligation of large feeding arteries. The goal is to reduce the volume of the malformation sufficiently to relieve high-output cardiac failure or hydrocephalus. Frequently hydrocephalus must be shunted because hemorrhage in and around the third ventricle and aqueduct has caused irrevocable damage. Proton beam therapy and other techniques that deliver radiation to induce endothelial proliferation and narrowing of the vessel walls may decrease the rate of hemorrhage in inoperable malformations (Ogilvy, 1990).

Supratentorial Malformations

Clinical Features. Among children with arteriovenous malformations in and around the cerebral hemispheres, the initial manifestation is intracranial hemorrhage in half and seizures in the other half. Recurrent vascular headache may precede the onset of hemorrhage and seizures or may develop concurrently. Headaches are usually unilateral but may not occur consistently on the same side. In some patients the headaches have a migraine quality: scintillating scotoma and unilateral throbbing pain. The incidence of such migrainelike headaches in patients with arteriovenous malformations does not appear to be greater than in the population at large. Probably the malformation provokes a migraine attack in people who are genetically predisposed (Mohr, 1984).

Most patients who have seizures have at least one focal seizure, but among seizures associated with arteriovenous malformations half are focal and half are generalized. No specific location of the malformation is associated with a higher incidence of seizures. However, small superficial malformations, especially in the centroparietal region, are associated with the highest incidence of hemorrhage (Graf et al, 1983). Hemorrhage may be only subarachnoid or may dissect into the brain parenchyma.

Diagnosis. MRI and contrast-enhanced CT provide excellent visualization of the malformation in most children. Four-vessel arteriography is required to define all arterial and venous channels.

Treatment. The photon knife is becoming the standard of treatment for small malformations. Other options for management include surgical excision and embolization. Superficial malformations are more accessible for direct surgical excision than those deep in the midline. In considering treatment modes the physician must balance the decision to do something against the decision to do nothing based on the likelihood of further bleeding and the morbidity of intervention.

COCAINE ABUSE

Intracranial hemorrhage has been associated with use of cocaine, especially crack, in young adults (Mangiardi et al, 1988). The hemorrhages may be subarachnoid or intracerebral and are thought to be caused by sudden transitory increases in systemic blood pressure.

◆ Infectious Disorders

Infections of the brain and meninges increase intracranial pressure by causing cerebral edema, obstructing the flow and reabsorption of cerebrospinal fluid, and impairing venous outflow. Symptoms of increased intracranial pressure are frequently the initial manifestations of bacterial and fungal infections and may also be the initial manifestations of viral encephalitis. However, viral infections are more likely to be manifested as seizures, personality change, or decreased consciousness and therefore are discussed in Chapter 2.

BACTERIAL MENINGITIS

The offending organism and the clinical features of bacterial meningitis vary with age (Table 4–7). Therefore it is useful to discuss the syndromes of bacterial meningitis by age group: newborn, infancy, early childhood, and school age.

Meningitis in the Newborn

Meningitis occurs in 1 live birth per 2500 and accounts for up to 4% of neonatal deaths. It is a consequence of septicemia, and target organs other than the brain are infected. The two risk factors that correlate best with sepsis and meningitis are low birth weight and maternal infection.

An early-onset and a late-onset pattern of meningitis have been identified in newborns. In early-onset meningitis the infection is acquired at the time of delivery and the responsible organisms are almost always *Escherichia coli* or group B *Streptococcus*. The child becomes symptomatic during the first week, and the mortality rate is 20% to 50%. In late-onset meningitis the infection is acquired postnatally and symptoms may begin as early as the fourth day post partum but usually begin after the first week. Newborns requiring intensive care are specifically at risk for late-onset meningitis because infection is introduced by instrumentation. The responsible organisms are not only *E. coli* and group B *Streptococcus,* but also enterococci, gram-negative enteric bacilli *(Pseudomonas* and *Klebsiella),* and *Listeria monocytogenes.* The mortality rate is 10% to 20%.

Clinical Features. Newborns infected in utero or during delivery may experience respiratory distress and shock within 24 hours of birth. Other features that may be associated with septicemia include hyperthermia, hypothermia, jaundice, hepatomegaly, lethargy, anorexia, and vomiting.

In meningitis of late onset the clinical manifestations are variable. Initial symptoms are usually nonspecific and include lethargy, disturbed feeding, and irritability. As the meningitis worsens, hyperthermia is present in 61%, respiratory distress or apnea in 54%, and seizures in 40%. Bulging of the fontanelle occurs in only 28% and nuchal rigidity in 15%. Shock is the usual cause of death.

Diagnosis. The diagnosis of septicemia and meningitis in the newborn is often difficult to establish on the basis of symptoms. Lumbar puncture must be prompted by the first suspicion of septicemia. Even in the absence of infection the cerebrospinal fluid of high-risk newborns contains an average of 8.4 leukocytes/mm^3 with a range of zero to 32. Sixty percent are polymorphonuclear leukocytes. The protein concentration has a mean value of 90 mg/dl (0.9 g/L), with a range from 20 to 170 mg/dl (0.2 to 1.7 g/L). In newborns with meningitis the leukocyte count is usually in the thousands and protein concentration may vary from less than 30 mg/dl (0.3 g/L) to more than 1000 mg/dl (10 g/L). A gram-stained smear of cerebrospinal fluid permits identification of an organism in less than half of cases. Even when the smear is positive, identification may be inaccurate.

Treatment. Treatment is initiated with the first suspicion of sepsis. Laboratory confirmation is not required. The choice of initial antibiotic coverage varies but usually includes ampicillin and either gentamicin or cefotaxime (Committee on Infectious Disease, 1988). All antibiotics are administered intravenously in divided doses (Table 4–8). If an organism is grown on culture, specific therapy is initiated.

E. coli is best treated with ampicillin and cefotaxime, group B *Streptococcus* with penicillin or ampicillin, and *Klebsiella pneumoniae* with cefotaxime and an aminoglycoside. *Pseudomonas* is difficult to eradicate, and combined intravenous and intrathecal therapy may be required. Carbenicillin and gentamicin are preferred for intravenous use.

Neonatal meningitis is treated for at least 2 weeks beyond the time the cerebrospinal fluid becomes sterile. Two days after antibiotic therapy is

---

Table 4–7 ◆ Most Common Organisms Responsible for Bacterial Meningitis

Newborn
1. Group B *Streptococcus*
2. *Escherichia coli*
3. Other Enterobacteriaceae
4. *Listeria monocytogenes*

Infancy and Preschool
1. *Haemophilus influenzae*
2. *Streptococcus pneumoniae*
3. *Neisseria meningitidis*
4. *Mycobacterium tuberculosis*

School Age
1. *Streptococcus pneumoniae*
2. *Neisseria meningitidis*
3. *Mycobacterium tuberculosis*

Table 4–8 ◆ Antibiotic Dosages for Newborns

Drug	Dosage
Ampicillin	150-200 mg/kg/day IV (q8h)
Carbenicillin	300 mg/kg/day IV (q8h)
Cefotaxime	100-150 mg/kg/day IV (q8h)
Gentamicin	
<1 week	5 mg/kg/day IV (q12h)
>1 week	7.5 mg/kg/day IV (q8h)
Penicillin G	250,000-400,000 units/kg/day IV (q8h)

discontinued, the cerebrospinal fluid should be cultured again. If the culture is positive for bacteria, a second course of therapy is indicated.

Citrobacter diversus infections often result in a hemorrhagic necrosis of the brain with liquefaction of the cerebral white matter and abscess formation (Foreman et al, 1984). These abscesses are readily identified on CT. Surgical drainage is seldom indicated and could cause further damage to the overlying preserved cortex.

Although the overall mortality rate for neonatal bacterial meningitis is less than 50%, significant neurologic sequelae are immediately evident in 50% of survivors. The more common sequelae include mental and motor disabilities, hydrocephalus, convulsive disorders, deafness, and vision loss. Even when the head circumference is normal, follow-up CT is essential to exclude underlying hydrocephalus.

Meningitis in Infants and Young Children

For children from 6 weeks to 3 months of age, group B *Streptococcus* remains a leading cause of meningitis, while *E. coli* becomes less common. Other important organisms are *Streptococcus pneumoniae, L. monocytogenes,* and *Salmonella. Haemophilus influenzae* first appears after 3 months and becomes the predominant organism, along with *S. pneumoniae* and *Neisseria meningitidis,* up to age 5.

Clinical Features. The onset of meningitis may be insidious or fulminating. The typical clinical findings include fever, irritability, and neck stiffness. A bulging fontanelle is noted in young infants. Headache, vomiting, and lethargy are the initial manifestations after the fontanelle has closed. Seizures generally occur during the first 24 hours and may be the first manifestations. Once seizures have occurred, the state of consciousness declines. Seizures can be focal or generalized and may be difficult to control. The overall incidence of seizures in children with

meningitis is 30%, but the rate is higher with *H. influenzae.*

Examination reveals a sick and irritable child who resists being touched or moved. Ophthalmoscopic findings are usually normal or only minimal papilledema. Focal neurologic signs are unusual except in tuberculous meningitis or in cases when abscess formation has occurred.

The rapidity with which neurologic function declines depends on the severity of cerebral edema and cerebral vasculitis. Death may ensue from brainstem compression caused by transtentorial herniation. Peripheral vascular collapse can result from brainstem herniation, endotoxic shock, or adrenal failure. Sixty percent of children with meningococcemia have a characteristic petechial or hemorrhagic rash. The rash, although generalized, is most prominent below the waist.

Neck stiffness, characterized by limited mobility and pain on attempted flexion of the head, is caused by meningeal irritation. Other signs of meningeal irritation are those of Kernig and Brudzinski. Both are tested with the patient supine. The *Kernig sign* is marked by pain and resistance to extending the knee with the leg flexed at the hip; the *Brudzinski sign* is spontaneous flexion at the hips when the neck is passively flexed. These signs of meningeal irritation can be noted in subarachnoid hemorrhage as well as in infectious meningitis.

Diagnosis. Lumbar puncture and examination of the cerebrospinal fluid are essential for the diagnosis of bacterial meningitis. However, since bacterial meningitis is often associated with septicemia, cultures of the blood, urine, and nasopharynx are indicated as well. The peripheral white blood cell count, especially immature granulocytes, is usually increased. Peripheral leukocytosis is much more common in bacterial than in viral infections but does not rule out viral meningitis. Platelet count is important because some infections are associated with thrombocytopenia. Blood glucose concentration must be measured concurrently for proper evaluation of the cerebrospinal fluid concentration of glucose. Serum electrolytes, especially sodium, should be measured as well. Inappropriate antidiuretic hormone secretion is present in the majority of patients with acute bacterial meningitis. A tuberculin skin test should be administered to every child at risk for tuberculous meningitis.

Lumbar puncture must be performed as quickly as possible when bacterial meningitis is suspected. Generalized increased intracranial pressure is always part of acute bacterial meningitis and is not a contraindication to lumbar puncture. Information to be derived from the procedure includes opening and closing pressures, appearance, white blood cell count with differential count, red blood cell count, concentrations of glucose and protein, Gram stain, and culture. The characteristic findings are increased pressure, a cloudy appearance, a cellular response of several thousand polymorphonuclear leukocytes, a reduction in the concentration of glucose to less than half of that in the plasma, and an elevated protein concentration. However, the classic findings of bacterial meningitis may vary with the organism, the timing of the lumbar puncture, the prior use of antibiotics, and the immunocompetence of the host.

Treatment. Dexamethasone, 0.15 mg/kg every 6 hours for 4 days, should be administered immediately. Children treated with dexamethasone become afebrile more quickly and have an improved neurologic outcome and a lower incidence of postmeningitic deafness (Lebel et al, 1988; Odio et al, 1991).

Ampicillin and chloramphenicol had been the standard initial therapy for infants and children younger than 5 years of age in whom bacterial meningitis was suspected before identification of the offending organism, because these two antibiotics cover the three organisms that account for the majority of cases (Table 4–7). However, newer cephalosporins (cefotaxime, ceftriaxone, and cefuroxime) are now considered as effective as ampicillin and chloramphenicol in the initial treatment of meningitis and are acceptable alternatives (Committee on Infectious Disease, 1988; Schaad et al, 1990). Gram stain identification is useful but can be misleading, and the final choice of antibiotic therapy should await the results of culture and antibiotic sensitivity.

There are several special cases in the choice of initial antimicrobials to treat bacterial meningitis. Meningitis in children with a ventricular shunt in place is usually caused by a staphylococcal species, and nafcillin may be added to the preceding choices or given alone if gram-positive cocci are present on smear. Meningitis secondary to chronic sinusitis or dental infection is frequently caused by anaerobic and aerobic organisms. Penicillin G and chloramphenicol are therefore reasonable choices for initial therapy, although cefotaxime may be needed for some gram-negative organisms not covered by chloramphenicol. Meningitis following trauma is usually caused by *S. pneumoniae,* whereas meningitis following neurosurgical procedures may be due to either streptococcal or staphylococcal organisms. Gram-negative organisms may be responsible as well, and a combination of penicillin G and cefotaxime is recommended.

Once a specific organism is identified, an appropriate antibiotic or combination of antibiotics is chosen (Table 4–9).

The outcome for infants and children with bacterial meningitis depends on the infecting organism and the speed with which appropriate antibiotic therapy is initiated. Ten percent of children have persistent bilateral or unilateral hearing loss following bacterial meningitis, and 4% have neurologic deficits. The incidence of hearing loss is 31% following infection with *S. pneumoniae* and 6% with *H. influenzae.* Hearing loss occurs early and is probably not related to the choice of antibiotic. Children with neurologic deficits are at risk for epilepsy (Pomeroy et al, 1990).

Meningitis in Older Children

H. influenzae, S. pneumoniae, and *N. meningitidis* account for most cases of bacterial meningitis in previously healthy school-age children in the United States (Bonadio et al, 1990), whereas *Mycobacterium tuberculosis* is a leading cause of meningitis in economically deprived populations. The symptoms of bacterial meningitis in school-age children do not differ substantially from those encountered in preschool children. The reader is referred to the prior section on clinical features and treatment.

Penicillin G is the treatment of choice for *S. pneumoniae* or *N. meningitidis.*

Tuberculous Meningitis

Worldwide, tuberculosis remains a leading cause of morbidity and death in children. In the United States it represents less than 5% of bacterial meningitis in children but occurs with higher frequency where sanitation is poor. Children are infected by inhalation of the organism from adults. Tuberculosis occurs first in the lungs and is then disseminated to other organs within 6 months.

Clinical Features. The peak incidence of tuberculous meningitis is between 6 months and 2 years of age. First symptoms tend to be more insidious than with other bacterial meningitides, but

Table 4–9 ◆ Antibiotic Dosages for Children

Drug	Dosage
Ampicillin	200-300 mg/kg/day IV (q6h)
Cefotaxime	200 mg/kg/day IV (q6h)
Ceftriaxone	80-100 mg/kg/day IV (q12h)
Chloramphenicol	75-100 mg/kg/day IV (q6h)
Penicillin G	250,000 units/kg/day IV (q6h)
Vancomycin	40-60 mg/kg/day IV (q6h)

they sometimes progress in a fulminating fashion. Most often, fever develops first and the child becomes listless and irritable. Irritability may be caused in part by headache, which is a common feature. Vomiting and abdominal pain are sometimes associated. Headache and vomiting increase in frequency and severity and are accompanied by signs of meningismus during the second week after onset of fever.

Cerebral infarction occurs in 30% to 40% of affected children. Seizures may occur early but more often appear after meningismus is established. Consciousness declines progressively, and focal neurologic deficits are noted. Most common are cranial neuropathies and hemipareses. Papilledema occurs relatively early in the course. Without treatment, death is invariable within 3 to 5 weeks.

Diagnosis. Tuberculosis must be considered in any child with a household contact. General use of tuberculin skin testing in children is critical to early detection. In the early stages children with tuberculous meningitis may have only fever. The peripheral white blood cell count is generally elevated to between 10,000 and 20,000 cells/mm³. Hyponatremia and hypochloremia are frequently present because of inappropriate secretion of antidiuretic hormone. The cerebrospinal fluid is usually cloudy and increased in pressure. The leukocyte count in the cerebrospinal fluid may range from 10 to 250 cells/mm³ and rarely exceeds 500. Lymphocytes predominate. The glucose concentration declines throughout the course of the illness and is generally less than 35 mg/dl (1.8 mmol/L). Conversely, the protein concentration increases steadily and is usually greater than 100 mg/dl (1 g/L).

Smears of cerebrospinal fluid stained by acid-fast technique generally demonstrate the bacillus. Recovery of the organism from the cerebrospinal fluid is not always successful even when guinea pig inoculation is used.

Cranial CT is useful to show basilar enhancement, cerebral infarction, hydrocephalus, and tuberculoma (Curless and Mitchell, 1991).

Treatment. The prognosis for survival and for neurologic recovery is enhanced by early treatment. Once a child's skin test is positive for the organism, isoniazid therapy is initiated even if the child is asymptomatic. Complete neurologic recovery is unlikely once the child becomes comatose. Mortality rates of 20% are recorded even when treatment is initiated early.

The drugs currently recommended for treatment of tuberculous meningitis include isoniazid, 20 mg/kg/day orally up to 500 mg/day; streptomycin, 20

mg/kg/day intramuscularly up to 1 g/day; and rifampin, 15 mg/kg/day orally up to 600 mg/day. Streptomycin and rifampin are continued for 8 weeks after clinical and laboratory improvement have been established. Isoniazid is continued for 2 years.

The use of corticosteroids to reduce inflammation had been controversial but is now considered appropriate treatment to reduce inflammation and cerebral edema.

Communicating hydrocephalus is a common complication of tuberculous meningitis because of impaired reabsorption of cerebrospinal fluid. The size of the ventricles must be assessed by CT at periodic intervals and whenever unexplained deterioration of mental function occurs. Before the infection is brought under control, communicating hydrocephalus may be treated by repeated lumbar punctures and acetazolamide. In many cases obstructive hydrocephalus develops later, and the children in these cases require a surgical shunt.

Brain Abscess

The factors commonly predisposing to pyogenic brain abscess in children are meningitis, chronic otitis media, mastoiditis, and congenital heart disease (Sáez-Llorens et al, 1989). Brain abscesses in the newborn are almost always the result of meningitis caused by *C. diversus* and other species of Enterobacteriaceae. Pyogenic abscesses in children younger than 5 months but beyond the neonatal period are uncommon and most often occur in children with hydrocephalus and shunt infection. The organisms most often responsible are species of *Staphylococcus*.

After 5 months of age congenital heart disease accounts for half of all cases of pyogenic brain abscess (Wong et al, 1989). The infecting organisms are diverse, and many abscesses contain a mixed flora. Coagulase-positive *S. aureus* and anaerobic *Streptococcus* are the organisms most frequently recovered. In up to 20% of cases no organism can be recovered.

Clinical Features. The clinical features of brain abscess, like any other space-occupying lesion, depend on the age of the child and the location of the mass. Encapsulation of the abscess is preceded by a period of cerebritis characterized by fever, headache, and lethargy. Seizures may also occur, but in the absence of seizures the initial symptoms may not be severe enough to arouse suspicion of cerebral infection. If the period of cerebritis is not recognized, the initial clinical manifestations are the same as with other mass lesions. Infants have abnormal head growth, a bulging fontanelle, failure to thrive, and sometimes seizures. Older children show signs of increased intracranial pressure and focal neurologic dysfunction. Fever is present in only 60% of cases, and meningeal irritation is relatively uncommon. Therefore, on the basis of clinical features alone, pyogenic brain abscess is difficult to differentiate from other mass lesions such as brain tumor. About 80% of abscesses are in the cerebral hemispheres. Hemiparesis, hemianopia, and seizures are the usual clinical features. Cerebellar abscess most often results from chronic otitis and is manifest as nystagmus and ataxia.

Diagnosis. The combination of headache and papilledema, with or without focal neurologic dysfunction, suggests the possibility of a mass lesion and leads to CT. Most abscesses appear as an area of decreased density surrounded by a rim of intense enhancement referred to as a ring lesion. This ring lesion, although characteristic, does not establish the diagnosis. Malignant brain tumors may have a similar appearance (Figure 4–7). Ring enhancement occurs during the late stages of cerebritis, just before capsule formation. After the capsule forms, the diameter of the ring decreases and the center becomes more hypodense. Multiple abscesses may be present.

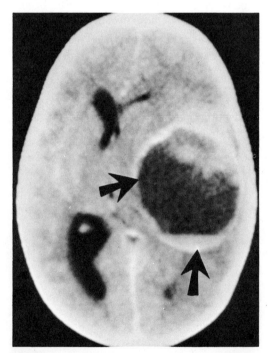

Figure 4–7 Ring enhancement surrounding a malignant tumor. A large cavity with a mural nodule is surrounded by a ring of contrast enhancement (arrows). The mass is producing falx herniation.

Treatment. The development of CT has altered the management of cerebral abscess. Previously, surgical drainage was initiated as soon as abscess formation was identified. Now even encapsulated abscesses are treated medically and the progress is followed with serial scans (Johnson et al, 1988).

The initial step in treatment is to reduce brain swelling by the use of corticosteroids. This is followed by an intravenous antibiotic regimen that generally includes a penicillinase-resistant penicillin such as methicillin, 300 mg/kg/day, and chloramphenicol, 100 mg/kg/day. This combination is selected for its effectiveness against *Staphylococcus* and mixed gram-negative organisms. If an organism can be identified by culture of spinal fluid or blood, more specific antibiotic therapy is selected. In general, penicillin G is preferable to ampicillin if penicillin-sensitive organisms are recovered.

If medical therapy does not resolve the abscess, surgical drainage is necessary. Even in such cases, prolonged medical therapy before surgery increases the success of total excision.

Subdural and Epidural Empyema

Meningitis in infants and sinusitis in older children are the most common factors causing infection in the subdural space. The subdural space is sterile in children with bacterial meningitis but can become contaminated by organisms if a subdural tap is performed before the subarachnoid space is sterilized with antibiotics or by secondary thrombophlebitis of perforating cerebral veins. In older children subdural and epidural abscesses are usually caused by penetrating head injuries or chronic mastoiditis.

Infections of the subdural space are difficult to contain and may extend over an entire hemisphere.

Clinical Features. Subdural empyema produces increased intracranial pressure because of mass effect, cerebral edema, and vasculitis. Vasculitis leads to thrombosis of cortical veins, resulting in focal neurologic dysfunction as well as increased intracranial pressure. Children with subdural infections are very sick. They have headache, fever, vomiting, seizures, and states of decreasing consciousness. Unilateral and alternating hemipareses are common. Children who are comatose have papilledema.

Diagnosis. Subdural empyema should be suspected in children with meningitis whose condition declines after an initial period of recovery or in children who continue to have increased intracranial pressure of uncertain cause. Examination of the cerebrospinal fluid may not be helpful; sometimes the fluid is normal. The usual abnormality is a mixed cellular response, generally less than 100 cells/mm³, with a lymphocytic predominance. The glucose concentration is normal, and the protein concentration is only mildly elevated.

CT is particularly helpful in demonstrating a subdural or epidural abscess. The infected collection appears as a lens-shaped mass of increased lucency just beneath the skull. A shift of midline structures is generally present.

In infants subdural puncture can provide a specimen of the abscess for identification of the organism. Subdural puncture can also be used to drain much of the abscess.

Treatment. The child with subdural or epidural empyema must be treated with corticosteroids to decrease intracranial pressure, antibiotics to eradicate the organisms, and anticonvulsants for seizures. Surgical drainage of subdural empyema had been considered an absolute necessity; it now appears that some can be treated medically, using CT to monitor progress (Leys et al, 1986).

FUNGAL INFECTIONS

Fungi exist in two forms: molds and yeasts. Molds are filamentous and divided into segments by hyphae. Yeasts are unicellular organisms surrounded by a thick cell wall and sometimes a capsule. Several fungi exist as yeast in tissue but are filamentous when grown in culture. Such fungi are said to be dimorphic. The common fungal pathogens are listed in Table 4–10.

Fungal infections of the central nervous system may result in acute, subacute, or chronic meningitis; solitary or multiple abscesses; and granulomas (Bell, 1981). Fungal infections of the nervous system are most common in children who are immunosuppressed, especially those with leukemia or acidosis. Fungal infections also occur in children who are immunocompetent. *Cryptococcus neofor-*

Table 4–10 ◆ Common Fungal Pathogens

Yeast Forms
1. *Cryptococcus neoformans*
2. *Candida*

Dimorphic Forms
1. *Histoplasma capsulatum*
2. *Blastomyces dermatitidis*
3. *Coccidioides immitis*

Mold Forms
1. *Aspergillus* species

mans and *Coccidioides immitis* are the leading causes of fungal meningitis in immunocompetent children.

Cryptococcal Meningitis

C. neoformans is carried by birds, especially pigeons, and is widely disseminated in soil. Human infection is acquired by inhalation. The organism is disseminated in the blood but has a predilection for the central nervous system. It is an important cause of subacute and chronic meningoencephalitis.

Clinical Features. Cryptococcal meningitis is uncommon before age 10, and perhaps only 10% of cases occur before age 20. Males are affected more often than females. Most children with cryptococcal meningitis are immunocompetent.

First symptoms are usually insidious; chronic headache is the major feature. The headache waxes and wanes but eventually becomes continuous and associated with nausea, vomiting, and lethargy. Body temperature may remain normal, especially in older children and adults, but younger children often have low-grade fever. Personality and behavioral changes are relatively common. The child becomes moody, listless, and sometimes frankly psychotic. Increased intracranial pressure is characterized by blurred vision, diplopia, and papilledema. Seizures and focal neurologic dysfunction are not early features but are signs of vasculitis, hydrocephalus, and granuloma formation.

Diagnosis. The diagnosis of cryptococcal meningitis is often missed even when suspected. The cerebrospinal fluid may be normal but more often demonstrates an increased opening pressure and a lymphocytic leukocytosis that generally averages fewer than 100 cells/mm³. The protein concentration is almost always elevated, generally greater than 100 mg/dl (1 g/L), and the glucose concentration is usually less than 40 mg/dl (2 mmol/L). Rapid diagnosis is possible if the fungus can be demonstrated in cerebrospinal fluid by the India ink technique. The cryptococcus is the only encapsulated fungus to invade the central nervous system and has a characteristic appearance on smear. However, the organism is not usually present in the lumbar subarachnoid space and must be obtained from cerebrospinal fluid at the base of the brain. This can be achieved either by removing large volumes of cerebrospinal fluid by lumbar puncture or by cisternal puncture.

Diagnosis has been made easier by the development of a latex agglutination test that reacts to the polysaccharide capsule of the organism. The test is reasonably accurate but may produce false-negative results, and serologic studies do not replace the actual demonstration of the organism. The latex agglutination technique can also be performed on the cerebrospinal fluid; titers of 1:8 or greater are considered significant and support the diagnosis of cryptococcal meningitis.

Treatment. Amphotericin B is the drug of choice for the treatment of cryptococcal meningitis (Bell, 1981). It is given intravenously diluted with 5% dextrose and water in a drug concentration no greater than 1 mg/10 ml of fluid. Nephrotoxicity is the limiting factor in achieving desirable blood levels. The intravenous regimen is generally the same for all fungal infections of the nervous system and is summarized in Table 4–11. The total dose varies with the response and the side effects but is usually in the range of 1500 to 2000 mg/1.7 m² of body surface.

The toxic effects include chills, fever, nausea, and vomiting. Anemia and nephrotoxicity must be monitored with frequent blood counts and urinalyses. Renal impairment is manifested by the appearance of cells or casts in the urine, elevated blood urea nitrogen concentration, and decreased creatinine clearance. When renal impairment occurs, the drug must be discontinued and restarted at a lower dose.

Patients who do not tolerate amphotericin can be treated with flucytosine or miconazole. Flucytosine is rarely effective alone but must be used in combination with low-dose amphotericin B. It is given orally at a dosage of 100 to 150 mg/kg/day in four divided doses. The intravenous dosage of miconazole is 30 mg/kg/day in three divided doses over a 30-minute period of infusion.

Seriously ill patients, treated late in the course of the disease, should also be given intrathecally administered amphotericin B and miconazole.

The efficacy of therapy can be followed by demonstrating a decline of the agglutination titer in the cerebrospinal fluid. Periodic CT is necessary to monitor for the development of hydrocephalus.

Table 4–11 ◆ Dosage Schedule for Amphotericin B

Mild Cases
1. 0.1 mg/kg/day infused intravenously over 4-6 hours
2. Slowly increased up to 1.0 mg/kg/day as tolerated

Severe Cases
1. 0.25 mg/kg/day infused intravenously over 4-6 hours
2. Slowly increased up to 1.0 mg/kg/day as tolerated

Coccidioidomycosis

C. immitis is endemic in the San Joaquin Valley of California and all southwestern states. Infection is by inhalation; almost 90% of individuals become infected within 10 years of moving into an endemic area. Only 40% of patients become symptomatic; the other 60% are identified only by skin test.

Clinical Features. Malaise, fever, cough, myalgia, and chest pain follow respiratory infection. The pulmonary infection is self-limited. The fungus is disseminated from the lung to other organs in only 1 person in 400. The dissemination rate is considerably higher in infants than in older children and adults.

Coccidioidal meningitis is almost always caused by hematogenous spread from lung to meninges but sometimes occurs by direct extension following infection of the skull. Symptoms of meningitis develop 2 to 4 weeks after respiratory symptoms begin. The major features are headache, apathy, and confusion. These symptoms may persist for weeks or months without concurrent seizures, meningismus, or focal neurologic disturbances. If the meningitis is allowed to become chronic, hydrocephalus eventually develops because the basilar meningitis prevents reabsorption of cerebrospinal fluid.

Diagnosis. Coccidioidal meningitis should be suspected in patients living in endemic areas when headache develops following an acute respiratory infection. Skin hypersensitivity among individuals living in an endemic area is not helpful, since a large percentage of the population is exposed and has a skin test positive for the organism. The cerebrospinal fluid generally demonstrates increased pressure and a lymphocytic cellular response of 50 to 500 cells/mm³. Eosinophils are frequently present as well. The protein concentration ranges from 100 to 500 mg/dl (1 to 5 g/L), and the glucose concentration is less than 35 mg/dl (1.8 mmol/L). The diagnosis is confirmed by isolation of the fungus, but this is often difficult to accomplish. Complement-fixing antibodies appear in the blood and cerebrospinal fluid. A positive serologic test in the cerebrospinal fluid is diagnostic, but false-negative results are possible.

Treatment. Amphotericin B is the drug of choice for coccidioidal meningitis. It must be administered both intravenously (Table 4–11) and intrathecally. The initial intrathecal dose is 0.1 mg for the first three injections and is then increased to 0.25 to 0.5 mg three or four times each week. Treatment must be prolonged, and some recommend that weekly intrathecal injections be continued indefinitely. Adverse reactions to intrathecal administration include aseptic meningitis and pain in the back and legs.

Miconazole may be administered intravenously and intrathecally to patients unable to tolerate high doses of amphotericin B. Ketoconazole, a synthetic antifungal agent, has excellent activity against *C. immitis* in culture but penetrates the cerebrospinal fluid poorly. It is not recommended for systemic treatment of coccidioidal meningitis.

Candidal Meningoencephalitis

Candida is a common inhabitant of the mouth, vagina, and intestinal tract. Ordinarily it causes no symptoms; however, it can multiply and become an important pathogen in children who are immunosuppressed, taking multiple antibiotics, suffering from debilitating diseases, and being treated with long-term vascular catheters. The most common sites of infection are the mouth (thrush), skin, and vagina. Candidal meningitis is almost unheard of in normal, nonhospitalized children.

Clinical Features. *Candida* reaches the brain and other organs by vascular dissemination. The brain is less often involved than other organs, and the prominent manifestations of candidal sepsis include fever, lethargy, and vomiting. Hepatosplenomegaly and arthritis may be present.

Cerebral involvement can be in the form of meningitis, abscess formation, or both. When meningoencephalitis is present, the clinical manifestations are fever, vomiting, meningismus, papilledema, and seizures leading to states of decreased consciousness. In some individuals a single large cerebral abscess forms that is manifested as focal neurologic dysfunction and papilledema.

Diagnosis. Cerebral candidiasis should be suspected when unexplained fever develops in children with risk factors for disseminated disease. The organism can be isolated from blood, joint effusion fluid, or cerebrospinal fluid. When meningitis is present, a predominantly neutrophilic response is present in the cerebrospinal fluid associated with a protein concentration that is generally 100 mg/dl (1 g/L). The glucose concentration is only slightly reduced. Children who have a candidal abscess rather than meningitis are likely to have normal or near-normal cerebrospinal fluid. Instead a mass lesion resembling a pyogenic abscess or tumor is demonstrated on CT.

Treatment. When candidal infections develop in children because of indwelling vascular catheters, the catheter must be removed. Amphotericin B and flucytosine are used together and thought to have a synergistic effect. Dosages are the same as for other fungal infections, and the drugs should be administered for 6 to 12 weeks, depending on the efficacy of therapy and presence of adverse reactions.

Other Fungal Infections

Histoplasmosis is endemic in the central United States and causes pulmonary infection. Miliary spread is unusual. Neurologic histoplasmosis may take the form of leptomeningitis, focal abscess, or multiple granulomas. Blastomycosis is primarily a disease of North America. It reaches the brain by hematogenous spread from the lungs and produces multiple abscesses that give the appearance of metastatic disease on CT. Cellular response in the cerebrospinal fluid is markedly increased when fungi produce meningitis and may be normal or only mildly increased when abscess formation occurs. Amphotericin B is the mainstay of therapy for fungal infections; miconazole is used in combination with amphotericin B against *Histoplasma capsulatum*.

◆ Idiopathic Intracranial Hypertension (Pseudotumor Cerebri)

The term "pseudotumor cerebri" is used to characterize increased intracranial pressure in the absence of mass lesion or hydrocephalus. The syndrome may have an identifiable, specific underlying cause or may be idiopathic. A specific cause can usually be found in children younger than 6 years, whereas most idiopathic cases occur after age 11. Between 6 and 11 years of age, half of cases are idiopathic and half are symptomatic (Couch et al, 1985).

Some causes of pseudotumor are listed in Table 4–12. A cause-and-effect relationship has not been established in all of these conditions. The most frequent causes are otitis media, head trauma, the use of certain drugs and vitamins, and feeding following malnutrition.

Idiopathic intracranial hypertension is primarily a disorder of the second and third decades. Women are more often affected than men, but in children both sexes are affected equally (Baker et al, 1989). Brain volume is enlarged because of increased cerebral blood volume, cerebral edema, or both. Reabsorption of cerebrospinal fluid is thought to be impaired, but hydrocephalus does not occur.

Clinical Features. Headache is the most common manifestation but is not invariable. Other frequent symptoms are diplopia, caused by abducens nerve palsy, and transient visual obscurations (Giu-

Table 4–12 ◆ Secondary Pseudotumor Cerebri

Drugs
1. Corticosteroid withdrawal
2. Nalidixic acid
3. Oral contraceptives
4. Tetracycline
5. Vitamin A

Systemic Disorders
1. Guillain-Barré syndrome
2. Iron deficiency anemia
3. Leukemia
4. Polycythemia vera
5. Protein malnutrition
6. Systemic lupus erythematosus

Head Trauma

Infections
1. Otitis media
2. Sinusitis

Metabolic
1. Adrenal insufficiency
2. Diabetic ketoacidosis (treatment)
3. Galactosemia
4. Hyperadrenalism
5. Hyperthyroidism
6. Hypoparathyroidism
7. Menarche
8. Pregnancy

seffi et al, 1991). Some children have nausea, vomiting, neck stiffness, tinnitus, paresthesias, and ataxia (Round and Keane, 1988). Most are not acutely ill, and mentation is normal.

Neurologic examination is unremarkable except for papilledema and abducens nerve palsy. No signs of focal neurologic dysfunction are observed. The major concern is for vision. If the syndrome is left untreated, some children have progressive papilledema and optic atrophy. Loss of vision may be rapid and severe (Baker et al, 1989). Early diagnosis and treatment are therefore essential to preserve vision.

Diagnosis. Pseudotumor cerebri is a diagnosis of exclusion. If a child has headache and papilledema, an enhanced CT scan or MRI is needed to exclude a mass lesion or hydrocephalus. Results of imaging studies are usually normal in children with pseudotumor cerebri. In some the ventricles are small and the normal sulcal markings may be obliterated by the increased cerebral volume.

Underlying causes of pseudotumor cerebri must be excluded by careful history and physical examination. Ordinarily these are easily identified.

Treatment. The goals of therapy are to relieve headache and preserve vision. A single lumbar puncture, with the closing pressure reduced to half of the opening pressure, is sufficient to reverse the process in most cases. The mechanism by which this is effective is unknown, but a transitory change in cerebrospinal fluid dynamics seems to be sufficient to readjust the pressure.

Children with pseudotumor cerebri are commonly treated with acetazolamide, 10 mg/kg/day, following the initial lumbar puncture. Whether this is an important addition to lumbar puncture is not clear. If symptoms return, lumbar puncture should be repeated on subsequent days. Serial lumbar punctures are rarely needed.

Occasionally children continue to have increased intracranial pressure and evidence of progressive optic neuropathy despite the use of lumbar puncture and acetazolamide. In such patients studies should be repeated to look for a cause other than idiopathic pseudotumor cerebri. If none is found, a 2-week course of dexamethasone is appropriate. If this fails to relieve symptoms, optic nerve fenestration or lumboperitoneal shunt may be needed (Johnston et al, 1988).

References

Allen GS, Ahn HS, Preziosi TJ, et al: Cerebral arterial spasm— A controlled trial of nimodipine in patients with subarachnoid hemorrhage. N Engl J Med 308:619, 1983.

Baker RS, Baumann RJ, Buncic JR, et al: Idiopathic intracranial hypertension (pseudotumor cerebri) in pediatric patients. Pediatr Neurol 5:5-11, 1989.

Bell WE: Treatment of fungal infections of the central nervous system. Ann Neurol 9:417, 1981.

Bonadio WA, Mannenbach M, Krippendorf R: Bacterial meningitis in older children. AJDC 144:463, 1990.

Cairncross G, Laperriere NJ: Low-grade gliomas: To treat or not to treat? Reply. Arch Neurol 47:1139, 1990.

Cohen ME, Duffner PK: Ependymomas. In Cohen ME, Duffner PK, eds: Brain Tumors in Children. Raven Press, New York, 1984, p 136.

Committee on Infectious Disease: Treatment of bacterial meningitis. Pediatrics 81:904, 1988.

Couch R, Camfield PR, Tibbles JAR: The changing picture of pseudotumor cerebri in children. Can J Neurol Sci 12:48, 1985.

Curless RG, Mitchell CD: Central nervous system tuberculosis in children. Pediatr Neurol 7:270, 1991.

Cutler RWP, Spertell RB: Cerebrospinal fluid: A selective review. Ann Neurol 11:1, 1982.

Dohrmann GJ, Farwell JR, Flannery JT: Ependymomas and ependymoblastomas in children. J Neurosurg 45:273, 1976.

Dropcho EJ, Wisoff JH, Walker RW, et al: Supratentorial malignant gliomas in childhood: A review of fifty cases. Ann Neurol 22:355, 1987.

Duffner PK, Cohen ME, Myers MH, et al: Survival of children with brain tumors: SEER program, 1973–1980. Neurology 36:597, 1986.

Dykes FD, Dunbar B, Lazarra A, et al: Posthemorrhagic hydrocephalus in high-risk preterm infants: Natural history, management and long-term outcome. J Pediatr 114:611, 1989.

Ellenbogen RG, Winston KR, Kupsky WJ: Tumors of the choroid plexus in children. Neurosurgery 25:327, 1989.

Emery JR, Peabody JL: Head position affects intracranial pressure in newborn infants. J Pediatr 103:950, 1983.

Fenichel GM, Webster DL, Wong WKT: Intracranial hemorrhage in the term newborn. Arch Neurol 41:30, 1984.

Fishman RA: Cerebrospinal Fluid in Disease of the Nervous System. WB Saunders, Philadelphia, 1980.

Foreman SD, Smith EE, Ryan NJ, et al: Neonatal *Citrobacter* meningitis: Pathogenesis of cerebral abscess formation. Ann Neurol 16:655, 1984.

Giuseffi V, Wall M, Siegel PZ, et al: Symptoms and disease associations in idiopathic intracranial hypertension (pseudotumor cerebri): A case-control study. Neurology 41:239, 1991.

Gower DJ, Baker AL, Bell WO, et al: Contraindications to lumbar puncture as defined by computed cranial tomography. J Neurol Neurosurg Psychiatry 50:1071, 1987.

Graf CJ, Perret GE, Torner JC: Bleeding from cerebral arteriovenous malformation as part of their natural history. J Neurosurg 58:331, 1983.

Graus F, Walker RW, Allen JC: Brain metastases in children. J Pediatr 103:558, 1983.

Harsh GR, Edwards MSB, Wilson CB: Intracranial arachnoid cysts in children. J Neurosurg 64:835, 1986.

Hill A, Perlman J, Volpe JJ: Relationship of pneumothorax to occurrence of intraventricular hemorrhage in the premature newborn. Pediatrics 69:144, 1982.

Johnson DL, Markle BM, Wiedermann BL, et al: Treatment of intracranial abscesses associated with sinusitis in children and adolescents. J Pediatr 113:15, 1988.

Johnston I, Besser M, Morgan MK: Cerebrospinal fluid diversion in the treatment of benign intracranial hypertension. J Neurosurg 69:195, 1988.

Kassell NF, Torner JC: The international cooperative study on timing of aneurysm surgery—An update. Stroke 15:566, 1984.

Kreusser KL, Tarby TJ, Kovnar E, et al: Serial lumbar punctures for at least temporary amelioration of neonatal posthemorrhagic hydrocephalus. Pediatrics 75:719, 1985.

Lazzara A, Ahmann P, Dykes F, et al: Clinical predictability of intraventricular hemorrhage in preterm infants. Pediatrics 65:30, 1980.

Le Roux PD, Jardine DS, Loeser JD: Pediatric intracranial pressure monitoring in hypoxic and nonhypoxic brain injury. Child Nerv Syst 7:34, 1991.

Lebel MH, Freij BJ, Syrogiannopoulos GA, et al: Dexamethasone therapy for bacterial meningitis: Results of two double-blind, placebo controlled trials. N Engl J Med 319:964, 1988.

Leys D, Destee A, Petit H, et al: Management of subdural intracranial empyemas should not always require surgery. J Neurol Neurosurg Psychiatry 49:635, 1986.

Mangiardi JR, Daras M, Geller ME, et al: Cocaine-related intracranial hemorrhage: Report of nine cases and review. Acta Neurol Scand 77:177, 1988.

Marrow PJ, Dransfield DA, Mott SM, et al: Posthemorrhagic hydrocephalus: Use of an intravenous-type catheter for cerebrospinal fluid drainage. AJDC 145:1141, 1991.

McCarton-Daum C, Danziger A, Ruff H, et al: Periventricular low density as a predictor of neurobehavioral outcome in very low-birthweight infants. Dev Med Child Neurol 25:559, 1983.

McMenamin JB, Shackleford GD, Volpe JJ: Outcome of neonatal intraventricular hemorrhage with periventricular echodense lesions. Ann Neurol 15:285, 1984.

Mohr JP: Neurological manifestations and factors related to therapeutic decisions. In Wilson CB, Stein BM, eds: Intracranial Arteriovenous Malformations. Williams & Wilkins, Baltimore, 1984, p 1.

Naidich TP, McLone DG, Radkowski MA: Intracranial arachnoid cysts. Pediatr Neurosci 12:112, 1986.

Odio CM, Faingezicht I, Paris M, et al: The beneficial effects of early dexamethasone administration in infants and children with bacterial meningitis. N Engl J Med 324:1525, 1991.

Ogilvy CS: Radiation therapy for arteriovenous malformations: A review. Neurosurgery 26:725, 1990.

Packer RJ, Sutton LN, Rosenstock JG, et al: Pineal region tumors of childhood. Pediatrics 74:97, 1984.

Palma L, Russo A, Mercuri S: Cystic cerebral astrocytomas in infancy and childhood: Long-term results. Child's Brain 10:79, 1983.

Philip AGS, Allen WC, Tito AM, et al: Intraventricular hemorrhage in preterm infants: Declining incidence in the 1980s. Pediatrics 84:797, 1989.

Pomeroy SL, Holmes SJ, Dodge PR, et al: Seizures and other neurologic sequelae of bacterial meningitis in children. N Engl J Med 323:1651, 1990.

Round R, Keane JR: The minor symptoms of increased intracranial pressure: 101 patients with benign intracranial hypertension. Neurology 38:1461, 1988.

Sáez-Llorens XJ, Umama MA, Odio CM, et al: Brain abscess in infants and children. Pediatr Infect Dis 8:449, 1989.

Schaad UB, Suter S, Gianella-Borradori A, et al: A comparison of ceftriaxone and cerfuroxime for the treatment of bacterial meningitis in children. N Engl J Med 322:141, 1990.

Scher MS, Wright FA, Lockman LA, et al: Intraventricular hemorrhage in the fullterm neonate. Arch Neurol 39:769, 1982.

Schulte FJ, Herrmann HD, Muller D, et al: Pineal region tumors of childhood. Eur J Pediatr 146:233, 1987.

Schut L, Packer RJ, Sutton LE: Medulloblastomas/primitive neuroectodermal tumors in children. Int Pediatr 4:172, 1989.

Shaw EG: Low-grade gliomas: To treat or not to treat? A radiation oncologist's viewpoint. Arch Neurol 47:1138, 1990.

Shinnar S, Gammon K, Bergman EW Jr, et al: Management of hydrocephalus in infancy: Use of acetazolamide and furosemide to avoid cerebrospinal fluid shunts. J Pediatr 107:31, 1985.

Steer CR: Barbiturate therapy in the management of cerebral ischemia. Dev Med Child Neurol 24:219, 1982.

Tomita T, McLone DG, Yasue M: Cerebral primitive neuroectodermal tumors in childhood. Neuro-oncology 6:233, 1988.

Vannucci RC: Current and potentially new management strategies for perinatal hypoxic-ischemic encephalopathy. Pediatrics 85:961, 1990.

Volpe JJ: Intraventricular hemorrhage in the premature infant—Current concepts. Parts I and II. Ann Neurol 25(3):109, 1989.

Weibers DO, Whisnant JP, O'Fallon WM: The natural history of unruptured intracranial aneurysms. N Engl J Med 304:696, 1981.

Weisberg LA: Cerebral computed tomography in the diagnosis of supratentorial astrocytoma. Comput Tomogr 4:87, 1980.

Williamson WD, Desmond MM, Wilson GS, et al: Survival of low-birthweight infants with neonatal intraventricular hemorrhage: Outcome in the preschool years. AJDC 137:1181, 1983.

Wong T-T, Lee L-S, Wang H-S, et al: Brain abscesses in children: A cooperative study of 83 cases. Child Nerv Syst 5:19, 1989.

Psychomotor Retardation and Regression

The differential diagnosis of psychomotor retardation (developmental delay) is quite different from that of psychomotor regression. Slow progress in the attainment of developmental milestones may be the result of either a static (Table 5–1) or a progressive (Table 5–2) encephalopathy. In contrast, the loss of developmental milestones previously attained is almost always evidence of a progressive disease of the nervous system. In the differential diagnosis of progressive diseases of the nervous system, diseases that start during infancy are somewhat different from those that begin during childhood (Tables 5–2 and 5–3).

◆ Developmental Delay

Delayed achievement of developmental milestones is one of the more common problems evaluated by child neurologists. Two questions must be asked: (1) Is delay restricted to specific areas of development or is it global? (2) Is there only developmental delay, or is there also developmental regression?

The second question is often difficult to answer in regard to infants. Even in static encephalopathies, new symptoms such as involuntary movements and seizures may occur as the child gets older. Many progressive diseases of the nervous system can be manifested by delayed acquisition of milestones without other neurologic deficits. However, once it is clear that milestones previously achieved have been lost or that focal neurologic deficits are evolving, a progressive disease of the nervous system must be considered.

The Denver Developmental Screening Test (DDST) is an efficient and reliable method for assessing development in the physician's office. It rapidly assesses four different components of development: personal-social, fine motor adaptive, language, and gross motor. The results can be amplified by several psychometric tests, but the DDST in combination with neurologic assessment provides sufficient information to initiate further diagnostic studies.

LANGUAGE DELAY

Normal infants and children have a remarkable facility for acquiring language. Infants and young children who are concurrently exposed to two languages usually learn both. Vocalization of vowels occurs in the first month, and laughing and squealing are well established by 5 months. At 6 months infants begin articulating consonants, usually M, D, and B. Parents translate these as "mama," "dada," and bottle or baby, although this is cer-

Table 5–1 ◆ Diagnosis of Developmental Delay: No Regression

Predominant Speech Delay
1. Hearing loss
2. Infantile autism

Predominant Motor Delay
1. Ataxia (see Chapter 10)
2. Hemiplegia (see Chapter 11)
3. Hypotonia (see Chapter 6)
4. Paraplegia (see Chapter 12)

Global Delay
1. Cerebral malformations
2. Chromosomal disturbances
3. Intrauterine infection
4. Perinatal disorders
5. Progressive encephalopathies (see Table 5–2)

Table 5–2 ◆ Progressive Encephalopathy: Onset Before Age 2

Acquired Immunodeficiency Syndrome Encephalopathy

Aminoacidurias
1. Homocystinuria
2. Maple syrup urine disease
   a. Intermediate form
   b. Thiamine-responsive form
3. Phenylketonuria

Hypothyroidism

Lysosomal Enzyme Disorders
1. Glycoprotein degradation disorders
   a. Mannosidosis type I
   b. Fucosidosis types I and II
   c. Sialidosis type II (infantile form)
2. Mucolipidoses
   a. Type II (I-cell)
   b. Type IV
3. Mucopolysaccharidoses
   a. Type I (Hurler)
   b. Type II (Sanfilippo)
4. Sphingolipidoses
   a. Gaucher disease type II (glucosylceramide lipidosis)
   b. GM$_1$ gangliosidosis types I and II
   c. GM$_2$ gangliosidosis (Tay-Sachs, Sandhoff)
   d. Globoid cell leukodystrophy (Krabbe)
   e. Metachromatic leukodystrophy (sulfatide lipidoses)
   f. Multiple sulfatase deficiency
   g. Niemann-Pick type A (sphingomyelin lipidosis)

Mitochondrial Disorders
1. Mitochondrial myopathy, encephalopathy, lactic acidosis, stroke (see Chapter 11)
2. Progressive infantile poliodystophy (Alper)
3. Subacute necrotizing encephalomyelopathy (Leigh)
4. Trichopoliodystrophy (Menkes)

Neurocutaneous Syndromes
1. Chédiak-Higashi syndrome
2. Neurofibromatosis
3. Tuberous sclerosis

Other Genetic Disorders of Gray Matter
1. Infantile ceroid lipofuscinosis (Santavuori)
2. Infantile neuroaxonal dystrophy
3. Lesch-Nyhan disease
4. Rett syndrome

Other Genetic Disorders of White Matter
1. Alexander disease
2. Galactosemia: transferase deficiency
3. Neonatal adrenoleukodystrophy (see Chapter 6)
4. Pelizaeus-Merzbacher disease
5. Spongy degeneration of infancy (Canavan–Van Bogaert)

Progressive Hydrocephalus

tainly not the infant's intention. These first attempts at vowels and consonants are automatic and sometimes occur even in deaf children. In the months that follow, the infant imitates many speech sounds, babbles and coos, and finally learns the specific use of mama and dada by 1 year of age. Receptive skills are always more highly developed than expressive skills because it is necessary to decode language before it can be encoded. By 2 years of age children have learned to combine at least two words, understand more than 250 words, and follow many simple verbal directions.

Hearing Impairment

The major cause of isolated delay in speech development is a hearing impairment (see Chapter 17). Hearing loss may occur concomitantly with global developmental retardation. Examples of the latter are rubella embryopathy, cytomegalic inclusion disease, neonatal meningitis, kernicterus, and several genetic disorders. Hearing loss need not be profound; it can be insidious, yet delay speech de-

velopment. The loss of high-frequency tones inherent in telephone conversation prevents the clear distinction of many consonants that we learn to fill in through experience; infants do not have experience in supplying missing sounds.

The hearing of any infant with isolated delay in speech development should be tested by formal audiometry. Crude testing in the office by slamming objects and ringing bells is inadequate. Hearing loss should be suspected in children with global retardation caused by disorders ordinarily associated with hearing loss or in retarded children who fail to imitate sounds. Other clues to hearing loss in children are excessive gesturing and staring at the lips of people who are talking.

Infantile Autism

Infantile autism was originally described as a form of psychosis resulting from abnormal mother-child bonding. It is now defined as a behavioral disorder caused by abnormal brain development from many different causes (Minshew and Payton,

Table 5–3 ◆ Progressive Encephalopathy:
Onset After Age 2

Infectious Diseases
1. Subacute sclerosing panencephalitis

Lysosomal Enzymes Disorders
1. Glycoprotein degradation disorders
   a. Aspartylglycosaminuria
   b. Mannosidosis type II
2. Mucopolysaccharidoses types II and VII
3. Sphingolipidoses
   a. Gaucher disease type III (glucosylceramide lipidosis)
   b. GM_2 gangliosidosis (juvenile Tay-Sachs)
   c. Globoid cell leukodystrophy (late-onset Krabbe)
   d. Metachromatic leukodystrophy (late-onset sulfatide lipidoses)
   e. Niemann-Pick type C (sphingomyelin lipidosis)

Other Genetic Disorders of Gray Matter
1. Ceroid lipofuscinosis
   a. Late infantile (Bielschowsky-Jansky)
   b. Juvenile
2. Heller syndrome
3. Huntington disease
4. Mitochondrial disorders
   a. Late-onset poliodystrophy
   b. Myoclonic epilepsy and ragged-red fibers (MERRF)
5. Xeroderma pigmentosum

Other Genetic Disorders of White Matter
1. Adrenoleukodystrophy
2. Alexander disease
3. Cerebrotendinous xanthomatosis

1988a,b). For example, some children with tuberous sclerosis and the fragile X syndrome display autistic behavior (Tuchman, 1991).

Clinical Features. The major diagnostic criteria are failure of language development, severe impairment of interpersonal relationships, a restricted repertoire of activities, and the beginning of symptoms before 3 years of age. Failure of language development is the feature most likely to bring autistic infants to medical attention and is the best predicter of outcome. The worst outcomes are associated with failure to develop language by age 5. The IQ is less than 70 in most children with autism. Autistic children show no affection to their parents or other care providers but treat people as if they were inanimate objects. Some children show a morbid preoccupation with spinning objects, stereotyped behavior such as rocking and spinning, and relative insensitivity to pain.

Diagnosis. Infantile autism is a clinical diagnosis and cannot be confirmed by laboratory tests. Infants with profound hearing impairment may display autistic behavior, and hearing must always be tested.

Treatment. Some aspects of the severely aberrant behavior can be improved by behavior modification techniques. However, despite the best program of treatment, these children function in a moderately to severely retarded range, even though some individuals have islands of normal ability (idiot savant).

DELAYED MOTOR DEVELOPMENT

Infants with delayed gross motor development but normal language and social skills are often hypotonic and may have a neuromuscular disease (see Chapter 6). Isolated delay in motor function may also be caused by ataxia (see Chapter 10), mild hemiplegia (see Chapter 11), and mild paraplegia (see Chapter 12). Many such children have a mild form of cerebral palsy, sufficient to delay the achievement of motor milestones but not severe enough to cause a recognizable disturbance of cognitive function during infancy. Mild disturbances in cognitive function are more often detected when the child enters school.

GLOBAL DEVELOPMENTAL DELAY

Most infants with global developmental delay have a static encephalopathy, usually as a result of antenatal or perinatal disturbances. However, a small percentage of infants with developmental delay and no evidence of regression have an underlying genetic disease. An exhaustive search to determine an underlying cause in every infant who is developing slowly but who has no evidence of developmental regression has a poor cost-benefit ratio. Factors that increase the likelihood of finding a progressive disease are summarized in Figure 5–1.

Chromosomal Disturbances

Abnormalities in chromosome structure or number are the single most common cause of severe mental retardation but still make up only one third of the total. Abnormalities of autosomal chromosomes are always associated with infantile hypotonia (see Chapter 6). In addition, there are usually multiple minor face and limb abnormalities, which in themselves are not unusual but assume diagnostic significance in combination. Clinical features that suggest chromosomal aberrations are summarized in Table 5–4, and the major chromosome syndromes are presented in Table 5–5.

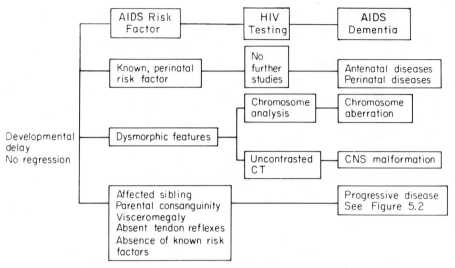

Figure 5–1 Evaluation of infants with development delay but no evidence of psychomotor regression.

With one exception, chromosomal aberrations causing developmental retardation are readily diagnosed by standard culture techniques. The exception, fragile X syndrome, identified by a secondary constriction in band Xq27, requires specialized techniques that must be requested beforehand. The defect is transmitted as an X-linked recessive trait and occurs in approximately 1 per 1000 males and 1 per 500 females (Butler et al, 1991). The phenotype includes mental retardation, hyperactivity, and a short attention span; a long face in which the forehead is prominent, the midface hypoplastic, the chin enlarged, and the ears are large and malformed; testicular enlargement in 80% of postpubertal men; and plantar and simian creases. Affected males are moderately retarded, and up to one third of carrier females are mildly retarded.

The phenotype is not sufficiently expressed in infancy to alert physicians but should be considered whenever a family has a history of mental retardation.

Cerebral Malformations

Approximately 3% of all children have at least one major malformation that "seriously interferes with viability or physical well-being" (Kalter and Warkany, 1983). The etiologic factors responsible for these malformations have been identified in no more than 20% of cases. Many intrauterine diseases cause destructive changes that result in malformation in the brain. The exposure of an embryo to infectious or toxic agents during the first weeks after conception can disorganize the delicate sequencing of neural development at a time when the brain is incapable of generating a cellular response. Alcohol, lead, prescription drugs, and substances of abuse have all been implicated in the production of cerebral malformations. Although a cause-and-effect relationship is difficult to establish in an individual case, maternal cocaine use is probably responsible for vascular insufficiency and infarction of many organs, including the brain (Dominguez et al, 1991).

Table 5–4 ◆ Clinical Indications for Chromosome Analysis

Genitourinary
1. Ambiguous genitalia
2. Polycystic kidney

Head and Neck
1. High nasal bridge
2. Hypertelorism or hypotelorism
3. Microphthalmia
4. Mongoloid slant (non-Asian)
5. Occipital scalp defect
6. Small mandible
7. Small or fish mouth (hard to open)
8. Small or low-set ears
9. Upward slant of eyes
10. Webbed neck

Limbs
1. Abnormal dermatoglyphics
2. Low-set thumb
3. Overlapping fingers
4. Polydactyly
5. Radial hypoplasia
6. Rocker-bottom feet

Table 5–5 ◆ Selected Autosomal Syndromes

Defect	Features*
5p monosomy	Characteristic "cri du chat" cry
	Moonlike face
	Hypertelorism
	Microcephaly
10p trisomy	Dolichocephaly
	"Turtle's beak"
	Osteoarticular anomalies
Partial 12p monosomy	Microcephaly
	Narrow forehead
	Pointed nose
	Micrognathia
18 trisomy	Pointed ears
	Micrognathia
	Occipital protuberance
	Narrow pelvis
	Rocker-bottom feet
21 trisomy	Hypotonia
	Round flat (mongoloid) facies
	Brushfield spots
	Flat nape of neck

Modified from de Grouchy J, Turleau J: Autosomal disorders. In Emery AEH, Rimoin DL (eds): Principles and Practice of Medical Genetics, Second Edition. Churchill Livingstone, New York, 1990, p 247.
*Growth retardation and mental retardation are features of all autosomal chromosome disorders.

Cerebral malformations should be suspected in any retarded child who is dysmorphic, has malformations of other organs, or has an abnormality of head size and shape (see Chapter 18). In such children non-contrast-enhanced computed tomography (CT) or magnetic resonance imaging (MRI) may be helpful in identifying a major malformation.

Intrauterine Infections

The three most commonly identified intrauterine infections are toxoplasmosis, cytomegalic inclusion disease, and rubella embryopathy. As demonstrated in animal models, maternal viral infections early in pregnancy may cause malformations of the embryo without leaving traditional pathologic evidence of viral infection.

Toxoplasmosis

Toxoplasma gondii is a protozoan that is estimated to infect 1 per 1000 live births in the United States each year. The symptoms of toxoplasmosis in the mother usually go unnoticed (Wilson and Remington, 1987). Transplacental transmission of toxoplasmosis is possible only if primary maternal infection occurs during pregnancy. The rate of placental transmission is highest during the last trimester, but fetuses infected at that time are least likely to have later symptoms. The transmission rate is lowest during the first trimester, but fetuses who are infected at that time have the most serious sequelae.

Clinical Features. About 25% of infected newborns have multisystem involvement (fever, rash, hepatosplenomegaly, jaundice, and thrombocytopenia) at birth. Neurologic dysfunction is manifested as seizures, altered states of consciousness, and increased intracranial pressure. The triad of hydrocephalus, chorioretinitis, and intracranial calcification is the hallmark of congenital toxoplasmosis in older children. About 8% of infected newborns, asymptomatic at birth, later show neurologic sequelae, especially psychomotor retardation.

Diagnosis. The Sabin-Feldman dye test had been the standard for diagnosis, but another useful serologic test for the diagnosis of congenital toxoplasmosis in the newborn is an enzyme-linked immunosorbent assay (ELISA) that demonstrates IgM-specific antibody to *Toxoplasma* in umbilical cord blood (Wilson and Remington, 1987). The demonstration of IgM-specific antibody is essential to prove active infection in the newborn. IgG-specific antibody appears in the newborn's serum by passive transfer from the mother and does not indicate active infection. Persistence of IgG-specific antibody correlates with active infection.

In older children the diagnosis requires not only serologic evidence of prior infection, but also compatible clinical features.

Treatment. A method for diagnosis and prenatal treatment of congenital toxoplasmosis has been tested (Daffos et al, 1988). When maternal acute infection is recognized by seroconversion, fetal blood and amniotic fluid are cultured and fetal blood is tested for *Toxoplasma*-specific IgM. The mother is then treated with spiramycin; if fetal infection is documented, pyrimethamine and either sulfadoxine or sulfadiazine are added to the regimen. Of 15 fetuses with congenital toxoplasmosis carried to term, only two had chorioretinitis during infancy.

In newborns with clinical evidence of toxoplasmosis, pyrimethamine (Daraprim), 0.5 mg/kg, and sulfadiazine, 25 mg/kg, are administered orally every 12 hours for 21 days. Because pyrimethamine is a folic acid antagonist, folic acid, 0.1 mg/kg/day, is also given. The peripheral platelet count must be monitored regularly. Prednisone, 1 to 2 mg/kg/day, should be added to the therapy in newborns with high protein concentrations in cerebrospinal fluid or chorioretinitis. The 21-day course of pyrimethamine and sulfadiazine is repeated every 3 or 4 months during the first year.

Cytomegalic Inclusion Disease

The cytomegalovirus is a member of the herpesvirus group and produces chronic infection characterized by long periods of latency punctuated by intervals of reactivation. It is transmitted by adults during sexual activity and produces an inapparent infection of the cervix. Pregnancy may cause reactivation of maternal infection, and cytomegalovirus can be cultured from the urine in 1% to 2% of liveborn infants in the United States. Fortunately, fewer than 0.05% of newborns with viruria have symptoms of cytomegalic inclusion disease.

Clinical Features. Cytomegalic inclusion disease is difficult to differentiate from other intrauterine infections on the basis of clinical examination alone. The typical clinical presentation includes skin rash, hepatosplenomegaly, jaundice, chorioretinitis, and microcephaly with cerebral calcification. Cytomegalic inclusion disease can also be manifested as microcephaly without evidence of systemic infection.

Diagnosis. Isolation of cytomegalovirus from the urine or cerebrospinal fluid indicates active infection in the newborn. In infants with developmental delay and microcephaly, the diagnosis of cytomegalic inclusion disease is made by serologic demonstration of prior infection and a consistent pattern of intracranial calcification.

Treatment. Several antiviral agents have been used to treat newborns with cytomegalic inclusion disease but none has been shown to have a beneficial effect on outcome. Ganciclovir, an agent used in the treatment of adult infections, has not yet been approved for use in children but is a candidate for clinical trials in neonatal cytomegalovirus infection (Yow, 1989).

Rubella Embryopathy

Clinical Features. Rubella embryopathy is a multisystem disease characterized by intrauterine growth retardation, cataracts, chorioretinitis, congenital heart disease, sensorineural deafness, hepatosplenomegaly, jaundice, anemia, thrombocytopenia, and rash (Desmond et al, 1967). Neurologic dysfunction is manifested as lethargy,

hypotonia, and seizures. Seizures may be delayed until 3 months of age.

Diagnosis. Rubella embryopathy should not be considered a cause of psychomotor retardation unless the newborn has other symptoms of rubella infection.

Treatment. No treatment is available for active infection. Fortunately, this disorder has almost disappeared since the introduction of routine immunization of children.

Perinatal Disorders

Perinatal infection, asphyxia, maternal drug use, and trauma are the major perinatal events that result in psychomotor retardation (see Chapter 1). The important infectious diseases are bacterial meningitis (see Chapter 4) and herpes encephalitis (see Chapter 1). Although the overall mortality rate of bacterial meningitis is now less than 50%, significant neurologic sequelae are noted almost immediately in 50% of survivors. The most common sequelae are mental and motor disabilities, hydrocephalus, epilepsy, deafness, and visual loss. Psychomotor retardation may be the only or the most prominent sequela. Progressive mental deterioration can occur if meningitis causes a secondary hydrocephalus.

◆ Progressive Encephalopathies of Infancy

Three questions must be answered in the history and physical examination before laboratory diagnosis is initiated:

1. Are the clinical features referable only to the central nervous system, or is there evidence of multiorgan involvement, that is, hepatosplenomegaly (Figure 5–2)?

2. If the disease is limited to the central nervous system, are peripheral nerves also involved? An early sign of peripheral neuropathy in infancy is loss of the ankle tendon reflex. More advanced neuropathy is manifested as distal weakness and hypotonia, and subclinical neuropathy is shown by electrophysiologic studies (see Chapters 6, 7, and 9).

3. Does the disease affect primarily the gray matter or the white matter? Early features of gray matter disease are personality change, seizures, and dementia. White matter disease is characterized by focal neurologic deficits and blindness. Whether the process begins in the gray matter or the white matter, eventually clinical features of dysfunction

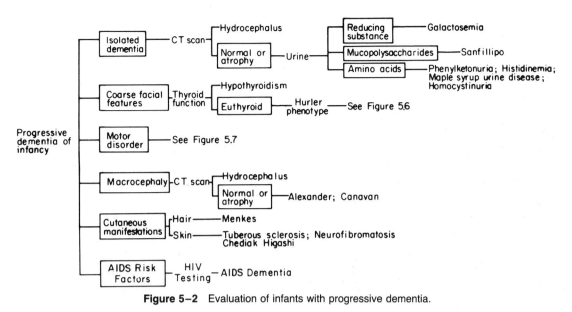

Figure 5–2 Evaluation of infants with progressive dementia.

develop in both. Early in the course of primary diseases of gray matter, the electroencephalogram (EEG) usually shows abnormalities that are sometimes characteristic. Cortical atrophy can be demonstrated by CT, and if the brainstem is involved, brainstem auditory evoked responses may be abnormal. MRI demonstrates cerebral demyelination with remarkable clarity (Figure 5–3). Visual evoked responses and motor conduction velocities are useful in documenting demyelination, even subclinical, in the optic and peripheral nerves, respectively.

ACQUIRED IMMUNODEFICIENCY SYNDROME ENCEPHALOPATHY

Acquired immunodeficiency syndrome (AIDS) is a human retroviral disease caused by the lentivirus subfamily designated as human immunodeficiency virus (HIV). HIV is spread in adults by sexual contact, intravenous drug abuse, and blood transfusion. Most pediatric AIDS cases result from transplacental or perinatal transmission of HIV from mothers who are intravenous drug users and prostitutes. The mother may be asymptomatic when the infection is noted in the child. Approximately 30% of children born to AIDS-infected mothers show evidence of infection during the first year (European Collaborative Study, 1988; Italian Multicentre Study, 1988). Fewer cases involve children receiving blood products, such as premature newborns and hemophiliacs.

Clinical Features. As a rule, the earlier the onset of symptoms, the worse the outcome. Children with AIDS fail to thrive and have an increased incidence of bacterial infections, but only 10% acquire opportunistic infections (Novick and Rubenstein, 1987). The most common opportunistic

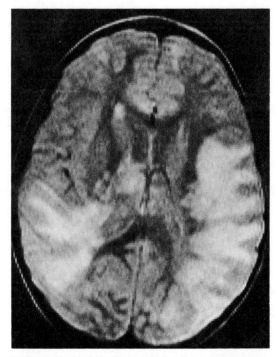

Figure 5–3 Krabbe disease. Magnetic resonance image demonstrating extensive demyelination of cerebral hemispheres.

infections are *Pneumocystis carinii* pneumonia, disseminated candidiasis, and disseminated *Mycobacterium avium intracellulare*. Toxoplasmosis, a common complication in adults with AIDS, is uncommon in pediatric AIDS. An immunocompromised state should be suspected in every child with an opportunistic infection.

The possible spectrum of neurologic outcome in children infected with HIV includes a static encephalopathy resulting from other prenatal and perinatal risk factors associated with drug abuse in the mother; opportunistic infection of the nervous system; HIV infection of the brain, causing a subacute encephalopathy; and HIV infection of the spinal cord, causing a transverse myelitis (see Chapter 12) (Butler et al, 1991; Hittelman, 1991). AIDS experts now believe that the disease will develop in all children with HIV infection.

AIDS encephalopathy may be subacute or indolent and is not necessarily associated with failure to thrive or opportunistic infections. The onset of encephalopathy may occur from 2 months to 5 years after exposure to the virus. Ninety percent of affected infants show symptoms by 18 months of age. The encephalopathy is characterized by progressive loss of developmental milestones, microcephaly, dementia, and spasticity. Other features in less than 50% of children are ataxia, pseudobulbar palsy, involuntary movement disorders, myoclonus, and seizures. Death usually occurs a few months after the onset of AIDS encephalopathy.

Diagnosis.   Criteria for the diagnosis of AIDS include (1) opportunistic infections, recurrent bacterial infections, or lymphoid interstitial pneumonitis, (2) appropriate risk factors, (3) defective cell-mediated immunity, (4) polyclonal hypergammaglobulinemia, and (5) positive antibody titer. Treatable infections (cryptococcal meningitis, *Candida* meningitis) must be excluded before HIV encephalitis is diagnosed.

The cerebrospinal fluid abnormalities are minimal and vary from patient to patient. Protein concentration is 50 to 100 mg/dl (0.5 to 1 g/L) and glucose concentration is normal or slightly decreased, but monocytic pleocytosis is uncommon. In some children progressive calcification of the basal ganglia is seen on CT.

The mortality rate in symptomatic children is 100%, but not all newborns with positive antibody titers become symptomatic.

Treatment.   Oral zidovudine (azidothymidine, AZT), 180 mg/m² every 6 hours, improves neurologic development in children with HIV infection (McKinney et al, 1991). Continuous intravenous infusion of AZT may actually improve cog-

nition (DeCarli et al, 1991). Bone marrow suppression is the only important evidence of toxicity.

In symptomatic children an intravenous infusion of immune globulin, 400 mg/kg/28 days, decreases the frequency of bacterial infections (NICHHD Intravenous Immunoglobulin Study Group, 1991).

AMINOACIDURIAS

Disorders of amino acid metabolism initially produce symptoms of gray matter dysfunction (mental retardation, seizures) and also have a profound effect on myelination.

Homocystinuria

Homocystinuria can be caused by three different genetic defects. The defect associated with mental retardation is almost complete deficiency of the enzyme cystathionine beta-synthase (Figure 5–4). Transmission is by autosomal recessive inheritance. Heterozygotes have partial deficiencies. Cystathionine beta-synthase catalyzes the condensation of serine and homocysteine to form cystathionine. When the enzyme is deficient, the concentrations of homocysteine, homocystine, and methionine in the blood and urine are elevated. It is hypermethioninemia that is detected in newborn screening programs.

Clinical Features.   Affected individuals appear normal at birth. Global developmental delay is usually the first clinical manifestation, and intelligence declines progressively with age in untreated children. Most eventually function in the mildly retarded range, but at least 20% have normal intelligence. Thromboembolism affecting large arteries, small arteries, and veins is a life-threatening complication of homocystinuria caused by hyperhomocysteinemia (Clarke et al, 1991). Emboli may occur in infancy or be delayed until adult life. Occlusion of the coronary or carotid arteries can lead to sudden death or severe neurologic handicap. Thromboembolism is the first clue to diagnosis in 15% of cases (Mudd et al, 1985). Dislocation of the lens, an almost constant feature of homocystinuria, typically occurs between 2 and 10 years of age but may be delayed until adult life. Ninety-seven percent of patients have lens dislocation by age 40. Older children have osteoporosis. The spine is affected first and most severely, resulting in scoliosis and sometimes vertebral collapse. Many children are tall and thin and have a Marfan syndrome habitus. This habitus does not develop until middle or late childhood and serves as a clue to diagnosis in fewer than 40% of cases.

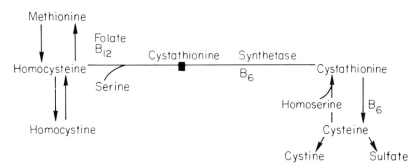

Figure 5–4 Metabolic disturbance in homocystinuria. Absence of cystathionine beta-synthase (cystathionine synthetase) blocks the metabolism of homocysteine, causing the accumulation of homocystine and methionine. (Reprinted from Fenichel GM: Neonatal Neurology, 2nd edition. Churchill Livingstone, New York, 1985. By permission.)

The diagnosis should be suspected in any infant with isolated and unexplained developmental delay, since disease-specific features may not appear until later childhood. The presence of either thromboembolism or lens dislocation strongly suggests homocystinuria.

Diagnosis. Rapid screening can be performed by adding 1 ml of a 5% aqueous solution of sodium cyanide to 1 ml of urine. After the solution is left for 5 minutes at room temperature, 3 to 5 drops of a 5% aqueous solution of sodium nitroprusside is added. If homocystine is present in the urine, the solution turns a deep red. Definitive diagnosis is made by demonstrating a deficiency of cystathionine beta-synthase either in the liver or in cultured fibroblasts.

Treatment. The administration of pyridoxine, 500 to 1000 mg/day, reduces or eliminates the biochemical abnormalities in one third of patients. An equal number are not pyridoxine responsive, and the remainder have an intermediate response. Folate must be given concomitantly. Most patients who respond to pyridoxine probably have a low-level or mutant form of cystathionine beta-synthase activity that is enhanced by the addition of cofactor.

The most widely used dietary treatment for homocystinuria is methionine restriction and cystine supplementation. When initiated in the newborn, this approach prevents mental retardation and may decrease the incidence of lens dislocation. The efficacy of diet in preventing thromboembolic events or osteoporosis has not been determined. Newborns who are pyridoxine responsive should be treated with both methionine restriction and pyridoxine.

Maple Syrup Urine Disease (Intermediate)

The three major branched-chain amino acids are leucine, isoleucine, and valine. In the course of their metabolism they are first transaminated to alpha-ketoacids and then further catabolized by oxidative decarboxylation (see Figure 1–4). Deficiency of the enzyme branched-chain ketoacid dehydrogenase, which is responsible for oxidative decarboxylation, is associated with at least three phenotypes: classic, intermittent, and intermediate maple syrup urine disease (Danner and Elsas, 1989). The classic and intermittent form are characterized by acute encephalopathies with ketoacidosis (see Chapters 1 and 10). The intermediate form is manifested as progressive mental retardation without ketoacidosis. The levels of dehydrogenase enzyme activity in the intermediate and intermittent forms are approximately the same (5% to 40% of normal), whereas activity in the classic form is zero to 2% of normal. Phenotypic difference between the intermediate and intermittent forms may be related to protein intake. Some infants with the intermediate form are thiamine responsive. The enzyme defect in these cases may be unique.

Clinical Features. Infants with intermediate maple syrup urine disease are normal at birth, slow in achieving milestones, and hyperactive. They generally function in the moderately retarded range of intelligence. Physical development is normal except for coarse, brittle hair. The urine may have the odor of maple syrup. Acute mental changes, seizures, and focal neurologic deficits do not occur.

Diagnosis. Preliminary screening is accomplished by demonstration of either a yellow precipitate when 0.2 ml of a 0.5% solution of 2,4-dinitrophenylhydrazine in 2N hydrochloride, or a navy blue color when 5 to 10 drops of a 5% to 10% solution of ferric chloride, is added to 1 ml of urine. Definitive diagnosis requires the demonstration of branched-chain ketoacids and amino acids in the blood and urine.

Treatment. All infants with intermediate maple syrup urine disease should be put on a protein-restricted diet. In addition, a trial of thiamine, 100 mg/day, is given to determine whether the biochemical error is thiamine responsive. If 100 mg is not effective, daily dosages up to 1 gm of thiamine should be tried before the condition is designated as thiamine refractory.

Phenylketonuria

Phenylketonuria is a disorder of phenylalanine metabolism caused by partial or total deficiency of the hepatic enzyme phenylalanine hydroxylase. The deficiency is transmitted by autosomal recessive inheritance and occurs in approximately 1 per 16,000 live births. Because phenylalanine cannot be adequately hydroxylated to tyrosine, phenylalanine accumulates and is transaminated to phenylpyruvic acid (Figure 5–5). Phenylpyruvic acid is oxidized to phenylacetic acid, which is excreted in the urine and causes a musty odor.

Clinical Features. Affected children are normal at birth and would not be detected in the absence of compulsory mass screening. The screening test detects hyperphenylalaninemia, which is not synonymous with phenylketonuria (Table 5–6). Blood phenylalanine and tyrosine concentrations must be precisely determined in every newborn whose abnormality is detected by the screening test to differentiate classic phenylketonuria from other conditions. In newborns with classic phenylketonuria, hyperphenylalaninemia develops 48 to 72 hours after initiation of milk feeding. Blood phenylalanine concentrations are 20 mg/dl (1200 μmol/L) or greater, and serum tyrosine levels are less than 5 mg/dl (275 μmol/L). When blood phenylalanine concentrations reach 15 mg/dl (900 μmol/L), phenylalanine spills over into the urine and the addition of ferric chloride solution (5 to 10 drops of FeCl to 1 ml of urine) produces a green color.

Untreated infants appear normal during the first months, but the skin may have a musty odor because of phenylacetic acid in the sweat. Developmental delay is sometimes manifested by the third month and always before the end of the first year. By the beginning of the second year, developmental regression is evident. Behavioral disturbances characterized by hyperactivity and aggressiveness are common; focal neurologic deficits are unusual. Approximately 25% of affected infants have seizures. Some have infantile spasms and hypsarrhythmia; others have tonic-clonic seizures. Infants with phenylketonuria frequently have blond hair, pale skin, and blue eyes owing to diminished pigment production. Eczema is common. These skin changes are the only nonneurologic manifestations of phenylketonuria.

Diagnosis. Benign variants of phenylketonuria are generally characterized by blood phenylalanine levels less than 25 mg/dl (1500 μmol/L), and frequently less than 15 mg/dl (900 μmol/L), and a normal concentration of tyrosine. The malignant forms of phenylketonuria result from disturbances in tetrahydrobiopterin. Seizures are the initial symptom and are followed by mental retardation and motor deficits. Progressive calcification of the basal ganglia occurs in untreated children (Woody et al, 1989).

Transitory tyrosinemia is estimated to occur in 2% of full-term newborns and in 25% of premature newborns. It is caused by a transitory deficiency of the enzyme p-hydroxyphenylpyruvic acid. It is a benign condition and can be distinguished from phenylketonuria because the blood concentrations of both tyrosine and phenylalanine are elevated.

Treatment. Experts agree that a phenylalanine-restricted diet should be started immediately in newborns with a blood phenylalanine concentration of 30 mg/dl (1800 μmol/L) or greater; some recommend diet therapy at a concentration of 20 mg/dl (1200 μmol/L). After 3 months of therapy a 3-day challenge of phenylalanine, 180

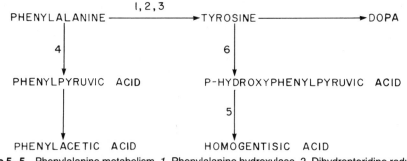

Figure 5–5 Phenylalanine metabolism. *1.* Phenylalanine hydroxylase. *2.* Dihydropteridine reductase. *3.* Tetrahydrobiopterin. *4.* Phenylalanine transaminase. *5.* p-Hydroxyphenylpyruvic acid. *6.* Tyrosine transaminase.

Table 5–6 ◆ Differential Diagnosis of
Hyperphenylalaninemia

Classic Phenylketonuria
1. Complete hydroxylase deficiency (zero to 6%)

Benign Variants
1. Partial hydroxylase deficiency (6% to 30%)
2. Transitory hydroxylase deficiency
3. Phenylalanine transaminase deficiency
4. Other

Malignant Variants
1. Dihydropteridine reductase deficiency
2. Tetrahydrobiopterin synthesis deficiency

Tyrosinemia
1. Transitory tyrosinemia
2. Tyrosinosis

Liver Disease
1. Galactose-1-phosphate uridyltransferase deficiency

mg/kg/day, is indicated to distinguish mild variants from classic phenylketonuria. Children with phenylketonuria have a blood phenylalanine concentration of 20 mg/dl (1200 μmol/L) or greater and need to continue restricted diets. Those with a blood concentration lower than 20 mg/dl (1200 μmol/L) probably have a benign variant and do not require further dietary restriction of phenylalanine. The goal of therapy is to maintain blood phenylalanine concentrations between 5 and 10 mg/dl (300 and 600 μmol/L). Diet therapy should be continued through adolescence to prevent intellectual deterioration (Azen et al, 1991).

Tetrahydrobiopterin is a cofactor for the enzymes phenylalanine hydroxylase, tyrosine hydroxylase, and tryptophan hydroxylase. Deficiency of tetrahydrobiopterin can be due to defective recycling or defective synthesis. In infants with cofactor deficiency a phenylalanine-restricted diet reduces the blood phenylalanine concentration but does not prevent neurologic deterioration. For these children tetrahydrobiopterin administration is the therapy of choice (Hoganson et al, 1984).

HYPOTHYROIDISM

Congenital hypothyroidism resulting from thyroid dysgenesis occurs in 1 per 4000 live births. The cause is unknown, but the occasional familial occurrence in siblings has suggested either a genetic basis or an underlying maternal factor. Early diagnosis and treatment are imperative to ensure a favorable outcome. Fortunately, newborn screening is universal in the United States and detects virtually all cases.

Clinical Features. Affected infants are usually asymptomatic at birth. Clinical features evolve insidiously during the first weeks post partum, and their significance is not always appreciated. Frequently the gestation lasts more than 42 weeks and birth weight is greater than 4 kg. Early clinical features include a wide-open posterior fontanelle, constipation, jaundice, poor temperature control, and umbilical hernia. The tongue is sometimes large, which makes feeding difficult. Edema of the eyes, hands, and feet may be present at birth but is often unrecognized in early infancy.

Diagnosis. Radiographs of the long bones demonstrate delayed maturation, and radiographs of the skull show excessive numbers of wormian bones. A definitive diagnosis relies on the demonstration of low serum concentrations of thyroxine (T_4) and high serum concentrations of thyroid-stimulating hormone (TSH).

Treatment. Once the diagnosis of congenital hypothyroidism is confirmed, treatment can be initiated with sodium-1-thyroxine, 24 to 50 μg/day. Most, if not all, of the sequelae of congenital hypothyroidism can be prevented by early treatment (Fisher and Foley, 1989). The ultimate intelligence of the hypothyroid infant declines with each month of delay.

DISORDERS OF LYSOSOMAL ENZYMES

Lysosomes are cytoplasmic vesicles containing enzymes that degrade the products of cellular catabolism. When lysosomal enzymes are deficient, abnormal storage of materials occurs. One or several organs may be affected. Mental retardation and regression are features of many lysosomal storage diseases. In some, such as acid lipase deficiency (Wolman disease) and ceramide deficiency (Farber lipogranulomatosis), mental retardation occurs, but it is neither a prominent nor the initial feature. Such disorders are omitted from this discussion.

Mucopolysaccharidoses
Type I (Hurler Syndrome)

Mucopolysaccharidoses are discussed first because the "Hurler phenotype" is common to many lysosomal disorders (Figure 5–6). The Hurler syndrome results from absence of the lysosomal hydrolase alpha-L-iduronidase. The defect is transmitted by autosomal recessive inheritance (Neufeld and Muenzer, 1989). Dermatan sulfate and heparan sulfate cannot be fully degraded and appear in the urine. Mucopolysaccharides are stored in the cornea, collagen, and leptomeninges, and gangliosides are stored in cortical neurons.

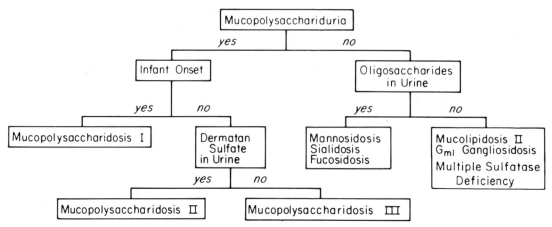

Figure 5–6 Evaluation of infants with a Hurler phenotype.

Clinical Features.   Affected children are normal during the first year. In the second year development is arrested and slow regression occurs. Motor dysfunction affects the corticospinal tracts and peripheral nerves. A distinctive Hurler phenotype evolves (Table 5–7). Clouding of the cornea is present in all cases, sometimes causing complete blindness. Facial features become coarse. The child has progressive hepatosplenomegaly, umbilical hernia, and skeletal deformities that produce dwarfism, kyphoscoliosis, and limited movement of the joints. The skeletal deformities, termed dysostosis multiplex, produce characteristic radiographic features: hypoplasia of the lateral clavicle, rounding and sometimes hypoplasia of the thoracolumbar vertebral bodies, flaring of the pelvis with hypoplasia of the acetabula, broadening of the ribs, and widening of the diaphyses of long bones. The skull loses its convolutional markings, the sella turcica is enlarged, and the orbits are shallow. Communicating hydrocephalus may result from thickening of the leptomeninges. Death usually occurs by age 10.

Diagnosis.   The diagnosis is suggested by the physical and radiographic appearance, the presence of vacuolated lymphocytes, and mucopolysacchariduria. A simple screening test is the appearance of a metachromatic spot when a drop of urine is placed on paper impregnated with toluidine blue. Definitive diagnosis requires the demonstration of enzyme deficiency in leukocytes or cultured fibroblasts.

Treatment.   No treatment is available.

Mucopolysaccharidosis Type III

The type III disorder is distinct from other mucopolysaccharidoses because only heparan sulfate is stored in viscera and appears in the urine. Gangliosides are stored in neurons. Four different, but related, enzyme deficiencies have been implicated. All are transmitted by autosomal recessive inheritance.

Clinical Features.   The Hurler phenotype is not prominent, but hepatomegaly is present in two thirds of cases. Dwarfism does not occur. The major feature is neurologic deterioration characterized by delayed motor development beginning toward the end of the second year, followed by an interval of arrested mental development and progressive dementia. Hyperactivity and sleep disorders are relatively common between the ages of 2 and 4. Most affected children are severely retarded by age 11 and dead before age 20. However, considerable variability exists, and type III disease should be considered even when the onset of mental regression occurs after age 5.

Diagnosis.   The diagnosis should be suspected in infants and children with progressive psychomotor regression and a screening test positive for mucopolysacchariduria. The presence of heparan sulfate, but not dermatan sulfate, in the urine is presumptive evidence of the disease. Specific diagnosis requires the demonstration of enzyme deficiency in cultured fibroblasts.

Treatment.   No treatment is available.

Table 5–7 ◆ Hurler Phenotype

1. Abdominal hernia
2. Coarse facial features
3. Corneal opacity
4. Deafness
5. Dysostosis multiplex
6. Mental retardation
7. Stiff joints
8. Visceromegaly

Glycoprotein Degradation Disorders

Glycoprotein degradation disorders are rare and resemble mild forms of mucopolysaccharidoses (Beaudet and Thomas, 1989).

Mannosidosis Type I

The deficient enzyme in mannosidosis is alpha-D-mannosidase. Type I has an infantile onset and type II a juvenile onset.

Clinical Features. All patients have mental retardation, dysostosis multiplex, hepatosplenomegaly, and coarse facial features. Deafness, corneal opacities, and recurrent bacterial infection are not constant features. Progression is rapid, and death occurs between 3 and 10 years of age.

Diagnosis. The diagnosis is suspected in infants with a Hurler phenotype but without mucopolysacchariduria (Figure 5–6). Vacuolated lymphocytes are present in the peripheral blood. Demonstration of mannosidase deficiency in leukocytes or fibroblasts provides definitive diagnosis.

Treatment. No treatment is available.

Fucosidosis Types I and II

Fucosidosis is caused by deficiency of the lysosomal enzyme alpha-L-fucosidase. Two clinical types are recognized; both have their onset during infancy. Type II progresses more slowly and allows longer survival.

Clinical Features. The onset of psychomotor retardation and regression occurs between 3 and 18 months in type I and between 1 and 2 years in type II. In both types a Hurler phenotype (Table 5–7) develops, except that corneal opacities are not present and skeletal abnormalities are restricted to the spine. Infants with fucosidosis type II survive to early adult life. A distinctive feature is that patients with type I experience increased sweating whereas those with type II have anhidrosis and angiokeratoma.

Diagnosis. The diagnosis is suspected in infants with a Hurler phenotype but without mucopolysacchariduria (Figure 5–6). Vacuolated lymphocytes are present in the peripheral blood. Demonstration of fucosidase deficiency in leukocytes or fibroblasts provides definitive diagnosis.

Treatment. No treatment is available.

Sialidosis Type II

Type II sialidosis is a rare disorder caused by a deficiency of the glycoprotein-specific alpha-neuraminidase (sialidase). Three different clinical syndromes are associated with sialidosis: a congenital form (I) with hydrops fetalis, an infantile form (II) with Hurler phenotype, and a juvenile form (III) characterized only by myoclonus and a cherry-red spot of the macula (Table 5–8).

Clinical Features. Infants with sialidosis type II look like they have a mucopolysaccharidosis. Toward the end of the first decade, ataxia, myoclonus, and seizures develop, sometimes associated with a cherry-red spot of the macula. Mental retardation is present, but progressive dementia is not a feature.

Diagnosis. Vacuolated lymphocytes are present in the peripheral blood, and the urine contains oligosaccharides. Definitive diagnosis requires demonstration of the enzyme deficiency in cultured fibroblasts.

Treatment. No treatment is available.

Mucolipidoses
Mucolipidosis Type II (I-Cell Disease)

Mucolipidosis type II is caused by partial or complete deficiency of several acid hydrolases. It resembles Hurler syndrome except that symptoms appear earlier, the neurologic deterioration is more rapid, and mucopolysacchariduria is not present.

Clinical Features. Affected newborns are small for gestational age and may have hyperplastic gums. Coarsening of facial features and limitation of joint movements occur within the first months. The complete Hurler phenotype is present within the first year except that corneal opacification is not seen in all cases. Death from congenital heart failure usually occurs before age 5.

Diagnosis. I-cell disease should be considered in infants with Hurler phenotype and a screening test negative for mucopolysacchariduria (Figure 5–6). Definitive diagnosis requires the demonstration of enzyme deficiency in cultured fibroblasts.

Treatment. No treatment is available.

Mucolipidosis Type IV

Mucolipidosis type IV is transmitted by autosomal recessive inheritance in Ashkenazi Jews.

Table 5–8 ◆ Lysosomal Enzyme Disorders with a Cherry-Red Spot

---

1. Cherry-red spot myoclonus (see Chapter 1)
2. Farber lipogranulomatosis
3. GM$_1$ gangliosidosis
4. GM$_2$ gangliosidosis
5. Metachromatic leukodystrophy
6. Niemann-Pick disease
7. Sialidosis type III

The suspected defect is deficiency of the enzyme ganglioside sialidase. Gangliosides, phospholipids, and acidic mucopolysaccharides accumulate in many tissues.

Clinical Features. Symptoms appear during infancy. Developmental delay and visual impairment caused by corneal clouding and retinal degeneration are the major features (Amir et al, 1987). Mental retardation is profound. There are no typical facial features, skeletal abnormalities, or visceromegaly. Longevity of affected children has not been established.

Diagnosis. Mucolipidosis type IV should be suspected in Jewish children with psychomotor delay or regression and corneal clouding. The electroretinogram usually shows a reduction in amplitude or absence of the retinal potential. Diagnosis is confirmed by the demonstration of ganglioside storage in cultured fibroblasts.

Treatment. Corneal transplant may be useful to restore vision, but no treatment is available for the mental deterioration.

Sphingolipidoses
Gaucher Disease Type II (Glucosylceramide Lipidosis)

Type II Gaucher disease, caused by a deficiency of the enzyme glucocerebrosidase, is transmitted by autosomal recessive inheritance. Type I, the most common form of Gaucher disease, does not affect the nervous system. Type II is an acute and devastating infantile disorder affecting the brain and viscera. Type III, like type II, is characterized by neurovisceral storage, but the onset is in childhood and the course is slow.

Clinical Features. Infants with Gaucher disease type II usually have symptoms of neurovisceral dysfunction before 6 months of age, and frequently before 3 months of age. The initial symptoms are motor regression and cranial nerve dysfunction. Children are first hypotonic and then spastic. Head retraction is an early and characteristic sign that probably is due to meningeal irritation. Difficulties in sucking and swallowing, trismus, and oculomotor palsies are typical. Mental deterioration is rapid, but seizures are uncommon. Splenomegaly is more prominent than hepatomegaly, and jaundice is unusual. Hypersplenism results in anemia, thrombocytopenia, and leukopenia. Death usually occurs during the first year and always by the second.

Diagnosis. The presence of Gaucher cells in the reticuloendothelial system establishes the diagnosis. These cells are altered macrophages measuring 20 to 100 μm. The cytoplasm has the appearance of wrinkled tissue paper, and the nucleus is eccentric. The cells are best identified from bone marrow aspirate stained by periodic acid–Schiff (PAS) reaction. Heterozygotes can be identified by a partial decrease in enzyme activity in leukocytes. No reliable method for prenatal diagnosis has been established.

Treatment. Efforts to treat the disease by enzyme replacement are still experimental. Splenectomy may improve the hematologic abnormalities but does not provide long-term relief of symptoms.

GM₁ Gangliosidosis Type I

GM₁ gangliosidosis types I and II are caused by deficiency of the lysosomal enzyme beta-galactosidase. Ganglioside GM₁ is stored in the brain and viscera. Both the early (I) and late (II) infantile forms are transmitted by autosomal recessive inheritance.

Clinical Features. Difficulty in feeding and failure to thrive are noted shortly after birth. Edema of the limbs may be present as well. Psychomotor development is first slow and then regresses. Affected newborns are poorly responsive, hypotonic, and hypoactive. The Hurler phenotype is present (Table 5–7), except that the cornea is clear and a cherry-red spot of the macula is present in 50% of patients (Table 5–8). Symptoms are rapidly progressive, and many infants die within 1 year. Those who survive the first year are in a vegetative state.

Diagnosis. Infantile GM₁ gangliosidosis can be distinguished from Hurler syndome by the absence of mucopolysacchariduria and the presence of a cherry-red spot. Definitive diagnosis requires demonstration of the enzyme deficiency in leukocytes, cultured fibroblasts, or serum.

Treatment. No treatment is available.

GM₁ Gangliosidosis Type II

Clinical Features. Infants with type II GM₁ gangliosidosis are normal during the first year, but symptoms of motor incoordination then develop. Ataxia, dysarthria, and strabismus are the initial manifestations. These are followed by mental regression, lethargy, spasticity, and seizures. The Hurler phenotype is not present: corneal clouding and hepatosplenomegaly do not occur, and skeletal radiographs demonstrate only mild beaking of vertebral bodies and metacarpal bones.

Diagnosis. Diagnosis requires demonstration of the deficient enzyme in leukocytes, cultured fibroblasts, or serum.

Treatment. No treatment is available.

GM₂ Gangliosidosis (Tay-Sachs Disease)

Tay-Sachs disease is transmitted by autosomal recessive inheritance and is caused by deficiency of the enzyme hexosaminidase A. Gene frequency is 1:30 in Ashkenazi Jews and 1:300 in gentiles. The central nervous system is the only affected organ.

Clinical Features. The onset of symptoms is between 3 and 6 months of age. An abnormal startle reaction (Moro reflex) to noise or light is characteristically the first symptom. Motor regression begins between 4 and 6 months of age. The infant may be brought for medical attention because of either delayed achievement of motor milestones or loss of milestones previously attained. A cherry-red spot of the macula is present in almost every patient but is not specific for Tay-Sachs disease, since it can be seen in several storage diseases and in central retinal artery occlusion (Table 5–8) (Kivlin et al, 1985). The cherry-red spot develops as retinal ganglion cells in the parafoveal region accumulate stored material, swell, and burst. The red color of the normal fundus can then be seen. Optic atrophy and blindness follow.

By 1 year of age the infant is severely retarded, unresponsive, and spastic. During the second year the head enlarges and seizures develop. Most children die by 5 years of age.

Diagnosis. The diagnosis should be strongly suspected in any Jewish child with psychomotor retardation and a cherry-red spot of the macula. Definitive diagnosis requires the demonstration of deficient activity of hexosaminidase A in white blood cells or serum. Heterozygotes can be detected by the same assay. Prenatal diagnosis is possible by amniocentesis.

Treatment. No treatment is available.

GM₂ Gangliosidosis (Sandhoff Disease)

Sandhoff disease is a rare disorder of neurovisceral storage that occurs in non-Jewish children. It is transmitted by autosomal recessive inheritance and is caused by deficiency of both hexosaminidase A and B.

Clinical Features. The clinical features and course of Sandhoff disease are identical to those of Tay-Sachs disease. The only difference is that organs other than the central nervous system are sometimes involved. Moderate hepatosplenomegaly may be present, and occasionally patients have bony deformities similar to those of infantile GM₁ gangliosidosis.

Diagnosis. The disease should be suspected in every non-Jewish infant with a Tay-Sachs phenotype. Peripheral lymphocytes are not vacuolated, but foamy histocytes may be present in the bone marrow. The disease is diagnosed in patients and carriers by demonstration of hexosaminidase deficiency in leukocytes, cultured fibroblasts, or serum. Prenatal diagnosis can be made by the detection of N-acetylglucosaminyl oligosaccharides in amniotic fluid (Warner et al, 1986).

Treatment. No treatment is available.

Globoid Cell Leukodystrophy (Krabbe Disease)

Krabbe disease is a rapidly progressive demyelinating disorder of infants caused by deficient activity of the enzyme galactosylceramidase (galactosylceramide beta-galactosidase). A juvenile and an adult form of the disease also occur. The defect is transmitted by autosomal recessive inheritance.

Clinical Features. The median age of onset is 4 months with a range of 1 to 7 months (Hagberg, 1984). Initial symptoms are irritability and hyperreactivity to stimuli. These are followed by progressive hypertonicity in the skeletal muscles. Unexplained low-grade fever is common. Psychomotor development is arrested and then regresses. Within 2 to 4 months the infant is in a permanent position of opisthotonos and has lost all previously achieved milestones. Tendon reflexes become hypoactive and disappear. Startle myoclonus and seizures develop. The infant becomes blind, and before 1 year 90% are either dead or in a chronic vegetative state.

Several variant forms of globoid leukodystrophy with different clinical features are described: infantile spasm syndrome (see Chapter 1), focal neurologic deficits (see Chapters 10 and 11), and polyneuropathy (see Chapter 7). The juvenile form is discussed later in this chapter.

Diagnosis. MRI demonstrates diffuse demyelination of the cerebral hemispheres (Figure 5–3). Motor nerve conduction velocity of peripheral nerves is usually prolonged, and the protein content of cerebrospinal fluid is elevated. Definitive diagnosis requires the demonstration of deficient activity of galactosylceramide beta-galactosidase in leukocytes or cultured fibroblasts.

Treatment. No treatment is available.

Metachromatic Leukodystrophy (Sulfatide Lipidoses)

Metachromatic leukodystrophy is a disorder of central and peripheral myelin metabolism caused by deficient activity of the enzyme arylsulfatase A. The disease is transmitted by autosomal recessive inheritance. Several clinical presentations are recognized. Because peripheral neuropathy is a prominent feature of the late infantile form of metachromatic leukodystrophy, the condition is discussed in Chapter 7. The juvenile form affects primarily the brain and is discussed later in this chapter.

Multiple Sulfatase Deficiency

Multiple sulfatase deficiency is a rare disorder characterized by deficiency of several sulfatases (arylsulfatase A, arylsulfatase B, iduronate sulfatase, N-acetylgalactosamine 6-sulfate sulfatase, and heparan-N-sulfatase) and the accumulation of sulfatides, glycosaminoglycans, sphingolipids, and steroid sulfates in tissue and body fluids (Soong et al, 1988).

Clinical Features.   Development during the first year is normal, but in the second year developmental arrest and regression occur. Ataxia and speech disturbances are also noted during the second year. Neurologic deterioration is progressive. The appearance suggests a mucopolysaccharidosis: short stature, microcephaly, and facial dysmorphism. Retinal degeneration can occur as well and suggests a neuronal ceroid lipofuscinosis (Harbord et al, 1991).

Diagnosis.   Sulfatase activity is deficient, but not absent, in cultured skin fibroblasts and leukocytes. If only arylsulfatase A is measured, an improper diagnosis of juvenile sulfatide lipidosis may be considered because peripheral neuropathy is not present. However, the facial dysmorphism is not consistent with either the infantile or the juvenile form of sulfatide lipidosis.

Treatment.   No treatment is available.

Niemann-Pick Disease Type A (Sphingomyelin Lipidosis)

Caused by a deficiency in the enzyme sphingomyelinase, Niemann-Pick disease type A is transmitted by autosomal recessive inheritance. Several phenotypes affecting children and adults are described.

Clinical Features.   The acute infantile form appears during the first months of life with feeding difficulty, failure to thrive, and hepatomegaly. Splenomegaly occurs later and is not prominent. A cherry-red spot is present in 50% of cases (Table 5–8). Psychomotor regression, characterized by postural hypotonia and loss of reactivity to the environment, occurs during the first year but may be overlooked because of the child's failure to thrive. With time, emaciation, a tendency for opisthotonos, exaggerated tendon reflexes, and blindness develop. Seizures are uncommon.

Diagnosis.   The diagnosis is suggested by the clinical course (Figure 5–7). Vacuolated histiocytes are present in the bone marrow and vacuolated lymphocytes in the peripheral blood. Definitive diagnosis requires the demonstration of sphingomyelinase deficiency in leukocytes or cultured fibroblasts.

Treatment.   No treatment is available.

MITOCHONDRIAL DISORDERS

Mitochondrial disorders involve pyruvate metabolism and respiratory complexes. Figure 8–5 depicts the five respiratory complexes, and Table 8–7 lists the disorders assigned to abnormalities in each of these complexes.

Subacute Necrotizing Encephalomyelopathy (Leigh Disease)

Leigh disease is a progressive poliodystrophy primarily affecting neurons of the brainstem, thalamus, basal ganglia, and cerebellum. The pathology is similar to Wernicke encephalopathy, but the mammillary bodies are spared. The pathologic features can be caused by more than one enzyme deficiency in pyruvate metabolism or by abnormalities in respiratory chain complexes I and IV (Moraes et al, 1991). Usually the disease is transmitted by autosomal recessive inheritance, but X-linked inheritance occurs as well (Livingstone et al, 1984).

Clinical Features.   Onset occurs during the first year in 60%, during the second year in 20%, and after infancy in 20%. Children who have symptoms in early infancy tend to have a steadily progressive course with severe disability and death. The initial symptoms are some combination of developmental delay, failure to thrive because of poor feeding or vomiting, hypotonia, and seizures. Symptoms are made worse by intercurrent infection or ingestion of a heavy carbohydrate meal. Three typical, but not constant, features during infancy are respiratory disturbances, abnormal ocular motility, and hypotonia. Respiratory disturbances are at first episodic and can be characterized by Cheyne-Stokes breathing, ataxic breathing, or central hyperventilation. Respiratory distress is the usual cause of death. Ocular motility dysfunction varies from nystagmus to ophthalmoplegia. Hypotonia results from a combination of peripheral neuropathy and disturbed cerebellar function.

Children with onset of symptoms during the second year have similar symptoms, but the course is

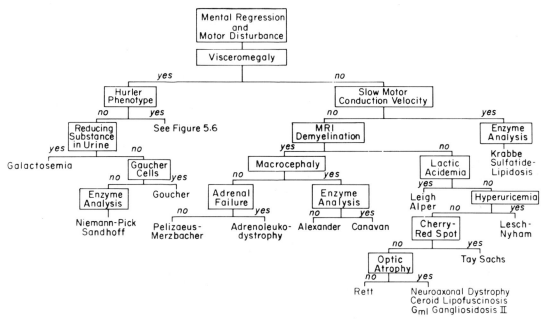

Figure 5–7 Evaluation of infants with progressive mental regression and motor disturbances.

less rapidly progressive and symptoms are more intermittent with exacerbations at time of infection.

Diagnosis. Blood concentrations of lactate and pyruvate are usually elevated and rise even higher at the time of clinical exacerbation. Lesions in the brainstem and around the third ventricle may be visualized on CT and MRI scans, and the interpeak latency of waves V to III is prolonged on brainstem auditory evoked response. Motor nerve conduction velocities are usually slowed. When peripheral neuropathy is present, the protein content of the cerebrospinal fluid is elevated. Studies should search for cytochrome-oxidase deficiency (Coster et al, 1991) and for disturbances in pyruvate utilization: deficiencies in pyruvate decarboxylase, multiple carboxylases, and pyruvate dehydrogenase. Muscle biopsy specimens have been useful for enzyme analysis in several patients.

Treatment. Patients with disorders of pyruvate utilization are less likely to have acute exacerbations of illness on a carbohydrate-restricted diet. Calories should be provided primarily as lipid. Large doses of thiamine are helpful in some patients.

Oral acetazolamide is useful when the disorder is transmitted by X-linked recessive inheritance (Evans et al, 1978). The mechanism of action is unknown. Whether acetazolamide is also effective in cases transmitted by autosomal recessive inheritance is not clear.

Progressive Infantile Poliodystrophy (Alper Disease)

Alper disease was described originally as a progressive degeneration of cerebral gray matter and probably encompassed several disease processes. Deficiencies in pyruvate carboxylase activity and respiratory chain complexes I and IV have been identified in familial cases of progressive infantile poliodystrophy associated with mitochondrial myopathy (Moraes et al, 1991). A transmissible agent may be responsible for some sporadic cases; a poliodystrophy has been serially transmitted to hamsters with brain tissue from an affected child (Manuelidis and Rorke, 1989).

Clinical Features. The onset of symptoms is either during infancy or childhood. Symptoms with infantile onset tend to be sporadic and are characterized first by delay in the achievement of developmental milestones and then by either myoclonic or tonic-clonic seizures. Status epilepticus can be the first manifestation of the seizure diathesis. Prolonged seizures are sometimes followed by transient hemiplegia. Psychomotor regression becomes evident, and blindness may occur.

Diagnosis. Definitive diagnosis can be made only by postmortem examination. However, an elevated blood concentration of lactate should be a clue to disturbed pyruvate utilization and should prompt investigation of mitochondrial enzymes in liver and skeletal muscle. A carbohydrate load in the form of an oral glucose tolerance test may raise the blood lactate concentration to two or three times normal and worsen symptoms.

Treatment.   A low-carbohydrate diet is recommended for children with disorders of pyruvate utilization. However, no specific treatment has proved effective in Alper disease.

Trichopoliodystrophy (Menkes Syndrome)

Menkes syndrome is believed to be a primary defect in intestinal transport of copper. The symptoms are attributed to a secondary deficiency of copper-dependent enzymes, especially cytochrome *c* oxidase. Some patients demonstrate enzyme deficiency in muscle, brain, and liver mitochondria; others show decreased copper concentration only in the brain (Nooijen et al, 1981).

Clinical Features.   The inital symptoms usually develop in the first 3 months. Development is first arrested and then regresses. The infant becomes lethargic and less reactive. Myoclonic seizures, provoked by stimulation, are an early and almost constant feature. By the end of the first year the infant is in a chronic vegetative state, and most die before 18 months.

The appearance of the scalp hair and eyebrows is almost pathognomonic. The hair is sparse, poorly pigmented, and wiry. The shafts break easily, forming short stubble (kinky hair). Radiographs of the long bones suggest osteogenesis imperfecta. Other facial abnormalities include abnormal fullness of the cheeks, a high-arched palate and micrognathia. Fullness of the cheeks also occurs in cerebrohepatorenal syndrome (see Chapter 6) in which mitochondrial abnormalities are present as well.

Diagnosis.   In infants with clinical features of Menkes disease the diagnosis can be established by the microscopic appearance of the hair shaft and by the demonstration of decreased plasma concentrations of copper.

Treatment.   One patient, treated from an early age with intramuscular copper histidine and oral D-penicillamine, developed much less severe neurologic dysfunction than did his maternal uncle (Nadal and Baerlocher, 1988).

NEUROCUTANEOUS SYNDROMES
Chédiak-Higashi Syndrome

Chédiak-Higashi syndrome is a rare disorder transmitted by autosomal recessive inheritance.

Clinical Features.   Affected children are born with deficient pigment of the skin and hair. Areas of skin depigmentation form bizarre patterns that resemble giant fingerprints. Recurrent infections are prominent during infancy.

Neurologic symptoms evolve during the first 2 years. These include developmental retardation, seizures, and severe peripheral neuropathy. Symptoms of autonomic dysfunction, increased perspiration and failure to produce overflow tears, are common and may suggest dysautonomia.

Diagnosis.   The diagnosis is primarily clinical, based on the combination of neurologic dysfunction and pigmentary changes. Examination of the peripheral blood smear is confirmatory. The nuclei of polymorphonuclear leukocytes are pyknotic, and their cytoplasm contains large oval and fusiform granules that stain for myeloperoxidase.

Treatment.   No treatment is available.

Neurofibromatosis Type 1

The neurofibromatoses are divided into a peripheral (neurofibromatosis type 1) and a central type (neurofibromatosis type 2) (NIH Consensus Development Conference, 1988). Both are transmitted by autosomal dominant inheritance and show considerable variation in expression. The abnormal gene in located on chromosome 17. Almost 50% of patients with neurofibromatosis type 1 (NF-1) are new mutations (Listernick and Charrow, 1990). New mutations are associated with increased paternal age.

Neurofibromatosis type 2 (NF-2) is characterized by bilateral acoustic neuromas as well as other intracranial and intraspinal tumors (see Chapter 17).

Clinical Features.   NF-1 is believed to be the most common single-gene disorder of the nervous system, affecting 1 in 4000 individuals. Mild cases are characterized by café au lait spots and subcutaneous neurofibromas. Axillary freckles are common.

Patients with severe cases have developmental and neoplastic disorders of the nervous system. No more than 10% of patients with NF-1 are retarded. Those who are retarded are more likely to have seizures than developmental delay as their first manifestation. Nevertheless, neurofibromatosis should be suspected in any infant with psychomotor retardation and café au lait spots.

Diagnosis.   Two or more of the following features are considered diagnostic: (1) six café au lait spots greater than 5 mm in diameter in prepubertal individuals, or greater than 15 mm in postpubertal individuals, (2) two or more neurofibromas or one plexiform neurofibroma, (3) freckling in the axillary or inguinal region, (4) optic glioma, (5) two or more iris hamartomas (Lisch nodules), (6) a distinctive osseous lesion such as sphenoid dysplasia or thinning of long bones, and (7) a first-degree relative with NF-1.

Treatment. Management is primarily symptomatic: anticonvulsant drugs for seizures, surgery for accessible tumors, and orthopedic procedures for bony deformities. Routine MRI studies to screen for optic gliomas in nonsymptomatic children were not recommended by the NIH Consensus Development Conference (1988).

Tuberous Sclerosis

Tuberous sclerosis is transmitted by autosomal dominant inheritance and has variable phenotypic expression.

Clinical Features. The most common initial symptom of neurologic dysfunction during infancy is seizures, especially infantile spasms (see Chapter 1). Some infants have evidence of developmental delay before the onset of seizures. The delay is often insufficient to prompt medical consultation. Most children with tuberous sclerosis who are mentally retarded eventually have seizures, and all children who have intractable seizures during the first year will be mentally retarded.

Life expectancy is shortened by the disease. The causes of death during childhood are renal disease, cardiovascular disorders, brain tumors, and status epilepticus (Shepherd et al, 1991).

Diagnosis. Tuberous sclerosis should be suspected in infants with developmental delay when hypopigmented areas are present in the skin. These hypochromic nevi are usually lance shaped or oval and are scattered on the trunk and limbs. Only 18% of patients have "characteristic" leaf-shaped hypochromic nevi. Depigmented areas are readily delineated by illumination with a Wood light.

In late infancy and early childhood, café au lait spots develop and an isolated raised plaque in the skin over the lower back or buttocks (shagreen patch) is present by 15 years in 50% of affected children. During childhood, adenoma sebaceum (actually angiokeratomas) appears on the face, usually in a butterfly distribution. Other organ involvement includes retinal tumors, rhabdomyoma of the heart, renal tumors, and cysts of the kidney, bone, and lung. Seizures and mental retardation are due to disturbed histogenesis of the brain. Neurons are decreased in number, and astrocytes are large and bizarrely shaped. Glial tumors are common in the subependymal region and may cause obstructive hydrocephalus.

Treatment. Anticonvulsants are helpful in reducing seizure frequency but rarely provide complete control. The mental retardation is not reversible. Genetic counseling is an important aspect of patient management. Although the disease is transmitted by autosomal dominant inheritance, gene expression is so variable that neither parent may

appear affected. Sporadic cases were thought to be common. However, 25% of parents without personal or family history of tuberous sclerosis are shown to be affected by careful history and physical examination, including Wood light examination of the skin, funduscopic examination, renal ultrasound, and cranial CT (Cassidy et al, 1983).

OTHER GENETIC DISORDERS OF GRAY MATTER
Infantile Neuronal Ceroid Lipofuscinosis (Santavuori Disease)

In this group of genetic disorders, lipopigment is deposited in neurons and some visceral tissues. These disorders are usually classified by age at onset and rapidity of progression. The more common types occur after age 2 (see "Progressive Encephalopathies of Childhood" later in this chapter). The early infantile type (Santavuori disease) occurs primarily in Finnish people and is believed transmitted by autosomal recessive inheritance.

Clinical Features. Onset is usually in the second year but may be in the first. Visual impairment and myoclonus are initial features. Rapid deterioration, characterized by psychomotor regression, hypotonia, ataxia, and hyperkinesia, follows. Seizures are not prominent.

Total blindness develops between the ages of 2 and 3 years. The macula has degenerated and has a brownish color, the optic disk is atrophic, and the peripheral retina is hypopigmented.

Diagnosis. Antemortem diagnosis can be established by ultrastructural studies of leukocytes, skin, or conjunctiva. Between 15% and 21% of lymphocytes or monocytes contain granular, osmiophilic membrane-bound cytoplasmic inclusions (Baumann and Markesbery, 1982). Skin and conjunctival biopsies reveal similar granular inclusions in endothelial and neuronal cells.

Treatment. Seizures and myoclonus should be treated with a combination of valproate, clonazepam, and phenobarbital (see Chapter 1). No treatment for the underlying metabolic error is available.

Infantile Neuroaxonal Dystrophy

Infantile neuroaxonal dystrophy (Seitelberger disease) is a disorder of axon terminals transmitted by autosomal recessive inheritance. It shares many pathologic features with Hallervorden-Spatz disease (see Chapter 14) and may be an infantile form.

Clinical Features. Affected children usually develop normally during the first year, but most do not walk independently. Toward the end of the first year, motor regression is evidenced by clumsiness and frequent falling. The infant is first hypotonic and hyporeflexic. Muscle atrophy may be present as well. At this stage a peripheral neuropathy is suspected, but motor nerve conduction velocity and the protein content of the cerebrospinal fluid are normal (Aicardi and Castelein, 1979).

After the initial phase of hypotonia, symptoms of cerebral degeneration become prominent. Increasing spastic quadriparesis, optic atrophy, involuntary movements, and mental regression are evident. By 2 years of age most children are severely handicapped. They deteriorate to a vegetative state, and death usually occurs by age 10.

Diagnosis.   The cerebrospinal fluid is usually normal. Electromyography demonstrates a denervation pattern consistent with anterior horn cell disease. Motor nerve conduction velocities are normal. The EEG is not characteristic and may be normal.

A definitive diagnosis requires the demonstration of neuroaxonal spheroids in peripheral nerve endings, conjunctiva, or brain. Neuroaxonal spheroids are large eosinophilic spheroids, caused by axonal swelling, throughout the gray matter. They are not unique to neuroaxonal dystrophy and are also seen in Hallervorden-Spatz disease, infantile GM$_2$ gangliosidosis, Niemann-Pick disease type C, and several other neurodegenerative conditions.

Treatment.   No treatment is available.

Lesch-Nyhan Disease

Lesch-Nyhan disease is caused by deficiency of the enzyme hypoxanthine guanine phosphoribosyltransferase. It is transmitted by X-linked inheritance.

Clinical Features.   Affected newborns appear normal at birth, except for mild hypotonia (Watts et al, 1982). Delayed motor development and poor head control are present during the first 3 months. These are followed by progressive limb rigidity and torticollis or retrocollis. The progression of neurologic disturbance is insidious, and many affected patients are thought to have cerebral palsy. During the second year, facial grimacing, corticospinal tract dysfunction, and involuntary movements (usually chorea but sometimes athetosis) develop.

It is not until after age 2, and sometimes considerably later, that affected children begin biting their fingers, lips, and cheeks. Compulsive self-mutilation is characteristic, but not invariable, and causes severe disfigurement. Often wrapping the hands or removing teeth is necessary to prevent further harm. In addition to self-directed aggressive behavior, aggressive behavior toward caretakers may be present. Mental retardation is constant but of variable severity. Intelligence is difficult to evaluate because of behavioral and motor disturbances.

Diagnosis.   Uric acid concentrations are increased in the blood and urine. Indeed, some parents note a reddish discoloration of diapers caused by uric acid. Definitive diagnosis requires the demonstration that hypoxanthine guanine phosphoribosyltransferase activity is absent in erythrocytes or cultured fibroblasts.

Treatment.   Allopurinol decreases the urinary concentration of uric acid and prevents the development of nephropathy. Self-mutilatory behavior may be abated by the use of levodopa or tetrabenazine (Jankovic et al, 1988). However, no treatment is available to prevent progressive degeneration of the nervous system.

Rett Syndrome

Rett syndrome occurs only in girls, and the prevalence is estimated to be 1:10,000. Most cases are sporadic, but two families with more than one affected sibling have been reported (Moeschler et al, 1988), suggesting a genetic mode of transmission. X-linked dominant inheritance with lethality in male fetuses is suspected.

Clinical Features.   Affected girls are normal during the first year. Developmental arrest usually begins at 12 months but may appear as early as 5 months or as late as 18 months. Within a few months rapid developmental regression occurs and is characterized by loss of language skills, decreased use of the hands, gait ataxia, and autistic behavior. Head growth is arrested with eventual microcephaly. Dementia is usually severe. Although affected girls are unable to sustain interest in the environment, stimulation produces an exaggerated, stereotyped reaction consisting of jerking movements of the trunk and limbs with episodes of disorganized breathing and apnea, followed by hyperpnea (Glaze et al, 1987). During these episodes circumoral cyanosis and diffuse perspiration may occur. Similar episodes may also occur without stimulation but not during sleep. Such episodes are frequently interpreted as seizures, although it is not clear that they are epileptic in nature. Typical tonic-clonic seizures, partial complex seizures, or myoclonic seizures occur in most children between the ages of 2 and 4.

A characteristic feature of the syndrome is loss of purposeful hand movements before the age of 3. They are replaced by stereotyped activity that looks like hand wringing or washing. Repetitive blows to the face are another form of stereotyped hand movement.

The initial rapid progression is followed by a continued slow progression of neurologic deterioration. Spastic paraparesis and quadriparesis are frequent endpoints.

Diagnosis.   Diagnosis is based entirely on the clinical features. Laboratory tests are not helpful. The Rett Syndrome Diagnostic Criteria Work Group (1988) established the diagnostic criteria that are summarized in Table 5–9.

Treatment.   Seizures often respond to standard anticonvulsant drugs. Because of the observation of increased beta-endorphin levels in affected girls, naltrexone, 1 to 2 mg/kg/day, has been tried and found effective in some patients for relieving the respiratory symptoms and decreasing seizure frequency (Myer et al, 1988). It has no effect on long-term outcome.

OTHER GENETIC DISORDERS OF WHITE MATTER
Alexander Disease

Alexander disease is a rare disorder thought to involve astrocytes (Borret and Becker, 1985). All cases are sporadic, and a genetic basis is only suspected. Rosenthal fibers are the hallmark of disease. These are rod-shaped or round bodies that stain red with hematoxylin and eosin and black with myelin stains. They appear as small granules within the cytoplasm of astrocytes. Rosenthal fibers are scattered diffusely in the cerebral cortex and the white matter but have a predilection for the subpial, subependymal, and perivascular regions.

Clinical Features.   Rosenthal fibers are pathologic features of three clinical syndromes. First and most common is the *infantile form*, which affects primarily males. The onset may be anytime from birth to early childhood. These infants demonstrate arrest and regression of psychomotor development, enlargement of the head owing to megalencephaly, spasticity, and seizures. Optic atrophy does not occur. Death usually occurs by the second or third year.

The *juvenile form* is characterized by bulbar symptoms, and the *adult form* has a course that suggests multiple sclerosis.

Diagnosis.   The cerebrospinal fluid is normal. The disease should be suspected in infants with macrocephaly and MRI evidence of progressive leukodystrophy. Definitive diagnosis relies entirely on the demonstration of Rosenthal fibers by postmortem examination.

Treatment.   No treatment is available.

Galactosemia: Transferase Deficiency

Three separate inborn errors of lactose metabolism are known to produce galactosemia in the newborn, but only galactose-1-phosphate uridyltransferase deficiency produces mental retardation. The defect is transmitted by autosomal recessive inheritance.

Clinical Features.   Affected newborns appear normal, but cataracts have already begun to develop. The initial symptoms are provoked by the first milk feeding and include failure to thrive, vomiting, diarrhea, jaundice, and hepatomegaly. During this time some newborns have clinical features of increased intracranial pressure, probably resulting from cerebral edema. The combination of a tense fontanelle and vomiting suggests a primary intracranial disturbance and can delay the diagnosis and treatment of the metabolic error.

Diagnosis.   Galactosemia should be considered in any newborn with vomiting and hepatomegaly, especially when cataracts are present. The best time to test the urine for reducing substances (by use of Clinitest tablets) is after feeding. Specific tests for glucose (Testape, Clinistix) show no abnormalities. Most cases of galactosemia in newborns are detected by routine screening tests.

Table 5–9 ◆ Diagnostic Criteria for Rett Syndrome

Necessary Criteria

1. Apparently normal prenatal and perinatal period and development in first 6 months
2. Normal head circumference at birth and deceleration of head growth between 5 months and 4 years
3. Loss of acquired purposeful hand movements between 6 and 30 months
4. Development of stereotyped hand movements
5. Severe progressive dementia
6. Appearance of gait apraxia and truncal apraxia and ataxia between 1 and 4 years of age

Supportive Criteria

1. Breathing dysfunction
2. Electroencephalographic abnormalities and seizures
3. Growth retardation and hypotrophic small feet
4. Spasticity and dystonia
5. Peripheral vasomotor disturbances
6. Scoliosis

Exclusion Criteria

1. Intrauterine growth retardation or microcephaly at birth
2. Organomegaly or signs of storage disease
3. Retinopathy or optic atrophy
4. Evidence of an identifiable, acquired neurologic disease

Treatment. Symptoms are reversed by providing a lactose-free diet. However, for optimal intellectual outcome the diet therapy must be initiated early.

Unfortunately, in some children with galactosemia mental retardation develops even when diet therapy is adequate (Lo et al, 1984). In such children the achievement of developmental milestones is delayed during the first year and intellectual function is moderately retarded by age 5. After age 5, truncal ataxia develops and progresses in severity. Associated with ataxia is a coarse resting tremor of the limbs. Because of the restricted diet, cataracts and hepatomegaly are not present. The enzyme deficiency in children who deteriorate neurologically does not appear different from the deficiency in those who respond favorably to lactose-free diets.

Pelizaeus-Merzbacher Disease

Pelizaeus-Merzbacher disease is a rare demyelinating encephalopathy transmitted by X-linked recessive inheritance. It is caused by defective biosynthesis of proteolipid protein, a structural protein composing half of the myelin sheath protein (Gencic et al, 1989). An infantile and a neonatal onset phenotype are caused by defects of the proteolipid protein. A transitional form between the two is also described. Whether the neonatal form is transmitted by autosomal dominant or X-linked inheritance is not known (Begleiter and Harris, 1989).

Clinical Features. The first symptoms of the neonatal form suggest spasmus nutans (see Chapter 15). The neonate has an intermittent nodding movement of the head and pendular nystagmus. Chorea or athetosis develops, psychomotor development is arrested by the third month, and regression follows. Limb movements become ataxic and tone becomes spastic, first in the legs and then in the arms. Optic atrophy and seizures are a late occurrence. Death occurs by 5 to 7 years of age.

When the onset of disease is at the end of the first month or later, the symptoms are the same as in the neonatal form but the course is longer and survival to adult life is relatively common.

Diagnosis. MRI shows diffuse demyelination of the hemispheres with sparing of scattered small areas (Shimomura et al, 1988). Postmortem examination is required for definitive diagnosis. Diffuse demyelination of the cerebral and cerebellar hemispheres is present but patches of normal myelin remain. Nerve cells and axons appear normal. When survival is prolonged, myelin is completely absent in the cerebral hemispheres.

Treatment. No treatment is available.

Spongy Degeneration of Infancy (Canavan–Van Bogaert Disease)

Canavan–Van Bogaert disease, transmitted by autosomal recessive inheritance, is associated with a deficiency of the enzyme aspartoacylase. The mechanism by which the enzyme deficiency causes disease is not known (Echenne et al, 1989; Gascon et al, 1990).

Clinical Features. Psychomotor arrest and regression occur during the first 6 months post partum. Clinical manifestations include decreased awareness of the environment, difficulty in feeding, irritability, and hypotonia. The initial flaccidity is eventually replaced by spasticity. A characteristic posture with leg extension, arm flexion, and head retraction is assumed, especially when the child is stimulated. Macrocephaly is noted by 6 months of age. The head continues to enlarge throughout infancy and reaches a plateau by the third year. Optic atrophy leading to blindness is noted between 6 and 10 months of age.

Diagnosis. Abnormal excretion of N-acetylaspartic acid can be detected in the urine, and aspartoacylase activity in cultured fibroblasts is less than 40% of normal. MRI shows diffuse symmetric leukoencephalopathy even before neurologic symptoms are evident. Demyelination of peripheral nerves does not occur, and the cerebrospinal fluid is normal.

Treatment. No treatment is available.

PROGRESSIVE HYDROCEPHALUS

Clinical Features. Progressive dilation of the ventricular system may be a consequence of congenital malformations, infectious diseases, intracranial hemorrhage, or connatal tumors. Whatever the cause, the clinical features of increasing intracranial pressure are much the same. Head circumference enlarges, anterior fontanelle feels full, and the child becomes lethargic, has difficulty feeding, and vomits. Ataxia and spastic gait are common.

Diagnosis. Progressive hydrocephalus is often insidious in premature newborns with intraventricular hemorrhage, especially when delayed progression follows initial arrest. Hydrocephalus should always be suspected in newborns and infants with excessive head growth; the diagnosis is readily confirmed by CT.

Treatment. Ventriculoperitoneal shunt is the usual procedure to relieve hydrocephalus in newborns and small infants with primary dilation of the lateral ventricles (see Chapter 18).

◆ Progressive Encephalopathies of Childhood (Onset After Age 2)
INFECTIOUS DISEASES

Infectious diseases are an uncommon cause of progressive dementia in childhood. Tuberculosis and several fungal species may produce a chronic meningitis characterized by personality change and some decline in higher intellectual function. *Cryptococcus* infection is especially notorious for its long, indolent course. However, the major features of these infections are fever and headache. Chronic meningitis is not a serious consideration in the differential diagnosis of isolated psychomotor regression.

In contrast, chronic viral infections, especially HIV, may produce a clinical picture similar to many genetic disorders in which dementia is a prominent feature.

Subacute Sclerosing Panencephalitis

Subacute sclerosing panencephalitis (SSPE) is a form of chronic measles encephalitis that was at one time endemic in several parts of the world but has almost disappeared in countries that require routine measles immunization. In a nonimmunized population the average age at onset is 8 years. As a rule, children with SSPE have experienced natural infection with the rubeola virus at an early age, half before age 2. A concomitant infection with a second virus at the time of initial exposure to measles and immunosuppression are additional risk factors for SSPE. In the United States incidence rates have been highest in rural areas, especially in the southeastern states and the Ohio River valley.

Clinical Features. The first symptoms of disease are personality change and declining school performance. Personality change may be aggressive behavior or withdrawal, and psychologic rather than medical services may be sought. However, retinal examination during this early stage already demonstrates pigmentary changes in the macula. Generalized seizures, usually myoclonic, develop next. An EEG at this time shows the characteristic pattern of periodic bursts of spike-wave complexes (approximately every 5 to 7 seconds) occurring synchronously with the myoclonic jerk. After the onset of seizures the child shows a rapid neurologic deterioration characterized by spasticity, dementia, and involuntary movements. Within 1 to 6 years from the onset of symptoms the child is in a chronic vegetative state.

Diagnosis. The diagnosis can be suspected from the clinical course and characteristic EEG. Confirmation requires demonstration of an elevated antibody titer against rubeola, usually associated with elevated gammaglobulin concentrations, in the cerebrospinal fluid. The cerebrospinal fluid is otherwise normal. Plasma rubeola antibody titers are also markedly elevated.

A similar progressive disorder of the nervous system may occur in children who were born with rubella embryopathy (chronic rubella panencephalitis).

Treatment. No drug is effective in treating the disease, but it can be prevented by measles immunization.

LYSOSOMAL ENZYMES DISORDERS
Glycoprotein Degradation Disorders
Aspartylglycosaminuria

Aspartylglycosaminuria is a rare condition that occurs primarily in Finland. The defect, a deficiency of the enzyme *N*-aspartyl-beta-glucosaminidase, is transmitted by autosomal recessive inheritance.

Clinical Features. Affected individuals are healthy in early infancy but later have recurrent infection, diarrhea, and inguinal hernia (Beaudet and Thomas, 1989). During early childhood the facial features become coarse and hepatomegaly occasionally develops. Lens opacities occur after age 10. Speech may be delayed, but mental development is otherwise normal until age 5. Afterward a slowly progressive regression of mental and motor skills results in severe retardation and generalized weakness.

Diagnosis. Vacuolated lymphocytes are present in the peripheral blood of most patients, and a mild form of dysostosis multiplex is demonstrated radiographically. The urine does not contain mucopolysaccharides but does contain oligosaccharides. For a definitive diagnosis the demonstration of enzyme deficiency in leukocytes or cultured fibroblasts is necessary.

Treatment. No treatment is available.

Mannosidosis Type II

Clinical Features. The late-onset, juvenile and adult form of mannosidosis is characterized by normal early development followed by mental regression during childhood or adolescence. Dysostosis multiplex is not a prominent feature, but deafness occurs in all cases.

Diagnosis. Vacuolated lymphocytes are present in peripheral blood. The urine contains oligosaccharides but not mucopolysaccharides. Definitive diagnosis requires demonstration of deficient activity of beta-mannosidase in cultured fibroblasts.

Treatment.   No treatment is available.

Mucopolysaccharidoses

The mucopolysaccharidoses result from deficiencies of enzymes involved in the catabolism of dermatan sulfate, heparan sulfate, or keratin sulfate. There are at least seven major types of mucopolysaccharidoses. Four of these, types I, II, III, and VII, affect the nervous system and produce mental retardation. Types I and III have their onset in infancy and are discussed in the prior section. Types II and VII ordinarily have their onset in childhood following 2 or more years of normal development (Figure 5–8).

Mucopolysaccharidosis Type II (Hunter Syndrome)

Clinical Features.   Patients with the Hunter syndrome have a Hurler phenotype (Table 5–7) but lack corneal clouding (Neufeld and Muenzer, 1989). This syndrome also differs from other mucopolysaccharidoses in that transmission is by X-linked recessive inheritance. A rare subtype is transmitted by autosomal recessive inheritance. Iduronate sulfatase is the deficient enzyme; dermatan sulfate and heparan sulfate are stored in the viscera and appear in the urine.

The Hurler phenotype may develop rapidly or evolve slowly during childhood and may not be recognized until the second decade or later. A prominent feature is the appearance of a nodular, ivory-colored lesion on the back, usually around the shoulders and upper arms. Mental regression, caused by neuronal storage of gangliosides, is slowly progressive, but many patients come to medical attention because of chronic hydrocephalus. Affected children survive into adult life. The accumulation of storage materials in collagen causes the entrapment of peripheral nerves, especially the median and ulnar.

Diagnosis.   Diagnosis is suggested by the presence of mucopolysacchariduria with equal excretion of dermatan sulfate and heparan sulfate. Definitive diagnosis requires the demonstration of enzyme deficiency in cultured fibroblasts or serum. Prenatal diagnosis is accomplished by detecting iduronate sulfatase activity in amniotic fluid.

Treatment.   Nerve entrapment and hydrocephalus can be relieved by appropriate surgical procedures. No treatment is available for the underlying storage disease.

Mucopolysaccharidosis Type VII (Sly Disease)

Sly disease is a rare disorder caused by deficiency of the enzyme beta-glucuronidase. It is transmitted by autosomal recessive inheritance.

Clinical Features.   The patient has an incom-

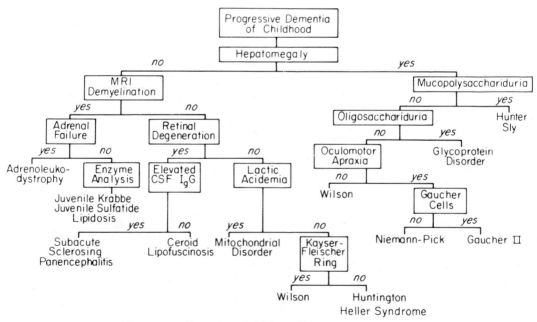

Figure 5–8   Evaluation of children with progressive dementia.

plete Hurler phenotype with hepatosplenomegaly, inguinal hernias, and dysostosis multiplex as the major features (Bernsen et al, 1987). Corneal clouding does not occur, and the face, although unusual, is not typical of the Hurler phenotype. Psychomotor retardation develops after age 2, but not in all cases.

Diagnosis. Both dermatan sulfate and heparan sulfate are present in the urine, causing a screening test to be positive for mucopolysacchariduria. Specific diagnosis requires the demonstration of beta-glucuronidase deficiency in leukocytes or cultured fibroblasts.

Treatment. No treatment is available.

Sphingolipidoses
Gaucher Disease, Type III
(Glucosylceramide Lipidosis)

The late-onset type of Gaucher disease, like other types, is caused by deficiency of the enzyme glucocerebrosidase and transmitted by autosomal recessive inheritance.

Clinical Features. Age at onset ranges from early childhood to adult life. Hepatosplenomegaly usually precedes neurologic deterioration. The most common neurologic manifestations are seizures and mental regression (Nishimura and Barranger, 1980). Mental regression varies from mild memory loss to severe dementia. Myoclonus and myoclonic seizures develop in many patients. Some combination of spasticity, ataxia, and cranial nerve dysfunction may be present as well. Vertical oculomotor apraxia, as described in Niemann-Pick disease, may occur in late-onset Gaucher disease as well.

Diagnosis. Gaucher cells are present in the bone marrow and are virtually diagnostic. Confirmation requires the demonstration of deficient glucocerebrosidase activity in hepatocytes or leukocytes.

Treatment. No treatment is available.

GM₂ Gangliosidosis (Juvenile Tay-Sachs Disease)

The juvenile form of Tay-Sachs disease, like the infantile form, is caused by deficiency of *N*-acetyl-beta-hexosaminidase. The enzymatic basis of the phenotypic variability is incompletely understood (Specola et al, 1990).

Clinical Features. There is no ethnic predilection. Affected children appear normal until age 3 years, but then dysarthria, language retardation, and gait disturbances develop. The gait is first ataxic and then spastic. Progressive dementia follows, and death usually occurs within the first de-

cade. Seizures and involuntary movements may occur in some patients.

Diagnosis. Enzyme deficiency is demonstrated in leukocytes and fibroblasts.

Treatment. No treatment is available.

Globoid Cell Leukodystrophy (Late-Onset Krabbe Disease)

Globoid cell leukodystrophy is caused by deficiency of the enzyme galactosylceramide beta-galactosidase. The defect is transmitted by autosomal recessive inheritance. The onset of symptoms in late infancy and in adolescence can occur in the same family (Verdru et al, 1991). The severity of enzyme deficiency is similar in all phenotypes from early infancy to adolescence.

Clinical Features. Neurologic deterioration usually begins between the ages of 2 and 6 but may start as early as the second year or as late as adolescence. The major features are mental regression, cortical blindness, and generalized or unilateral spasticity. The inital manifestation is more often progressive spasticity than dementia. Unlike the infantile form, the juvenile form is not characterized by peripheral neuropathy and the protein content of the cerebrospinal fluid is normal. Progressive neurologic deterioration results in a vegetative state.

Diagnosis. MRI demonstrates diffuse demyelination of the cerebral hemispheres. Definitive diagnosis requires demonstration of enzyme deficiency in leukocytes or cultured fibroblasts.

Treatment. No treatment is available.

Metachromatic Leukodystrophy (Late-Onset Sulfatide Lipidosis)

The juvenile form of sulfatide lipidosis, like the infantile form, is caused by a deficiency of the enzyme arylsulfatase A and transmitted by autosomal recessive inheritance. The percentage of residual arylsulfatase A activity is the same in the infantile and juvenile forms, and the reason for the phenotypic difference remains unexplained.

Clinical Features. The onset of symptoms is generally between 5 and 10 years but may be delayed to adolescence or occur as early as late infancy. The early-onset juvenile form is clinically different from the infantile form despite the age overlap. No clinical symptoms of peripheral neuropathy occur, progression is slow, and the protein content of the cerebrospinal fluid is normal (Haltia et al, 1980).

Mental regression, speech disturbances, and clumsiness of gait are the prominent initial features. The dementia usually progresses slowly over

3 to 5 years but sometimes progresses rapidly to a vegetative state. A delay of several years may separate the onset of dementia from the appearance of other neurologic disturbances. Ataxia may be an early and prominent manifestation. A spastic quadriplegia eventually develops in all affected children, and most have seizures. Death usually occurs during the second decade.

Diagnosis. The juvenile form can overlap in age with a late-onset form that usually is manifest as psychosis or dementia (Alves et al, 1986). MRI demonstrates demyelination in the cerebral hemispheres. Motor nerve conduction velocities may be normal early in the course. Definitive diagnosis requires demonstration of arylsulfatase A deficiency in leukocytes or cultured fibroblasts.

Treatment. No treatment is available.

Niemann-Pick Disease Type C (Sphingomyelin Lipidosis)

The chronic neuronopathic form of Niemann-Pick disease is similar to the acute infantile form except that onset is usually after age 2, progression is slower, and there is no specific racial predilection. Sphingomyelinase is the deficient enzyme in all forms of Niemann-Pick disease. The defect is transmitted by autosomal recessive inheritance.

Clinical Features. Three phenotypes are distinguished by age at onset and predominant symptoms (Fink et al, 1989). (1) The early-onset form is characterized by organomegaly and rapidly progressive hepatic dysfunction during the first year, often in the first 6 months. Developmental delay is noted during the first year, and neurologic deterioration (ataxia, vertical gaze apraxia, dementia) occurs between 1 and 3 years of age. (2) The delayed-onset form is more common than the other two and has the most stereotyped clinical features. Early development is normal. Mild intellectual impairment is noted at 2 years, cerebellar ataxia at 3 years, and apraxia of vertical gaze at 4 years or later. Oculomotor apraxia, in which the eyes move reflexively but not voluntarily, is unusual in children (see Chapter 15). Vertical gaze apraxia is particularly uncommon and always suggests Niemann-Pick disease type C. Dementia, seizures, dysphagia, and dystonia develop after age 6 and cause severe disability by the end of the second decade. Organomegaly is seldom prominent early in the course. (3) The late-onset form begins in adolescence or adult life and is similar to the delayed-onset form except that the progression is considerably slower.

Diagnosis. Examination of bone marrow reveals two unusual storage cells. One is large and vacuolated, the other smaller. Both contain dark, granular material. Definitive diagnosis requires demonstration of sphingomyelinase deficiency in leukocytes or cultured fibroblasts. Heterozygote detection and prenatal diagnosis are possible.

Treatment. No treatment is available.

OTHER DISORDERS OF GRAY MATTER
Ceroid Lipofuscinosis

Several disorders characterized by dementia and blindness are now considered to be forms of ceroid lipofuscinosis (Boustany and Kolodny, 1989). When these disorders were first described, different eponymic designations were used, depending on age at onset. The common pathologic feature is the accumulation of autofluorescent lipopigments, ceroid and lipofuscin, within the brain, retina, and some visceral tissues. Childhood-onset disease is thought to be transmitted by autosomal recessive inheritance, but some adult-onset disorders are transmitted as an autosomal dominant trait.

An early infantile form was described in the previous section. In addition, there are an infantile or childhood form (Bielschowsky-Jansky), a juvenile form (Spielmeyer-Vogt-Sjögren), and several adult forms.

Late Infantile Type (Bielschowsky-Jansky)

Clinical Features. Age at onset is 2 to 4 years. Seizures rather than blindness are the initial feature. The seizures are myoclonic, akinetic, and tonic-clonic and are usually refractory to anticonvulsant drugs. Severe ataxia develops, owing in part to seizures and in part to motor system deterioration. This is followed by myoclonus, involuntary movements, and dementia. Dementia sometimes precedes the first seizure.

Ophthalmoscopic findings are abnormal before visual symptoms occur. They include attenuation of vessels, early optic atrophy, and pigmentary degeneration of the macula. The loss of motor, mental, and visual function is relentlessly progressive, and within months the child is in a chronic vegetative state. Death is usually in the first decade.

Diagnosis. Antemortem diagnosis is accomplished by skin and conjunctival biopsy (Santavuori et al, 1991). Curvilinear inclusions are observed by electron microscopy within the cytoplasm of endothelial and neuronal cells. In addition, azurophilic granules are present in neutrophilic leukocytes stained by the Giemsa method.

Treatment. Seizures are difficult to control but may respond in part to a combination of valproate, clonazepam, and phenobarbital (see Chapter 1). No treatment is available for the underlying metabolic error.

Juvenile Type (Spielmeyer-Vogt-Sjögren Disease)

Clinical Features. The mean age at onset of the juvenile type is 6 years with a range from 4 to 9. Unlike patients with the late infantile type, these children frequently have decreasing visual acuity. Ophthalmoscopic examination reveals attenuation of retinal vessels, a patchy retinal atrophy that resembles retinitis pigmentosa, mild optic atrophy, and a granular discoloration of the macula that may have a bull's-eye appearance with a dull red spot in the center.

The dementia is characterized by declining school performance and behavioral disturbances. Delusions and hallucinations are common. Blindness and dementia are the only symptoms for many years. Late in the course, speech becomes slurred and Parkinson-like rigidity develops. Myoclonic jerks and tonic-clonic seizures begin some years after onset but are not usually severe. Death usually occurs within 15 years of onset.

Diagnosis. Antemortem diagnosis is reasonably certain because of the characteristic retinal changes and is confirmed by skin and conjunctival biopsy. Fingerprint bodies are present in the cytoplasm of several cell types. The electroretinogram demonstrates depression or absence of retinal potentials early in the course. Leukocytes in the peripheral blood are frequently abnormal. Translucent vacuoles are present in lymphocytes, and azurophilic granules occur in neutrophils.

Treatment. No treatment is available for the underlying metabolic defect. Seizures usually respond to standard anticonvulsant drugs.

Heller Syndrome

Heller syndrome has not been established as a genetic disease. It was originally described as a progressive dementia of childhood affecting males and females between the ages of 1 and 4 years. The early-onset female cases are now believed to be Rett syndrome.

Clinical Features. Probably Heller syndrome has a male predominance. Affected children develop normally to at least 30 months of age. Dementia progresses for 1 to 3 years and results in profound mental retardation with marked autistic features but no effect on motor skills (Burd et al, 1989).

Diagnosis. The diagnosis is based on clinical symptoms. The syndrome is differentiated from Rett syndrome by the age at onset, male predominance, and lack of motor disturbances and from infantile autism by the age at onset. All other causes of progressive dementia of childhood must be excluded (Table 5–3).

Treatment. No treatment is available.

Huntington Disease

Huntington disease is a chronic degenerative disease of the nervous system transmitted by autosomal dominant inheritance. It is believed that all cases are traceable to a single family. There are no new mutations. The prevalence is 5 to 10: 100,000.

Clinical Features. The age at onset is usually between 35 and 55 years but may be as early as 2 years. Approximately 10% of affected individuals show symptoms before 20 years of age and 5% before 14 years (Myers et al, 1985). When Huntington disease begins in childhood, the father is the affected parent in 83% of cases and may be asymptomatic when the child is born. Extrachromosomal organelles, such as mitochondria, are inherited exclusively from the mother and may delay the expression of the gene when the mother is the affected individual.

The initial manifestations are usually progressive dementia and behavioral disturbances (Menkes, 1988). Declining school performance often brings the child to medical attention. Rigidity, with loss of facial expression and associative movements, is more common than choreoathetosis and hyperkinesis, especially in early-onset cases. Cerebellar dysfunction occurs in approximately 20% of cases and can be a major cause of disability. Ocular motor apraxia may also be present (see Chapter 15). Seizures, which are rare in adult-onset cases, are present in 50% of affected children. The course in childhood is relentlessly progressive, and the average duration from onset to death is 8 years.

Diagnosis. Diagnosis requires evidence of disease in one of the parents. Atrophy of the caudate nucleus and cerebral cortex is characteristically seen on CT and MRI, and either study can be used to follow the progress of the disease.

Treatment. Rigidity may be temporarily relieved with levodopa, bromocriptine, and amantadine. Neuroleptics are useful for behavioral control, but no treatment is available for the dementia.

Mitochondrial Encephalomyopathies

The mitochondrial encephalomyopathies are a diverse group of disorders with defects in oxidative metabolism. Three such disorders are described in the section on progressive encephalopathies of infancy. Later onset mitochondrial disorders are characterized by progressive external ophthalmoplegia or myopathy. However, a late-onset form of poliodystrophy and a syndrome of myoclonic epilepsy associated with ragged-red fibers in skeletal muscle cause childhood dementia as the initial manifestation. Genetic transmission is by maternal inheritance.

Late-Onset Poliodystrophy

Clinical Features. The clinical features are similar to those of progressive infantile poliodystrophy except that the onset of dementia is delayed until 6 years of age or later. The dementia may be preceded by years of intermittent vomiting, lethargy, and headaches. Generalized tonic-clonic seizures can precede the onset of dementia or at least bring the child, who is already demonstrating poor school performance, to medical attention. The subsequent course is variable and probably depends on the underlying defect in mitochondrial metabolism. In many children myopathy develops; others have spasticity and blindness.

Diagnosis. Many children with mitochondrial enzyme defects have an increased blood concentration of lactate. However, the blood lactate concentration may vary with diet, and a glucose-lactate tolerance test is useful to screen for disturbances in mitochondrial function. An ordinary glucose tolerance test is administered except that both blood lactate and glucose concentrations are measured concurrently. Lactate levels do not rise significantly in normal children but may reach two or three times the upper limit of normal in children with defective mitochondrial metabolism. The elevated glucose concentration is slow in returning to normal.

When myopathy is present in addition to dementia, muscle biopsy usually demonstrates ragged-red fibers (see Figure 8–6).

Treatment. Children with defects in mitochondrial enzymes should be placed on a low-carbohydrate, high-fat diet. Although this does not cure the underlying defect, it helps to relieve symptoms caused by lactic acidosis. No other treatment is available.

Myoclonic Epilepsy and Ragged-Red Fibers (MERRF)

Cytochrome oxidase deficiency (complex IV) associated with a point deletion of mitochondrial DNA has been identified in one family (Lombes et al, 1989). Deficiencies in complexes I and IV are reported in another family (see Figure 8–5).

Clinical Features. Clinical heterogeneity is common even among members of the same family. Onset may be anytime during childhood or up until the fourth decade (Silva et al, 1987). An insidious decline in school performance is often the initial feature, but generalized tonic-clonic seizures or myoclonus may be the symptoms that first prompt medical consultation. The seizures may be induced by flickering light or watching television. Brief myoclonic twitching develops, often induced by action (action myoclonus), that may interfere with hand movement and posture. Ataxia is a constant feature as the disease progresses, and this may be due to action myoclonus rather than cerebellar dysfunction. Some patients have hearing loss, short stature, and endocrine dysfunction.

Neurologic deterioration is progressive and may include spasticity, sensory loss, and central hypoventilation. Clinical evidence of myopathy is not always present.

Diagnosis. Blood concentrations of pyruvate and lactate may be increased. EEG shows slowing of the background rhythms and a photoconvulsive response. Ragged-red fibers are seen on muscle biopsy (see Figure 8–6).

Treatment. Anticonvulsant drug therapy may provide seizure control early in the course but often fails as the disease progresses. Glucose loads should be avoided. No treatment is available for the underlying defect.

Xeroderma Pigmentosum

Xeroderma pigmentosum is a genetic disorder characterized by defective deoxyribonucleic acid (DNA) repair. Ten genetic subtypes have been defined. Group A is the most common form and is associated with neurologic deterioration (Robbins et al, 1991).

Clinical Features. A photosensitive dermatitis develops during the first year, and skin cancer may develop as well. Progressive psychomotor retardation and poor head growth leading to microcephaly are noted after age 3. Sensorineural hearing loss and spinocerebellar degeneration may develop after age 7. Approximately one third of patients are short in stature.

Diagnosis. The typical skin rash associated with neurologic deterioration in both the central and peripheral nervous system suggests the diagnosis, which is confirmed by the demonstration of abnormal DNA repair in cultured fibroblasts.

Treatment. No treatment is available. Radiation must be avoided.

OTHER DISEASES OF WHITE MATTER
Adrenoleukodystrophy

Adrenoleukodystrophy is a progressive demyelination of the central nervous system associated with adrenal cortical failure. It is transmitted by X-linked inheritance. Affected children have an impaired ability to oxidize very-long-chain fatty acids, especially hexacosanoic acid, because of deficiency of a peroxisomal acyl coenzyme A (CoA) synthetase. Very-long-chain fatty acids accumulate in tissues and plasma. Many cases previously designated as Schilder disease were probably the juvenile form of adrenoleukodystrophy.

Clinical Features. Clinical expression varies considerably. Neurologic deterioration precedes clinical evidence of adrenal insufficiency in 85% of cases (Moser and Moser, 1984). Melanoderma may be the only feature of adrenal disease and then in only isolated areas of the skin and mucosal surfaces. In rare instances, when adrenal failure is early and prominent, the subsequent neurologic manifestations may be attributed to adrenal failure and not recognized as a coexisting problem.

The onset of neurologic manifestations can occur anytime during childhood and may even be delayed until adult life. Most affected boys are 5 to 10 years of age. The first symptoms are usually an alteration in behavior ranging from a withdrawn state to aggressive outbursts. Poor school performance follows invariably and may lead parents to seek psychologic services. Neurologic deterioration is then relentlessly progressive and includes disturbances of gait and coordination, loss of vision and hearing, and ultimate deterioration to a vegetative state. Seizures are a late manifestation.

Diagnosis. The protein concentration of cerebrospinal fluid is generally increased. CT reveals hypodensities near the trigones of the lateral ventricles with contrast enhancement around the edges. MRI is more sensitive than CT, and T_2-weighted images demonstrate high signal intensity in the periventricular white matter even in asymptomatic individuals (Aubourg et al, 1989). Adrenal insufficiency may be documented in asymptomatic children by demonstrating a subnormal response to the stimulation by adrenocorticotropic hormone (ACTH). However, up to 15% have a normal response, and definitive diagnosis requires a plasma assay of very-long-chain fatty acids. The assay also permits identification of carrier females and the prenatal diagnosis of affected fetuses by measuring long-chain fatty acid concentrations in amniocytes.

Treatment. Corticosteroids reverse clinical symptoms of adrenal insufficiency, and a diet enriched with erucic acid and oleic acid may halt or slow the progression of demyelination (Rizzo et al, 1989).

Cerebrotendinous Xanthomatosis

Cerebrotendinous xanthomatosis is a rare disorder transmitted as an autosomal recessive trait. Deficiency of a liver mitochondrial enzyme blocks the oxidation of cholesterol to bile acids, causing the accumulation of cholestanol and bile alcohols in serum and the storage of sterols in all tissues, but especially the central nervous system (Peynet et al, 1991).

Clinical Features. Dementia begins in early childhood but is insidious in its progression so that affected children seem mildly retarded rather than actively deteriorating. By age 15, cataracts are present and tendinous xanthomas begin to form. They are small at first and may go unnoticed until adult life. Progressive spasticity and ataxia develop during adolescence, and the patient becomes incapacitated in early adult life. A demyelinating neuropathy may be present as well. Speech and swallowing are impaired, and death occurs from brainstem dysfunction or myocardial infarction.

Diagnosis. The triad of cataracts, tendon xanthomas, and progressive neurologic deterioration establishes the diagnosis, but all three features are not expressed completely until late in the course. Definitive diagnosis requires the demonstration of increased concentration of cholestanol in plasma or xanthomas.

Treatment. Oral chenodeoxycholic acid, lovastatin, and simvastin decrease cholestanol plasma and tissue concentrations by expanding the deficient bile pool. However, the biochemical improvement does not have a clinical benefit.

References

Aicardi J, Castelein P: Infantile neuroaxonal dystrophy. Brain 102:727, 1979.

Alves D, Pires MM, Guimaraes A, et al: Four cases of late onset metachromatic leukodystrophy in a family: Clinical, biochemical and neuropathological studies. J Neurol Neurosurg Psychiatry 49:1417, 1986.

Amir N, Zlotogora J, Bach G: Mucolipidosis type IV: Clinical spectrum and natural history. Pediatrics 79:953, 1987.

Aubourg P, Sellier N, Chaussain JL, et al: MRI detects cerebral involvement in neurologically asymptomatic patients with adrenoleukodystrophy. Neurology 39:1619, 1989.

Azen CG, Koch R, Friedman EG, et al: Intellectual development in 12-year-old children treated with phenylketonuria. Am J Dis Child 145:35, 1991.

Baumann RJ, Markesbery WR: Santavuori disease: Diagnosis by leukocyte ultrastructure. Neurology 32:1277, 1982.

Beaudet AL, Thomas GH: Disorders of glycoprotein degradation: Mannosidosis, fucosidoses, sialidosis, and aspartyl-glycosaminuria. In Scriver CR, Beaudet AL, Sly WS, et al (eds): The Metabolic Basis of Metabolic Disorders, 6th Edition. New York, McGraw-Hill, 1989, p 1603.

Begleiter ML, Harris DJ: Autosomal recessive form of connatal Pelizaeus-Merzbacher disease. Am J Med Genet 33:311, 1989.

Bernsen PLJA, Wevers RA, Gabreels FJM, et al: Phenotypic expression in mucopolysaccharidosis VII. J Neurol Neurosurg Psychiatry 50:699, 1987.

Borrett D, Becker LE: Alexander's disease: A disease of astrocytes. Brain 108:367, 1985.

Boustany RM, Kolodny EH: The neuronal ceroid lipofuscinosis: A review. Rev Neurol 145:105, 1989.

Burd L, Fisher W, Kerbeshian J: Pervasive disintegrative disorder: Are Rett syndrome and Heller dementia infantilis subtypes? Dev Med Child Neurol 31:609, 1989.

Butler C, Hittleman J, Hauger SB: Approach to neurodevelopmental and neurologic complications in pediatrics HIV infection. J Pediatr 119(suppl):S41, 1991.

Butler MG, Mangrum T, Gupta R, et al: A 15-item checklist for screening mentally retarded males for the fragile X syndrome. Clin Genet 39:347, 1991.

Cassidy SB, Pagon RA, Pepin M, et al: Family studies in tuberous sclerosis. JAMA 249:1302, 1983.

Clarke R, Daly L, Robinson K, et al: Hyperhomocysteinemia: An independent risk factor for vascular disease. N Engl J Med 324:1149, 1991.

Coster RV, Lombes A, DeVivo D, et al: Cytochrome c oxidase–associated Leigh syndrome: Phenotypic features and pathogenetic speculations. J Neurol Sci 104:97, 1991.

Daffos F, Forestier F, Capella-Pavlovsky M, et al: Prenatal management of 746 pregancies at risk for congenital toxoplasmosis. N Engl J Med 318:271, 1988.

Danner DJ, Elsas LJ: Disorders of branched chain amino acid metabolism. In Scriver CR, Beaudet AL, Sly WS, et al (eds): The Metabolic Basis of Metabolic Disorders, 6th Edition. New York, McGraw-Hill, 1989, p 671.

DeCarli C, Fugate L, Falloon J, et al: Brain growth and cognitive improvement in children with human immunodeficiency virus–induced encephalopathy after six months of continuous infusion zidovudine therapy. J Acquir Immune Defic Syndr 4:585, 1991.

Desmond MM, Wilson GS, Melnick JL, et al: Congenital rubella encephalitis. J Pediatr 71:311, 1967.

Dominguez R, Vila-Coro AA, Slopis JM, et al: Brain and ocular abnormalities in infants with in utero exposure to cocaine and other street drugs. Am J Dis Child 145:688, 1991.

Echenne H, Divry P, Vianey-Liaud C: Spongy degeneration of the neuraxis (Canavan–Van Bogaert disease) and N-acetylaspartic aciduria. Neuropediatrics 20:79, 1989.

European Collaborative Study: Mother-to-child transmission of HIV infection. Lancet 2:1039, 1988.

Evans OB, Kilroy AW, Fenichel GM: Acetazolamide in the treatment of pyruvate dysmetabolism syndromes. Arch Neurol 35:302, 1978.

Fink JK, Filling-Katz MR, Sokol J, et al: Clinical spectrum of Niemann-Pick disease type C. Neurology 39:1040, 1989.

Fisher DA, Foley BL: Early treatment of congenital hypothyroidism. Pediatrics 83:785, 1989.

Gascon GG, Ozand PT, Mahdi A, et al: Infantile CNS spongy degeneration—14 cases: Clinical update. Neurology 40:1876, 1990.

Gencic S, Abuelo M, Hudson LD: Pelizaeus-Merzbacher disease: An X-linked neurologic disorder of myelin metabolism with a novel mutation in the gene encoding proteolipid protein. Am J Hum Genet 45:435, 1989.

Glaze DG, Frost JD Jr, Zoghibi HY, et al: Rett's syndrome: Characterization of respiratory patterns and sleep. Ann Neurol 21:377, 1987.

Hagberg B: Krabbe's disease: Clinical presentation of neurologic variants. Neuropediatrics 15:11, 1984.

Haltia T, Palo J, Haltia M, et al: Juvenile metachromatic leukodystrophy: Clinical, biochemical, and neuropathological studies in nine new cases. Arch Neurol 37:42, 1980.

Harbord M, Buncic JR, Chuang SA, et al: Multiple sulfatase deficiency with early severe retinal degeneration. J Child Neurol 6:229, 1991.

Hittelman J: Neurodevelopmental aspects of HIV infection. In Kozlowski P, Vietze P, Wisniewski H (eds): Pediatric AIDS. Basel, S Karger, 1991, p 64.

Hoganson G, Berlow S, Kaufman S, et al: Biopterin synthesis defects: Problems in diagnosis. Pediatrics 74:1004, 1984.

Italian Multicentre Study: Epidemiology, clinical features, and prognostic factors of pediatric HIV infection. Lancet 2:1043, 1988.

Jankovic J, Caskey TC, Stout JT, et al: Lesch-Nyhan syndrome: A study of motor behavior and cerebrospinal fluid transmitters. Ann Neurol 23:466, 1988.

Kalter H, Warkany J: Congenital malformations: Etiologic factors and their role in prevention. N Engl J Med 308:424, 1983.

Kivlin JD, Sanborn GE, Myers GG: The cherry-red spot in Tay-Sachs and other storage diseases. Ann Neurol 17:356, 1985.

Listernick R, Charrow J: Neurofibromatosis type 1 in childhood. J Pediatr 116:845, 1990.

Livingstone IR, Gardner-Medwin D, Pennington RJT: Familial intermittent ataxia with possible X-linked recessive inheritance. J Neurol Sci 64:89, 1984.

Lo W, Packman S, Nash S, et al: Curious neurologic sequelae in galactosemia. Pediatrics 73:309, 1984.

Lombes A, Mendell JR, Nakase H, et al: Myoclonic epilepsy and ragged-red fibers with cytochrome oxidase deficiency: Neuropathology, biochemistry, and molecular genetics. Ann Neurol 26:20, 1989.

Manuelidis EE, Rorke LB: Transmission of Alper's disease (chronic progressive encephalopathy) produces experimental Creutzfeldt-Jacob disease in hamsters. Neurology 39:615, 1989.

McKinney RE, Maha MA, Connor EM, et al: A multicenter trial of zidovudine in children with advanced human immunodeficiency virus disease. N Engl J Med 324:1018, 1991.

Menkes JH: Huntington disease: Finding the gene and after. Pediatr Neurol 4:73, 1988.

Minshew NJ, Payton JB: New perspective in autism. I. The clinical spectrum of autism. Curr Probl Pediatr 18:561, 1988a.

Minshew NJ, Payton JB: New perspectives in autism. II. The differential diagnosis and neurobiology of autism. Curr Probl Pediatr 18:615, 1988b.

Moeschler JB, Charman CE, Berg SZ, et al: Rett syndrome: Natural history and management. Pediatrics 82:1, 1988.

Moraes CT, Schon EA, DiMauro S: Mitochondrial diseases: Toward a rational classification. In Appel SH (ed): Current Neurology, vol II, Mosby–Yearbook, St Louis, 1991, p 83.

Moser HW, Moser AE: Adrenoleukodystrophy: Survey of 303 cases; Biochemistry, diagnosis, and therapy. Ann Neurol 16:628, 1984.

Mudd SH, Skouby F, Levy HL, et al: The natural history of homocystinuria due to cystathionine β-synthase deficiency. Am J Hum Genet 37:1, 1985.

Myer EC, Morris DL, Brase DA, et al: Hyperendorphinism in Rett syndrome: Cause or result? Ann Neurol 24:340, 1988.

Myers RH, Cupples LA, Schoenfield M, et al: Maternal factors in transmission of Huntington's disease. Am J Hum Genet 37:511, 1985.

Nadal D, Baerlocher K: Menkes' disease: Long-term treatment with copper and D-penicillamine. Eur J Pediatr 147:621, 1988.

National Institute of Child Health and Human Development Intravenous Immunoglobulin Study Group: Immune globulin for the prevention of bacterial infections in children with human immunodeficiency virus infection. N Engl J Med 325:73, 1991.

National Institutes of Health Consensus Development Conference: Neurofibromatosis: Conference statement. Arch Neurol 45:575, 1988.

Neufeld EF, Muenzer J: The mucopolysaccharidoses. In Scriver CR, Beaudet AL, Sly WS, et al (eds): The Metabolic Basis of Metabolic Disorders, 6th Edition. New York, McGraw-Hill, 1989, p 1565.

Nishimura RN, Barranger JA: Neurologic complications of Gaucher's disease, type 3. Arch Neurol 37:92, 1980.

Nooijen JL, DeGroot CJ, VanDenHamer CJA, et al: Trace element studies in three patients and a fetus with Menkes' disease: Effect of copper therapy. Pediatr Res 15:284, 1981.

Novick BE, Rubinstein A: AIDS—the pediatric perspective. AIDS 1:3, 1987.

Peynet J, Laurent A, De Liege P, et al: Cerebrotendinous xanthomatosis: Treatments with simvastin, lovastatin, and chenodeoxycholic acid in 3 siblings. Neurology 41:434, 1991.

Rett Syndrome Diagnostic Criteria Work Group: Diagnostic criteria for Rett syndrome. Ann Neurol 23:425, 1988.

Rizzo WB, Leshner RT, Odone A, et al: Dietary erucic acid therapy for X-linked adrenoleukodystrophy. Neurology 39:1415, 1989.

Robbins JH, Brumback RA, Mendiones M, et al: Neurological disease in xeroderma pigmentosum: Documentation of a late onset type of the juvenile onset form. Brain 114:1335, 1991.

Santavuori P, Rapola J, Nuutila A, et al: The spectrum of Jansky-Bielschowsky disease. Neuropediatrics 22:92, 1991.

Shepherd CW, Gomez MR, Lie JT, et al: Causes of death in patients with tuberous sclerosis. Mayo Clin Proc 66:792, 1991.

Shimomura C, Matsui A, Choh H, et al: Magnetic resonance imaging in Pelizaeus-Merzbacher disease. Pediatr Neurol 4:124, 1988.

Silva MTG, Aicardi J, Goutieres JJ, et al: The syndrome of myoclonic epilepsy with ragged-red fibers: Report of a case and review of the literature. Neuropediatrics 18:200, 1987.

Soong B-W, Casamassima AC, Fink JK, et al: Multiple sulfatase deficiency. Neurology, 38:1273, 1988.

Specola N, Vanier MT, Goutiéres F, et al: The juvenile and chronic forms of GM_2 gangliosidosis: Clinical and genetic heterogeneity. Neurology 40:145, 1990.

Tuchman RE: Autism: Delineating the spectrum. Int Pediatr 6:161, 1991.

Verdru P, Lammens M, Dom R, et al: Globoid cell leukodystrophy: A family with both late-infantile and adult type. Neurology 41:1382, 1991.

Warner TG, Turner MW, Toone JR, et al: Prenatal diagnosis of infantile G_{m2} gangliosidosis type II (Sandhoff disease) by detection of N-acetylglucosaminyl-oligosaccharides in amniotic fluid with high-performance liquid chromatography. Prenat Diagn 6:393, 1986.

Watts RWE, Spellacy E, Gibbs DA: Clinical, post-mortem, biochemical and therapeutic observations on the Lesch-Nyhan syndrome with particular reference to the neurological manifestations. Q J Med 201:43, 1982.

Wilson CB, Remington JS: Toxoplasmosis. In Feigen RD, Cherry JD (eds): Textbook of Pediatric Infectious Disease, vol II, 2nd Edition. WB Saunders, Philadelphia, 1987, p 2067.

Woody RC, Brewster MA, Glasier C: Progressive intracranial calcification in dihydropteridine reductase deficiency prior to folinic acid therapy. Neurology 39:673, 1989.

Yow MD: Congenital cytomegalovirus disease: A NOW problem. J Infect Dis 159:163, 1989.

Hypotonic Infant

◆ Definitions

Tone is the resistance of muscle to stretch. Two kinds of tone are measured clinically: phasic and postural.

Phasic tone is a rapid contraction in response to a high-intensity stretch. It is examined by testing the tendon reflexes. When a hammer strikes the patellar tendon, the quadriceps muscle is stretched and the spindle apparatus, sensing the stretch, sends an impulse through the sensory nerve to the spinal cord. This information is transmitted to the alpha motor neuron, and the quadriceps muscle contracts (monosynaptic reflex).

Postural tone is a prolonged contraction in response to a low-intensity stretch. Gravity is the stimulus that provokes a steady, low-amplitude stretch on antigravity muscles. They respond with prolonged contraction. When postural tone is depressed, the infant is less able to maintain the body and limbs against gravity and is hypotonic.

The maintenance of normal tone requires an intact central and peripheral nervous system. Not surprisingly, therefore, hypotonia is a common symptom of neurologic dysfunction and is encountered in diseases of the brain, spinal cord, nerves, and muscles (Table 6–1). One anterior horn cell and all the muscle fibers that it innervates make up a *motor unit*. A primary disorder of the anterior horn cell body is a *neuronopathy,* a primary disorder of the axon or its myelin covering is a *neuropathy,* and a primary disorder of the muscle fiber is a *myopathy*. In infancy and childhood, diseases of the brain are far more common than diseases of the motor unit. The term *cerebral hypotonia* is used to encompass all causes of postural hypotonia related to cerebral disease or defect.

◆ Appearance of Hypotonia

When lying supine, all hypotonic infants look much the same regardless of the underlying cause or the location of abnormality within the nervous system (Figure 6–1). Spontaneous movement is lacking, the legs are fully abducted with the lateral surface of the thighs against the examining table, and the arms lie either extended at the sides of the body or flexed at the elbow with the hands beside the head. Pectus excavatum is present when the infant has long-standing weakness in the muscles of the chest wall. Infants who lie motionless eventually develop flattening of the occiput and loss of hair on the portion of the scalp that is in constant contact with the crib sheet. When the infant is placed in a sitting posture, the head falls forward, the shoulders droop, and the limbs hang limply.

Newborns who are hypotonic in utero may be born with dislocation of the hips, arthrogryposis, or both. Hip dislocation is a common feature of intrauterine hypotonia because the formation of a normal hip joint requires the forceful contraction of muscles to pull the head of the femur into the acetabulum. Arthrogryposis varies in severity from clubfoot, the most common manifestation, to symmetric flexion deformities of all limb joints. Joint contractures are believed to be a nonspecific consequence of intrauterine immobilization. However, among the several disorders that equally decrease fetal movement, some commonly produce arthrogryposis and others never do. The differential diagnosis of arthrogryposis is summarized in Table 6–2. Conditions caused by abnormality in the fetal brain or motor unit are also part of the differential diagnosis of infantile hypotonia.

The tone of infants who appear hypotonic at rest

Table 6–1 ◆ Differential Diagnosis of Infantile Hypotonia

Cerebral Hypotonia
1. "Benign" congenital hypotonia
2. Chromosome disorders
   a. Prader-Willi syndrome
   b. Trisomy
3. Chronic nonprogressive encephalopathy
   a. Cerebral malformation
   b. Perinatal distress
   c. Postnatal disorders
4. Peroxisomal disorders
   a. Cerebrohepatorenal syndrome (Zellweger)
   b. Neonatal adrenoleukodystrophy
5. Other genetic defects
   a. Familial dysautonomia
   b. Oculocerebrorenal syndrome (Lowe)
6. Other metabolic defects
   a. Acid maltase deficiency (see "Metabolic Myopathies")
   b. Infantile GM_1 gangliosidosis (see Chapter 5)

Spinal Cord Disorders
1. Hypoxic-ischemia myelopathy
2. Injuries

Spinal Muscular Atrophies
1. Acute infantile
2. Chronic infantile
3. Incontinentia pigmenti
4. Infantile neuronal degeneration
5. Neurogenic arthrogryposis

Polyneuropathies
1. Congenital hypomyelinating neuropathy
2. Giant axonal neuropathy (see Chapter 7)
3. Hereditary motor-sensory neuropathies (see Chapter 7)

Disorders of Neuromuscular Transmission
1. Infantile botulism
2. Familial infantile myasthenia
3. Transitory myasthenia gravis

Fiber-Type Disproportion Myopathies
1. Central core disease
2. Congenital fiber-type disproportion myopathy
3. Myotubular (centronuclear) myopathy
   a. Acute
   b. Chronic
4. Nemaline (rod) myopathy

Infantile Myositis

Metabolic Myopathies
1. Acid maltase deficiency
2. Cytochrome-c-oxidase deficiency
3. Carnitine deficiency
4. Phosphofructokinase deficiency
5. Phosphorylase deficiency

Muscular Dystrophies
1. Congenital muscular dystrophy
   a. Cerebroocular dystrophy
   b. Fukuyama type
   c. Leukodystrophy
2. Congenital myotonic dystrophy

can be further evaluated by the traction response, by vertical suspension, and by horizontal suspension.

TRACTION RESPONSE

The traction response is the most sensitive measure of postural tone and can be tested in premature newborns within an Isolette. The response is initiated by grasping the hands and pulling the infant to a sitting position. In a normal infant the head lifts from the surface immediately with the body. When the sitting position is attained, the head is held erect in the midline. During traction the examiner should feel the infant pulling back against traction and observe flexion at the elbow, knee, and ankle (Figure 6–2). A traction response is not present in premature newborns of less than 33 weeks' gestation. After 33 weeks the newborn has considerable head lag but the neck flexors consis-

tently respond to traction by lifting the head. At term only minimal head lag is present; when the sitting posture is attained, the head may continue

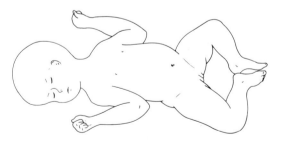

Figure 6–1 Hypotonia, with the infant at rest. The thighs are fully abducted (frog-leg position), and the arms lie in a flaccid position beside the head. (From Fenichel GM: Neonatal Neurology, 3rd edition. Churchill Livingstone, New York, 1990. By permission.)

Table 6–2 ◆ Differential Diagnosis of
Arthrogryposis

1. Cerebrohepatorenal syndrome
2. Cerebral malformations
3. Chromosomal disorders
4. Fetal, non–nervous system causes
5. Motor unit disorders
   a. Congenital cervical spinal atrophy
   b. Congenital fiber-type disproportion myopathy
   c. Congenital hypomyelinating neuropathy
   d. Congenital muscular dystrophy
   e. Genetic myasthenic syndromes
   f. Infantile neuronal degeneration
   g. Myotonic dystrophy
   h. Neurogenic arthrogryposis
   i. Phosphofructokinase deficiency
   j. Transitory neonatal myasthenia
6. Nonfetal causes

to lag or may become erect momentarily and then fall forward.

The presence of more than minimal head lag and of failure to counter traction by flexion of the limbs is abnormal and indicates hypotonia.

VERTICAL SUSPENSION

To perform vertical suspension, the examiner places both hands in the infant's axillae and, without grasping the thorax, lifts straight up. The muscles of the shoulders should be strong enough to press down against the examiner's hands and allow the infant to suspend vertically without falling

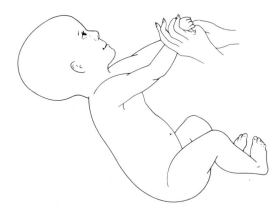

Figure 6–2 Normal traction response. The lift of the head is almost parallel to the lift of the body, and all limb joints show flexion. (From Fenichel GM: Neonatal Neurology, 3rd edition. Churchill Livingstone, New York, 1990. By permission.)

through. While the infant is in vertical suspension, the head is held erect in the midline and the legs are kept flexed at the knee, hip, and ankle. When a hypotonic infant is suspended vertically, the head falls forward, the legs dangle, and the infant may slip through the examiner's hands because of weakness in the shoulder muscles.

HORIZONTAL SUSPENSION

When suspended horizontally, a normal infant keeps the head erect, maintains the back straight, and demonstrates flexion at the elbow, hip, knee, and ankle. A healthy full-term newborn makes intermittent efforts to maintain the head erect, the back straight, and the limbs flexed against gravity. Hypotonic newborns and infants drape over the examiner's hands with the head and legs hanging limply.

◆ Approach to Diagnosis

The first step in diagnosis is to determine whether the site of disease is cerebral, spinal, or motor unit. More than one site may be involved (Table 6–3). The brain and the peripheral nerves are concomitantly involved in some lipid storage diseases, mitochondrial disorders, and familial dysautonomia. Both brain and skeletal muscles are abnormal in acid maltase deficiency and neonatal myotonic dystrophy. Newborns with severe hypoxic-ischemic encephalopathy may have hypoxic injury to the spinal cord as well. Several motor unit disorders produce sufficient hypotonia at birth to impair respiration and cause perinatal asphyxia (Table 6–4). Such infants also have cerebral hypotonia. Newborns with spinal cord injuries are frequently the product of long, difficult deliveries in which brachial plexus injuries and depressed cerebral function from asphyxia occur.

CLUES TO THE DIAGNOSIS OF CEREBRAL HYPOTONIA

Cerebral hypotonia in newborns usually does not pose diagnostic difficulty and can be identified by history and physical examination. Many clues to the diagnosis of cerebral hypotonia exist (Table 6–5), but most important is the presence of other abnormal brain functions: decreased consciousness and seizures. Cerebral malformation is the likely explanation for hypotonia in an infant with dysmorphic features or with malformations in other organs.

Table 6–3 ◆ Combined Cerebral and Motor Unit Hypotonia

1. Acid maltase deficiency
2. Familial dysautonomia
3. Giant axonal neuropathy
4. Hypoxic-ischemic encephalomyopathy
5. Infantile neuronal degeneration
6. Lipid storage diseases
7. Mitochondrial (respiratory chain) disorders
8. Neonatal myotonic dystrophy
9. Perinatal asphyxia secondary to motor unit disease

Table 6–4 ◆ Motor Unit Disorders with Perinatal Respiratory Distress

1. Acute infantile spinal muscular atrophy
2. Congenital hypomyelinating neuropathy
3. Congenital myotonic dystrophy
4. Familial infantile myasthenia
5. Neurogenic arthrogryposis
6. X-linked myotubular myopathy

A tightly fisted hand in which the thumb is constantly enclosed by the other fingers and does not open spontaneously *(fisting)* and adduction of the thigh so that the legs are crossed when the infant is suspended vertically *(scissoring)* are considered precursors of spasticity and indicate cerebral dysfunction. Postural reflexes may be elicited in newborns and infants with cerebral hypotonia even when spontaneous movement is lacking. In some acute encephalopathies, and especially in metabolic disorders, the Moro reflex may be exaggerated. The tonic neck reflex is an important indicator of cerebral abnormality if the responses are excessive and obligatory and persist beyond 6 months of age. When hemispheric damage is severe but the brainstem is intact, turning the head produces full extension of both ipsilateral limbs and tight flexion on the contralateral side. An obligatory reflex is one in which these postures are maintained

Table 6–5 ◆ Clues to Cerebral Hypotonia

1. Abnormalities of other brain function
2. Dysmorphic features
3. Fisting of the hands
4. Malformations of other organs
5. Movement through postural reflexes
6. Normal or brisk tendon reflexes
7. Scissoring on vertical suspension

Table 6–6 ◆ Clues to Motor Unit Disorders

1. Absent or depressed tendon reflexes
2. Failure of movement on postural reflexes
3. Fasciculations
4. Muscle atrophy
5. No abnormalities of other organs

as long as the head is kept rotated. Tendon reflexes are generally normal or brisk, and clonus may be present.

CLUES TO MOTOR UNIT DISORDERS

Disorders of the motor unit are not associated with malformations of other organs except for joint deformities and the maldevelopment of bony structures. The face sometimes looks dysmorphic when facial muscles are weak or when the jaw is underdeveloped.

Tendon reflexes are absent or depressed. Total loss of reflexes in muscles with residual movement is more likely caused by neuropathy than myopathy, whereas diminished reflexes consistent with the degree of weakness are more often encountered in myopathy than in neuropathy (Table 6–6). Muscle atrophy suggests motor unit disease but does not exclude the possibility of cerebral hypotonia. Failure of growth and even atrophy can be considerable in brain-damaged infants. The combination of atrophy and fasciculations is strong evidence for denervation. However, the observation of fasciculations in newborns and infants is often restricted to the tongue, and distinguishing fasciculations from normal random movements of the tongue is difficult unless atrophy is present.

Postural reflexes, such as the tonic-neck and positive supporting reaction, cannot be superimposed on weak muscles. The motor unit is the final common pathway of tone; limbs that will not move voluntarily cannot be moved reflexively.

◆ Cerebral Hypotonia

Hypotonia is a feature of almost every cerebral disorder in newborns and infants. This section does not deal with conditions in which the major symptoms are states of decreased consciousness, seizures, and progressive psychomotor retardation. Rather, the discussion is limited to conditions in which hypotonia is so prominent a feature that the examining physician may consider the possibility of motor unit disease.

BENIGN CONGENITAL HYPOTONIA

The term "benign congenital hypotonia" is retrospective and refers to infants who are hypotonic at birth or shortly thereafter and later have normal tone. It encompasses many different pathologic processes affecting the brain, the motor unit, or both. The majority of affected children have cerebral hypotonia. An increased incidence of mental retardation, learning disabilities, and other sequelae of cerebral abnormality is evident later in life, despite the recovery of normal muscle tone.

CHROMOSOME DISORDERS

Despite considerable syndrome diversity, common characteristics of autosomal chromosome aberrations in the newborn are dysmorphic features of the hands and face and profound hypotonia (see Table 5–4). For this reason chromosome studies are indicated for any hypotonic newborn with dysmorphic features of the hands and face, with or without other organ malformation (Table 6–7).

Prader-Willi Syndrome

The Prader-Willi syndrome is characterized by hypotonia, hypogonadism, mental retardation, short stature, and obesity. Approximately 50% of children with this syndrome have an interstitial deletion of the proximal long arm of chromosome 15 (Butler, 1990). Deoxyribonucleic acid (DNA) abnormalities of chromosome 15 are recognized even in individuals without chromosomal deletions.

Clinical Features.   Decreased fetal activity is recorded in 75% of affected pregnancies and is associated with a 10% incidence of congenital hip dislocation and a 6% incidence of clubfoot. At birth the hypotonia is profound and tendon reflexes are absent or greatly depressed. Feeding problems are invariable, and prolonged nasogastric tube feeding is common (Table 6–8). Cryptorchidism is present in 84% and hypogenitalism in 100%.

Both hypotonia and feeding difficulty persist until 8 to 11 months of age and are later replaced by

Table 6–7 ◆ Hypotonia and Dysmorphic Features

1. Cerebral dysgenesis
2. Cerebrohepatorenal syndrome
3. Congenital myotonic dystrophy
4. Chromosomal aberrations
5. Fiber-type disproportion myopathies
6. Neonatal adrenoleukodystrophy
7. Prader-Willi syndrome

Table 6–8 ◆ Difficulty of Feeding in the Alert Newborn

1. Congenital myotonic dystrophy
2. Familial dysautonomia
3. Genetic myasthenic syndromes
4. Hypoplasia of bulbar motor nuclei (see Chapter 17)
5. Infantile neuronal degeneration
6. Myophosphorylase deficiency
7. Neurogenic arthrogryposis
8. Prader-Willi syndrome
9. Transitory neonatal myasthenia

relatively normal muscle tone and insatiable hunger. Developmental milestones are delayed, and mental retardation is a constant feature. Minor abnormalities that become more obvious during infancy include a narrow bifrontal diameter of the skull, strabismus, almond-shaped eyes, enamel hypoplasia, and small hands and feet. Obesity is the rule during childhood. The combination of obesity and minor abnormalities of the face and limbs produces a resemblance among children with this syndrome.

Diagnosis.   The combination of hypotonia, difficulty feeding, and cryptorchidism in the newborn warrants chromosome analysis with special reference to chromosome 15. Other studies are not helpful, and if chromosomes are not studied, diagnosis is delayed until the development of obesity.

Treatment.   No specific treatment is available.

CHRONIC NONPROGRESSIVE ENCEPHALOPATHY

Cerebral dysgenesis may be due to known or unknown noxious environmental agents, chromosomal disorders, or genetic defects. In the absence of an acute encephalopathy, hypotonia may be the only symptom at birth or during early infancy. Hypotonia is usually worse at birth and gets better with time. Cerebral dysgenesis should be suspected when hypotonia is coupled with malformations in other organs or abnormalities in head size and shape. Magnetic resonance imaging (MRI) of the head is advisable when cerebral malformation is suspected. The identification of a cerebral malformation provides useful information not only for prognosis but also on the feasibility of aggressive therapy to correct malformations in other organs.

Brain injuries occur in the perinatal period and less commonly throughout infancy as a result of anoxia, hemorrhage, infection, and trauma. The sudden onset of hypotonia in a previously well newborn or infant, with or without signs of encephalopathy, should suggest a cerebral cause. The premature newborn who demonstrates a decline in spontaneous movement and tone may have an intraventricular hemorrhage. Hypotonia is an early feature of meningitis in full-term and premature newborns. Tendon reflexes may be diminished or absent during the acute phase.

PEROXISOMAL DISORDERS

Peroxisomes are subcellular organelles that participate in the biosynthesis of ether phospholipids and bile acids; the oxidation of very-long-chain fatty acids, prostaglandins, and unsaturated long-chain fatty acids; and the catabolism of phytanate, pipecolate, and glycolate (Wanders et al, 1989). Peroxide is generated in the course of several oxidation reactions and catabolized by the enzyme catalase. The chemical abnormalities usually associated with peroxisomal defects include elevated concentrations of very-long-chain fatty acids in tissue and plasma, secretion of abnormal bile acid precursors, hyperpipecolic acidemia and aciduria, and decreased concentrations of tissue plasmalogens. Table 6–9 lists the clinical features that suggest peroxisomal disorders; only mental retardation is an obligatory criterion (Naidu et al, 1988).

The three infantile syndromes of peroxisomal dysfunction are cerebrohepatorenal (Zellweger) syndrome, neonatal adrenoleukodystrophy, and infantile Refsum disease. The first two are manifested as infantile hypotonia and are discussed here. Infantile Refsum disease is manifested as impaired vision and hearing and is discussed in Chapter 16.

Cerebrohepatorenal Syndrome (Zellweger Syndrome)

Cerebrohepatorenal syndrome is a defect in peroxisomal biogenesis; the intrinsic protein membrane can be identified, but all matrix enzymes are missing (Santos et al, 1988). The defect is probably transmitted by autosomal recessive inheritance. Biochemical disturbances include nonspecific aminoaciduria, increased serum levels of iron and copper, alterations in bile acid synthesis, pipecolic acidemia, and the accumulation of very-long-chain fatty acids in ocular tissue.

Clinical Features. Affected newborns are poorly responsive and have severe hypotonia, arthrogryposis, and dysmorphic features. The arthrogryposis is characterized by limited extension of the fingers (*camptodactyly*) and flexion deformities of the knee and ankle. Suck and cry are weak, and

Table 6–9 ◆ Phenotypic Features of Peroxisomal Disorders

1. Aberrant bone calcification
2. Adrenal insufficiency (rare)
3. Dysmorphic features
4. Hepatomegaly with impaired function
5. Hypotonia
6. Impaired hearing
7. Psychomotor retardation
8. Renal cysts
9. Retinal pigmentary degeneration
10. Seizures

Modified from Naidu et al: Pediatr Neurol 4:5, 1988.

tendon reflexes diminished or absent. Characteristic craniofacial abnormalities include a pear-shaped head owing to a high forehead and an unusual fullness of the cheeks, widened sutures, micrognathia, a high-arched palate, flattening of the bridge of the nose, and hypertelorism. Abnormalities of other organs include biliary cirrhosis, polycystic kidneys, retinal degeneration, and cerebral malformation.

Seizures usually begin shortly after birth but may begin anytime during infancy. They are difficult to control. Death from aspiration, gastrointestinal bleeding, or liver failure usually occurs within 6 months and almost always within 1 year.

Diagnosis. Clinical diagnosis can be made on the basis of specific organ involvement. Muscle biopsy reveals large aggregates of mitochondria and increased lipid in subsarcolemmal intermyofibrillary spaces. Liver biopsy demonstrates biliary dysgenesis and iron storage.

Treatment. Experimental diet therapy has had limited success and is being refined and tested.

Neonatal Adrenoleukodystrophy

The neonatal form of adrenoleukodystrophy is transmitted by autosomal recessive inheritance. The childhood form, discussed in Chapter 5, is transmitted by X-linked inheritance.

Clinical Features. In some newborns with adrenoleukodystrophy the disease shows phenotypic resemblance to the cerebrohepatorenal syndrome. The initial clinical features are hypotonia and failure to thrive. Tendon reflexes are present and often brisk. Abnormal facial features, hepatomegaly, and retinitis pigmentosa are constant features (Aubourg et al, 1986). Progressive neurologic deterioration is characterized by seizures, blindness, psychomotor retardation, and spasticity. The adrenal glands are hypoplastic, but no symptoms of adrenal failure are present. Death usually occurs during early childhood.

Diagnosis. The diagnosis is established by demonstrating poor adrenal function and increased concentrations of very-long-chain fatty acids in the plasma. Increased concentrations of phytanic acid and trihydroxycoprostanic acid may be present.

Treatment. Dietary treatment has been attempted in the X-linked childhood form (see Chapter 5) but has not been reported in the neonatal form.

OTHER GENETIC DEFECTS
Familial Dysautonomia

Familial dysautonomia, the *Riley-Day syndrome,* was originally described as a genetic disorder transmitted by autosomal recessive inheritance in Ashkenazi Jews. Similar clinical syndromes also occur in non-Jewish infants; these are often sporadic and the mode of inheritance is not clear.

Clinical Features. In the newborn the important clinical features are meconium aspiration, poor or no suck reflex, and hypotonia (Axelrod et al, 1987). Hypotonia is caused by disturbances in the brain, the dorsal root ganglia, and the peripheral nerves. Tendon reflexes are hypoactive or absent. The feeding difficulty is unique to familial dysautonomia and provides a clue to diagnosis. Sucking and swallowing are normal separately but cannot be coordinated for effective feeding. Other clinical features that may be noted either in the newborn or later in infancy include pallor, temperature instability, absence of fungiform papillae of the tongue, diarrhea and abdominal distention, poor weight gain, lethargy, episodes of irritability, absence of corneal reflexes, a labile blood pressure, and failure to produce overflow tears.

Diagnosis. Diagnosis should be suspected from the constellation of clinical symptoms and can be confirmed by the pilocarpine or histamine test. The instillation of 1 drop of 0.0625% pilocarpine solution into the conjunctival sac has no effect on a normal pupil but causes immediate pupillary constriction in infants with dysautonomia. This reaction is an example of denervation hypersensitivity. An intradermal injection of 0.1 ml of histamine sulfate (1:10,000) produces an erythematous wheal followed by a painful flare that extends more than 5 cm and lasts for more than an hour in normal children. In infants with dysautonomia the same injection produces a wheal 2 to 3 cm in diameter with a sharp red border, but the flare, an axon reflex, is lacking.

Treatment. Treatment is directed at the symptoms. Bethanechol (Urecholine), 1 to 2 mg/kg/day orally, is thought to be helpful. Its use is based on the observation that injections of acetylcholine produce a transient relief of some symptoms. Longevity has increased because of improved treatment of symptoms.

Oculocerebrorenal Syndrome (Lowe Syndrome)

Oculocerebrorenal syndrome is transmitted by X-linked recessive inheritance. Partial expression in the form of minor lenticular opacities is seen in female carriers. The primary abnormality of this disease has not been established, but a mitochondrial disorder causing multiple organ dysfunction is likely (Gobernado et al, 1984).

Clinical Features. The important features at birth are hypotonia and hyporeflexia, sometimes associated with congenital cataracts and glaucoma. The differential diagnosis of cataracts in newborns and young infants is listed in Table 16–3. Features that appear later in infancy are mental retardation and a progressive disorder of the renal tubules resulting in metabolic acidosis, proteinuria, aminoaciduria, and defective acidification of the urine. Many infants die after failing to thrive. Others have mild symptoms, including growth retardation, borderline intellectual function, mild renal disturbances, and late-onset cataract formation. Life expectancy is normal in the milder cases.

Diagnosis. Diagnosis depends on recognition of the clinical constellation. MRI demonstrates diffuse and irregular foci of increased signal consistent with demyelination (Charnas and Bernar, 1988).

Treatment. Most patients require alkinization therapy, and many benefit from supplements of potassium, phosphate, calcium, and carnitine (Charnas et al, 1991).

OTHER METABOLIC DEFECTS

Inborn errors of metabolism, other than peroxisomal disorders, are seldom manifested by hypotonia alone. However, two disorders in the newborn period or early infancy are sometimes exceptions to the rule: acid maltase deficiency and generalized GM$_1$ gangliosidosis. Acid maltase deficiency, the more common of the two, produces a severe myopathy and is discussed with other metabolic myopathies. Generalized GM$_1$ gangliosidosis is discussed in Chapter 5.

◆ Spinal Cord Disorders
HYPOXIC-ISCHEMIC MYELOPATHY

Hypoxic-ischemic encephalopathy is an expected outcome in severe perinatal asphyxia (see Chapter 1). Affected newborns are hypotonic and areflexic. These features have been attributed exclusively to the cerebral injury but also may be caused by spinal cord dysfunction. Concurrent ischemic necrosis of gray matter occurs in the spinal cord as well as in the brain (Clancy et al, 1989). The spinal cord component is often found on postmortem examination but may also be demonstrated in nonfatal cases by electromyography (EMG).

SPINAL CORD INJURY

Only in the newborn does spinal cord injury enter the differential diagnosis of hypotonia. Injuries to the cervical spinal cord occur almost exclusively during vaginal delivery; approximately 75% are associated with breech presentation and 25% with cephalic presentation. Because the injuries are always associated with a difficult and prolonged delivery, decreased consciousness is common and hypotonia may be falsely attributed to asphyxia or cerebral trauma (Painter and Bergman, 1982). However, the presence of impaired sphincter function and loss of sensation below the midchest should suggest myelopathy.

Injuries in Breech Presentation

Traction injuries to the lower cervical and upper thoracic regions of the cord occur almost exclusively when the angle of extension of the fetal head exceeds 90%. Indeed, the risk of spinal cord injury to a fetus in breech position whose head is hyperextended is greater than 70%. In such cases delivery should always be by cesarean section. The tractional forces applied to the extended head are sufficient not only to stretch the cord but also to herniate the brainstem through the foramen magnum. In addition, the hyperextended position compromises the vertebral arteries as they enter the skull.

The spectrum of pathologic findings varies from edema of the cord without loss of anatomic continuity to massive hemorrhage (epidural, subdural, and intramedullary), which is most pronounced in the lower cervical and upper thoracic segments but may extend the entire length of the cord. Concurrent hemorrhage in the posterior fossa and laceration of the cerebellum may be present as well.

Clinical Features. Mild tractional injuries, in which there is edema of the cord but not intraparenchymal hemorrhage or loss of anatomic continuity, produce few or no clinical manifestations. The major feature is hypotonia, which may be falsely attributed to asphyxia.

Severe tractional injuries are accompanied by hemorrhage into the posterior fossa. Affected newborns are unconscious and atonic at birth. They have flaccid quadriplegia with diaphragmatic breathing. Most do not survive the neonatal period. Injuries restricted to the low cervical and high thoracic segments produce near-normal strength in the biceps muscles and weakness of the triceps muscles. The result is flexion of the arms at the elbow and flaccid paraplegia. Spontaneous movement and tendon reflexes in the legs are absent, but foot withdrawal from pinprick may occur as a spinal reflex. The infant has a distended bladder and dribbling of urine. Sensory levels are difficult to measure but may be deduced by the absence of sweating below the injury.

Diagnosis. Radiographs of the vertebrae show no abnormalities because bony displacement does not occur. MRI of the spine shows intraspinal edema and hemorrhage (Adams et al, 1988).

Unconscious newborns are generally thought to have intracerebral hemorrhage or asphyxia (see Chapter 2), and the diagnosis of spinal cord injury may not be considered until consciousness is regained and the typical motor deficits are observed. Even then, a neuromuscular disorder may be suspected. The disturbance in bladder function and the development of progressive spastic paraplegia should alert the physician to the correct diagnosis.

Treatment. The treatment of spinal cord traction injuries of the newborn is similar to the management of cord injuries in older children (see Chapter 12).

Injuries in Cephalic Presentation

Injuries in cephalic presentation are high cervical cord injuries caused by twisting of the neck during midforceps rotation when the trunk fails to rotate with the head. The risk is greatest when amniotic fluid is absent because of delay from time of membrane rupture to application of forceps. The spectrum of injury varies from intraparenchymal hemorrhage to complete transection. Transection usually occurs at the level of a fractured odontoid process with atlantoaxial dislocation.

Clinical Features. Newborns are flaccid and fail to breathe spontaneously. Those with milder injuries may have shallow, labored respirations, but all require assisted ventilation at birth. Most are unconscious at birth owing to edema in the brainstem. When consciousness is regained, eye movements, sucking, and the withdrawal reflex are the only movements observed. Tendon reflexes are at first absent but later become exaggerated if the child survives. The bladder becomes distended, and overflow incontinence occurs. Priapism may be present. Sensation is difficult to assess because the withdrawal reflex is present.

Death from sepsis or respiratory complications generally occurs in the first week. Occasionally children have survived for several years.

Diagnosis. Most children with high cervical cord injuries are thought to have neuromuscular disorders, especially infantile spinal muscular atrophy, because the limbs are flaccid but the eye movements are normal. EMG of the limbs should exclude that possibility. Radiographs of the cervical vertebrae usually do not show abnormalities, but MRI shows marked thinning or disruption of the cord at the site of injury (Lanska et al, 1990).

Treatment. Newborns with high cervical cord injuries are intubated and provided with respiratory assistance before the diagnosis is established. Further management of spinal cord transection is discussed in Chapter 12.

◆ Motor Unit Disorders
EVALUATION OF MOTOR UNIT DISORDERS

In the diagnosis of cerebral hypotonia in infants, the choice of laboratory tests varies depending on the disease entity. This is not the case with motor unit hypotonia. A battery of tests is available that readily defines the anatomy and cause of pathologic processes affecting the motor unit (Table 6–10). The sequence in which the tests are done is important.

Serum Creatine Kinase

Increased serum concentrations of creatine kinase reflect skeletal or cardiac muscle necrosis. Blood should be drawn for creatine kinase determination before the performance of EMG or muscle biopsy because either procedure elevates the serum concentration of creatine kinase. Laboratory reference values for the normal serum concentration are usually based on nonambulatory patients. Normal values tend to be higher in an ambulatory population, especially after exercise. The total concentration of creatine kinase and its isoenzymes

Table 6–10 ◆ Evaluation of Motor Unit Disorders

1. Serum creatine kinase
2. Electrodiagnosis
   a. Electromyography
   b. Nerve conduction studies
   c. Repetitive stimulation
3. Muscle biopsy
4. Nerve biopsy
5. Tensilon test

increases significantly with acidosis. Levels as high as 1000 IU/L may be recorded in severely asphyxiated newborns, but even normal newborns have a higher than normal concentration during the first 24 hours post partum (Warburton et al, 1981). A normal creatine kinase level in a hypotonic infant is strong evidence against a rapidly progressive myopathy, but it does not exclude fiber-type disproportion myopathies and some metabolic myopathies from the diagnosis. Conversely, a mild elevation in the creatine kinase concentration is sometimes encountered in rapidly progressive spinal muscular atrophies.

Electrodiagnosis

EMG is extremely useful in the diagnosis of infantile hypotonia when the study is performed by an experienced physician. It enables prediction of the final diagnosis in 82% of infants younger than 3 months of age with hypotonia or motor unit origin. Fewer than 5% of hypotonic infants with normal EMG findings show abnormalities on muscle biopsy (Packer et al, 1982). The needle portion of the study helps to distinguish myopathic from neuropathic processes. Myopathies are generally characterized by the appearance of brief, small-amplitude, polyphasic potentials (BSAPPs). Neuropathies are characterized by the presence of denervation potentials at rest (fibrillations, fasciculations, sharp waves) and motor unit potentials that are large, prolonged, and polyphasic. Studies of nerve conduction velocity are useful in distinguishing axonal from demyelinating neuropathies; demyelinating neuropathies cause greater slowing of conduction velocity. Repetitive nerve stimulation studies demonstrate disturbances in neuromuscular transmission.

Muscle Biopsy

Muscle biopsy should not be undertaken unless the tissue can be processed by histochemical techniques. The muscle selected for biopsy should be weak but still able to contract. When weakness is symmetric, the muscles of one limb should be studied by EMG and the muscles of the other limb reserved for biopsy. Adequate tissue can be obtained either by needle biopsy or by open biopsy, depending on the physician's preference.

Histochemical analysis is essential for the complete evaluation of muscle histology because special techniques are needed to demonstrate fiber types and storage materials. Human skeletal muscle can be arbitrarily divided into two fiber types on the basis of the intensity of reaction to myosin adenosine triphosphatase (ATPase) at pH 9.4. Type I fibers react weakly to ATPase, are characterized by oxidative metabolism, and serve a tonic function. Type II fibers react intensely to ATPase, utilize glycolytic metabolism, and serve a phasic function. Type I and II fibers are generally equal in number and randomly distributed in each fascicle. Disorders may be characterized by abnormalities in fiber type number, fiber type size, or both.

The important storage materials identified in skeletal muscle are glycogen and lipid. In most storage disorders vacuoles are present in the fibers that contain the abnormal material. The vacuoles are seen with light microscopy, and the specific material is identified by its histochemical reaction.

Nerve Biopsy

Sural nerve biopsy is indicated only in patients with electrodiagnostic evidence of sural neuropathy. Nerve biopsy is useful in differentiating axonal from demyelinating neuropathies and can be useful for diagnosis by demonstrating vasculitis, amyloid, and lipid storage products.

Tensilon Test

Edrophonium chloride (Tensilon) is a rapidly acting anticholinesterase that temporarily reverses weakness in patients with myasthenia. Ptosis and oculomotor paresis are the only functions that are reliably tested. Rare patients are supersensitive to Tensilon and may stop breathing because of depolarization of endplates or an abnormal vagal response. Equipment for mechanical ventilation should always be available when the test is performed. In newborns a subcutaneous injection of 0.15 mg/kg produces a response within 10 minutes. In infants the drug is given intravenously at a dose of 0.2 mg/kg and reverses weakness within 1 minute.

SPINAL MUSCULAR ATROPHIES

Spinal muscular atrophies are a heterogeneous group of disorders, usually genetic in origin and characterized by the degeneration of anterior horn cells in the spinal cord and motor nuclei of the brainstem. Symptoms begin at any age from the newborn period to adult life. Some spinal muscular atrophies are marked by a generalized distribution of weakness, and others affect specific muscle groups. Those that begin in infancy usually have generalized weakness and are manifested as infantile hypotonia. Infantile spinal muscular atrophy (Werdnig-Hoffmann disease) is one of the more common motor unit disorders causing infantile hypotonia.

Two clinical syndromes of infantile spinal muscular atrophy, both transmitted by autosomal inheritance, can be distinguished. One is an acute fulminating form that begins at birth or within the first 6 months, and the other is a chronic form that begins after 3 months of age. Both the acute and chronic forms are caused by a defect at the same site on chromosome 5 (Munsat et al, 1990). As a rule the course of disease within a kinship is consistent.

A male predominance of cases may be explained by the existence of an X-linked form that is phenotypically indistinguishable from the more prevalent form transmitted by autosomal recessive inheritance (Greenberg et al, 1988). Newborns with the X-linked form often have arthrogryposis at birth, and their weakness progresses rapidly to cause respiratory insufficiency and death.

Acute Infantile Spinal Muscular Atrophy

Clinical Features. In acute infantile spinal muscular atrophy, neuronal degeneration begins in utero and reduced fetal movement is sometimes noted during pregnancy. Affected newborns have a generalized weakness involving proximal more than distal muscles, hypotonia, and areflexia. At rest they assume the characteristic posture of hypotonia.

Newborns who are hypotonic in utero and weak at birth may have difficulty adapting to extrauterine life and experience postnatal asphyxia and encephalopathy. The majority breathe adequately at first and appear alert despite the generalized weakness because facial expression is relatively well preserved and extraocular movement is normal. Paradoxic respiration develops because intercostal paralysis and thoracic collapse occur before diaphragmatic movement is impaired. Despite intrauterine hypotonia, arthrogryposis is not present. Neurogenic arthrogryposis is probably a distinct entity and is described separately in this chapter.

When weakness begins in infancy, the decline in strength can be sudden or decremental. At times the child seems to improve because of normal cerebral development, but the progression of weakness is relentless. Atrophy and fasciculations may be observed in the tongue. After the gag reflex is lost, feeding becomes difficult and death results from aspiration and pneumonia. When weakness is present at birth, death occurs by 6 months of age. Infants in whom symptoms develop later may survive longer.

Diagnosis. The diagnosis is readily established by laboratory investigation. Serum concentration of creatine kinase is usually normal but may be mildly elevated in infants with rapidly progressive weakness. EMG studies demonstrate fibrillations and fasciculations at rest and an increased mean amplitude of motor unit potentials. Motor nerve conduction velocities may be slowed but are usually normal. The histopathologic findings in muscle establish the diagnosis. Routine histologic stains demonstrate groups of small fibers adjacent to groups of normal-sized or hypertrophied fibers. The diagnostic features of acute infantile spinal muscular atrophy are revealed by the myosin ATPase reaction. All hypertrophied fibers are type I. Fibers of medium and small size are a mixture of types I and II (Figure 6–3). The normal random arrangement of fiber types is replaced by type grouping, a sign of reinnervation in which large numbers of fibers of the same type are contiguous.

Treatment. No treatment is available for this disorder, nor is there a method for prenatal diagnosis.

Chronic Infantile Spinal Muscular Atrophy

Clinical Features. The chronic form of infantile spinal muscular atrophy begins after 3 months of age. Therefore, when weakness begins between 3 and 6 months, the physician cannot predict whether the course of illness will be acute or chronic. Initial weakness is usually symmetric and affects the proximal muscles of the legs, the arms, or all limbs. An unusual form that begins with neck weakness has also been described (Goutiéres et al, 1991). The infants manifest head droop and generalized weakness with respiratory insufficiency. They die by 3 years of age.

More typically, pelvic weakness is the initial symptom. Distal muscles are affected little or not at all during early infancy. Tendon reflexes of weak

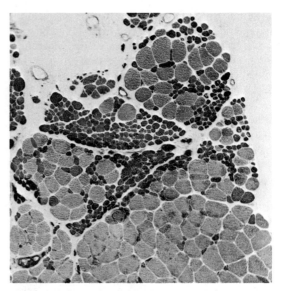

Figure 6–3 Infantile spinal muscular atrophy. The normal checkerboard pattern is lost. Groups of large type I fibers *(light shade)* are adjacent to groups of small type II fibers *(dark shade).* (ATPase reaction.) (From Fenichel GM: Neonatal Neurology, 3rd edition. Churchill Livingstone, New York, 1990. By permission.)

muscles are depressed or unobtainable. Facial muscles are not affected early in the course, and extraocular muscles are spared.

During infancy the weakness progresses slowly and is not life threatening. In some children the progression of weakness ceases and remains stable for many years, but eventually slow progression of weakness resumes. Improvement never occurs, and even during periods of stabilization the EMG continues to demonstrate fibrillations and fasciculations.

Contractures commonly develop during childhood. Pseudohypertrophy of the calves and gluteal muscles is common and may suggest Duchenne muscular dystrophy. As the plantar flexor muscles become weaker, the foot everts into an equinovarus posture. Some children have hand tremor. Death results from respiratory insufficiency. The mean age at death is 30 years.

Diagnosis. The serum concentration of creatine kinase is normal. EMG findings are identical to those described for the acute infantile form. Muscle biopsy demonstrates groups of small fibers adjacent to fibers of normal size. Type grouping is usually present, but type I fiber hypertrophy is not.

Treatment. Although there is no treatment for the underlying disease, physical therapy and other rehabilitative measures may prevent contractures and maintain function.

Incontinentia Pigmenti

Incontinentia pigmenti usually is manifested by neonatal seizures and is described fully in Chapter 1. It is characterized by the combination of typical skin lesions and cerebral malformations. Occasionally the skin lesions are associated with progressive anterior horn cell degeneration (Larsen et al, 1987).

Infantile Neuronal Degeneration

Clinical Features. Infantile neuronal degeneration is a rare disorder in which the typical features of infantile spinal muscular atrophy are combined with degenerative changes in the cerebellum, thalamus, and peripheral sensory nerves (Steiman et al, 1980). The defect is thought to be transmitted as an autosomal recessive trait because of three families with two or more affected siblings. All demonstrated hypotonia and areflexia, and one had arthrogryposis as well. The hypotonia is due primarily to denervation but probably has a cerebral component. In half of cases the symptoms are present at birth; in the other half they appear during early infancy. Dyspnea, weak cry, and difficulty in feeding are prominent features in the newborn, all of whom die within 5 months. The symptoms are the same when the onset is delayed until early infancy, but survival beyond 2 years of age is recorded.

Diagnosis. Infantile neuronal degeneration can be differentiated from infantile spinal muscular atrophy by electrophysiologic studies. Motor nerve conduction velocities are slow, and sensory nerve responses are absent or reduced.

Treatment. No treatment is available.

Neurogenic Arthrogryposis

The term "neurogenic arthrogryposis" was originally used to denote the association of arthrogryposis with infantile spinal muscular atrophy. Most cases are sporadic. Transmission occurs by autosomal recessive inheritance in some families and by X-linked inheritance in others. I am aware of two sets of identical twins in which one twin was born with neurogenic arthrogryposis and the other remained normal. This suggests that some sporadic cases may have nongenetic causes.

Several kindreds with neurogenic arthrogryposis transmitted as an autosomal dominant pattern have been reported (Fleury and Hageman, 1985). These kinships tend to have clinical or pathologic features that distinguish them from the sporadic cases and

the autosomal recessive group. Arthrogryposis may not occur in every affected family member, weakness or joint deformity may be limited to the legs or arms, and progression is minimal.

Clinical Features. In neurogenic arthrogryposis the most active phase of disease occurs in utero. Severely affected newborns have respiratory and feeding difficulties, and some die of aspiration. The less severely affected survive and have little or no progression of their weakness. Indeed, the respiratory and feeding difficulties lessen with time. Contractures are present in both proximal and distal joints. Micrognathia and a high-arched palate may be associated features, and a pattern of facial anomalies suggesting trisomy 18 is present in some newborns.

Newborns with respiratory distress may have a separate genetic error with a consistent phenotype in siblings (McWilliam et al, 1985; Schapira and Swash, 1985). The phenotype consists of minimal limb weakness and an unpredictable course in which long intervals of stability are expected.

Diagnosis. The diagnosis is suspected in newborns with arthrogryposis who have a normal serum concentration of creatine kinase and EMG findings compatible with a neuropathic process. Muscle histologic examination reveals the typical pattern of denervation and reinnervation. However, the histology may also have myopathic features: increased collagen and adipose tissue, structural derangements in medium-sized fibers, and fibrosis of the muscle spindle capsule.

Treatment. The joint deformities respond to physical therapy, and an intensive program of rehabilitation should be initiated as soon after birth as possible.

POLYNEUROPATHIES

Polyneuropathies are uncommon in childhood and even more uncommon during infancy. Table 6–11 lists the polyneuropathies that begin during infancy. They are divided into those that affect primarily the myelin (demyelinating) and those that affect primarily the axon (axonal). In newborns and infants the term "demyelinating" also includes disorders in which myelin has failed to form (hypomyelinating). Only congenital hypomyelinating neuropathy is commonly first manifested as infantile hypotonia. The initial symptom in the other conditions is more likely to be a progressive gait disturbance or psychomotor retardation. A complete discussion of the clinical approach to neuropathy can be found in Chapter 7.

Congenital Hypomyelinating Neuropathy

The term "congenital hypomyelinating neuropathy" encompasses several disorders with similar
clinical and pathologic manifestations. Sporadic
occurrence is the rule, but autosomal recessive inheritance is suggested by reports of disease in cou-
sins and in siblings of both sexes. Some cases,
especially those with a family history of the disease, may represent an infantile form of hereditary
motor and sensory neuropathy type III (Balestrini
et al, 1991) (see Chapter 7).

Clinical Features. The symptoms in the newborn are indistinguishable from those of acute infantile spinal muscular atrophy. Arthrogryposis
may be present (Charnas et al, 1988). Newborns
have progressive flaccid weakness and atrophy of
the skeletal muscles, a bulbar palsy that spares
extraocular motility, and areflexia. Respiratory insufficiency causes death during infancy.

Some children are not identified as abnormal
until late infancy, when they fail to meet motor
milestones (Harati and Butler, 1985). Examination
reveals diffuse weakness, distal atrophy, and areflexia. Weakness progresses slowly and is not life
threatening during childhood. Sensation remains
intact. These late-onset cases may represent de-
myelinating-remyelinating neuropathies with subsequent enlargement of the peripheral nerves.

Diagnosis. The serum concentration of creatine kinase is normal, EMG findings are consistent

with denervation, and motor nerve conduction velocities are extremely slow, usually less than 10
m/sec. The protein concentration of the cerebrospinal fluid is markedly elevated in almost every
case. Muscle biopsy reveals groups of atrophic fibers adjacent to groups of normal fibers, without
fiber hypertrophy.

Definitive antemortem diagnosis is established
by sural nerve biopsy, which reveals naked axons
without evidence of myelin formation (Vital et al,
1989). No evidence of inflammation or lipid storage is seen. However, the possibility of chronic
inflammatory demyelinating neuropathy cannot be
eliminated by laboratory investigation.

Treatment. Some infants with hypomyelinating neuropathies respond to treatment with oral
prednisone (Sladky et al, 1986). I have treated one
newborn who became normal, both clinically and
electrophysiologically, by 1 year of age. Myelination may have been only delayed and might have
progressed spontaneously even without treatment.
Some patients may have a form of chronic inflammatory demyelinating neuropathy (see Chapter 7).
Whatever the mechanism, every affected child
should be given a course of oral prednisone, 2 mg/
kg/day. Those who respond become stronger
within 4 weeks of starting therapy. Following the
initial response the children should be maintained
on alternate-day therapy, 0.5 mg/kg, for at least
1 year.

DISORDERS OF NEUROMUSCULAR TRANSMISSION
Infantile Botulism

Human botulism ordinarily results from eating
food contaminated by preformed exotoxin of the
organism *Clostridium botulinum*. The exotoxin
prevents the release of acetylcholine, producing a
cholinergic blockade of skeletal muscle and end
organs innervated by autonomic nerves. Infantile
botulism is an age-limited disorder in which *C.
botulinum* is ingested, colonizes the intestinal tract,
and produces toxin in situ. Dietary contamination
with honey or corn syrup accounts for less than
20% of cases (Spika et al, 1989). In most cases
the source of contamination is not defined.

Clinical Features. The clinical spectrum of
infantile botulism includes asymptomatic carriers
of organisms; mild hypotonia and failure to thrive;
severe, progressive, life-threatening paralysis; and
sudden infant death (Thompson et al, 1980). Infected infants are between 2 and 26 weeks of age
and usually live in a dusty environment adjacent
to construction or agricultural soil disruption. The
incidence is mainly between March and October.

Most infants have a prodromal syndrome of constipation and poor feeding. Progressive bulbar and skeletal muscle weakness and loss of tendon reflexes develop 4 to 5 days later. Typical features on examination include diffuse hypotonia, ptosis, dysphagia, weak cry, and dilated pupils that react sluggishly to light.

Infantile botulism is a self-limited disease generally lasting 2 to 6 weeks. Recovery is complete, but relapse occurs in as many as 5% of babies (Glauser et al, 1990).

Diagnosis.   The syndrome suggests postinfectious polyradiculoneuropathy (Guillain-Barré syndrome), infantile spinal muscular atrophy, or generalized myasthenia gravis. Clinical differentiation of infantile botulism from Guillain-Barré syndrome is difficult, and some reported cases of Guillain-Barré syndrome during infancy may actually have been infantile botulism. Infantile botulism differs from infantile spinal muscular atrophy by the early appearance of facial and pharyngeal weakness, the presence of ptosis and dilated pupils, and the occurrence of severe constipation. Infants with generalized myasthenia do not have dilated pupils, absent reflexes, or severe constipation.

Electrophysiologic studies provide the first clue to diagnosis. Repetitive stimulation between 20 and 50 Hz reverses the presynaptic block and produces an incremental increase in the size of the motor unit potentials in 90% of cases (Cornblath et al, 1983). The EMG demonstrates short-duration, low-amplitude motor unit potentials. The diagnosis is confirmed by the isolation of organisms from the stool.

Treatment.   The use of antitoxin and antibiotics does not influence the course of the disease. Indeed, gentamicin, an agent that produces presynaptic neuromuscular blockade, may worsen the condition. Intensive care is necessary throughout the period of profound hypotonia, and many infants require ventilator support. Sudden apnea and death are a constant danger.

Familial Infantile Myasthenia

Several genetic defects causing myasthenic syndromes have been identified (Table 6–12) (Misulis and Fenichel, 1989). All are presumed to be transmitted by autosomal recessive transmission except for the slow channel syndrome, which is transmitted as an autosomal dominant trait (see Chapter 7). Antibodies against the acetylcholine receptor protein (AChRP) are not detected in any of these syndromes.

Despite considerable phenotypic diversity, two clinical syndromes are recognized in the newborn:

Table 6–12 ◆ Genetic Myasthenic Syndromes

Presynaptic Defects
1. Abnormal acetylcholine release
2. Abnormal acetylcholine resynthesis or mobilization

Postsynaptic Defects
1. Endplate acetylcholinesterase deficiency
2. Impaired function of acetylcholine receptor
3. Reduced number of acetylcholine receptors
4. Slow channel syndrome

familial infantile myasthenia with respiratory or feeding difficulty at birth, and congenital myasthenia with predominantly ocular findings (see Chapter 15). Identification of the precise defect requires special laboratory techniques.

Clinical Features.   Presynaptic defects and some postsynaptic defects produce the clinical syndrome of familial infantile myasthenia. Respiratory insufficiency and feeding difficulty may be present at birth (Albers et al, 1984; Mora et al, 1987). Many affected newborns require mechanical ventilation. Ptosis and generalized weakness either are present at birth or develop during infancy. Arthrogryposis may also be present. Although facial and skeletal muscles are weak, extraocular motility is usually normal. Within weeks the infants become stronger and no longer need mechanical ventilation. However, episodes of weakness and life-threatening apnea occur repeatedly throughout infancy and childhood, sometimes even into adult life (Gieron and Korthals, 1985).

Diagnosis.   The diagnosis is established by the intravenous or subcutaneous injection of Tensilon, 0.15 mg/kg. The weakness and the respiratory distress are reversed almost immediately after intravenous injection and within 10 minutes of subcutaneous injection. Further confirmation can be accomplished by the demonstration of a decrement in the amplitude of successive motor unit potentials with repetitive nerve stimulation at low frequency.

Treatment.   Long-term treatment with neostigmine or pyridostigmine is needed to prevent sudden episodes of apnea at the time of intercurrent illness. Treatment should be continued throughout childhood. Because there is no evidence of immunopathy, no rational basis for thymectomy or immunosuppressive therapy exists.

Transitory Neonatal Myasthenia

A transitory myasthenic syndrome is observed in 10% to 15% of offspring of myasthenic mothers. The syndrome is believed to be due to the passive transfer of antibody directed against AChRP from the myasthenic mother to her normal fetus. Passive transfer of antibody from mother to fetus clearly occurs, but this does not fully explain why only a small percentage of newborns are affected or why symptoms are delayed. The severity of symptoms in the newborn correlates with the newborn's antibody concentration but not with the severity or duration of weakness in the mother (Morel et al, 1988).

Clinical Features. Difficulty feeding and generalized hypotonia are the major clinical features. Affected children are eager to feed, but their ability to suck fatigues quickly and nutrition is inadequate. The symptoms usually arise within hours of birth but can be delayed until the third day. Some newborns have had intrauterine hypotonia and are born with arthrogryposis. Weakness of cry and facial expression is present in 50%, but only 15% have limitation of extraocular movement and ptosis. Respiratory insufficiency is uncommon. Weakness becomes progressively worse in the first few days and then improves. The mean duration of symptoms is 18 days with a range of 5 days to 2 months. Recovery is complete, and transitory neonatal myasthenia does not develop into myasthenia later in life.

Diagnosis. The diagnosis of transitory neonatal myasthenia is accomplished by demonstrating high serum concentrations of AChRP antibody in the newborn and temporary reversal of weakness by the subcutaneous or intravenous injection of Tensilon, 0.15 mg/kg.

Treatment. Newborns with severe generalized weakness and respiratory distress should be treated with exchange transfusion. For those who are less impaired an intramuscular injection of 0.1% neostigmine methylsulfate before feeding sufficiently improves sucking and swallowing to allow adequate nutrition. The dose is progressively reduced as symptoms remit. Neostigmine may also be administered through a nasogastric tube at a dose 10 times the parenteral level.

FIBER-TYPE DISPROPORTION MYOPATHIES

Several "congenital myopathies" have been described that are manifested as neonatal hypotonia and are diagnosed only by muscle biopsy. The common feature is that type I fibers are greater in number, but smaller in size, than type II fibers (Figure 6–4). This fiber type predominance, in the absence of fiber degeneration, has led to the notion that fiber-type disproportion myopathies are not primary diseases of muscle but rather are developmental abnormalities of innervation. In some pa-

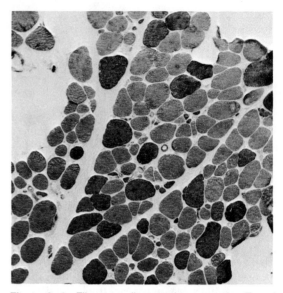

Figure 6–4 Fiber-type disproportion myopathy. Type I fibers *(light shade)* are more numerous than type II fibers *(dark shade)*. Type II fibers are generally larger in diameter than type I fibers. (ATPase reaction.) (From Fenichel GM: Neonatal Neurology, 3rd edition. Churchill Livingstone, New York, 1990. By permission.)

tients fiber-type disproportion is the only histologic abnormality; this finding is referred to as *congenital fiber-type disproportion myopathy*. Other patients have a unique histologic feature for which their form of fiber-type disproportion myopathy is named: central core disease, myotubular myopathy, or nemaline myopathy.

Central Core Disease

Central core disease is a rare but distinct genetic entity transmitted by autosomal dominant inheritance (Byrne et al, 1982).

Clinical Features. Mild hypotonia is noted immediately after birth or during the first month. Congenital dislocation of the hips is relatively common. Weakness is greater in proximal than in distal limb muscles. Tendon reflexes of weak muscles are depressed or absent. Extraocular motility, facial expression, and swallowing are normal. Some children become progressively weaker, have motor impairment, and develop kyphoscoliosis. In others weakness remains mild and never causes disability.

Diagnosis. The serum concentration of creatine kinase is normal, and EMG findings may be normal as well. More frequently the EMG suggests a myopathic process. Diagnosis depends on muscle biopsy. Sharply demarcated cores of closely packed myofibrils undergoing varying degrees of degeneration are present in the center of all type I fibers. Because of the tight packing of myofibrils, the cores are deficient in sarcoplasmic reticulum, glycogen, and mitochondria.

Treatment.   No treatment is available, nor is there a method for prenatal diagnosis.

Congenital Fiber-Type Disproportion Myopathy

The congenital fiber-type disproportion myopathies are a heterogeneous group of diseases that have similar patterns of muscle histology. The initial feature of all these diseases is infantile hypotonia (Sulaiman et al, 1983). Both sexes are involved equally. Most cases are sporadic, some are clearly transmitted by autosomal dominant inheritance, and others are familial but without a definite pattern of genetic transmission. Despite the label "congenital," an identical pattern of fiber-type disproportion may be present in patients who are asymptomatic at birth and first have weakness during childhood.

Clinical Features.   In newborns weakness may be mild or so severe that it causes respiratory insufficiency. Many had intrauterine hypotonia and demonstrate congenital hip dislocation, dysmorphic features, and joint contractures. Proximal muscles are weaker than distal muscles. Facial weakness, ptosis, and disturbance of ocular motility may be present. If axial weakness was present in infancy, kyphoscoliosis often develops during childhood. Tendon reflexes are depressed or absent. Intellectual function is normal.

Weakness is most severe during the first 2 years and then either improves or becomes relatively stable.

Diagnosis.   Muscle biopsy demonstration of type I fiber predominance and hypotrophy is essential for diagnosis. Other laboratory studies are not helpful. The serum concentration of creatine kinase may be slightly elevated or normal, and the EMG may be consistent with a neuropathic process, a myopathic process, or both. Nerve conduction velocities are normal.

Treatment.   Physical therapy should be initiated immediately, not only to relieve existing contractures but also to prevent new contractures from developing.

Myotubular (Centronuclear) Myopathy

Several clinical syndromes are included in the category myotubular (centronuclear) myopathy. Some are clearly transmitted by X-linked inheritance, others by autosomal dominant inheritance, and still others are sporadic and possibly transmitted by autosomal recessive inheritance (Kinoshite et al, 1975; Meyers et al, 1974; Pavone et al, 1980). The common histologic feature on muscle biopsy is an appearance that suggests the persistence of fetal myotubes (Sarnat et al, 1981).

Acute Myotubular Myopathy

Clinical Features.   The abnormal gene that causes acute myotubular myopathy has been mapped to the long arm of the X chromosome (Xq28) (Liechti-Gallati et al, 1991). It is manifested in the newborn as generalized hypotonia and respiratory distress. Decreased fetal movement during pregnancy and polyhydramnios are common. Sucking, swallowing, and tendon reflexes are depressed or absent. Ptosis, and sometimes complete ophthalmoplegia, may be present. Repeated episodes of apnea, asphyxia, and pneumonia usually lead to death during the neonatal period or in early infancy.

Diagnosis.   The serum concentration of creatine kinase is normal. The EMG may suggest a neuropathic process, a myopathic process, or both. Muscle biopsy reveals type I fiber predominance and hypotrophy, the presence of many internal nuclei, and a central area of increased oxidative enzyme and decreased myosin ATPase activity.

Treatment.   No treatment is available for this disorder, nor is there a method for prenatal diagnosis.

Chronic Myotubular Myopathy

Clinical Features.   Chronic myotubular myopathy may be transmitted by either autosomal dominant or autosomal recessive inheritance. In some patients the disease is manifested by hypotonia at birth; in others it comes to attention because of delayed motor development. Limb weakness may be predominantly proximal or distal. The axial and neck flexor muscles are weak as well. Ptosis, but not ophthalmoplegia, is sometimes present at birth. Infants have slowly progressive ophthalmoplegia, loss of facial expression, continuing weakness of limb muscles, and loss of tendon reflexes. Many patients have seizures and mental deficiency.

Diagnosis.   The serum concentration of creatine kinase is normal, and EMG findings are abnormal but do not establish the diagnosis. Muscle biopsy is essential for diagnosis, and histologic features are identical to those of the acute form.

Treatment.   No treatment is available, nor is there a method for prenatal diagnosis.

Nemaline (Rod) Myopathy

Nemaline myopathy is probably transmitted by autosomal dominant inheritance (Kondo and Yuasa, 1980). Penetrance is variable, and affected parents may be asymptomatic.

Clinical Features. Hypotonia is usually mild but can be so severe as to cause immediate respiratory insufficiency and neonatal death (Norton et al, 1983). Affected newborns often appear normal, and attention is not sought until infancy when achievement of motor milestones is delayed. The infant is hypotonic with greater weakness in proximal than distal muscles. Weakness of facial muscles causes a dysmorphic appearance in which the face appears long and narrow and the palate is high and arched. Axial weakness leads to scoliosis. Weakness is not progressive and tends to stabilize, but some residual handicap remains.

Diagnosis. The concentration of serum creatine kinase is either normal or only mildly elevated. EMG findings may be normal, and when abnormal they are not the basis for diagnosis. Muscle biopsy is essential for diagnosis. Multiple small rodlike particles, thought to be structural protein, are present within most, if not all, muscle fibers (Figure 6–5). Similar rodlike structures are a nonspecific histologic feature in some inflammatory myopathies, but only in nemaline myopathy is type I fiber predominance an associated feature.

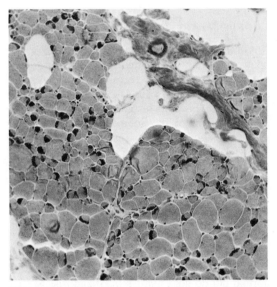

Figure 6–5 Nemaline (rod) myopathy. A spectrum of fiber sizes is present. The small fibers are all type I and contain rodlike bodies in a subsarcolemmal position. (Trichrome stain.) (From Fenichel GM: Neonatal Neurology, 3rd edition. Churchill Livingstone, New York, 1990. By permission.)

Treatment. No treatment is available, nor is there a method for prenatal diagnosis. Parents who have the abnormal gene but are not weak may have rod bodies and fiber-type predominance in their muscle.

MUSCULAR DYSTROPHIES
Congenital Muscular Dystrophy

The term "congenital muscular dystrophy" (CMD) is often used generically for any muscular disorder present at birth or shortly thereafter. These disorders are generally regarded as genetic disorders, but neither an abnormal gene nor an abnormal gene product has been identified. In the absence of a genetic marker the definition and classification of CMD rely wholly on clinical features (Table 6–1). A satisfying definition and classification of CMD are not possible at present, but for purposes of this discussion CMD may be defined by the following criteria (Fenichel, 1988):

1. Hypotonia, weakness, or arthrogryposis is present at birth.
2. The muscle biopsy is consistent with myopathy (i.e., spectrum of fiber sizes, degeneration of medium-sized muscle fibers, fat and collagen replacement of muscle fibers) and specifically excludes denervation.
3. Other myopathies of the newborn with recognizable clinical or pathologic features are excluded.

In most cases the defect appears to be transmitted by autosomal recessive inheritance; siblings are frequently affected, and many instances of parental consanguinity have been reported. Autosomal dominant transmission has been identified in two families.

Several phenotypes are considered variants of CMD, depending on the involvement of other organs, especially the brain and eye.

Clinical Features. Hypotonia and arthrogryposis are present at birth. The infant has generalized limb weakness; proximal muscles are affected earlier and more severely than distal muscles. Facial and neck weakness is common, but extraocular motility is normal. Tendon reflexes may be present or absent and are often difficult to test because of joint contractures. Contractures at birth may involve any joint, but torticollis and clubfoot are particularly common and congenital dislocation of the hips is often an associated feature.

Weakness progresses little or remains stable, but new joint contractures may continue to form at the ankles, hips, knees, and elbows. Muscles are not hypertrophied. Motor development is delayed because of weakness and contractures, but intelligence is normal.

Because approximately 15% of children with CMD die, a more severe form of the disease than that described in the preceding must be recognized. The neck muscles are especially weak and head control is impaired. Contractures are often absent at birth but may develop during infancy. Intercostal and diaphragmatic muscle weakness may be present at birth or develop during infancy. Chronic hypoventilation leading to respiratory failure is the usual cause of death.

Diagnosis. The serum concentration of creatine kinase may be normal or elevated in the newborn and tends to decline with age; however, it does not correlate with the severity of weakness. Elevated serum concentrations of creatine kinase can sometimes be demonstrated in siblings or parents. EMG findings are consistent with a myopathic process.

Muscle histologic appearance is characteristic. Features include a variation in fiber size with occasional central nucleation, extensive fibrosis and proliferation of adipose tissue, fibers undergoing regeneration and degeneration, and thickening of the muscle spindle capsule.

MRI is mandatory to look for demyelination or cerebral malformation.

Treatment. Physical therapy is important to prevent further contractures. Antenatal diagnosis is not available.

Fukuyama Type

A clinical syndrome of congenital muscular dystrophy associated with cerebral dysplasia is the second most prevalent form of muscular dystrophy in Japan (McMenamin et al, 1982b). The major feature is a disturbance of cellular migration to the cortex between the fourth and fifth gestational months, resulting in polymicrogyria, lissencephaly, and heterotopia. Other abnormalities may include fusion of the frontal lobes, hydrocephalus, periventricular cysts, optic nerve atrophy, hypoplasia of the pyramidal tracts, reduction in the number of anterior horn cells, and inflammation of the leptomeninges.

Myelination may be delayed. Computed tomography (CT) shows hypodensity of the centrum semiovale in 50% of children with Fukuyama-type CMD. The hypodensity is thought to represent delayed myelination rather than demyelination because the hypodensity becomes less prominent as the child gets older (Yoshioka et al, 1981). Autosomal recessive inheritance is suggested because males and females are affected equally, and several families with affected siblings and a history of parental consanguinity have been reported. However, the high prevalence of the disease in Japan, but not among ethnic Japanese living outside Japan, suggests that an environmental factor acting on a genetically predisposed population may be important.

Clinical Features. A history of spontaneous abortion is recorded for 25% of mothers who have affected children. At birth, affected newborns are hypotonic and have an expressionless face, a weak cry, and an ineffective suck. Weakness affects the proximal more than the distal limb muscles. Mild contractures of the elbow and knee joints may be present at birth or develop later. Tendon reflexes are usually absent. Pseudohypertrophy of the calves develops in half of cases.

Symptoms of cerebral involvement are present early in infancy. Febrile or nonfebrile generalized seizures are usually the first manifestation. Development is always globally delayed, and microcephaly is the rule. Weakness and atrophy are progressive and result in severe disability, cachexia, and death before 10 years of age.

Diagnosis. The serum concentration of creatine kinase is generally elevated, and EMG indicates a myopathy. Muscle biopsy demonstrates excessive proliferation of adipose tissue and collagen out of proportion to the degree of fiber degeneration. Typical CT or MRI abnormalities are dilation of the cerebral ventricles and subarachnoid space and lucency of cortical white matter.

Treatment. No treatment is available for this disorder, nor is there a method for prenatal diagnosis.

Leukodystrophy

Demyelination of the cerebral hemispheres is often associated with CMD in European children (Trevisan et al, 1991). However, the combination of leukodystrophy and migrational malformations as seen in Fukuyama-type CMD is unusual. Several affected sibling pairs have been reported, suggesting autosomal recessive inheritance.

Clinical Features. Affected newborns are hypotonic, and some have arthrogryposis as well. Feeding disturbances and apnea may be associated symptoms. Tendon reflexes are diminished or absent. Intelligence is normal at first, and some children never show clinical evidence of cerebral abnormality. Others have progressive dementia and epilepsy during childhood.

Diagnosis. The serum concentration of creatine kinase is elevated, and the EMG is consistent with a myopathic process. Nerve conduction velocity is normal. The electroencephalogram may demonstrate epileptiform activity. MRI is necessary for antemortem diagnosis and demonstrates abnormalities in the cerebral white matter.

Treatment. No treatment is available for this

disorder, nor is there a method for prenatal diagnosis.

Cerebro-ocular Dysplasia

Cerebro-ocular muscular dystrophy is characterized by the combination of CMD, cerebral malformations, and ocular anomalies. The cerebral and the muscle abnormalities are the same as in Fukuyama-type CMD. The major differences from Fukuyama-type CMD are the presence of ocular abnormalities and the occurrence of the syndrome in non-Japanese children (Echenne et al, 1986; Warburg, 1987).

Clinical Features.   Hypotonia and arthrogryposis are present at birth. Hydrocephalus occurs in most cases (see discussion of Warburg syndrome in Chapter 18). Several different cerebral malformations may be present: abnormal gyral patterns, heterotopias, hypomyelination, and agenesis of tracts. Ocular abnormalities include corneal clouding, cataracts, retinal dysplasia or detachment, and optic nerve hypoplasia.

Diagnosis.   All newborns with muscular dystrophy and eye-brain abnormalities, no matter how mild any one element may be, should be considered to have cerebroocular dysplasia.

Treatment.   No treatment is available, nor is there a method for prenatal diagnosis.

Neonatal Myotonic Dystrophy

Myotonic dystrophy is a multisystem disorder transmitted by autosomal dominant inheritance (see Chapter 7). The disease is caused by an unstable DNA region on chromosome 19 that can expand in successive generations and cause in the children a more severe disease than their parents had (Harley et al, 1992). Symptoms usually begin in young adult life and include weakness of the face and distal limb muscles, cataracts, multiple endocrinopathies, frontal baldness in males, and myotonia. Myotonia is a disturbance of the muscle membrane; it prevents normal relaxation after contraction.

Clinical Features.   A neonatal form of myotonic dystrophy sometimes occurs in the offspring of affected mothers. Women with myotonic dystrophy become weaker and have greater myotonia during pregnancy (Sarnat et al, 1976). Polyhydramnios is common. Labor is prolonged because of inadequate uterine contraction, and forceps assistance is frequently needed. Severely affected newborns have inadequate diaphragmatic and intercostal muscle function and are incapable of spontaneous respiration. In the absence of prompt intubation and mechanical ventilation, many die immediately after birth. The newborn's precarious ventilatory reserve is further complicated by perinatal asphyxia as a consequence of the prolonged and difficult delivery.

Prominent clinical features in the newborn include facial diplegia, in which the mouth is oddly shaped so that the upper lip forms an inverted V; generalized muscular hypotonia; joint deformities ranging from bilateral clubfoot to generalized arthrogryposis; and gastrointestinal dysfunction, including choking, regurgitation, aspiration, swallowing difficulties, and gastroparesis. Limb weakness in the newborn is more often proximal than distal. Tendon reflexes are usually absent in weak muscles. Myotonia is not elicited by percussion and may not be demonstrable on EMG. Cardiomyopathy contributes to early neonatal deaths. Congenital cataract has been reported only once. The long-term prognosis is poor, and affected children are mentally and physically handicapped.

Diagnosis.   The diagnosis of myotonic dystrophy in the newborn requires a diagnosis of myotonic dystrophy in the mother. She is likely to have many clinical features of the disease. If myotonia is not present on examination, it should be demonstrated by EMG. Myotonia is characterized by the repetitive firing of very-short-duration potentials that decline in frequency and amplitude.

Muscle biopsy of affected infants reveals an apparent maturational arrest that may be confused with myotubular myopathy (Sarnat and Silbert, 1976). Changes are most profound in muscles surrounding a fixed joint. The fibers are small and round, contain many internal nuclei, and are not completely filled with myofibrils (myotubes). Unlike myotubular myopathy, neonatal myotonic dystrophy demonstrates type II rather than type I fiber predominance.

Treatment.   The immediate treatment is intubation and mechanical ventilation. Fixed joints respond to physical therapy and casting. Gastroparesis may be alleviated by metoclopramide therapy (Bodensteiner and Grunow, 1984).

METABOLIC MYOPATHIES
Acid Maltase Deficiency (Pompe Disease)

Acid maltase is a lysosomal enzyme, present in all tissues, that hydrolyzes maltose and other branches of glycogen to yield glucose. It has no function in maintaining blood glucose concentrations. Three distinct clinical forms of deficiency are recognized: infantile, childhood (see Chapter 7), and adult. All are transmitted by autosomal recessive inheritance (Loonen et al, 1981).

Clinical Features.   The infantile form may begin immediately after birth but more usually appears during the second month. Profound generalized hypotonia without atrophy and congestive heart failure are the initial symptoms. Hypotonia is the result of glycogen storage in the brain, spinal cord, and skeletal muscles, causing mixed signs of cerebral and motor unit dysfunction: decreased awareness and depressed tendon reflexes. The mixed signs may be confusing, but the presence of cardiomegaly is almost diagnostic (see also "Carnitine Deficiency"). The electrocardiogram demonstrates abnormalities, including short PR intervals and high QRS complexes on all leads. Most patients die of cardiac failure by 1 year of age.

Diagnosis. Diagnosis is established by muscle biopsy. Large vacuoles containing glycogen are observed in muscle fibers. Definitive diagnosis requires the demonstration of deficient acid maltase activity in fibroblasts or other tissues.

Treatment. A high-protein diet has been found helpful in the childhood form of the disease but has not yet proved useful in the infantile form.

Carnitine Deficiency

Carnitine is an essential cofactor in the transfer of long-chain fatty acids across the inner mitochondrial membrane. Deficiencies of carnitine may occur as primary genetic defects or secondary to other disorders (see Table 2–5). Primary carnitine deficiency usually is manifested in young children as an encephalopathy (see Chapter 2) and in older children as progressive proximal weakness (see Chapter 7).

Clinical Features. There is a single report of an infant with only muscle symptoms of carnitine deficiency (Hart et al, 1978). The mother reported diminished fetal movements during pregnancy, and the child seemed limp at birth. Early motor milestones were achieved at the appropriate times, but walking was delayed. Congestive heart failure developed at 23 months. There was mild generalized hypotonia, and tendon reflexes were normal. During the next 7 months, progressive muscular weakness developed, tendon reflexes were lost, and death occurred following cardiac arrest.

Diagnosis. Primary muscle carnitine deficiency should be suspected in hypotonic infants with cardiomegaly. The other disorder that causes this combination is acid maltase deficiency. Muscle biopsy reveals vacuoles primarily in type I muscle. The vacuoles stain for lipid but not for glycogen. The presence of both lipid and glycogen storage should suggest a deficiency in one of the respiratory chain enzymes. Such deficiencies may produce secondary carnitine deficiency in muscle. Definitive diagnosis requires a demonstration of reduced levels of carnitine in muscle.

Treatment. Several patients with primary muscle carnitine deficiency, including the infant described previously, have been treated with L-carnitine. The results in other children have been variable. Nevertheless, a trial of L-carnitine, 100 mg/kg/day in three divided doses, is recommended in all cases of primary muscle carnitine deficiency.

Cytochrome-c-oxidase Deficiency

The electron transfer chain and oxidative phosphorylation are the principal sources of adenosine triphosphate (ATP) synthesis (see Figure 8–5). Deficiencies of mitochondrial enzymes that make up the electron transfer chain in skeletal muscle may be manifested as hypotonia in the newborn or infant and as exercise intolerance in older children. The defect in infantile hypotonia is usually a deficiency of complex IV (cytochrome-c-oxidase) (Oldfors et al, 1989). Deficiencies in other complexes may be present (Sengers et al, 1984). Most cases are sporadic. Both a fatal and a benign form of infantile cytochrome-c-oxidase deficiency are recognized (Zevianai et al, 1987). Early in their course these forms are indistinguishable, but in the benign form a spontaneous increase in cytochrome-c-oxidase activity associated with increased strength occurs during infancy. Different abnormalities in subunits of cytochrome-c-oxidase account for the phenotypic difference (Tritschler et al, 1991).

Clinical Features. Clinical features vary with the number of enzyme deficiencies, the percentage reduction in enzyme activity, and the presence of mitochondrial enzyme deficiencies in organs other than muscle. The typical syndrome is characterized by profound generalized weakness, causing difficulty in feeding, early respiratory failure, and death; severe lactic acidosis; and the *De Toni-Franconi-Debré syndrome* (glycosuria, proteinuria, phosphaturia, and generalized aminoaciduria). Onset is anytime within the first 6 months. Ptosis, ophthalmoplegia, and macroglossia may be present. Newborns with multiple enzyme deficiencies in multiple organs die within 6 months.

Diagnosis. A deficiency in respiratory chain enzymes should be suspected in any hypotonic infant with lactic acidosis. The serum concentration of creatine kinase is elevated, but EMG findings may be normal. Muscle biopsy reveals vacuoles, mainly in type I fibers, with abnormal glycogen and lipid accumulations. Mitochondria are large, increased in number, and abnormal in structure (ragged-red fibers).

Treatment. No effective treatment is available for infants with overwhelming disease caused by multiorgan enzyme deficiency. Coenzyme Q therapy may be tried, although the evidence supporting efficacy is not compelling (Nishikawa et al, 1989). The fatal and the benign form of the deficiency should be distinguished by immunohistochemical findings, and supportive care should be provided for newborns with the transitory form.

Phosphofructokinase Deficiency

The usual manifestations of muscle phosphofructokinase deficiency are cramps on exercise and myoglobinuria (see Chapter 8). Symptoms usually begin in childhood, and patients are otherwise asymptomatic. A neonatal form of phosphofructokinase deficiency has been reported in four children (Servidei et al, 1986). The defect is transmitted by autosomal recessive inheritance.

Clinical Features. The neonatal form is manifested as hypotonia, weakness, respiratory deficiency, and joint deformities. The tendon reflexes are diminished or absent. Cerebral and corneal abnormalities may be present. Death occurs during infancy or early childhood.

Diagnosis. The serum concentration of creatine kinase is normal. The EMG, at least late in the disease, is consistent with a myopathic process. Muscle biopsy is critical for diagnosis. Light microscopy reveals only nonspecific myopathy, but electron microscopy demonstrates an abnormal accumulation of subsarcolemmal and intramyofibrillary glycogen. Large cytoplasmic vacuoles, as in acid maltase deficiency, are not present. Phosphofructokinase activity is absent in skeletal muscle but present in red blood cells and fibroblasts.

Treatment. No treatment is available for this disorder.

Phosphorylase Deficiency

Myophosphorylase deficiency (McArdle disease) is characterized by exercise intolerance in young adults and progressive myopathy in middle life (see Chapter 8). A neonatal form of variable severity has been recognized (Cornelio et al, 1983; DiMauro and Hartlage, 1978). It is reported in siblings and probably transmitted, like the older onset form, by autosomal recessive inheritance. Indeed, the enzyme deficiency appears identical at all ages, and the reason for clinical heterogeneity is not understood.

Clinical Features. Newborns with myophosphorylase deficiency have difficulty with sucking and swallowing immediately post partum or in the early neonatal period. In some, weakness is so profound that it produces immediate respiratory insufficiency. In others, weakness is progressive over several months or years. The child appears alert and has normal cranial nerve function. The tongue and heart are not affected. Tendon reflexes are depressed or absent.

Diagnosis. The serum concentration of creatine kinase is elevated, and EMG findings are abnormal, with features of both neuropathy and myopathy. Muscle biopsy is diagnostic. Fibers vary in size from atrophic to normal and contain peripheral vacuoles that react intensely for glycogen. The glycogen concentration of muscle is greatly elevated, and phosphorylase activity cannot be detected.

Treatment. A high-protein diet is useful in older patients with phosphorylase deficiency but has not been tried in newborns.

◆ Infantile Myositis

There have been only 11 case reports of infantile myositis; three were newborns. Probably these do not represent a single nosologic entity (Roddy et al, 1986; Thompson, 1982).

Clinical Features. Affected newborns have difficulty breathing immediately after birth and require resuscitation or intubation. In others symptoms begin at 2 to 12 months of age. Infants are hypotonic and have diminished or absent tendon reflexes.

Diagnosis. The serum concentration of creatine kinase is markedly elevated, and the EMG is consistent with myopathy. Muscle biopsy reveals diffuse inflammation and considerable proliferation of connective tissue. Muscle fiber degeneration may be seen.

Treatment. A trial of prednisone is appropriate in infants with inflammatory myopathy. High doses of prednisone, 2 mg/kg/day, are initiated, changed to alternate-day doses after 1 week, and then rapidly tapered over 3 to 6 months, depending on the response.

References

Adams C, Babyn PS, Logan WJ: Spinal cord birth injury: Value of computed tomographic myelography. Pediatr Neurol 4:105, 1988.

Albers JW, Faulkner JA, Dorovini-Zis K, et al: Abnormal neuromuscular transmission in an infantile myasthenic syndrome. Ann Neurol 16:28, 1984.

Aubourg P, Scotto J, Rocchiccioli F, et al: Neonatal adrenoleukodystrophy. J Neurol Neurosurg Psychiatry 49:77, 1986.

Axelrod FB, Porges RF, Sein ME: Neonatal recognition of familial dysautonomia. J Pediatr 110:946, 1987.

Balestrini MR, Cavaletti G, D'Angelo A, et al: Infantile hereditary neuropathy with hypomyelination: Report of two siblings with different expressivity. Neuropediatrics 22:65, 1991.

Bodensteiner JB, Grunow JE: Gastroparesis in neonatal myotonic dystrophy. Muscle Nerve 7:486, 1984.

Butler MG: Prader-Willi syndrome: Current understanding of cause and diagnosis. Am J Med Genet 35:319, 1990.

Byrne E, Blumbergs PC, Hallpike JF: Central core disease: Study of a family with five affected generations. J Neurol Sci 53:77, 1982.

Charnas L, Bernar J: MRI findings and peripheral neuropathy in Lowe's syndrome. Neuropediatrics 19:7, 1988.

Charnas LR, Bernardini I, Rader D, et al: Clinical and laboratory findings in the oculocerebrorenal syndrome of Lowe, with special reference to growth and renal function. N Engl J Med 324:1318, 1991.

Charnas L, Trapp B, Griffin J: Congenital absence of peripheral myelin: Abnormal Schwann cell development causes lethal arthrogryposis multiplex congenita. Neurology 38:966, 1988.

Clancy RR, Sladky JT, Rorke LB: Hypoxic-ischemic spinal cord injury following perinatal asphyxia. Ann Neurol 25:185, 1989.

Cornblath DR, Sladky JT, Sumner AJ: Clinical electrophysiology of infantile botulism. Muscle Nerve 6:448, 1983.

Cornelio F, Bresolin N, DiMauro S, et al: Congenital myopathy due to phosphorylase deficiency. Neurology 33:1383, 1983.

DiMauro S, Hartlage P: Fatal infantile form of muscle phosphorylase deficiency. Neurology 28:1124, 1978.

Echenne B, Arthuis M, Billard C, et al: Congenital muscular dystrophy and cerebral CT scan abnormalities: Results of a collaborative study of the Société de Neurologie Infantile. J Neurol Sci 75:7, 1986.

Fenichel GM: Congenital muscular dystrophies. Neurol Clin 6:519, 1988.

Fleury P, Hageman G: A dominantly inherited lower motor neuron disorder presenting at birth with associated arthrogryposis. J Neurol Neurosurg Psychiatry 48:1037, 1985.

Gieron MA, Korthals JK: Familial infantile myasthenia: Report of three patients with follow-up to adulthood. Arch Neurol 42:143, 1985.

Glauser TA, Maguire HC, Sladky JT: Relapse of infant botulism. Ann Neurol 28:187, 1990.

Gobernado JM, Lousa M, Gimemo A, et al: Mitochondrial defects in Lowe's oculocerebrorenal syndrome. Arch Neurol 41:208, 1984.

Goutiéres F, Bogicevic D, Aicardi J: A predominantly cervical form of spinal muscular atrophy. J Neurol Neurosurg Psychiatry 54:223, 1991.

Greenberg F, Fenolio KR, Hejtmancik F, et al: X-linked infantile spinal muscular atrophy. AJDC 142:217, 1988.

Harati Y, Butler IJ: Congenital hypomyelinating neuropathy. J Neurol Neurosurg Psychiatry 48:1269, 1985.

Harley HG, Brook JD, Rundle SA, et al: Expansion of an unstable DNA region and phenotypic variation in myotonic dystrophy. Nature 355:545, 1992.

Hart ZH, Chang CH, DiMauro S, et al: Muscle carnitine deficiency and fatal cardiomyopathy. Neurology 28:147, 1978.

Kinoshite M, Satoyoshi E, Matsuo N: "Myotubular myopathy" and "Type I fiber atrophy" in a family. J Neurol Sci 26:575, 1975.

Kondo K, Yuasa T: Genetics of congenital nemaline myopathy. Muscle Nerve 3:308, 1980.

Lanska MJ, Roessmann U, Wiznitzer M: Magnetic resonance imaging in cervical cord birth injury. Pediatrics 85:760, 1990.

Larsen R, Ashwal S, Peckham N: Incontinentia pigmenti: Association with anterior horn cell degeneration. Neurology 37:446, 1987.

Licheti-Gallati S, Muller B, Grimm T, et al: X-linked centronuclear myopathy: Mapping the gene to Xq28. Neuromuscular Dis 1:239, 1991.

Loonen MCB, Busch HFM, Koster JF, et al: A family with different clinical forms of acid maltase deficiency (glycogenosis type II): Biochemical and genetic studies. Neurology 31:1209, 1981.

McMenamin JB, Becker LE, Murphy EG: Fukuyama-type congenital muscular dystrophy. J Pediatr 101:580, 1982.

McWilliam RC, Garder-Medwin D, Doyle D, et al: Diaphragmatic paralysis due to spinal muscular atrophy: An unrecognized cause of respiratory failure in infancy? Arch Dis Child 60:145, 1985.

Meyers KR, Golomb HM, Hansen JL, et al: Familial neuromuscular disease with "myotubes." Clin Genet 5:327, 1974.

Misulis KE, Fenichel GM: Genetic forms of myasthenia gravis. Pediatr Neurol 5:205, 1989.

Mora M, Lambert EH, Engel A: A synaptic vessel abnormality in familial infantile myasthenia. Neurology 37:206, 1987.

Morel E, Eymard B, Garabedian BV, et al: Neonatal myasthenia gravis: A new clinical and immunologic appraisal on 30 cases. Neurology 38:138, 1988.

Munsat TL, Skerry L, Korf B, et al: Phenotypic heterogeneity of spinal muscular atrophy mapping to chromosome 5q11.2-13.3 (SMA 5q). Neurology 40:1831, 1990.

Naidu S, Moser AE, Moser HW: Phenotypic and genotypic variability of generalized peroxisomal disorders. Pediatr Neurol 4:4, 1988.

Nishikawa Y, Takahashi M, Nakamura Y, et al: Long-term coenzyme Q_{10} therapy for a mitochondrial encephalomyopathy with cytochrome c oxidase deficiency: A ^{31}P NMR study. Neurology 39:399, 1989.

Norton P, Ellison P, Sulaiman AR, et al: Nemaline myopathy in the neonate. Neurology 33:351, 1983.

Oldfors A, Sommerland H, Holme E, et al: Cytochrome c oxidase deficiency in infancy. Acta Neuropathol 77:267, 1989.

Packer RJ, Brown MJ, Berman PH: The diagnostic value of electromyography in infantile hypotonia. AJDC 136:1057, 1982.

Painter MJ, Bergman I: Obstetrical trauma to the neonatal central and peripheral nervous system. Semin Perinatol 6:89, 1982.

Pavone L, Mollica F, Grasso A, et al: Familial centronuclear myopathy. Acta Neurol Scand 62:33, 1980.

Roddy SM, Ashwal S, Peckham N, et al: Infantile myositis: A case diagnosed in the neonatal period. Pediatr Neurol 2:241, 1986.

Santos MJ, Imanaka T, Shio H, et al: Peroxisomal membrane ghosts in Zellweger syndrome–aberrant organelle assembly. Science 239:1536, 1988.

Sarnat HB, O'Connor T, Byrne PA: Clinical effects of myotonic dystrophy on pregnancy and the neonate. Arch Neurol 33:459, 1976.

Sarnat HB, Roth SI, Jimenez JF: Neonatal myotubular myopathy: Neuropathy and failure of postnatal maturation of fetal muscle. Can J Neurol Sci 8:313, 1981.

Sarnat HB, Silbert SW: Maturational arrest of fetal muscle in neonatal myotonic dystrophy. Arch Neurol 33:466, 1976.

Schapira D, Swash W: Neonatal spinal muscular atrophy presenting as respiratory distress: A clinical variant. Muscle Nerve 8:661, 1985.

Sengers RCA, Trijbees JMF, Bakkeren JAJM, et al: Deficiency of cytochrome b and aa₃ in muscle from an infant with cytochrome oxidase deficiency. Eur J Pediatr 141:178, 1984.

Servidei S, Bonilla E, Diedrich RG, et al: Fatal infantile form of muscle phosphofructokinase deficiency. Neurology 36:1465, 1986.

Sladky JT, Brown MJ, Berman PH: Chronic inflammatory demyelinating polyneuropathy of infancy: A corticosteroid-responsive disorder. Ann Neurol 20:76, 1986.

Spika JC, Shaffer N, Hargrett-Bean N: Risk factors for infant botulism in the United States. AJDC 143:828, 1989.

Steiman GS, Rorke LB, Brown MJ: Infantile neuronal degeneration masquerading as Werdnig-Hoffmann disease. Ann Neurol 8:317, 1980.

Sulaiman A, Swick HM, Kindu D: Congenital fiber type disproportion with unusual clinico-pathologic manifestations. J Neurol Neurosurg Psychiatry 46:175, 1983.

Thompson CE: Infantile myositis. Dev Med Child Neurol 24:307, 1982.

Thompson JA, Glasgow LA, Warpinski JR, et al: Infant botulism: Clinical spectrum and epidemiology. Pediatrics 66:936, 1980.

Trevisan CP, Carollo C, Angelini C, et al: Congenital muscular dystrophy: Brain alterations in an unselected series of Western patients. J Neurol Neurosurg Psychiatry 54:330, 1991.

Tritschler HJ, Bonilla E, Lombes A, et al: Differential diagnosis of fatal and benign cytochrome c oxidase deficient myopathies of infancy: An immunohistochemical approach. Neurology 41:300, 1991.

Vital A, Vital C, Coquet M, et al: Congenital hypomyelination with axonopathy. Eur J Pediatr 148:470, 1989.

Wanders RJA, Heymans HSA, Schutgens RBH, et al: Peroxisomal disorders in neurology. J Neurol Sci 88:1, 1989.

Warburg M: Ocular malformations and lissencephaly. Eur J Pediatr 146:450, 1987.

Warburton D, Singer DB, Oh W: Effects of acidosis on the activity of creatine phosphokinase and its isoenzymes in the serum of newborn infants. Pediatrics 68:195, 1981.

Yoshioka M, Okuno T, Ito M, et al: Congenital muscular dystrophy (Fukuyama type)—repeated CT studies in 19 children. Computed Tomogr 5:81, 1981.

Zeviani M, Peterson P, Servidei E, et al: Benign reversible muscle cytochrome c oxidase deficiency: A second case. Neurology 37:64, 1987.

Flaccid Limb Weakness in Childhood

Most children with acute or chronic flaccid limb weakness have a disorder of the motor unit. Flaccid weakness of the legs may be the initial feature of disturbances in the lumbosacral region, but other symptoms of spinal cord dysfunction are usually present as well. For a child who has flaccid weakness of the legs but no impairment of the arms, the reader should refer to the differential diagnosis in Chapter 12. Cerebral disorders may cause flaccid weakness, but dementia (see Chapter 5) or seizures (see Chapter 1) are usually present concomitantly.

◆ Symptoms and Signs of Neuromuscular Disease

INITIAL COMPLAINT

Limb weakness in children is almost always noted first in the legs and then in the arms (Table 7–1). This is because many neuromuscular disorders affect the legs before the arms and because symptoms of mild leg weakness are more obvious than mild arm weakness, since they impair walking. In young children with neuromuscular disease, delayed development of motor skills may be an initial complaint or a prominent feature of the history. If the degree of motor delay is marginal and other developmental skills are normal, parents and grandparents may rationalize the delay by saying, "I do everything for him," or "His father was also a slow baby."

Older children are frequently referred for neurologic examination because they are unable to keep up with peers or because they tire easily. Those in whom exercise intolerance is due to persistent weakness are discussed in this chapter. A second group, who are normal when not exercising but "run out of energy" or have muscle cramps when they do exercise, probably have an underlying metabolic disorder; these patients are discussed in Chapter 8.

An abnormal gait is often the initial symptom of either proximal or distal leg weakness. With proximal weakness the pelvis is not stabilized and waddles from side to side as the child walks. Running is especially difficult and accentuates the hip waddle.

Toe-walking is commonly encountered in Duchenne muscular dystrophy because the pelvis is thrust forward to shift the center of gravity and the gastrocnemius muscle is replaced by collagen and fat. Toe-walking is seen also in upper motor neuron disorders that cause spasticity and in children who have tight heel cords but no identifiable neurologic disease. Muscular dystrophy is usually associated with hyporeflexia, and spasticity with hyperreflexia. However, tendon reflexes may be difficult to elicit when the tendon is tight for any reason.

Children with footdrop tend to lift the knee high in the air so the foot will clear the ground. The weak foot then comes down with a slapping motion (steppage gait).

Stumbling is an early complaint when there is distal weakness, especially weakness of the evertors and dorsiflexors of the foot, and is a later feature with proximal weakness. Falling is first noted when the child is walking on uneven surfaces. The child is thought to be clumsy, but after a while parents realize that the child is "tripping on nothing at all." One parent remarked that the child could "trip on a blade of grass."

Adolescents and adults, but usually not children with weakness, complain of specific disabilities. A young woman with proximal weakness may have difficulty keeping her arms elevated to groom her hair or rotating the shoulder to get into and out of

Table 7–1 ◆ Symptoms of Neuromuscular Disease

1. Abnormal gait
   a. Steppage
   b. Toe-walking
   c. Waddle
2. Easy fatigability
3. Frequent falls
4. Slow motor development
5. Specific disability
   a. Arm elevation
   b. Climbing stairs
   c. Hand grip
   d. Rising from floor

garments that have a zipper or hook in the back. Weakness in hand muscles is frequently spotted by teachers who become upset with the child's handwriting. Adolescents may notice difficulty in unscrewing jar tops or working with tools. Teachers report to parents when children are slower than classmates in climbing stairs, getting up from the floor, and skipping and jumping. Parents may report a specific complaint to the physician, but more often they say that the child's problem is an inability to keep up with other children.

A child whose limbs are weak may have weakness in the muscles of the head and neck as well. The physician should ask specifically about double vision, drooping of the eyelids, difficulty chewing and swallowing, loss of facial expression and facial strength (whistling, sucking, chewing, blowing), and the clarity and tone of speech. Weakness of neck muscles is frequently noticed when the child is a passenger in a car that suddenly accelerates or decelerates. The neck muscles are unable to stabilize the head, which snaps backward or forward.

PHYSICAL FINDINGS

The physician should begin the examination by watching the child sit, stand, and walk. To test the strength of proximal leg muscles, the physician should have the child sit on the floor and then rise without using the hands to push off. When pelvic muscles are weak, the child cannot rise from the floor without using the hands for assistance (Figure 7–1). With greater weakness the child uses the hands to climb up the legs (Gower sign). After observing gait, the examiner should have the child stand and walk first on toes and then on heels (Table 7–2).

During this period of observation and again during muscle strength testing, the physician should

look for atrophy or hypertrophy. Wasting of muscles in the shoulders is easily seen because bony prominences stand out even further. Wasting of hand muscles causes flattening of the thenar and hypothenar eminences. Wasting of the quadriceps muscles causes a tapering appearance to the thigh that is exaggerated when the patient is asked to tense the thigh by straightening the knee. Atrophy of the anterior tibial and peroneal muscles gives the anterior border of the tibia a sharp appearance, and atrophy of the gastrocnemius muscle diminishes the normal contour of the calf.

As individual muscles are examined for strength, they should also be palpated for texture and tenderness. The texture of normal muscle is quite different from the flabby texture of denervated muscle and the rubbery consistency of dystrophic muscle infiltrated with collagen and fat. Tenderness generally suggests an inflammatory process.

Loss of tendon reflexes occurs early in denervation, especially if the child has sensory neuropathy, but tends to parallel the degree of weakness in myopathy. Tendon reflexes are usually normal even during times of weakness in patients with myasthenia gravis and may be normal between episodes of recurrent weakness in metabolic myopathies.

Myotonia, a disturbance in muscle relaxation following contraction, is described in the section on myotonic dystrophy.

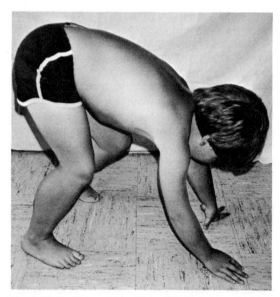

Figure 7–1 Gower sign. The child rises from the floor by pushing off with the hands to overcome proximal pelvic weakness.

Table 7–2 ◆ Signs of Neuromuscular Disease

Observation
1. Atrophy and hypertrophy
2. Fasciculations
3. Functional ability

Palpation
1. Muscle texture
2. Tenderness

Examination
1. Joint contractures
2. Myotonia
3. Strength
4. Tendon reflexes

◆ Progressive Proximal Weakness

Progressive proximal weakness in childhood is most often due to myopathy, usually a muscular dystrophy (Table 7–3). Juvenile spinal muscular atrophy is the only chronic denervating disease in which weakness is more proximal than distal. It is readily distinguished from myopathic disorders by electromyography (EMG) and muscle biopsy. Limb-girdle myasthenia is rare but is an important consideration because specific treatment is available (Table 7–4).

SPINAL MUSCULAR ATROPHIES

The juvenile form of spinal muscular atrophy *(Wohlfart-Kugelberg-Welander disease)* was initially thought to be genetically distinct from infantile spinal muscular atrophy (see Chapter 6). However, despite considerable phenotypic heterogeneity, most cases of infantile and juvenile spinal muscular atrophy are due to defects on chromosome 5 (Gilliam et al, 1990; Munsat et al, 1990). The only genetic distinction possible at this time is between an autosomal recessive and an autosomal dominant form of juvenile spinal muscular atrophy.

The prevalence of juvenile spinal muscular atrophy is estimated at 1.2 per 100,000 general population (Emery, 1991) but is higher in some inbred populations. In the overwhelming majority of cases the defect is transmitted by autosomal recessive inheritance.

Autosomal Recessive Type

In the autosomal recessive form, fetal movements are reported as normal and the child is normal at birth. Three clinical types of spinal muscular

atrophy are distinguished by age at onset. The severe type begins before 6 months of age and is described in Chapter 6. A mild type begins after 18 months, and an intermediate type II between 7 and 18 months. The age at onset does not consistently predict the degree of eventual disability, and the physician must be cautious when predicting outcome at the time of initial diagnosis.

Clinical Features. The initial symptom of the intermediate type is delayed motor development, and affected children are never able to stand alone. Gait instability caused by proximal weakness is the initial feature of the mild type. Calf hypertrophy may be present as well and suggests the erroneous diagnosis of Duchenne muscular dystrophy. The disease progresses very slowly, sometimes in a stepwise fashion, and often appears to be arrested. The progression of weakness may be either to the distal muscles of the legs or to the proximal muscles of the arms. The hands are affected last. The facial muscles may be weak, but extraocular motility is almost always spared. Ophthalmoplegia is so uncommon that such cases may prove genetically dis-

Table 7–3 ◆ Progressive Proximal Weakness

Spinal Cord Disorders (see Chapter 12)

Juvenile Spinal Muscular Atrophies
1. Autosomal recessive
2. Autosomal dominant
3. GM$_2$ Gangliosidosis (hexosaminidase A deficiency)

Myasthenic Syndromes
1. Familial limb-girdle
2. Myasthenia gravis (see Chapter 15)
3. Slow channel syndrome

Myopathies
1. Muscular dystrophies
   a. Duchenne and Becker dystrophies
   b. Facioscapulohumeral syndrome
   c. Limb-girdle dystrophy
2. Inflammatory myopathies
   a. Dermatomyositis
   b. Polymyositis
   c. Inclusion body myositis
3. Metabolic myopathies
   a. Acid maltase deficiency
   b. Carnitine deficiency
   c. Debrancher enzyme deficiency (see Chapter 8)
   d. Lipid storage myopathies
   e. Mitochondrial myopathies (see Chapter 8)
   f. Myophosphorylase deficiency (see Chapter 8)
4. Endocrine myopathies
   a. Adrenal cortex
   b. Parathyroid
   c. Thyroid

Table 7–4 ◆ Distinguishing Features in Proximal Weakness

	Neuronopathy	Myopathy	Myasthenia
Tendon reflexes	Absent	Depressed or absent	Normal
Electromyography	Fasciculations; denervation potentials; high-amplitude, long-duration, polyphasic motor units	Brief, small-amplitude polyphasic motor units	Normal
Nerve conduction studies	Normal or mildly slow	Normal	Abnormal repetitive stimulation
Creatine kinase concentration	Normal or mildly elevated	Elevated	Normal
Muscle biopsy	Group atrophy; group typing	Fiber necrosis; fatty replacement; excessive collagen	Normal replacement; excessive collagen

tinct. Tendon reflexes of weak muscles are absent or greatly diminished.

An exaggerated physiologic tremor of the hands is sometimes present. Its cause is unknown.

In some children the arms are more profoundly affected than the legs, and these children are likely to have facial weakness as well. Some children may have predominant leg weakness whereas their siblings have predominant arm weakness.

The pattern of progression in other family members provides a clue to prognosis but cannot be counted on to predict the future in any specific patient.

Diagnosis. The serum concentration of creatine kinase may be two to four times the upper limit of normal. Elevated concentrations of creatine kinase correlate directly with the duration of illness.

The most helpful investigation is the needle EMG, which shows spontaneous discharges (fasciculations, fibrillations, and positive sharp waves) in about half of patients. With exertion, motor unit potentials are consistently of large amplitude and often polyphasic, prolonged in duration, and reduced in number. Sensory nerve conduction is always normal, but motor nerve conduction velocity is occasionally prolonged late in the course.

Muscle biopsy reveals a pattern of denervation similar to that observed in infantile spinal muscular atrophy. Groups of atrophic fibers are adjacent to groups of fibers that are normal in size or hypertrophied. Hypertrophied fibers are always type I. In children with chronic denervation, "myopathic" changes may be seen as well. Because of sampling error, occasional biopsy specimens demonstrate only myopathic features. Therefore confirmation by muscle biopsy is not essential if the EMG results are clearly consistent with spinal muscular atrophy.

Treatment. Proper management of spinal muscular atrophy in children increases longevity and decreases disability. The goals are to maintain function and prevent contractures. Children who quickly take to a wheelchair develop disuse atrophy. Dietary counseling is usually needed to prevent obesity, which only increases the strain on weakened muscles. The prevention of contractures usually requires range of motion exercise and the early use of splints, especially at night.

Families should be provided with genetic counseling. Antenatal diagnosis and tests to detect the carrier state are not yet available.

Autosomal Dominant Type

Proximal spinal muscular atrophy transmitted by autosomal dominant inheritance may have either a juvenile or an adult onset. The juvenile and adult types were believed to be genetically distinct because families usually have complete concordance for age of onset. However, variability in age of onset from childhood to adult life has been reported in several families. More than 90% of patients with the juvenile form have their onset before the age of 5 years and 100% before the age of 10 (Pearn, 1978). A new dominant mutation would be impossible to distinguish from the autosomal recessive form.

Clinical Features. The pattern of weakness in the autosomal dominant type is somewhat more generalized than in the autosomal recessive type, but proximal muscles are still affected more severely than distal muscles. Symptoms progress slowly, and some patients report no worsening of weakness after adolescence. Most patients can walk and function well into middle and late adult life. Bulbar weakness is unusual and is mild when present. Extraocular muscles are not affected. Tendon reflexes are depressed or absent in weak muscles. Joint contractures are uncommon.

Diagnosis. The serum concentration of creatine kinase is normal or only mildly elevated. The EMG is the basis for diagnosis, as in the autosomal recessive type. Muscle biopsy provides further confirmation of diagnosis.

Treatment. Treatment is the same for the dominant and recessive forms. Genetic counseling should stress the complete penetrance of the phenotype. Antenatal diagnosis is not available. When the family has no history of spinal muscular atrophy, genetic counseling is difficult, but autosomal dominant inheritance should be considered if the onset occurs after 3 years of age.

GM₂ Gangliosidosis

The typical clinical expression of *hexosaminidase A deficiency* is Tay-Sachs disease (see Chapter 5). Several phenotypic variants of the enzyme deficiency with onset throughout childhood and adult life are described. All are transmitted by autosomal recessive inheritance. Most patients are of Ashkenazi Jewish origin. A juvenile-onset type occurs in which the initial manifestations mimic juvenile spinal muscular atrophy (Parnes et al, 1985).

Clinical Features. Weakness, wasting, and cramps of the proximal leg muscles begin after infancy and frequently not until adolescence. These are followed by distal leg weakness, proximal and distal arm weakness, and tremor. After motor neuron dysfunction is established, symptoms of cerebral degeneration (personality change, intermittent psychosis, dementia) become evident (Mantovani et al, 1985; Parnes et al, 1985).

Examination reveals a mixture of upper and lower motor neuron signs. The macula is usually normal and the cranial nerves are intact, with the exception of atrophy and fasciculations in the tongue. Fasciculations may be present in the limbs as well. Tendon reflexes may be absent or exaggerated, depending on the relative severity of upper and lower motor neuron dysfunction. Plantar responses are sometimes extensor and sometimes flexor. Tremor, but not dysmetria, is present in the outstretched arms, and sensation is intact.

In some patients cerebral dysfunction never develops and only motor neuron disease is present; adults with only dementia and psychosis have been reported. The course is variable and compatible with prolonged survival.

Diagnosis. The serum concentration of creatine kinase is normal or only mildly elevated. Motor and sensory nerve conduction velocities are normal, but needle EMG demonstrates neuropathic motor units. Autonomic neurons obtained by intestinal biopsy are distended by Sudan black-B-positive material and are indistinguishable from those in Tay-Sachs disease.

Definitive diagnosis is based on a severe deficiency or absence of hexosaminidase A activity in leukocytes or cultured fibroblasts.

Treatment. No treatment is available. Heterozygote detection is possible because enzyme activity is partially deficient. Prenatal diagnosis is possible.

MYASTHENIC SYNDROMES

Several patients who show electrophysiologic or pharmacologic evidence of myasthenia have been described as having proximal weakness and sometimes wasting. In many such patients the weakness responds to standard treatment for myasthenia gravis. Two genetic syndromes have this presentation: familial limb-girdle myasthenia and the slow channel syndrome.

Autoimmune myasthenia gravis sometimes begins in children as a progressive proximal weakness affecting primarily the limb-girdle musculature and sparing ocular motility (Fenichel, 1978). Weakness may not fluctuate with exercise. Muscles of facial expression may be affected, although other bulbar function is spared. Tendon reflexes are usually present but may be hypoactive. The clinical manifestations suggest limb-girdle dystrophy or polymyositis.

Familial Limb-Girdle Myasthenia

Familial limb-girdle myasthenia has been described in three families having two or more siblings affected with a similar disorder (Dobkin and Verity, 1978; Johns et al, 1973; McQuillen, 1966).

Clinical Features. In two of the families the children at 13 and 14 years of age developed progressive proximal weakness that later stabilized. In the third family, mild, nonprogressive proximal weakness was present from infancy. Ocular motility, facial expression, and bulbar function were spared, and tendon reflexes were present in every case. Family members whose weakness had started in infancy were not evaluated until adult life. At that time cardiomyopathy was also present.

Diagnosis. Limb weakness responds to the intravenous injection of edrophonium chloride (Tensilon). Repetitive stimulation causes a decremental response that can be reversed by the injection of Tensilon or other anticholinesterase medication. The EMG suggests myopathy because polyphasic action potentials of short duration are present. Muscle biopsy results were normal in some families and abnormal in others. The abnormalities were not helpful in diagnosis. The serum concentration of antibody to acetylcholine receptor protein was investigated in only one family and was normal.

Treatment.   Limb weakness in patients with familial limb-girdle myasthenia responds to treatment with anticholinesterase medication (see next section for dosage). Thymectomy and immunosuppressive therapy are not indicated because there is no evidence of an abnormal immune state. However, one patient who showed only a moderate response to anticholinesterase medication appeared to improve when corticosteroids were added to the therapy.

Slow Channel Syndrome

The slow channel syndrome has been described in three families and in two sporadic cases (Oosterhuis et al, 1987). Some individuals have EMG evidence of disease without clinical symptoms.

Clinical Features.   No symptoms are present at birth. Onset usually occurs during infancy but can be delayed until adult life. Weakness of the cervical and scapular muscles is often the initial feature. Other features, present in most patients, are exercise intolerance, ophthalmoparesis, and muscle atrophy. Ptosis, bulbar dysfunction, and leg weakness are less common. The syndrome progresses slowly, and many patients do not come to medical attention until after the first decade.

Diagnosis.   Weakness does not respond either to injection or to oral administration of anticholinesterase medication. Two patients were hypersensitive to Tensilon and responded with muscarinic side effects. Repetitive nerve stimulation at three stimuli per second produces an abnormal decremental response and a single nerve stimulation produces a repetitive muscle potential. Muscle biopsy demonstrates type I fiber predominance. Group

atrophy, tubular aggregates, and an abnormal endplate configuration are present in some specimens.

Treatment.   No treatment is available.

MUSCULAR DYSTROPHIES

The dystrophies are a group of genetic myopathies distinguished by mode of transmission, age at onset, and pattern of weakness (Table 7–5).

Duchenne and Becker Muscular Dystrophies

Duchenne and Becker muscular dystrophies are variable phenotypic expressions of a gene defect at the Xp21 site on the X chromosome. The range of phenotypes associated with the Xp21 gene site is expanding (Table 7–6). The abnormal gene product in both Duchenne and Becker muscular dystrophy is a reduced muscle content of the structural protein *dystrophin*. In boys with Duchenne muscular dystrophy the dystrophin content is less than 3% of normal, while in Becker muscular dystrophy the dystrophin content is 3% to 20% of normal (Hoffman et al, 1989). Duchenne dystrophy has a worldwide distribution with a mean incidence of 1 per 3500 male births (Emery, 1991). The phenotypic difference between the two dystrophies is that the Becker form has a later age at onset (after age 5), unassisted ambulation after age 15, and survival into adult life. The mildest form is *quadriceps myopathy,* characterized by slowly progressive weakness of the quadriceps muscle, calf enlargement, and elevated serum concentrations of creatine kinase.

Clinical Features.   Most children with Duchenne muscular dystrophy have gait disturbance before age 5 and many before age 3. Toe-walking and frequent falling are typical initial complaints. Some delay in achieving motor milestones is often

Table 7–5 ◆ Muscular Dystrophies

	Genetic Type	Age at Onset (yr)	Age at Disability (yr)	Pattern of Weakness
Duchenne	X-linked	0-5	10-15	Proximal
Becker	X-linked	5-15	15-25	Proximal
Limb-girdle	Autosomal recessive	10-30	20-40	Proximal
Facioscapulo-humeral	Autosomal dominant	10-30	30-50	Proximal arm, face
Myotonic	Autosomal dominant	10-30	30-50	Distal limbs, face
Scapuloperoneal	Autosomal dominant	20-30	30-50	Proximal arm, distal leg
Emery-Dreifuss	X-linked	5-15	25-50	Proximal arm, distal leg

Table 7–6 ◆ Phenotypes Associated With the Xp21 Gene Site

1. Becker muscular dystrophy
2. Duchenne muscular dystrophy
3. Familial X-linked myalgia and cramps (see Chapter 8)
4. McLeod syndrome (elevated serum creatine kinase concentration, acanthocytosis, and absence of Kell antigen)
5. Quadriceps myopathy

elicited in retrospect. Early symptoms are insidious and likely to be dismissed by both parents and physicians. Children may not be brought to medical attention until proximal weakness is sufficiently severe to cause difficulty in rising from the floor and an obvious waddling gait. At this stage, mild proximal weakness is present in pelvic muscles and the Gower sign (Figure 7–1) is present. The calf muscles are large and feel rubbery (Figure 7–2). The Achilles tendon is shortened, and the heels do not quite touch the floor. Tendon reflexes may still be present at the ankle and knee but are difficult to obtain.

The decline in motor strength is linear throughout childhood. Between 3 and 6 years of age, most children show some functional improvement because of cerebral maturation. Children of the same age vary widely in the severity of weakness. Most maintain their ability to walk and climb stairs until 8 years of age. Between ages 3 and 8 the child shows progressive contracture of the Achilles tendon and the iliotibial band, increased lordosis, a more pronounced waddling gait, and increased toe-walking. Gait is more precarious, and the child falls more often. Tendon reflexes at the knees and ankles are lost, and proximal weakness develops in the arms.

Considerable variability of expression occurs even within the Duchenne phenotype (Brooke et al, 1989). On average, functional ability declines rapidly after 8 years of age because of increasing muscle weakness and contractures. By 9 years of age some children require a wheelchair, but most can remain ambulatory until age 12 and may continue to stand in braces until age 16.

Scoliosis occurs in some boys and is not caused by early use of a wheelchair. Deterioration of vital capacity to less than 20% of normal leads to symptoms of nocturnal hypoventilation. The child frequently awakens and is afraid of sleep.

The immediate cause of death is not always clear, but respiratory insufficiency is a contributing factor in almost every case. Arrhythmia caused by cardiomyopathy can be documented in some boys.

In others with chronic hypoxia, intercurrent infection or aspiration produces respiratory arrest.

Diagnosis. Before 5 years of age the serum concentration of creatine kinase is 10 times the upper limit of normal. The concentration then declines with age at an approximate rate of 20% per year.

Mutation analysis using restriction fragment length polymorphism linkage studies is the standard for diagnosis, carrier detection, and fetal diagnosis (Bieber et al, 1989; Cole et al, 1988). Intragenic deletion can be identified in 70% of patients, and a higher percentage is expected with improved techniques. A small percentage of patients have intragenic duplications. Dystrophin analysis is useful to distinguish Duchenne from Becker dystrophy and can also be used for carrier detection (Clerk et al, 1991).

Treatment. Although Duchenne muscular dystrophy is not curable, it is treatable. Prednisone provides an increase in strength and function that can be maintained for up to 3 years (Fenichel et al, 1991).

Treatment goals are to maintain function, pre-

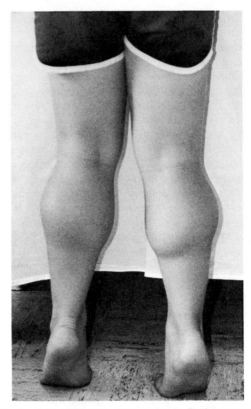

Figure 7–2 Enlarged calf muscles in Duchenne muscular dystrophy. Enlarged calves may be seen in other neuromuscular disorders.

vent contractures, and provide psychologic support not only for the child but also for the family. Every effort should be made to keep children standing and walking as long as possible. This is best accomplished by passive stretching exercises to prevent contractures, a lightweight plastic ankle-foot orthosis to maintain the foot in a neutral position during sleep, and the use of long-leg braces when walking becomes precarious. External appliances have not prevented scoliosis, but a recently developed surgical technique to wire the laminae together is effective in preventing scoliosis without the need for long-term immobilization.

Facioscapulohumeral Syndrome

Progressive facioscapulohumeral (FSH) weakness was originally considered a muscular dystrophy with autosomal dominant inheritance. Later, similar patterns of weakness were described in spinal muscular atrophy and polymyositis. It is now recognized that patients with genetic FSH weakness may have histologic evidence of myopathy, neuropathy, and inflammation. Therefore the term "facioscapulohumeral syndrome" is used to designate this entity that, although predominantly a dystrophy, has elements of denervation. The gene responsible for FSH syndrome has been localized to chromosome 4q35. The defect has complete penetrance but variable expression.

Clinical Features.   Weakness usually begins in the second decade. Initial involvement is often in the shoulder girdle with subsequent spread to the face, but the reverse also occurs. The progression of weakness is insidious, and diagnosis is often delayed. Family history of the syndrome may not be elicited because affected family members are unaware they have a problem. Patients eventually notice a change in facial expression. Late in the course, speech becomes indistinct and leg muscles are sometimes involved. Anterior tibial weakness is most prominent, but proximal weakness may occur as well. In patients with only minimal facial weakness, the combination of proximal weakness in the arms and distal weakness in the legs may suggest a scapuloperoneal syndrome. FSH syndrome and scapuloperoneal syndrome are probably variable expressions of the same genetic disease.

The course of FSH syndrome is variable. Many patients do not become disabled, and their life expectancy is normal. Others are confined to a wheelchair in adult life. In the infantile form, progression is always rapid and disability is always severe (see Chapter 17).

Retinal vascular abnormalities can be demonstrated by angiography in the majority of people with FSH syndrome and should be considered part of the phenotype (Fitzsimons et al, 1987). The most severe manifestations are retinal telangiectasia, exudation, and detachment *(Coates disease)*. Hearing loss and mental retardation may also be present.

Diagnosis.   The serum concentration of creatine kinase can be normal or increased to five times normal. The EMG may show denervation potentials, myopathic motor units, or both. Histologic changes are minimal in many limb muscles; the supraspinatus muscle yields the highest abnormal return (Bodensteiner and Schochet, 1986). Occasional fibers are noted undergoing degeneration, small angulated denervated fibers may be seen, and inflammatory cells may be present.

Treatment.   No treatment for the weakness is available. The retina should be carefully examined for Coates disease. Retinal telangiectasia can be treated by coagulation to prevent blindness.

Limb-Girdle Dystrophy

The term "limb-girdle dystrophy" is used to describe proximal muscle weakness beginning in the second or third decade and progressing slowly to severe disability after 20 years. Both sexes are affected, and although the disease occurs sporadically, autosomal recessive inheritance is suspected. Limb-girdle muscular dystrophy is not a single entity, and the term is often applied to any myopathy that cannot be otherwise categorized.

Clinical Features.   Patients with slowly progressive symmetric proximal weakness, with or without facial involvement, and diminished or absent tendon reflexes should be considered to have limb-girdle dystrophy if other specific entities can be excluded. Either the pelvic or the shoulder girdle muscles can be affected first.

Diagnosis.   The most common problem in differential diagnosis is distinguishing limb-girdle dystrophy from Becker muscular dystrophy, and indeed many males in whom limb-girdle dystrophy is diagnosed prove to have Becker muscular dystrophy when dystrophin is measured. The distinction between these two dystrophies is important for accurate genetic counseling. In addition to Duchenne and Becker muscular dystrophies, conditions to be considered in the differential diagnosis include juvenile spinal muscular atrophy, glycogen storage myopathies, endocrine myopathies, polymyositis, and inclusion body myositis.

The serum concentration of creatine kinase is elevated, but not to the extent seen in early Duchenne muscular dystrophy. EMG findings are consistent with a myopathy. Muscle histologic findings vary with the stage of disease. The earliest changes are variation in fiber size and increase in internal nuclei. Later, fiber splitting and an uneven distribution of mitochondria produce a "moth-eaten" appearance when histochemical reagents for oxidative enzymes are applied. Both fiber types are affected equally (Figure 7–3).

Treatment. The treatment goals in limb-girdle muscular dystrophy are the same as those for Duchenne muscular dystrophy. The only difference is that contractures are not as serious a problem.

INFLAMMATORY MYOPATHIES

The inflammatory myopathies are a heterogeneous group of disorders that together make up the most common form of acquired muscle disease. The annual incidence for hospital diagnosis of polymyositis is 5 per 1 million population. These occur in a bimodal age distribution with the childhood mode accounting for 21% of the total. The trough between the two distribution curves is 15 to 24 years of age.

The leading hypotheses concerning the patho-

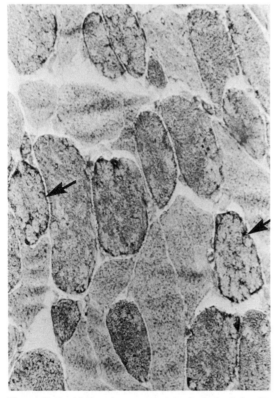

Figure 7–3 Moth-eaten appearance in limb-girdle dystrophy (DPNH reaction). The usual lacelike appearance of the mitochondria is replaced by mitochondrial clumping.

physiology of inflammatory myopathy are viral infection and immunopathy. The two are not mutually exclusive because viral infection may occur in a person whose immune state is abnormal and immune-mediated destruction of tissue may be generated by a viral infection (Whitaker, 1982). A progressive proximal myopathy occurs in adults with acquired immunodeficiency syndrome (AIDS), but cases have not yet been reported in children. However, concentrations of serum creatine kinase are elevated in children with AIDS treated with zidovudine (Walter et al, 1991). Acute infectious myositis is described in the section on acute generalized weakness. The conditions discussed in this section are considered idiopathic.

Dermatomyositis

Dermatomyositis is a systemic angiopathy in which the process of vascular occlusion and infarction accounts for all pathologic changes observed in muscle, connective tissue, skin, gastrointestinal tract, and small nerves. More than 30% of adults with dermatomyositis have an underlying malignancy, but cancer is not a factor in children. The childhood form of dermatomyositis is a relatively homogeneous disease that may have a single cause.

Clinical Features. Peak incidence is generally between the ages of 5 and 10 years, but an onset as early as 4 months has been reported. The presentation of illness may be insidious or fulminating. An insidious onset is characterized by fever, fatigue, and anorexia in the absence of rash or weakness. These symptoms may persist for weeks or months and suggest an underlying infection. In most children dermatitis precedes myositis. The characteristic rash is marked by an erythematous discoloration and edema of the upper eyelids that spread to involve the entire periorbital and malar regions. Erythema and edema of the extensor surfaces overlying the joints of the knuckles, elbows, and knees develop later. With time the skin appears atrophic and scaly.

The myopathy is characterized by proximal weakness, stiffness, and pain, which are most severe in the shoulder and pelvic girdle. Weakness becomes generalized, and flexion contractures develop rapidly and produce joint deformities. Tendon reflexes become increasingly difficult to obtain and finally disappear.

Calcinosis of subcutaneous tissue, especially under discolored areas of skin, occurs in 60% of children. When severe it produces an armorlike appearance (*calcinosis universalis*) on radiographs. In some children stiffness is the predominant initial symptom and skin and muscle symptoms are only minor.

In the past, gastrointestinal tract infarction was a leading cause of death. Ulcerations may extend the length of the bowel and are sometimes preceded by pneumatosis intestinalis as the vasculitis allows the submucosal dissection of intraluminal bowel gas. The mortality rate has fallen to less than 5% (Bowyer et al, 1982).

Diagnosis. The combination of fever, rash, myalgia, and weakness is compelling evidence for the diagnosis of dermatomyositis. The serum concentration of creatine kinase is usually elevated early in the course. At the time of active myositis the EMG shows abnormalities, including increased insertional activity, fibrillations, and positive sharp waves at rest and brief, small-amplitude polyphasic potentials with contraction. The diagnostic feature on muscle biopsy is perifascicular atrophy (Figure 7–4). Capillary necrosis usually starts at the periphery of the muscle fascicle and causes ischemia in the adjacent muscle fibers. The most profound atrophy occurs in fascicular borders that face large

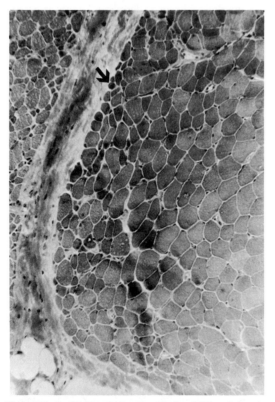

Figure 7–4 Perifascicular atrophy in childhood dermatomyositis (trichrome stain). The muscle fibers at the edge of each fascicle are atrophied.

connective tissue septa. Type I and type II fibers are affected equally.

Treatment. The inflammatory process is thought to be active for approximately 2 years. Corticosteroids may suppress the inflammatory response and provide symptomatic relief but do not cure the underlying disease. The best results are obtained when corticosteroids are started early in high doses and are maintained for long periods of time (Henriksson and Sandstedt, 1982).

Prednisone is initiated in a dosage of 2 mg/kg/day, not to exceed 100 mg/day. The response follows a predictable pattern. Temperature returns to normal within 48 hours. Serum concentrations of creatine kinase return to normal by the second week, and muscle strength increases simultaneously. When these occur, prednisone should be given on alternate days in the same dosage to reduce the frequency and severity of corticosteroid-induced side effects. Alternate day and every day therapy are equally effective if the doses are large and the treatment is maintained. As muscle strength increases, the original dosage of alternate day prednisone is tapered by 10% per month for 5 months. Further reductions are then at a rate of 5% per month. For most children the alternate day maintenance dosage needed for normal muscle strength and normal serum concentrations of creatine kinase is 25% of the starting dosage. The response of the skin rash to prednisone is variable: in some children the rash heals completely, but most will have some permanent scar of the disease.

Although most children demonstrate a dramatic improvement and seem normal in 3 months, prednisone must be continued for a full 2 years. If treatment is discontinued prematurely, relapse is invariable. Calcinosis and contractures are more likely to develop in children treated intermittently. Indeed, corticosteroids are useful in the treatment of calcinosis universalis. In addition to prednisone, a well-structured program of physical therapy is needed to prevent contractures.

Eighty percent of children with dermatomyositis have a favorable outcome if high-dose prednisone is started within 4 months of the onset of symptoms. Children who do not respond immediately to high-dose prednisone should be started on oral methotrexate, 10 to 20 mg/m^2, given twice weekly. Regular monitoring of liver function and white blood cell count is required. If medication fails, plasmapheresis is a reasonable alternative.

Once the disease becomes inactive, reactivation is unlikely. However, late progression or recurrence may occur and should be treated with an additional 1-year course of corticosteroids.

Polymyositis

Polymyositis without evidence of other target organ involvement is uncommon before puberty. Polymyositis has been reported in several infants, some affected from birth (see Chapter 6). Children with systemic lupus erythematosus may have myalgia and arthralgia as early symptoms but generally do not have muscle weakness at onset. Skin, joint, and systemic manifestations are usually well established before the onset of myopathy. Polymyositis in adolescence is similar to the disorder in adult life except that malignancy is not a causative factor.

Clinical Features.   Polymyositis begins as a symmetric proximal weakness that develops insidiously and progresses to moderate handicap within weeks to months. The patient may have prolonged periods of stability or even remission that suggest the diagnosis of limb-girdle muscular dystrophy because of the slow progress. Tendon reflexes are present early in the course and become hypoactive as muscle bulk is lost. Cardiorespiratory complications are less common in childhood than in adult polymyositis.

Diagnosis.   The serum concentration of creatine kinase is not invariably elevated, but the EMG almost always shows abnormalities that typically include both myopathic and neuropathic features. Muscle biopsy may show several different patterns of abnormality, and perivascular inflammation may not be present. Instead, features of myopathy, denervation, or both may be observed (Mastaglia and Ojeda, 1985).

Treatment.   The same treatment schedule suggested for childhood dermatomyositis should be used for children with polymyositis. Unfortunately, the response to corticosteroids is far less predictable in polymyositis than in dermatomyositis. Children who do not respond to corticosteroids should be treated with methotrexate.

Inclusion Body Myositis

Inclusion body myositis is an insidiously progressive myopathy with characteristic clinical and histologic features (Lotz et al, 1989). The onset ordinarily occurs after 50 years of age, but childhood onset is recognized as well (Riggs et al, 1989).

Clinical Features.   Males are affected more often than females. Painless weakness occurs first in the proximal muscles of the pelvis. The progression of weakness is slow. The biceps and triceps muscles are affected next, but the interval between leg and arm weakness may be as long as 10 years. Dysphagia, fatigue, myalgia, and paresthesias may occur later in the course. Tendon reflexes are reduced or absent.

Diagnosis.   The serum concentration of creatine kinase is normal or only mildly elevated. EMG shows abnormal spontaneous electrical activity: increased insertion activity and fibrillations. Short-duration motor units and polyphasic potentials are the rule, but long-duration motor units are also observed. Motor and sensory conduction velocities are normal unless a concomitant neuropathy is present.

Light microscopy characteristically shows muscle fibers with single or multiple vacuoles rimmed with basophilic material, predominantly endomysial mononuclear inflammatory cells in necrotic or nonnecrotic fibers, and atrophic fibers. Electron microscopy demonstrates filamentous inclusions, usually adjacent to vacuoles.

Therapy.   The weakness seldom responds to corticosteroid or immunosuppresive therapy. Progressive debilitation results in death from cardiac or respiratory failure.

METABOLIC MYOPATHIES
Acid Maltase Deficiency

The initial symptoms of acid maltase deficiency may occur in infancy, childhood, or adult life. The enzyme defect appears to be the same regardless of the age at onset, and different ages of onset may occur within the same family (Loonen et al, 1981). Why the age at onset varies so widely is unknown. The defect is always transmitted by autosomal recessive inheritance.

Clinical Features.   Infants with acid maltase deficiency have glycogen storage in both skeletal and cardiac muscle. Death from cardiac failure occurs during infancy (see Chapter 6).

In the childhood form, only skeletal muscle is involved and the main clinical feature is slowly progressive proximal limb weakness. Tendon reflexes are hypoactive or unobtainable. Occasionally children have mild hypertrophy of the calves simulating Duchenne muscular dystrophy. The illness progresses steadily, leading to disability and respiratory insufficiency by 20 years of age. The later the onset of symptoms, the longer and more benign the course.

Diagnosis.   The diagnosis of acid maltase deficiency depends on the demonstration of glycogen storage by muscle biopsy and the absence of acid maltase in muscle or fibroblasts.

Treatment.   No treatment is available.

Other Carbohydrate Myopathies

McArdle disease and debrancher enzyme deficiency are sometimes manifested as slowly progressive proximal weakness and must at least be considered in the differential diagnosis. The usual initial symptom of these disorders, however, is exercise intolerance, and for this reason they are discussed in Chapter 8.

Muscle Carnitine Deficiency

Carnitine is an essential cofactor in the transfer of long-chain fatty acids across the inner mitochondrial membrane and modulates the ratio of acyl to acylcoenzyme A (Breningstall, 1990). Carnitine deficiency causes a failure in the production of energy for metabolism and the storage of triglycerides. It occurs (1) in newborns receiving total parenteral alimentation, (2) in several systemic disorders (see Table 2–5), (3) as the result of several genetic disorders of organic acid metabolism, (4) in children treated with valproate, (5) and as a primary genetic defect of the cellular carnitine transporter (DeVivo and Tein, 1990).

The primary genetic defect is transmitted by autosomal recessive inheritance. Clinical manifestations may be restricted to skeletal muscle or may include systemic symptoms resembling Reye syndrome (see Chapter 2).

Clinical Features.   The major clinical feature of muscle carnitine deficiency is the childhood onset of progressive proximal weakness, affecting the legs before and more severely than the arms. Occasional patients have recurrent attacks of myoglobinuria and cardiomyopathy. The cardiomyopathy is not manifested clinically but is recognized on electrocardiography (EKG) and echocardiography.

Diagnosis.   The serum concentration of creatine kinase is elevated. EMG findings may suggest a neuropathic process early in the course and then may become consistent with myopathy. Muscle biopsy reveals a vacuolar myopathy with lipid storage mainly in type I fibers and a reduced carnitine content.

Treatment.   Dietary therapy with L-carnitine is effective and safe. Diarrhea is the major side effect. The usual dosage is 100 mg/kg/day in three or four divided doses.

Other Lipid Myopathies

Patients with progressive proximal weakness during childhood, lipid storage in muscle, and normal carnitine content have been described. Such patients have in common a disturbance of mitochondrial fatty acid oxidations. Some have obvious morphologic abnormalities of mitochondria (Askansas et al, 1985); in others only biochemical abnormalities can be identified (Carroll et al, 1986). These disorders are genetically heterogeneous and difficult to distinguish from the mitochondrial myopathies.

Clinical Features.   Progressive proximal weakness begins anytime from early childhood to adolescence. The legs are affected first and then the arms. Exercise intolerance is noted, and in some cases the ingestion of fatty foods leads to nausea and vomiting. The pattern and progression of weakness may simulate Duchenne muscular dystrophy even to the presence of calf hypertrophy. Limb weakness is steadily progressive, and cardiomyopathy may develop.

Diagnosis.   The serum concentration of creatine kinase is markedly elevated. EMG findings are abnormal and consistent with a myopathic process. Muscle biopsy is critical to diagnosis. Type I muscle fibers contain fatty droplets. Carnitine and carnitine palmitoyl transferase levels are normal.

Treatment.   Propranolol has improved some patients' strength (Martyn et al, 1981). The mechanism of action is unknown. Patients with fat intolerance may show improvement on a diet free of long-chain fatty acids.

ENDOCRINE MYOPATHIES

Progressive proximal limb weakness may occur in patients with hyperthyroidism, hypothyroidism, hyperparathyroidism, hypoparathyroidism, hyperadrenalism, or hypoadrenalism.

Clinical Features.   Patients with endocrine myopathy usually show systemic signs of endocrine disease before the onset of weakness. However, weakness is the initial feature in some patients, especially those with primary or secondary hypoparathyroidism or thyroid disorders. Weakness is much more prominent in the legs than the arms. Tendon reflexes, even in weak muscles, are normal or diminished but generally are not absent.

Diagnosis.   The serum concentration of creatine kinase is typically normal. EMG is not useful for diagnosis; it may show normal results, myopathy, or neuropathy. Many endocrinopathies produce both neuropathy and myopathy. In Cushing disease and in hyperparathyroidism, muscle histologic studies reveal type II fiber atrophy. Other conditions demonstrate nonspecific myopathic changes that vary with the severity of endocrinopathy.

Treatment. In all endocrine myopathies, weakness is reversed by treating the underlying endocrinopathy.

◆ Progressive Distal Weakness

Progressive distal weakness in childhood is most often due to neuropathy (Table 7–7). Among the slowly progressive neuropathies of childhood, hereditary disorders are far more common than acquired disorders. The only common acquired neuropathy is postinfectious polyradiculoneuropathy (Guillain-Barré syndrome), in which weakness evolves rapidly.

Table 7–7 ◆ Progressive Distal Weakness

Spinal Cord Disorders (see Chapter 12)

Motor Neuron Diseases
1. Juvenile amyotrophic lateral sclerosis
2. Spinal muscular atrophies
   a. Genetic forms
   b. Nonfamilial Asian (see Chapter 13)

Neuropathies
1. Hereditary motor sensory neuropathies (HMSN)
   a. HMSN I: Charcot-Marie-Tooth
   b. HMSN II: neuronal Charcot-Marie-Tooth
   c. HMSN III: Déjérine-Sottas
   d. HMSN IV: Refsum
2. Other genetic neuropathies
   a. Familial amyloid neuropathy (see Chapter 9)
   b. Giant axonal neuropathy
   c. Pyruvate dehydrogenase deficiency
      (see Chapter 10)
   d. Sulfatide lipidoses: metachromatic leukodystrophy
   e. Other leukodystrophies
3. Neuropathies with systemic diseases
   a. Drug-induced
   b. Systemic vasculitis
   c. Toxins
   d. Uremia
4. Idiopathic neuropathy
   a. Chronic axonal neuropathy
   b. Chronic demyelinating neuropathy

Myopathies
1. Hereditary distal myopathies
2. Myotonic dystrophy

Scapulo(humeral)Peroneal Syndrome
1. Bethlem myopathy
2. Emery-Dreifuss syndrome
3. Scapulohumeral syndrome with dementia
4. Scapuloperoneal neuronopathy

DIAGNOSIS IN NEUROPATHY

The typical presentation of neuropathy in children is progressive symmetric distal weakness affecting the legs and then the arms. When sensation is disturbed, dysesthesias consisting of tingling, "pins and needles," or burning sensations of the feet are felt. The weakness and sensory loss move from distal to proximal in a glove-and-stocking distribution. Tendon reflexes are lost early in the course of disease, especially when sensory fibers are affected.

An important first step in diagnosis is to determine the primary site of the disorder: cell body (anterior horn cell), nerve axon, or myelin. This is accomplished by electrodiagnosis (Table 7–8). In primary disorders of the cell body (neuronopathy) an EMG of resting muscle demonstrates fibrillations and fasciculations. With voluntary contraction the number of motor unit potentials is reduced but the amplitude is normal or increased because of collateral reinnervation. Motor conduction nerve velocity is normal or only slightly diminished, and the amplitude of sensory action potentials is normal. In axonopathies the EMG shows fibrillations at rest and motor unit potentials that are reduced in number but normal or increased in amplitude. High-amplitude potentials may be polyphasic. Motor nerve conduction velocity is normal or mildly reduced, and the amplitude of sensory action potentials may also be reduced. Demyelinating neuropathies are characterized by marked slowing of motor conduction velocity and reduced amplitude of sensory evoked potentials. EMG findings may be normal early in the course of disease.

JUVENILE AMYOTROPHIC LATERAL SCLEROSIS

The term "juvenile amyotrophic lateral sclerosis" describes a group of rare hereditary diseases characterized by some combination of upper and lower motor neuron dysfunction (Hamida et al, 1990). Genetic transmission may be by autosomal recessive or dominant inheritance. Onset usually occurs in the second decade, and progression is slow. The clinical features are some combination of spastic paraplegia and wasting of the hands or peroneal atrophy. Bulbar and pseudobulbar palsy may also be present. There is clinical overlap between these conditions, the hereditary spinal muscular atrophies, and familial spastic paraplegia (see Chapter 12). Many of the hereditary motor neuron diseases may prove to have a similar genetic defect or abnormal gene product.

Table 7–8 ◆ Electrodiagnosis in Neuropathy

	Neuronopathy	Axonal	Demyelinating
Fasciculations	+ + +	+ + +	+
Denervation potentials	+ + +	+ + +	+
Reduced number of motor units	+ + +	+ + +	0
High-amplitude potentials	+ + +	+ + +	0
Slow motor velocity	0	+	+ + +
Reduced sensory potentials	0	+	+ + +

0, absent; +, rare; + + +, common.

SPINAL MUSCULAR ATROPHY

The distal form of spinal muscular atrophy is genetically heterogeneous. Sometimes the disease is segmental and affects only the arms or only the feet. The trait may be transmitted by autosomal dominant or recessive inheritance. Severe and mild forms that may be genetically distinct exist for each type of inheritance (Harding and Thomas, 1980; Pearn et al, 1978).

Clinical Features.   The disease usually begins with weakness and wasting in the anterior compartment of the legs associated with pes cavus deformities of the feet. Tendon reflexes may be preserved. The clinical picture is indistinguishable from hereditary motor sensory neuropathy type I (HMSN I). In the severe autosomal recessive form, weakness progresses to involve the proximal muscles of the legs and sometimes the hands. Weakness in the arms varies from family to family but shows concordance within an individual family. Approximately 25% of patients have scoliosis.

In some families the weakness begins in the hands and either is confined to the arms or affects the legs later and less severely. A genetic basis for segmental spinal muscular atrophy affecting only the arms was established in one set of identical twin brothers (Tandan et al, 1990). However, whether transmission is by autosomal recessive inheritance or dominant inheritance with incomplete penetrance is unknown.

The onset of distal spinal muscular atrophies is always before age 20. Except in the severe autosomal recessive form the prognosis is generally good. Progression of weakness is slow and sometimes appears to be arrested. Distinguishing between mild and severe autosomal recessive forms is possible only when other family members are affected. The course of disease runs true within each family.

Diagnosis.   Electrodiagnosis is critical to distinguish these disorders from peripheral neuropathies. Motor nerve conduction velocity is normal despite total denervation of the small muscles of the foot. Sensory evoked potentials are also normal. The serum concentration of creatine kinase is usually normal but may be mildly elevated. Muscle biopsy results demonstrate nonspecific changes of denervation, and the sural nerve is normal.

Treatment.   No treatment is available, nor is there a method for antenatal diagnosis.

HEREDITARY MOTOR AND SENSORY NEUROPATHY

The term "hereditary motor and sensory neuropathy" (HMSN) encompasses several genetic neuropathies that previously had been known by a variety of eponyms. As a group, their incidence is estimated to be 10 per 100,000 population (Emery, 1991). Almost half of patients with idiopathic polyneuropathies are found to have HMSN when detailed family histories are taken and other family members are examined (Dyck et al, 1981).

Hereditary Motor and Sensory Neuropathy Type 1: Charcot-Marie-Tooth Disease

HMSN I is a dominantly inherited hypertrophic neuropathy with prominent peroneal atrophy. In most cases the abnormal gene is on chromosome 17 (Timmerman et al, 1990). However, in some cases the gene is localized to chromosome 1 and in others to neither 17 nor 1. An identical, much rarer syndrome is also transmitted by X-linked inheritance (Ionasescu et al, 1988). The *Roussy-Lévy syndrome* is also included in this classification. Clinical expression varies considerably, and clinical examination, including electrodiagnosis, may be needed to demonstrate the phenotype in parents.

Clinical Features.   The initial symptoms are either foot deformities or gait disturbances, beginning usually in the second decade or later but sometimes in early infancy (Vanasse and Dubowitz, 1981). Dysesthesias are never an early symptom, although some patients, because of foot deformity, may complain of pain from pressure by shoes. Pes cavus is typical, and hammertoes may be present. These deformities are caused by weakness of the intrinsic foot muscles and result in foreshortening of the foot and elevation of the arch. The initial gait disturbance is usually described as clumsiness, especially in running.

HMSN I is not a severe disorder in childhood. Examination reveals pes cavus, weakness of the peroneal muscles, and diminished reactivity of the Achilles tendon reflex (Hagberg and Lyon, 1981). With time the anterior tibial, as well as the peroneal, muscles become weak, producing footdrop. The gastrocnemius and soleus muscles may be involved as well. Eventually, usually after 20 years of age, weakness spreads to the proximal muscles of the legs and the hands. Scoliosis is present in only a minority of patients. Cramps with exercise and fasciculations are present in weak muscles. Sensation is generally normal.

Peripheral nerves are enlarged in adults but not in children. The enlargement is caused by repeated episodes of demyelination and remyelination.

Diagnosis. Diagnosis relies on characteristic clinical findings and a family history of the disease. Motor nerve conduction velocities are less than 50% of normal in affected individuals. The cerebrospinal fluid protein content is usually normal in children but may be elevated in adults. Muscle histologic appearance reveals nonspecific changes of denervation; myopathic changes may also be present in older individuals. "Onion bulb" formation is noted in peripheral nerves that have undergone repeated episodes of demyelination and remyelination but is not pathognomonic.

Treatment. No specific treatment is available, but proper foot care may minimize discomfort and maximize function. Shoes should be roomy and soft to prevent rubbing against bony prominences. Footwear that is molded to the shape of the foot is especially useful. When footdrop is present, a lightweight plastic ankle-foot orthosis that fits into the patient's own shoe not only lifts the foot but also prevents turning and injury of the ankle.

Hereditary Motor and Sensory Neuropathy Type II: Charcot-Marie-Tooth Disease, Neuronal Type

HMSN II is transmitted by autosomal dominant inheritance and clinically resembles HMSN I, except that symptoms are considerably milder. Because the pathologic process is primarily axonal rather than demyelinating, motor nerve conduction

velocities are either normal or only mildly prolonged (Berciano et al, 1986).

Clinical Features. The peak age at onset is during the second decade. Onset in early childhood may represent a genetically distinct form that is transmitted by autosomal recessive inheritance (Ouvrier et al, 1981).

Distal weakness begins in the legs and can be asymmetric. The hands are affected later. Tendon reflexes are generally absent at the ankle but may be preserved at the knee and elbow. Most children have distal sensory loss. In some children all modalities are affected; others experience loss of pain or vibration and position sense. Progression of symptoms is slow, and disability does not occur until middle adult life.

Diagnosis. The cerebrospinal fluid protein content is normal as is the serum concentration of creatine kinase. Motor conduction velocity is 60% or more of normal. The EMG demonstrates a denervation pattern in affected muscles.

Treatment. No specific treatment is available.

Hereditary Motor and Sensory Neuropathy Type III: Déjérine-Sottas Disease

HMSN III is a demyelinating and remyelinating neuropathy transmitted by autosomal recessive inheritance. Many cases are sporadic. Parenteral consanguinity is a factor in many families. However, the heterozygote parent has no evidence of neuropathy either by clinical examination or by electrodiagnosis (Dyck, 1984). Some infants with congenital hypomyelinating neuropathy (see Chapter 6) may actually have a severe form of HMSN III (Balestrini et al, 1991).

Clinical Features. Slow motor development and hypotonia are common during the first year. Weakness begins distally in the limbs and progresses to involve the proximal muscles by the second decade. Sensory ataxia is present in all patients (Ouvrier et al, 1987). Clubfoot and scoliosis are associated findings. Distal sensory loss of all modalities is readily demonstrated on examination. Tendon reflexes are absent. Peripheral nerves enlarge, and the great auricular, the median, and the ulnar nerves are frequently palpable. Associated findings in some patients include miosis, sluggish pupillary responses to light, nystagmus, and choreiform movements of the fingers.

Diagnosis. The cerebrospinal fluid protein content is generally elevated in proportion to the severity of weakness. Motor nerve conduction velocities are markedly prolonged, and sensory potentials are reduced in amplitude. Sural nerve biopsy demonstrates massive interstitial hypertrophy and marked onion bulb formation. These typical findings are not pathognomonic and are seen in HMSN I as well. Because of overlap in the clinical, electrodiagnostic, and pathologic features of HMSN I and HMSN III, the two disorders are differentiated primarily by their mode of genetic transmission (Hagberg and Lyon, 1981).

Treatment.   No treatment is available.

Hereditary Motor and Sensory Neuropathy Type IV: Refsum Disease

Refsum disease is an inborn error of phytanic acid metabolism reported mainly from Scandinavia, Great Britain, Germany, and France. Autosomal recessive transmission is suspected because of a high incidence of consanguinity in affected families and no evidence of disease in parents (Refsum, 1984). In fibroblasts derived from homozygotes the rate of phytanic acid oxidation is 3% of that in control samples; in heterozygotes the rate is 50%.

Clinical Features.   Age at onset varies from the first to the third decade but is sometimes difficult to determine because initial symptoms are insidious. The cardinal clinical manifestations are retinitis pigmentosa, chronic or recurrent polyneuropathy, and cerebellar ataxia. Retinitis pigmentosa is a constant finding and is indispensable for diagnosis. Night blindness is often the first symptom. The neuropathy is hypertrophic, symmetric, and distal, affecting both motor and sensory fibers. Vibration and position sense are more diminished than are pain and temperature. Tendon reflexes become progressively hyporesponsive and are finally lost. The ataxia may be of cerebellar origin; nystagmus and intention tremor are sometimes present but could be caused by sensory neuropathy. Other symptoms include progressive loss of hearing, cataracts, cardiomyopathy, ichthyosis, and pes cavus.

The course is variable; there may be steady progression, long periods of stability, or remissions and exacerbations. The patient may die suddenly from cardiac arrhythmia as a consequence of cardiomyopathy.

Diagnosis.   The protein content of the cerebrospinal fluid is elevated to between 100 and 700 mg/dl (1 and 7 g/L). Motor and sensory nerve conduction velocities are markedly reduced. EMG results are consistent with denervation. Electroretinography demonstrates a severe abnormality of the photoreceptors of the retina, involving both rods and cones. Definitive diagnosis requires demonstration of reduced oxidation of phytanic acid in cultured fibroblasts. Antenatal diagnosis is accomplished by measuring phytanic acid oxidation in amniotic cells.

Treatment.   Phytanic acid is not produced endogenously and must be derived completely from diet. Exacerbations of disease correlate well with blood levels of phytanic acid. Treatment is a combination of diet and plasma exchange (Gibberd et al, 1979). This has proved successful in preventing progression of symptoms and in reversing symptoms already present.

OTHER GENETIC NEUROPATHIES
Giant Axonal Neuropathy

Giant axonal neuropathy is a rare disorder transmitted by autosomal recessive inheritance. It is possibly an inborn error of enzyme-linked sulfhydryl-containing enzymes (Tandan et al, 1987). Both central and peripheral axons are affected.

Clinical Features.   Males and females are affected equally, and 6 of 19 cases have been from consanguineous marriages (Donaghy et al, 1988). Affected children are pale and thin and have curly scalp hair. Gait impairment usually begins by 3 years of age but can appear later. Some children are asymptomatic at birth and then have generalized hypotonia as the initial manifestation. Symmetric distal atrophy of leg muscles is a constant early feature. Vibratory and proprioceptive sensations in the legs are profoundly impaired, and tendon reflexes are decreased or absent.

Central involvement may result in cerebellar dysfunction, dementia, optic atrophy, and cranial neuropathies.

Diagnosis.   Sural nerve biopsy reveals enlarged axons filled with disrupted neurofilaments that are surrounded by a thin or fragmented myelin sheath. Mainly the large myelinated nerve fibers are affected. Magnetic resonance imaging of the brain may demonstrate increased signal intensity of the white matter.

Treatment.   No treatment is available.

Sulfatide Lipidosis: Metachromatic Leukodystrophy

Metachromatic leukodystrophy is an inherited disorder of myelin metabolism caused by defective activity of the enzyme arylsulfatase A. The gene defect is transmitted by autosomal recessive inheritance. Three forms are recognized: late infantile, juvenile, and adult. The late infantile form is the most common. Juvenile- and adult-onset cases affect primarily the brain and are difficult to distinguish from each other (see Chapter 5). Heterozygosity and homozygosity of two alleles account for the different forms of the disease (Polten et al, 1991). Only the late infantile form is discussed in this section.

Clinical Features.   After a period of normal development, gait disburbances develop, usually by 2 years of age but sometimes not until age 4. Initial examination reveals distal weakness of the feet with loss of the Achilles tendon reflex. Progressive weakness of all limbs results in generalized hypotonia and hyporeflexia. Later, brain function deteriorates and dementia, spasticity, and blindness develop.

Diagnosis.   The protein content of the cerebrospinal fluid is elevated, and motor nerve conduction velocities are reduced at the time of initial leg weakness. The diagnosis is confirmed by demonstrating the absence of arylsulfatase A in white blood cells. Prenatal diagnosis is possible by analysis of arylsulfatase A in amniocytes.

Treatment.   Bone marrow transplantation early in the course of the disease may slow the course (Krivit et al, 1990). No other treatment is available.

Other Leukodystrophies

Peripheral neuropathy occurs in *globoid cell leukodystrophy* (Krabbe disease) but is not as prominent a feature as in metachromatic leukodystrophy. Krabbe disease is manifested in infancy by psychomotor retardation and irritability rather than flaccid weakness (see Chapter 5). Tendon reflexes may be absent or hyperactive, and motor nerve conduction velocity is reduced in half of cases. Cerebrospinal fluid protein concentration is elevated.

Cockayne syndrome is characterized by progeria, small stature, ataxia, retinitis pigmentosa, deafness, and mental retardation (see Chapter 16). A primary segmental demyelinating neuropathy is present in 10% to 20% of cases but is not an initial symptom (Ohnishi et al, 1987). The neuropathy is manifest as hyporeflexia and reduced motor nerve conduction velocity.

Other disorders of lipid metabolism in which demyelinating neuropathy is present, but not an important feature, include Niemann-Pick disease, Gaucher disease, and Farber disease.

NEUROPATHIES WITH SYSTEMIC DISEASE
Drug-Induced Neuropathy

Several drugs that are used widely in children, such as chloramphenicol and phenytoin, are capable of producing a polyneuropathy (Ouvrier et al, 1990a). However, the neuropathy is usually subclinical and is detected only by electrodiagnosis or because of loss of the Achilles tendon reflex. Drugs that commonly produce clinical evidence of motor and sensory neuropathy are isoniazid, nitrofurantoin, vincristine, and zidovudine.

Isoniazid

Clinical Features.   The initial symptoms are numbness and paresthesias of the fingers and toes. If therapy is continued, superficial sensation is diminished in a glove-and-stocking pattern. Distal limb weakness follows and is associated with tenderness of the muscles and burning dysesthesias. The Achilles tendon reflex is diminished or absent.

Diagnosis.   Isoniazid neuropathy should be suspected whenever neuropathy develops in a child taking the drug.

Treatment.   Isoniazid interferes with pyridoxine metabolism and produces neuropathy by causing a pyridoxine deficiency state. The administration of pyridoxine along with isoniazid prevents neuropathy without interfering with antituberculous activity. The longer that symptoms are allowed to progress, the longer the time until recovery. Although pyridoxine can prevent the development of neuropathy, it has little effect on the speed of recovery once neuropathy is established.

Nitrofurantoin

Clinical Features.   Nitrofurantoin neuropathy most often occurs in patients with impaired renal function. High blood concentrations of the drug produce an axonal neuropathy. The initial symptoms are usually paresthesias, followed within a few days or weeks by glove-and-stocking sensory loss and weakness of distal muscles. Pure motor neuropathy is occasionally present.

Diagnosis.   Nitrofurantoin neuropathy should be suspected in any child who has neuropathy and is taking the drug. It may be difficult to distinguish from uremic neuropathy.

Treatment.   Recovery is usually complete when the drug is stopped. Occasional patients have gone on to complete paralysis and death despite discontinuation of nitrofurantoin.

Vincristine

Clinical Features.   Neuropathy is an expected complication of vincristine therapy (Casey et al, 1973). The Achilles tendon reflex is lost first; later, other tendon reflexes become less reactive and may be lost. The first symptoms are paresthesias, often starting in the fingers rather than the feet and then progressing to mild loss of superficial sensation, but not position sense. Weakness follows sensory loss and is evidenced by clumsiness in the hands and cramps in the feet. Distal muscles are affected more than proximal muscles, and extensors more than flexors. Weakness may progress rapidly with loss of ambulation in a few weeks. The initial weakness may be asymmetric and suggests mononeuropathy multiplex.

Diagnosis. Electrodiagnostic findings are consistent with axonal neuropathy; fibrillations and fasciculations are seen on the EMG, but motor nerve conduction velocity is normal.

Treatment. The neuropathy is dose related, and usually the patient recovers 1 to 3 months after the drug is discontinued.

Zidovudine

Postnatal infection of children with the human immunodeficiency virus (HIV) was caused by contamination of the blood supply before screening was implemented. Children with hemophilia were especially at risk. AIDS can cause neuropathy as can its treatment with zidovudine.

Toxins

Several heavy metals, inorganic chemicals, and insecticides produce polyneuropathies in children (Ouvrier et al, 1990a). In adults heavy metal poisoning is generally caused by industrial exposure, agricultural exposure, or attempted homicide. Small children who have a single accidental ingestion are more likely to have acute symptoms of systemic disease or central nervous system dysfunction than a slowly progressive neuropathy. Sometimes, progressive distal weakness is an early sign in older children addicted to sniffing glue or gasoline. Even in these cases symptoms of central nervous system dysfunction are usually present.

Uremia

Some degree of neuropathy occurs at one time or another in many children undergoing long-term periodic hemodialysis. Uremic neuropathy is more common in males than females, but the reason for the sex bias is unknown.

Clinical Features. The earliest symptoms may be muscle cramps in the hands and feet, burning feet, or restless legs. Loss of the Achilles tendon reflex can be demonstrated at the onset. After the initial sensory symptoms the disorder progresses to a severe distal, symmetric, mixed motor, and sensory polyneuropathy affecting the legs more

than the arms. The rate of progression is variable and may be fulminating or may evolve over several months.

A pure motor neuropathy develops in a small proportion of uremic patients. Symptoms begin after hemodialysis is started and may be initiated by septicemia. The rapid progression of distal weakness in all limbs does not respond to dialysis but may be reversed by renal transplantation.

Diagnosis. Uremia produces an axonal neuropathy, but chronic renal failure causes segmental demyelination that is out of proportion to axonal changes. (Ouvrier et al, 1990b). Therefore the determination of motor nerve conduction velocity is used widely to monitor the severity of neuropathy. Slow conduction velocities are present even before clinical symptoms occur. Reductions in creatine clearance are highly correlated with slowing of the conduction velocity.

Treatment. Early neuropathy can be reversed by dialysis. Patients with severe neuropathy rarely recover fully despite adequate treatment.

Systemic Vasculitis and Vasculopathy

Polyneuropathy and mononeuropathy multiplex are relatively common neurologic complications of vasculitis in adults but not in children. Children with lupus erythematosus are generally sicker than adults, but peripheral neuropathy is not a prominent feature of their disease. When neuropathy is present, it is not an initial feature.

IDIOPATHIC NEUROPATHY
Chronic Axonal Neuropathy

Clinical Features. Most axonal neuropathies are either hereditary or toxic. Glue sniffing is an example of a toxic cause. Some children have a progressive axonal neuropathy for which no cause can be determined. Most often the initial symptom is progressive weakness of the feet, with or without sensory impairment. Parents and siblings should undergo electrodiagnostic studies to be certain that they do not have the disorder (Dyck et al, 1981).

Diagnosis. The EMG demonstrates fibrillations and fasciculations, but motor nerve conduction velocity is normal or only mildly delayed. The protein content of the cerebrospinal fluid is normal.

Treatment. Children with idiopathic axonal neuropathy usually have a slowly progressive weakness that does not respond to corticosteroids. However, occasional patients do respond, and a 2-month trial of prednisone is indicated in patients with subacute progression of disease. These responsive cases may be variants of chronic inflammatory demyelinating neuropathy, in which both axonal involvement and demyelination are present.

Chronic Inflammatory Demyelinating Polyradiculoneuropathy

Acquired demyelinating neuropathies occur in both an acute and a chronic form. The acute form is called *Guillain-Barré syndrome* and is described in the section that follows (Table 7–9). The chronic form is called *chronic inflammatory demyelinating polyradiculoneuropathy* (CIDP). The acute and chronic forms may be difficult to distinguish from each other at the onset of symptoms but are identified by their subsequent course.

CIDP, like the Guillain-Barré syndrome, is generally believed to be immune mediated. However, although a clear relationship exists between the Guillain-Barré syndrome and a preceding viral infection, the provocative stimulus for CIDP is unknown.

Clinical Features. CIDP affects adults more often than children but may be present even at birth (see Chapter 6). The initial symptoms are usually weakness and paresthesias in the distal portions of the limbs; only rarely does motor involvement occur alone. Facial weakness occurs in only 13% of cases. Mandatory criteria for diagnosis are (1) progressive or relapsing motor and sensory dysfunction of more than one limb, of a peripheral nerve nature, developing over at least 2 months, and (2) areflexia or hyporeflexia, usually affecting all four limbs (American Academy of Neurology, 1991). In 65% of patients the course is steadily progressive or stepwise, and in the remaining 35% it is characterized by recurrent episodes of acute polyradic-

Table 7–9 ◆ Acute Generalized Weakness

Infectious Disorders
1. Acute infectious myositis
2. Acute inflammatory polyradiculoneuropathy (Guillain-Barré syndrome)
3. Enterovirus infections

Metabolic Disorders
1. Acute intermittent porphyria (see Chapter 9)
2. Hereditary tyrosinemia (see Chapter 9)

Neuromuscular Blockade
1. Botulism
2. Tick paralysis

Periodic Paralysis
1. Familial hyperkalemic
2. Familial hypokalemic
3. Familial normokalemic

uloneuropathy with only partial or complete recovery between episodes (McCombe et al, 1987). Whichever the course, progression occurs for at least 6 months and sometimes several years.

Diagnosis. This diagnosis should not be considered if there is a family history of a similar disorder, a pure sensory neuropathy, other organ involvement, or abnormal storage of material in nerves. The protein content of the cerebrospinal fluid is always greater than 0.45 g/L, and a small number of mononuclear cells may be present. Motor nerve conduction velocity is less than 70% of the lower limit of normal in at least two nerves. Sural nerve biopsy shows features of demyelination. Cellular infiltration of the nerve is uncommon, and evidence of vasculitis excludes the diagnosis of CIDP.

Acquired demyelinating neuropathies in children can be differentiated from familial demyelinating neuropathies by electrodiagnosis. Acquired neuropathies demonstrate a multifocal disturbance of conduction velocity, whereas in hereditary disorders conduction is uniformly slowed throughout the length of the nerve (Miller et al, 1985).

Treatment. Prednisone had been considered the treatment of choice, but high-dose intravenous human immune globulin may be more effective in some patients, especially if given during the first year of illness (Van Doorn et al, 1990, 1991; Vettaikorumakankav et al, 1991). The recommended dosage is 400 mg/kg/day infused over 8 hours for 5 days. Diphenhydramine should be given concurrently to reduce allergic reactions. The clinical response is often immediate. Forty percent of patients require repeated infusions.

Prednisone should be initiated at a dosage of 2 mg/kg/day, not to exceed 100 mg, for 5 days and then changed to alternate day therapy. Initial improvement is expected within 2 months and a clinical plateau within 6 months. Patients who respond to prednisone frequently have a relapse when prednisone is withdrawn. Because of the relapsing nature of the disease, low-dose corticosteroid therapy should continue for several years.

The outcome is more favorable in children than in adults and full recovery is the rule, although some children have relapses in adult life (McCombe et al, 1987).

MYOPATHIES
Hereditary Distal Myopathies

Three clinical forms of hereditary distal myopathy have been described: two are transmitted by dominant inheritance and one by recessive inheritance. One of the dominant forms occurs in infancy (Bautista et al, 1978) and the other in young adults (Markesbery et al, 1974). The recessive form begins during adolescence or later (Barohn et al, 1991). Sporadic cases with onset in early adult life are also reported. In one family the father had late-onset oculopharyngeal dystrophy and his son had an infantile-onset distal myopathy (Fukuhara et al, 1982). Which hereditary distal myopathies are genetically distinct has not been determined. Some of the autosomal dominant forms may be variants of myotonic dystrophy.

Infantile-Onset Dominant Form

Clinical Features. Hereditary distal myopathy with onset in infancy begins anytime during the first 2 years. The first signs are footdrop and weakness in the hand extensor muscles. Little or no progression occurs throughout the remainder of childhood. Occasionally children demonstrate pseudohypertrophy of the calves, scoliosis, or pes cavus.

Diagnosis. The creatine kinase concentration is usually normal, but EMG demonstrates brief, small-amplitude polyphasic potentials, occasional fibrillations, and myotonia. Muscle biopsy reveals fiber-type disproportion in which type I fibers are more numerous, but smaller, than type II fibers.

Treatment. No treatment is available.

Adult-Onset Dominant Form

Clinical Features. Adult-onset hereditary distal myopathy usually begins after age 20 and frequently not until middle age. The first symptoms are weakness of the hands and feet with slow progression throughout adulthood.

Diagnosis. The serum concentration of creatine kinase is usually elevated, and the EMG reveals brief, small-amplitude polyphasic potentials. Muscle histologic findings are variable and generally include fiber size variation, central nuclei, and vacuoles. Both fiber types are affected.

Treatment. No treatment is available.

Autosomal Recessive Form (Miyoshi Myopathy)

Clinical Features. Onset of the autosomal recessive form of hereditary distal myopathy occurs between 15 and 25 years of age. Weakness and atrophy in the gastrocnemius muscle are the initial features, with relative sparing of the anterior compartment. The ankle jerk reflex is lost, but other tendon reflexes are normal. Slowly progressive weakness is the rule with eventual involvement of the quadriceps muscle. However, ambulation is usually preserved.

Diagnosis. The serum creatine kinase concentration is at least 10 times the upper limit of normal, EMG findings are consistent with a myopathy, and muscle biopsy shows a chronic active myopathy without vacuoles.

Treatment. Immunosuppressive therapy does not effect the course of disease.

Myotonic Dystrophy

Myotonic dystrophy is a multisystem disorder transmitted by autosomal dominant inheritance with variable penetrance. An unstable fragment of desoxyribonucleic acid is detected on chromosome 19 in all patients, and the size of the defective fragment correlates with disease severity (Buxton et al, 1992). The onset of symptoms is usually during adolescence or later. A neonatal form, which occurs in children born to mothers with myotonic dystrophy, is described in Chapter 6.

Clinical Features. The major features are myotonia (a disturbance in muscle relaxation after contraction), weakness in the face and distal portion of the limbs, cataracts, frontal baldness, and multiple endocrinopathies. The pattern of muscle atrophy in the face is so stereotyped that all patients with the disease have a similar facies. The face is long and thin because of wasting of the temporal and masseter muscles, and the neck is thin because of atrophy of the sternocleidomastoid muscles. The eyelids and corners of the mouth droop, and the lower part of the face sags, producing the appearance of sadness.

Although medical treatment is rarely sought before adolescence, myotonia is usually present in childhood and can be detected by the EMG, if not by clinical examination. Myotonia is demonstrated by percussion of muscle, usually the thenar eminence, which dimples and remains dimpled at the site of percussion. In addition, the thumb abducts and remains in that position for several seconds. The physician can also detect myotonia by shaking hands with the patient. The patient has difficulty in letting go and releases the grip in part by flexing the wrist to force the flexors of the fingers open.

Some patients have little or no evidence of muscle weakness, only cataracts, frontal baldness, or endocrine disturbances. However, when muscle weakness is present before age 20, it is likely to be relentlessly progressive, causing severe distal weakness in the hands and feet by adult life. Smooth and cardiac muscle involvement may be present and is characterized by disturbed gastrointestinal motility. Endocrine disturbances include testicular atrophy, infertility in women, hyperinsulinism, adrenal atrophy, and disturbances in growth hormone secretion.

Diagnosis.   The diagnosis of myotonic dystrophy is usually based on clinical features and family history. EMG studies demonstrate myotonia (the appearance of motor unit potentials that wax and wane in amplitude and frequency), myopathic potentials, and involvement of peripheral large-diameter motor and sensory fibers (Jamal et al, 1986).

Studies of muscle histology reveal a combination of internal nuclei and type I fiber atrophy. In addition, some fibers contain fibrils that are oriented in the wrong plane (ringed fibers) and have undergone degeneration (sarcoplasmic masses). The serum concentration of creatine kinase is elevated.

Treatment.   Myotonia frequently responds to drugs that stabilize membranes: quinidine, procainamide, phenytoin, and carbamazepine. However, it is weakness, for which no treatment is available, and not myotonia that disables the patient. Braces for footdrop are usually required as the disease progresses.

SCAPULO(HUMERAL)PERONEAL SYNDROMES

Progressive weakness and atrophy affecting the proximal muscles of the arms and the distal muscles of the legs may result from neuronopathy or myopathy, but many patients have features of both nerve and muscle disease. Dominantly inherited scapulo(humeral)peroneal syndromes and facioscapulohumeral syndrome are probably the same or similar genetic disorders.

Bethlem Myopathy

Bethlem myopathy is a form of muscular dystrophy transmitted by autosomal dominant inheritance (Mohire et al, 1988).

Clinical Features.   The onset of scapulohumeropelvic weakness is in infancy or early childhood. The neck and trunk are involved, but the face is spared. Weakness progresses slowly and usually does not produce disability or shorten life span. Contractures form in the elbows, fingers, ankles, and knees but spare the spine. Tendon reflexes are normal or depressed. Cardiomyopathy does not occur.

Diagnosis.   The serum concentration of creatine kinase is normal or slightly elevated, EMG is usually myopathic, and muscle biopsy reveals a nonspecific myopathy.

Treatment.   Physical therapy for contractures is the only treatment available.

Emery-Dreifuss Muscular Dystrophy

Emery-Dreifuss muscular dystrophy is transmitted by X-linked recessive inheritance and is manifested between the ages of 5 and 15 years (Merlini et al, 1986). A disorder identical to Emery-Dreifuss syndrome but with transmission by autosomal dominant inheritance has also been described (Fenichel et al, 1982).

Clinical Features.   The earliest feature of disease is the development of contractures in the flexors of the elbows, the Achilles tendon, and the extensors of the hand. This is followed by weakness and wasting in the biceps and triceps muscles and then the deltoid and other shoulder muscles. The peroneal muscles are severely affected. Calf hypertrophy does not occur. The progression of symptoms is slow, and the condition usually stabilizes by 20 years of age. In some patients, however, weakness progresses into adult life and ambulation is lost. In all patients a cardiomyopathy leading to permanent atrial paralysis develops. Bradycardia and syncope may precede muscle weakness or be delayed until the third decade. The arrhythmia, if not treated by use of a permanent pacemaker, may be the cause of stroke and death.

Diagnosis.   The EMG may demonstrate features of denervation and myopathy in the same patient or may show myopathy in one sibling and neuropathy in another. The most prominent feature on muscle biopsy is type I fiber atrophy. This histologic pattern is seen in many congenital myopathies in which it is uncertain whether the primary disease is in nerve or muscle (see Chapter 6).

Treatment.   No treatment is available for the muscle weakness and wasting, but cardiac arrhythmia should be treated early by implantation of a permanent pacemaker.

Scapulohumeral Syndrome with Dementia

Scapulohumeral syndrome with dementia is transmitted by X-linked inheritance (Bergia et al, 1986).

Clinical Features.   Affected children appear normal until 5 years of age and then have mental deterioration, recognized first as a learning disability and then as mental retardation. Weakness and atrophy of the scapular or humeral muscles and peroneal muscles follow shortly thereafter. Contractures do not develop in affected muscles, and pseudohypertrophy is not present. Symptomatic cardiomyopathy occurs during adolescence and proves fatal.

Diagnosis. Scapulohumeral syndrome with dementia is distinguished from Emery-Dreifuss dystrophy by the absence of contractures and the presence of mental deterioration. EMG demonstrates a mixed myopathic-neuropathic pattern, and muscle biopsy reveals excessive internal nuclei and fiber splitting. The concentration of serum creatine kinase is elevated.

Treatment. No treatment is available for the underlying disease. Fatalities may be prevented only by heart transplantation.

Scapuloperoneal Syndrome

Clinical Features. Scapuloperoneal syndrome is most often transmitted by autosomal dominant inheritance and is probably the same disease as facioscapulohumeral dystrophy. The onset of symptoms is usually during adult life but can be as early as the first decade. Weakness begins in the muscles around the shoulder, in the anterior compartment of the legs, or in both simultaneously. Some spread to the proximal muscles of the legs occurs, and the face may be involved. Tendon reflexes are lost early. The rate of progression is slow.

Diagnosis. The concentration of serum creatine kinase is usually normal or only slightly elevated. EMG may show mixed features of myopathy and neuropathy. Muscle biopsy usually shows mild features of denervation or type I atrophy.

Treatment. No treatment is available.

◆ Acute Generalized Weakness

The sudden onset or rapid evolution of generalized flaccid weakness, in the absence of symptoms of encephalopathy, is always due to disorders of the motor unit. Among the disorders listed in Table 7–9, acute inflammatory demyelinating polyradiculoneuropathy (Guillain-Barré syndrome) is by far the most common.

The combination of acute weakness and rhabdomyolysis, as evidenced by myoglobinuria, indicates that muscle is degenerating rapidly. This may occur in some disorders of carbohydrate metabolism (see Chapter 8), after intense and unusual exercise, in some cases of infectious and idiopathic polymyositis, and in intoxication with alcohol and cocaine (Roth et al, 1988). Death from renal failure is a possible outcome in patients with rhabdomyolysis.

INFECTIOUS DISEASE
Acute Infectious Myositis

Acute myositis in children most often follows influenza or other respiratory infections.

Clinical Features. Ordinarily, prodromal respiratory symptoms persist for 1 to 7 days before the onset of severe symmetric muscle pain and weakness, which may lead to severe disability within 24 hours (McKinley and Mitchell, 1976). Proximal muscles are more severely affected than distal muscles, but generalized weakness may be present. The muscles are tender to palpation. Tendon reflexes are present.

Diagnosis. The serum concentration of creatine kinase is elevated, usually more than 10 times the upper limit of normal.

Treatment. Spontaneous resolution of the myositis occurs almost immediately. Bed rest is required for 2 to 7 days until pain subsides, after which the patient recovers completely.

Acute Inflammatory Demyelinating Polyradiculoneuropathy (Guillain-Barré Syndrome)

Guillain-Barré syndrome is an acute, monophasic demyelinating neuropathy that is generally believed to be immunologically mediated. More than half of patients describe an antecedent viral infection. Respiratory tract infections are most common, and the remainder are mainly gastrointestinal infections. Enteritis caused by specific strains of *Campylobacter jejuni* is the inciting disease in up to 18% of cases (Mishu et al, in press).

Clinical Features. Diagnostic criteria for Guillain-Barré syndrome were developed in response to the increased incidence of cases following the swine flu vaccination program of 1976 (Asbury, 1981). The natural history of the disease in children is substantially the same as in adults (Kleyweg et al, 1989). The clinical features are so stereotyped that the diagnosis is established without laboratory confirmation. This is important because the characteristic laboratory features of Guillain-Barré syndrome may not be present at the onset of clinical symptoms.

The two essential features of Guillain-Barré syndrome are progressive motor weakness involving more than one limb and areflexia. Weakness is frequently preceded by insidious sensory symptoms that are usually ignored. These consist of fleeting dysesthesias and muscle tenderness in limbs that are soon to become paralytic. Weakness progresses rapidly, and approximately 50% of patients reach a nadir by 2 weeks, 80% by 3 weeks, and the rest by 4 weeks. The weakness may be ascending or descending but is relatively symmetric qualitatively, if not quantitatively. Tendon reflexes are absent in all weak muscles and can be absent even before the muscle is weak. Bilateral facial weakness occurs in as many as half of cases. Autonomic dysfunction, characterized by arrhythmia, labile blood pressure, and gastrointestinal dysfunction, may be present as well.

Recovery of function usually begins 2 to 4 weeks after progression stops. In children recovery is almost always complete. The prognosis is best when recovery begins early. Respiratory paralysis develops in 20% to 30% of children with Guillain-Barré syndrome. If the patient's respiratory function can be supported during the critical time of profound paralysis, complete recovery can be expected.

Diagnosis. The concentration of protein in the cerebrospinal fluid is elevated after the first week of symptoms. During the first week the cerebrospinal fluid commonly contains 10 or fewer mononuclear leukocytes per cubic millimeter; however, these rapidly disappear and none are found in subsequent weeks. Electrophysiologic evidence of segmental demyelination is present in 50% of patients during the first 2 weeks of illness and in 85% during the third week (Albers and Kelly, 1989).

Treatment. Respiratory function must be carefully monitored in children with Guillain-Barré syndrome. If vital capacity falls rapidly to less than 50% of normal, an endotracheal tube should be inserted. Most children who require respiratory support need that support for several weeks, and many require tracheostomy. Adequate control of respiration should prevent death from the disorder. Corticosteroids are not helpful because, although they may produce some initial improvement, they tend to prolong the course. Plasma exchange with albumin is recommended to shorten the course in children whose condition is so severe that they cannot walk without assistance (Epstein and Sladky, 1990). The results are best if the exchange is started within 2 weeks of the onset of symptoms.

Enterovirus Infections

Poliovirus, coxsackievirus, and the echovirus group are small RNA viruses that inhabit the intestinal tract of humans. They are neurotropic and produce paralytic disease by destroying the motor neurons of the brainstem and spinal cord. Of this group, poliovirus causes the most severe and dev-

astating disease. Coxsackievirus and echoviruses are more likely to cause aseptic meningitis, although they produce an acute paralytic syndrome similar to poliomyelitis.

Clinical Features. Enterovirus infections occur in epidemics during the spring and summer. The most common manifestation of poliovirus infection is a brief illness characterized by fever, malaise, and gastrointestinal symptoms. Aseptic meningitis occurs in more severe cases. The extreme situation is paralytic poliomyelitis. It begins with fever, sore throat, and malaise lasting 1 to 2 days. After a brief period of apparent well-being, fever recurs in association with headache, vomiting, and signs of meningeal irritation. Pain in the limbs or over the spine is an antecedent symptom of limb paralysis. Flaccid muscle weakness develops rapidly thereafter. The pattern of muscle weakness varies, but it is generally asymmetric. One arm or leg is affected more than other limbs.

Bulbar polio may occur with or without spinal cord disease and is life threatening. Affected children have prolonged episodes of apnea and require respiratory assistance. Several motor cranial nerves may be involved as well, but the extraocular muscles are spared.

The introduction of inactivated poliomyelitis vaccine in 1954, followed by the use of attenuated live poliomyelitis vaccine in 1960, has almost abolished the disease. Nearly all recently reported cases are vaccine related. Paralytic poliomyelitis develops in approximately 1 healthy child in 12 million immunized with trivalent oral polio vaccine. Most cases occur following the first immunization (Nkowane et al, 1987).

Diagnosis. The diagnosis can be suspected from clinical findings and confirmed by isolation and viral typing from stool and nasopharyngeal specimens. The cerebrospinal fluid initially demonstrates a polymorphonuclear reaction with the cell count ranging from 50 to 200/mm³. After a week, lymphocytes predominate; after 2 to 3 weeks the total cell count decreases. The protein content is elevated early and remains elevated for several months.

Treatment. No treatment, other than supportive care, is available.

NEUROMUSCULAR BLOCKADE

A fulminating form of myasthenia gravis in which generalized weakness progresses to respiratory distress within 12 to 18 hours has been described in infants. Bulbar and limb paralyses are present. There have been no recent reports, and earlier cases may have been infantile botulism (see later discussion).

Children treated for prolonged periods with neuromuscular blocking agents for assisted ventilation may remain in a flaccid state for days or weeks after the drug is discontinued (Benzing et al, 1990). This is especially true in newborns, who often receive several drugs that block the neuromuscular junction.

Botulism

Clostridium botulinum produces a toxin that interferes with the release of acetylcholine at the neuromuscular junction. An infantile form of botulism is described in Chapter 6, but most cases occur after infancy in people who eat food, usually preserved at home, contaminated with the organism (Cherington, 1974).

Clinical Features. The first symptoms are blurred vision, diplopia, dizziness, dysarthria, and dysphagia, which have their onset 12 to 36 hours after the ingestion of toxin. Some patients have only bulbar signs; in others, flaccid paralysis develops in all limbs. Patients with generalized weakness have ophthalmoplegia, but the pupillary response is usually spared. Tendon reflexes may be present or absent.

Diagnosis. Repetitive supermaximal nerve stimulation at a rate of 20 to 50 stimuli per second produces an incremental response characteristic of a presynaptic defect. The electrical abnormality evolves with time and may not be demonstrable in all limbs on any given day.

Treatment. Botulism can be fatal because of respiratory depression. Treatment relies primarily on supportive care, which is similar to the management of Guillain-Barré syndrome. Antitoxin does not influence the course of disease. Guanidine hydrochloride, a drug that enhances the release of acetylcholine from nerve terminals, may offer some benefit at an average dosage of 250 mg every 6 hours in adults. In both children and adults the dose should be titrated to the degree of weakness. Recovery is prolonged when paralysis has been severe, but all patients recover completely.

Tick Paralysis

The female of several species of North American ticks elaborates a salivary gland toxin that induces paralysis (Swift and Ignacio, 1975).

Clinical Features. The clinical syndrome is similar to Guillain-Barré syndrome. A severe generalized flaccid weakness develops rapidly and is sometimes associated with bifacial palsy. Tendon reflexes are usually absent or greatly depressed. Dysesthesias may be present at the onset of weakness, but loss of sensation cannot be demonstrated on examination.

Diagnosis. The cerebrospinal fluid protein concentration is normal. Electrophysiologic studies demonstrate slowing of conduction velocities. The possibility of tick paralysis should be considered during the spring and summer in any child who has Guillain-Barré syndrome and a normal protein content in the cerebrospinal fluid.

Treatment. Strength returns quickly once the tick is removed. However, the tick may be hard to find, since it is frequently hidden in body hair.

PERIODIC PARALYSES

The periodic paralyses are usually classified in relation to serum potassium: hyperkalemic, hypokalemic, or normokalemic. In addition, periodic paralysis may be primary (genetically transmitted) or secondary. Secondary hypokalemic periodic paralysis is caused by urinary or gastrointestinal loss of potassium. Urinary loss accompanies primary hyperaldosteronism, licorice intoxication, amphotericin B therapy, and several renal tubular defects. Gastrointestinal loss most often occurs with severe chronic diarrhea, prolonged gastrointestinal intubation and vomiting, and a draining gastrointestinal fistula. Either urinary or gastrointestinal loss, or both, may occur in children with anorexia nervosa who overuse diuretics or induce vomiting. Hypokalemic periodic paralysis is also seen with thyrotoxicoses, especially in Asians. Secondary hyperkalemic periodic paralysis is associated with renal or adrenal insufficiency.

Familial Hyperkalemic Periodic Paralysis

Familial hyperkalemic periodic paralysis is transmitted by autosomal dominant inheritance and occurs with equal frequency in both sexes. It is caused by a defect of the gene encoding the sodium channel on chromosome 17 (Fontaine et al, 1992). Myotonia of the eyelids, face, and hands is sometimes an associated symptom, and such cases are referred to as *paramyotonia congenita* (de Silva et al, 1990).

Clinical Features. The onset of weakness is in early childhood and sometimes in infancy. As in hypokalemic periodic paralysis, attacks may be provoked by rest shortly after exercise. However, only moderate exercise is required. Weakness begins with a sensation of heaviness in the back and leg muscles. Sometimes the patient can delay the paralysis by walking or moving about. In infants and small children the attacks are characterized by an episode of floppiness in which the child lies around and can not move. In older children and adults both mild and severe attacks may occur. Mild attacks last for less than an hour and do not produce complete paralysis. More than one mild attack may occur in a day. Severe attacks are similar to the complete flaccid paralysis seen in hypokalemic periodic paralysis and may last for several hours. Residual weakness may persist after several severe attacks.

Diagnosis. Myotonia in patients with hyperkalemic periodic paralysis is mild and sometimes is demonstrated only on exposure to cold. To do this, the examiner lays a towel soaked in ice water over the patient's eyes for a few minutes. After the towel is removed, the patient is asked to look upward briefly and then to look down quickly. When the eyelids are myotonic, the lids cannot come down quickly and a rim of sclera is exposed.

During attacks the serum concentration of potassium increases but may not increase sufficiently to be abnormal. When potassium concentrations are high, EKG demonstrates changes consistent with hyperkalemia. The oral administration of potassium chloride just after exercise in the fasting state provokes an attack. During the attack the muscles are electrically silent.

Treatment. Acute attacks seldom require treatment, since they are brief. Daily administration of acetazolamide may prevent recurrence of attacks (Hoskins and Vroom, 1975). The reason that acetazolamide prevents both hyperkalemic and hypokalemic periodic paralysis is unknown, but the effect is apparently through stabilization of the muscle membrane.

Familial Hypokalemic Periodic Paralysis

Familial hypokalemic periodic paralysis is transmitted by autosomal dominant inheritance with decreased penetrance in women.

Clinical Features. The onset of symptoms occurs before 16 years of age in 60% of cases and by 20 years of age in the remainder. Attacks of paralysis are at first infrequent but then may occur several times a week. Factors that trigger an attack include rest after exercise (therefore many attacks occur early in the morning), a large meal with high carbohydrate content, emotional or physical stress, alcohol ingestion, and exposure to cold. Before and during the attack the patient may have excessive thirst and oliguria. The weakness begins with a sensation of aching in the proximal muscles. Sometimes only the proximal muscles are affected; at other times there is complete paralysis so that the

patient cannot even raise the head. Facial muscles are rarely affected, and extraocular muscles are never disturbed. Respiratory distress does not occur. When the weakness is most extreme, the muscles feel swollen and the tendon reflexes are absent. Most attacks last 6 to 12 hours and some for the whole day. Strength recovers rapidly, but after several attacks residual weakness may be present.

Diagnosis. During the attack, serum potassium concentrations may fall to 1.5 mEq/L (1.5 mmol/L) and EKG changes occur, including bradycardia, flattening of T waves, and prolongation of the PR and QT intervals. The muscle is electrically silent and not excitable. Attacks can be provoked by the oral administration of glucose, 2 g/kg, with 10 to 20 units of crystalline insulin given subcutaneously. The serum potassium concentration falls, and an attack of paralysis is initiated within 2 to 3 hours.

Treatment. Acute attacks in patients with good renal function are treated by repeated oral doses of potassium. In adolescents 5 to 10 g is used. Smaller amounts should be considered for younger children. Daily use of acetazolamide is beneficial in many families to prevent attacks, lithium gluconate may be useful in refractory cases (Confavreux et al, 1991).

Familial Normokalemic Periodic Paralysis

Several families reported in the literature have an autosomal dominant inherited periodic paralysis in which no alteration in serum concentration of potassium can be detected. These may represent hyperkalemic periodic paralysis in which the flux of potassium into the serum was insufficient to be detected.

References

Albers JW, Kelly JJ Jr: Acquired inflammatory demyelinating polyneuropathies: Clinical and electrodiagnostic features. Muscle Nerve 12:435, 1989.

American Academy of Neurology: Ad Hoc Subcommittee of AIDS Task Force: Research criteria for diagnosis of chronic inflammatory demyelinating polyneuropathy (CIDP). Neurology 41:617, 1991.

Asbury AK: Diagnostic considerations in Guillain-Barré syndrome. Ann Neurol 9:1, 1981.

Askansas V, Engel WK, Kwan HH, et al: Autosomal dominant syndrome of lipid neuromyopathy with normal carnitine: Successful treatment with long-chain fatty-acid-free diet. Neurology 35:66, 1985.

Balestrini MR, Cavaletti G, D'Angelo A, et al: Infantile hereditary neuropathy with hypomyelination: Report of two siblings with different expressivity. Neuropediatrics 22:65, 1991.

Barohn RJ, Miller RG, Griggs RC: Autosomal recessive distal dystrophy. Neurology 41:1365, 1991.

Bautista J, Rafel E, Castilla A, et al: Hereditary distal myopathy with onset in early infancy. J Neurol Sci 37:149, 1978.

Benzing G III, Iannaccone ST, Bove KE, et al: Prolonged myasthenic syndrome after one week of muscle relaxants. Pediatr Neurol 6:190, 1990.

Berciano J, Combarros O, Figols J, et al: Hereditary motor and sensory neuropathy type II. Brain 109:897, 1986.

Bergia B, Sybers HD, Butler IJ: Familial lethal cardiomyopathy with mental retardation and scapuloperoneal muscular dystrophy. J Neurol Neurosurg Psychiatry 49:1423, 1986.

Bieber FR, Hoffman EP, Amos JA: Dystrophin analysis in Duchenne muscular dystrophy: Use in fetal diagnosis and in genetic counseling. Am J Hum Genet 45:362, 1989.

Bodensteiner JB, Schochet SS: Facioscapulohumeral muscular dystrophy: The choice of a biopsy site. Muscle Nerve 9:544, 1986.

Bowyer SL, Blane CE, Sullivan DB, et al: Childhood dermatomyositis: Factors predicting functional outcome and development of dystrophic calcification. J Pediatr 103:882, 1982.

Breningstall GN: Carnitine deficiency syndromes. Pediatr Neurol 6:75, 1990.

Brooke MH, Fenichel GM, Griggs RC, et al: Duchenne muscular dystrophy: Patterns of clinical progression and effects of supportive therapy. Neurology 39:475, 1989.

Buxton J, Shelbourne P, Davies J, et al: Detection of an unstable fragment of DNA specific to individuals with myotonic dystrophy. Nature 355:547, 1992.

Carroll JE, Brooke MH, Villadiego A, et al: "Dystrophic" lipid myopathy in two sisters. Arch Neurol 43:128, 1986.

Casey EB, Jellife AM, LeQuesne PM, et al: Vincristine neuropathy: Clinical and electrophysiological observations. Brain 96:69, 1973.

Cherington M: Botulism. Arch Neurol 30:432, 1974.

Clerk A, Rodilo E, Heckmatt JZ, et al: Characterisation of dystrophin in carriers of Duchenne muscular dystrophy. J Neurol Sci 102:197, 1991.

Cole CG, Walker A, Coyne A, et al: Prenatal testing for Duchenne and Becker muscular dystrophy. Lancet 1:262, 1988.

Confavreux C, Garassus P, Vighetto A, et al: Familial hypokalemic periodic paralysis: Prevention of paralytic attacks with lithium gluconate. J Neurol Neurosurg Psychiatry 54:87, 1991.

de Silva SM, Kuncl RW, Griffin JW, et al: Paramyotonia congenita or hyperkalemic periodic paralysis? Clinical and electrophysiological features of each entity in one family. Muscle Nerve 13:21, 1990.

DeVivo DC, Tein I: Primary and secondary disorders of carnitine metabolism. Pediatrics 5:134, 1990.

Dobkin BH, Verity MA: Familial neuromuscular disease with type I fiber hypoplasia, tubular aggregates, cardiomyopathy, and myasthenic features. Neurology 28:1135, 1978.

Donaghy M, Brett EM, Ormerod EC, et al: Giant axonal neuropathy: Observations on a further patient. J Neurol Neurosurg Psychiatry 51:991, 1988.

Dyck PJ: Inherited neuronal degeneration and atrophy affecting peripheral motor, sensory, and autonomic neurons. In Dyck PJ, Thomas PK, Lambert EH, Bunge R, eds: Peripheral Neuropathy. WB Saunders, Philadelphia, 1984, p 1600.

Dyck PJ, Oviatt KF, Lambert EH: Intensive evaluation of referred unclassified neuropathies yields improved diagnosis. Ann Neurol 10:222, 1981.

Emery AEH: Population frequencies of inherited neuromuscular diseases—a world survey. Neuromusc Dis 1:19, 1991.

Epstein MA, Sladky JT: The role of plasmapheresis in childhood Guillain-Barré syndrome. Ann Neurol 28:65, 1990.

Fenichel GM: Clinical syndromes of myasthenia gravis in infancy and childhood. Arch Neurol 35:97, 1978.

Fenichel GM, Florence J, Pestronk A, et al: Long-term use of prednisone therapy in the treatment of Duchenne muscular dystrophy. Neurology, 41:1874, 1991.

Fenichel GM, Sul YC, Kilroy AW, et al: An autosomal-dominant dystrophy with humeropelvic distribution and cardiomyopathy. Neurology 32:1399, 1982.

Fitzsimons RB, Gurwin EB, Bird AC: Retinal vascular abnormalities in facioscapulohumeral muscular dystrophy: A general association with genetic and therapeutic implications. Brian 110:631, 1987.

Fontaine B, Trofatter J, Rouleau GA, et al: Different gene loci for hyperkalemic and hypokalemic periodic paralysis. Neuromuscular Dis 1:235, 1992.

Fukuhara N, Kumamoto T, Tsubaki T, et al: Oculopharyngeal muscular dystrophy and distal myopathy: Intrafamilial difference in the onset and distribution of muscular involvement. Acta Neurol Scand 65:458, 1982.

Gibberd FB, Page NGR, Billimoria JD, et al: Heredopathia actactica polyneuritiformis (Refsum's disease) treated by diet and plasma-exchange. Lancet 1:575, 1979.

Gilliam TC, Brzustowicz LM, Castilla LH, et al: Genetic homogeneity between acute (SMA I) and chronic (SMA II & III) forms of spinal muscular atrophy. Nature 345:823, 1990.

Hamida MB, Hentati F, Hamida CB: Hereditary motor system diseases (chronic juvenile amyotrophic lateral sclerosis): Conditions combining a bilateral pyramidal syndrome with limb and bulbar amyotrophy. Brain 113:347, 1990.

Hagberg B, Lyon G: Pooled European series of hereditary peripheral neuropathies in infancy and childhood. Neuropediatrie 12:9, 1981.

Harding AE, Thomas PK: Hereditary distal spinal muscular atrophy: A report on 34 cases and a review of the literature. J Neurol Sci 45:337, 1980.

Henriksson K-G, Sandstedt P: Polymyositis—treatment and prognosis. Acta Neurol Scand 65:280, 1982.

Hoffman EP, Kunkel LM, Angelini C, et al: Improved diagnosis of Becker muscular dystrophy by dystrophin testing. Neurology 39:1011, 1989.

Hoskins B, Vroom FQ: Hyperkalemic periodic paralysis: Effects of potassium, exercise, glucose and acetazolamide on blood chemistry. Arch Neurol 32:519, 1975.

Ionasescu VV, Trofatter J, Haines JL, et al: X-linked recessive Charcot-Marie-Tooth neuropathy: Clinical and genetic study. Muscle Nerve 15:368, 1992.

Jamal GA, Weir AI, Hansen S, et al: Myotonic dystrophy: A reassessment by conventional and more recently introduced neurophysiological techniques. Brain 109:1279, 1986.

Johns TR, Campa J, Adelman L: Familial myasthenia with "tubular aggregates" treated with prednisone [Abstract]. Neurology 23:426, 1973.

Kleyweg RP, Van Der Meché FGA, Loonen MCB, et al: The natural history of the Guillain-Barré syndrome in 18 children and 50 adults. J Neurol Neurosurg Psychiatry 52:853, 1989.

Krivit W, Shapiro E, Kennedy W, et al: Treatment of late infantile metachromatic leukodystrophy by bone marrow transplantation. N Engl J Med 322:28, 1990.

Loonen MCB, Busch HFM, Koster JF, et al: A family with different clinical forms of acid maltase deficiency (glycogenosis type II): Biochemical and genetic studies. Neurology 31:1209, 1981.

Lotz BP, Engle AG, Nishano H, et al: Inclusion body myositis: Observations in 40 patients. Brain 112:727, 1989.

Mantovani JF, Vidgoff J, Cass M: Brain dysfunction in an adolescent with the neuromuscular form of hexosaminidase deficiency. Dev Med Child Neurol 27:664, 1985.

Markesbery WR, Griggs RC, Leach RP, et al: Late onset hereditary distal myopathy. Neurology 24:127, 1974.

Martyn C, Jellinek EH, Webb JN: Lipid storage myopathy: Successful treatment with propranolol. Br Med J 282:1997, 1981.

Mastaglia FL, Ojeda VJ: Inflammatory myopathies parts 1 and 2. Ann Neurol 17:215, 1985; 18:317, 1985.

McCombe PA, Pollard JD, McLeod JG: Chronic inflammatory demyelinating polyradiculoneuropathy: A clinical and electrophysiological study of 92 cases. Brain 110:1617, 1987.

McKinley IA, Mitchell A: Transient acute myositis in childhood. Arch Dis Child 51:135, 1976.

McQuillen M: Familial limb-girdle myasthenia. Brain 89:121, 1966.

Merlini L, Granata C, Dominici P, et al: Emery-Dreifuss muscular dystrophy: Report of five cases in a family and review of the literature. Muscle Nerve 9:481, 1986.

Miller RG, Gutmann L, Lewis RA, et al: Acquired versus familial demyelinative neuropathies in children. Muscle Nerve 8:205, 1985.

Mishu B, Tauxe RV, Griffin PM, et al: *Campylobacter jejuni* infection and Guillain-Barré syndrome. Neurology. In press.

Mohire MD, Tandan R, Fries TJ, et al: Early-onset benign autosomal dominant limb-girdle myopathy with contractures (Bethlem myopathy). Neurology 38:573, 1988.

Munsat TL, Skerry L, Korf B, et al: Phenotypic heterogeneity of spinal muscular atrophy mapping to chromosome 5q11.2-13.3 (SMA 5q). Neurology 40:1831, 1990.

Nkowane BH, Wassilak SGF, Orenstein WA: Vaccine associated paralytic poliomyelitis: United States: 1973 through 1984. JAMA 257:1335, 1987.

Ohnishi A, Mitsudome A, Murai Y: Primary segmental demyelination in the sural nerve in Cockayne's syndrome. Muscle Nerve 10:163, 1987.

Oosterhuis HJGH, Newson-Davies J, Wokke JHJ, et al: The slow channel syndrome: Two new cases. Brain 110:1061, 1987.

Ouvrier RA, McLeod JG, Conchin TE: The hypertrophic forms of hereditary motor and sensory neuropathy: A study of hypertrophic Charcot-Marie-Tooth disease (HMSN type I) and Déjérine-Sottas disease (HMSN type III) in childhood. Brain 110:121, 1987.

Ouvrier RA, McLeod JG, Morgan GJ, et al: Hereditary motor and sensory neuropathy of neuronal type with onset in early childhood. J Neurol Sci 51:181, 1981.

Ouvrier R, McLeod JG, Pollard J: Toxic neuropathies. In Peripheral Neuropathy in Childhood. International Review of Child Neurology Series. Raven Press, New York, 1990a, p 167.

Ouvrier R, McLeod JG, Pollard J: Neuropathies in systemic disease. In Peripheral Neuropathy in Childhood. International Review of Child Neurology Series. Raven Press, New York, 1990b, p 181.

Parnes S, Karpati G, Carpenter S, et al: Hexosaminidase-A deficiency presenting as atypical juvenile-onset spinal muscular atrophy. Arch Neurol 42:1176, 1985.

Pearn JH: Autosomal dominant spinal muscular atrophy: A clinical and genetic study. J Neurol Sci 38:263, 1978.

Pearn JH, Hudson P, Walton JN: A clinical and genetic study of adult-onset spinal muscular atrophy: The autosomal recessive form as a discrete entity. Brain 101:591, 1978.

Polten A, Fluharty AL, Fluharty CB, et al: Molecular basis of different forms of metachromatic leukodystrophy. N Engl J Med 324:18, 1991.

Refsum S: Clinical and genetic aspects of Refsum disease. In Dyck PJ, Thomas PK, Lambert EH, Bunge R, eds: Peripheral Neuropathy. WB Saunders, Philadelphia, 1984, p 1680.

Riggs JE, Schochet SS, Gutman L, et al: Childhood onset inclusion body myositis mimicking limb-girdle muscular dystrophy. J Child Neurol 4:283, 1989.

Roth D, Alarcon FJ, Fernandez JA, et al: Acute rhabdomyolysis associated with cocaine intoxication. N Engl J Med 319:673, 1988.

Speer MC, Pericak-Vance MA, Yamaoka L, et al: Presymptomatic and prenatal diagnosis on myotonic dystrophy by genetic linkage studies. Neurology 40:671, 1990.

Sunohara N, Arahata K, Hoffman EP, et al: Quadriceps myopathy: Forme fruste of Becker muscular dystrophy. Ann Neurol 28:634, 1990.

Swift TR, Ignacio OJ: Tick paralysis: Electrophysiologic studies. Neurology 25:1130, 1975.

Tandan R, Little BW, Emery ES, et al: Childhood giant axonal neuropathy: Case report and review of the literature. J Neurol Sci 82:205, 1987.

Tandan R, Sharma KR, Bradley WG, et al: Chronic segmental spinal muscular atrophy of upper extremities in identical twins. Neurology 40:236, 1990.

Timmerman V, Raeymaekers P, De Jonghe P, et al: Assignment of the Charcot-Marie-Tooth neuropathy type 1 (CMT 1a) gene to 17p11.2-p12. Am J Hum Genet 47:680, 1990.

van Doorn PA, Brand A, Strengers PFW, et al: High-dose intravenous immunoglobulin treatment in chronic inflammatory demyelinating polyneuropathy: A double-blind, placebo-controlled, crossover study. Neurology 40:209, 1990.

van Doorn PA, Vermeulen M, Brand A, et al: Intravenous immunoglobulin treatment in patients with chronic inflammatory demyelinating polyneuropathy: Clinical and laboratory characteristics associated with improvement. Arch Neurol 48:217, 1991.

Vanasse M, Dubowitz V: Dominantly inherited peroneal muscular atrophy (hereditary motor and sensory neuropathy type I) in infancy and childhood. Muscle Nerve 4:26, 1981.

Vettaikorumakankav V, Kandt RS, Lewis DV Jr, et al: Chronic demyelinating polyradiculopathy of childhood: Treatment with high-dose intravenous immunoglobulin. Neurology 41:828, 1991.

Walter EB, Drucker RP, McKinney RE: Myopathy in human immunodeficiency virus–infected children receiving long-term zidovudine therapy. J Pediatr 119:152, 1991.

Whitaker JN: Inflammatory myopathy: A review of etiologic and pathogenetic factors. Muscle Nerve 5:573, 1982.

Cramps, Muscle Stiffness, and Exercise Intolerance

A cramp is an involuntary painful contraction of a muscle or part of a muscle. Cramps can occur in normal children during and after vigorous exercise and after excessive loss of fluid or electrolytes. Such cramps are characterized on electromyography (EMG) by the repetitive firing of normal motor unit potentials. Stretching the muscle relieves the cramp, and it is generally believed, although without evidence, that muscle stretching before exercise may prevent cramps. Muscle that is partially denervated is particularly susceptible to cramping not only during exercise, but also during sleep. Night cramps may awaken patients with neuronopathies, neuropathies, or root compression. Cramps during exercise occur also in patients with several different disorders of muscle energy metabolism. These cramps differ from other cramps in that they are not detected by electrodiagnostic examination.

Muscle stiffness and spasms are sometimes called cramps by patients but are actually prolonged contractions of several muscles that are able to impose postures. Such contractions may or may not be painful. When painful, they lack the explosive character of cramps (Layzer, 1985). Prolonged contractions occur when muscles fail to relax (myotonia) or when motor unit activity is continuous (Table 8–1). Prolonged, painless muscle contractions occur also in dystonia and in other movement disorders (see Chapter 14).

Many normal children, especially preadolescent boys, complain of pain in their legs at night and sometimes during the day, especially after a period of increased activity. These pains are not true cramps. The muscle is not in spasm, the pain is diffuse and aching in quality, and the discomfort lasts for an hour or longer. Stretching the muscle does not relieve the pain. This is not a symptom of neuromuscular disease and, for want of better

understanding, is usually referred to as *growing pains*. Symptoms are relieved by mild analgesics or heat.

Exercise intolerance is a relative term for an inability to maintain exercise at an expected level. The causes of exercise intolerance considered in this chapter are fatigue and muscle pain. Fatigue is a normal consequence of exercise and occurs in everyone at some level of activity. In general, weak children become fatigued more quickly than children who have normal strength. Many children with exercise intolerance and cramps, but no permanent weakness, have a defect in an enzyme needed to produce energy for muscular contraction (Table 8–2). Several such inborn errors of metabolism have been defined, and others are yet to be defined. Even when the full spectrum of biochemical tests is available, the metabolic defect cannot be identified in some children in whom cramps

Table 8–1 ◆ Diseases with Abnormal Muscle Activity

Continuous Motor Unit Activity
1. Neuromyotonia
2. Paroxysmal ataxia and myokymia (see Chapter 10)
3. Schwartz-Jampel syndrome
4. Stiffman syndrome
5. Thyrotoxicosis

Cramps-Fasciculation Syndrome

Myotonia Congenita

Systemic Disorders
1. Hypoadrenalism
2. Hypocalcemia (tetany)
3. Strychnine poisoning
4. Thyroid disease
5. Uremia

Table 8–2 ◆ Diseases with Decreased Muscle Energy

1. Carnitine palmitoyl transferase deficiency
2. Defects of carbohydrate utilization
   a. Lactate dehydrogenase deficiency
   b. Myophosphorylase deficiency
   c. Phosphofructokinase deficiency
   d. Phosphoglycerate kinase deficiency
   e. Phosphoglycerate mutase deficiency
3. Mitochondrial (respiratory chain) myopathies
4. Myoadenylate deaminase deficiency

develop after exercise and in whom there is clear-cut evidence of muscle disease.

Myasthenia gravis is a disorder characterized by exercise intolerance, but it is not covered in this chapter because the usual initial symptoms are either isolated cranial nerve disturbances (see Chapter 15) or limb weakness (see Chapters 6 and 7).

Conditions that produce some combination of cramps and exercise intolerance can be divided into three groups: diseases with abnormal muscle activity, diseases with decreased energy for muscle contraction, and myopathies. As a rule, the first and third groups are symptomatic at all times, whereas the second group is symptomatic only with

Table 8–3 ◆ Electromyography in Muscle Stiffness

Normal Between Cramps (or may be myopathic)
1. Brody disease
2. Defects of carbohydrate metabolism
3. Defects of lipid metabolism
4. Mitochondrial myopathies
5. Myoadenylate deaminase deficiency
6. Tubular aggregates

Silent Cramps
1. Brody disease
2. Defects of carbohydrate metabolism
3. Tubular aggregates

Continuous Motor Activity
1. Neuromyotonia
2. Schwartz-Jampel syndrome
3. Stiffman syndrome

Myotonia
1. Myotonia congenita
2. Myotonic dystrophy
3. Schwartz-Jampel syndrome

Myopathy
1. Emery-Dreifuss muscular dystrophy
2. Rigid spine syndrome
3. Trilaminar myopathy
4. X-linked myalgia

exercise. The first group requires EMG for diagnosis.

EMG should be the initial diagnostic test in patients with muscle stiffness that is not due to spasticity or rigidity. It usually leads to the correct diagnosis (Table 8–3).

◆ Abnormal Muscle Activity
CONTINUOUS MOTOR UNIT ACTIVITY

Continuous motor unit activity (CMUA) is caused by the uncontrolled release of acetylcholine (ACh) packets at the neuromuscular junction. The EMG features of CMUA are repetitive muscle action potentials in response to a single nerve stimulus; high-frequency bursts of motor unit potentials of normal morphology that start and stop abruptly; and rhythmically firing doublets, triplets, and multiplets. During long bursts the potentials decline in amplitude. This activity is difficult to distinguish from normal voluntary activity. CMUA is seen in a heterogeneous group of disorders characterized clinically by some combination of muscular pain, fasciculations, myokymia, contractures, and cramps (Table 8–4) (Valli et al, 1983).

Disorders with CMUA can be subdivided into syndromes in which the primary defect is believed to be within the spinal cord (stiffman syndrome) and those in which the primary defect is believed to be within the peripheral nerve (neuromyotonia). Neuromyotonia is also called *Isaac syndrome* and *quantal squander syndrome*. These disorders may be sporadic or familial in occurrence. When familial, they are usually transmitted by autosomal dominant inheritance.

Neuromyotonia

The primary abnormality in neuromyotonia is in the nerve or the nerve terminal. Most childhood cases are sporadic in occurrence, but some are transmitted by autosomal dominant inheritance (Ashizawa et al, 1983; McGuire et al, 1984).

Clinical Features. The clinical triad includes involuntary muscle twitching (fasciculations or myokymia), muscle cramps or stiffness, and myotonia. Excessive sweating is frequently associated with the muscle stiffness. The age at onset is anytime from birth to adult life.

The initial symptoms are muscle twitching and cramps brought on by exercise. Later these symptoms occur also at rest and even during sleep. The cramps may affect only distal muscles, causing painful posturing of the hands and feet. As a rule the legs are affected more severely than the arms.

Table 8–4 ◆ Abnormal Muscle Activity

1. *Fasciculations:* Spontaneous, random twitching of a group of muscle fibers
2. *Fibrillation:* Spontaneous contraction of a single muscle fiber; not visible through the skin
3. *Myotonia:* Disturbance in muscle relaxation following voluntary contraction or percussion
4. *Myokymia:* Repetitive fasciculations causing a quivering or undulating twitch
5. *Neuromyotonia:* Continuous muscle activity characterized by muscle rippling, muscle stiffness, and myotonia

These disorders are not progressive and do not lead to permanent disability. Attacks of cramping become less frequent and less severe with age.

In some children cramps and fasciculations are not as prominent as stiffness, which causes abnormal limb posturing associated frequently with excessive sweating. The legs are more often affected than the arms, and the symptoms suggest dystonia (see Chapter 14). Limb posturing may begin in one foot and remain asymmetric for months. Most cases are sporadic.

Muscle mass, muscle strength, and tendon reflexes are normal. Fasciculations are sporadic and are noted only after prolonged observation.

Diagnosis. Some adult-onset cases are associated with malignancy, but this is never the case in children. EMG demonstrates CMUA, fasciculations, and sometimes myotonia. The continuous activity persists during sleep and during general and spinal anesthesia. It is progressively diminished by more distal nerve blocks and is abolished by curare.

Treatment. Carbamazepine and phenytoin, at usual anticonvulsant doses, are both effective in reducing or abolishing symptoms.

Schwartz-Jampel Syndrome

The Schwartz-Jampel syndrome (osteochondromuscular dystrophy) is a hereditary disorder, probably transmitted by autosomal recessive inheritance, but possibly also by autosomal dominant inheritance (Pascuzzi et al, 1990). It is characterized by short stature, skeletal abnormalities, and persistent muscular contraction and hypertrophy.

Clinical Features. Infants have progressive skeletal deformities, including hip dislocation, coxa vara or coxa valga, pectus carinatum, vertebral flattening, basilar impression, and dwarfism. The constellation of skeletal deformities suggests the Morquio syndrome (osteochondrodystrophy). CMUA is most prominent in the face and produces

a characteristic triad that includes narrowing of the palpebral fissures (blepharophimosis), pursing of the mouth, and puckering of the chin. Blepharospasm is provoked by striking or even blowing on the eyelids (see Chapter 14). CMUA in the limbs produces stiffness of gait and exercise intolerance. Motor development during the first year is slow, but intelligence is normal.

Diagnosis. EMG demonstrates CMUA. Initial reports suggested incorrectly that the abnormal activity seen on EMG and expressed clinically was myotonia. Myotonia may be present, but CMUA, generated in the nerve and abolished by curare, is responsible for the facial and limb symptoms. The serum concentration of creatine kinase can be mildly elevated. The muscle histologic appearance is usually normal but may demonstrate variation in fiber size and an increased number of central nuclei.

Treatment. Muscle stiffness is diminished by phenytoin or carbamazepine. Early treatment with relief of muscle stiffness reduces the severity of subsequent muscle deformity.

Stiffman Syndrome

Stiffman syndrome is a sporadic condition of adult life that is now considered an autoimmune disease (Blum and Jankovic, 1991; McEvoy, 1991). It is extremely rare in children. A genetic form, transmitted by autosomal dominant inheritance, has been described in children, but it is actually startle disease (see Chapter 1) and should not be considered part of the stiffman syndrome.

Clinical Features. Following an initial period of aching and tightness in the truncal muscles, involuntary painful spasms occur without spinal deformity. The spasms are triggered by startle and by emotional upset and are relieved by sleep. Proximal limb muscles and bulbar muscles may be involved later. The patient becomes so rigid that he or she tends to walk or stand in a hyperextended position. Tendon reflexes are active or hyperactive, and no evidence of muscle atrophy is found.

Diagnosis. Individuals with stiffman syndrome and their relatives have an increased incidence of several organ-specific autoimmune disorders, especially insulin-dependent diabetes. Antibodies against glutamic acid decarboxylase and pancreatic islet cells are present in the serum and cerebrospinal fluid of many patients.

Treatment. Diazepam had been the mainstay of treatment and is useful for symptomatic relief of the spasms. Prednisone and plasma exchange have been partially successful in treating the underlying disease.

CRAMPS-FASCICULATION SYNDROME

The clinical features of cramps-fasciculation syndrome, including the response to carbamazepine, are identical to neuromyotonia except that CMUA is not seen on EMG (Tahmoush et al, 1991). They are probably the same syndrome.

MYOTONIA CONGENITA

Myotonia congenita is a genetic disorder characterized by muscle stiffness and hypertrophy. Dystrophy does not occur, although families with features of both myotonic dystrophy and myotonia congenita have been reported. In 19% of families, clear evidence of autosomal dominant inheritance is present. A smaller percentage is definitely transmitted by autosomal recessive inheritance, but most cases are sporadic and cannot be classified genetically (Kuhn et al, 1979). In general, the autosomal recessive form has a later onset and more severe myotonia than the dominant form. However, the overlap of clinical features is considerable, and the pattern of genetic transmission cannot be determined with certainty unless several family members are affected.

Clinical Features. Clinical features are stereotyped. After rest, muscles are stiff and difficult to move. With activity the stiffness disappears and movement may be normal. One patient played Little League baseball and could not sit while he was waiting to bat for fear that he would be unable to get up. The autosomal dominant type is frequently present from birth or infancy, and the CMUA produces generalized hypertrophy, which gives the infant a Herculean appearance. The tongue, face, and jaw muscles are sometimes involved. Stiffness is painless and is exacerbated by exposure to cold. Percussion myotonia is present. Muscle mass, strength, and tendon reflexes are normal.

Diagnosis. Diagnosis is established by EMG. Repetitive discharges at rates of 20 to 80 cps are recorded when the needle is first inserted into the muscle and again on voluntary contraction. Two types of discharges are seen: a biphasic spike potential of less than 5 ms and a positive wave of less than 50 ms. The amplitude and frequency of potentials wax and wane, producing a characteristic sound. No evidence of dystrophy is demonstrated. The serum concentration of creatine kinase is normal. Muscle biopsy specimens in patients with either the dominant or recessive form do not contain type IIb fibers.

Treatment. Myotonia does not always require treatment but sometimes can be relieved by phenytoin or carbamazepine at ordinary anticonvulsant doses. Tocainide, starting at 200 mg twice a day and incrementally raised to 400 mg three times a day, is reported to improve the stiffness markedly in children with the recessive form of the disease (Teasley et al, 1990).

Acetazolamide was effective in relieving symptoms in one kindred with myotonia congenita transmitted by autosomal dominant inheritance (Trudell et al, 1987). It is not clear whether this is a unique kindred or whether acetazolamide will prove useful in other patients with myotonia.

SYSTEMIC DISORDERS
Hypoadrenalism

A small percentage of patients with Addison disease complain of cramps and pain in truncal muscles. At times, paroxysmal cramps occur in the lower torso and legs and cause the patient to double up in pain. The symptoms are relieved by hormone replacement.

Hypocalcemia and Hypomagnesemia

Tetany caused by dietary deficiency of calcium is rare in modern times except in newborns fed cow's milk. Hypocalcemic tetany is more likely to result from hypothyroidism or hyperventilation-induced alkalosis.

The initial symptom of tetany is tingling around the mouth and in the hands and feet. With time the tingling increases in intensity and becomes generalized. This is followed by spasms in the muscles of the face, hands, and feet. The hands assume a typical posture in which the fingers are extended, the wrist is flexed, and the thumb is adducted. Fasciculations and laryngeal spasm may be present. Percussion of the facial nerve, either just anterior to the ear or over the cheek, produces contraction of the muscles innervated by that branch of the nerve.

A similar syndrome is encountered with magnesium deficiency. In addition to the tetany, encephalopathy occurs.

The cramps associated with hypocalcemia and hypomagnesemia are reversed by restoring the proper concentration of serum electrolytes.

Strychnine Poisoning

Strychnine is sometimes used as an adulterant in cocaine because it is a white odorless powder that is readily available as rat poison (Shannon, 1988). It is a competitive antagonist of glycine, a central nervous system inhibitory neurotransmitter.

The clinical features of poisoning are apprehension, nausea, muscle twitching, extensor spasm, opisthotonos, and seizures. Excessive muscle contraction causes myoglobinuria and lactic acidosis. Intravenous diazepam reduces spasms and can prevent death.

Thyroid Disease

Muscle aches, cramps, and stiffness occur as initial manifestations in up to half of patients with hypothyroidism. Stiffness is worse in the morning, especially on cold days, and is probably caused by slowing of both muscular contraction and relaxation. This is different from myotonia, in which only relaxation is affected. Indeed, the stiffness of hypothyroidism is made worse by activity and may be painful, whereas myotonia is relieved by activity and is painless. The slowing of muscular contraction and relaxation is sometimes demonstrated when tendon reflexes are tested. The response tends to "hangup."

Percussion of a muscle produces a localized knot of contraction called *myoedema*. This localized contraction lasts for up to 1 minute before slowly returning to normal.

Myokymia, CMUA of the face, tongue, and limbs, and muscle cramps develop occasionally in patients with thyrotoxicosis.

All of the neuromuscular symptoms of hypothyroidism and hyperthyroidism can be reversed by restoring the euthyroid state.

Uremia

Uremia is a known cause of polyneuropathy (see Chapter 7). However, 50% of patients complain of nocturnal leg cramps and flexion cramps of the hands even before clinical evidence of polyneuropathy is present (Nielsen, 1986). Excessive use of diuretics may be the triggering factor. Muscle cramps occur also in approximately one third of patients undergoing hemodialysis (Neal et al, 1981). Monitoring with EMG during dialysis documents a buildup of spontaneous discharges, which after several hours, usually toward the end of dialysis treatment, culminate in repetitive high-voltage discharges associated with clinical cramps. Because standard dialysis fluid is slightly hypotonic, many nephrologists have attempted to treat the cramps by administering hypertonic solutions. Either sodium chloride or glucose solutions relieve cramps in most patients. The cramps apparently result from either extracellular volume contraction or hypoosmolarity. Similar cramps occur in children with severe diarrhea or vomiting.

◆ Decreased Muscle Energy

Three sources for replenishing adenosine triphosphate (ATP) during exercise are available: the phosphorylation of adenosine diphosphate (ADP) to ATP by phosphocreatine (PCr); glycogen and lipids within the exercising muscles; and glucose and triglycerides brought to the exercising muscles by the blood. A fourth and less efficient source is derived from ADP via an alternate pathway using adenylate kinase and deaminase (Figure 8–1). PCr stores are the main source from which ATP is replenished during intense activity of short duration. During the first 30 seconds of intense endurance exercise, PCr is decreased by 35% and muscle glycogen stores are reduced by 25%. Exercise lasting longer than 30 seconds is associated with the mobilization of substantial amounts of carbohydrate and lipid (Bonen et al, 1989).

The glucose required to sustain a single powerful contraction can be provided by the breakdown of muscle glycogen (glycogenolysis) and the anaerobic metabolism of glucose to pyruvate (glycolysis) (Figure 8–2). Anaerobic glycolysis is an inefficient mechanism for producing energy and is not satisfactory for endurance exercise. Endurance requires that pyruvate generated in muscle by glycolysis be metabolized aerobically in the mitochondria. Oxidative metabolism produces high levels of energy for every molecule of glucose metabolized (Figure 8–3).

The central compound of oxidative metabolism in mitochondria is acetylcoenzyme A (acetyl-CoA). Acetyl-CoA is derived from pyruvate, fatty acids, and amino acids. When exercise is prolonged, fatty acids become an important substrate to maintain muscular contraction. Acetyl-CoA is oxidized through the Krebs cycle and releases hydrogen ions that reduce nicotinamide adenine dinucleotide (NAD). These reduced compounds then enter a sequence of oxidation-reduction steps in the respiratory chain that liberate energy. Energy is stored as ATP. This process of liberating and storing energy is called oxidation-phosphorylation coupling.

The production of energy for muscular contraction is therefore impaired by disorders that prevent the delivery of glucose or fatty acids, the oxidation process in the mitochondria, or the creation of ATP.

ISCHEMIC EXERCISE TEST

The ischemic exercise test is the first step in the diagnosis of muscle energy disorders and should be performed by every patient who develops

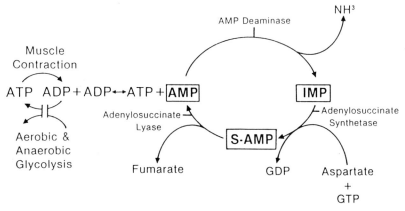

Figure 8–1 Metabolic pathway using myoadenylate deaminase. (From Ashwal S, Peckham N: Pediatr Neurol 1:185, 1985.)

cramps on exercise (Figure 8–4). Instructions for the procedure are outlined in Table 8–5.

In most normal individuals, serum lactate concentrations are raised more than 20 mg/dl (2 mmol/L) and serum ammonia concentrations are raised more than 100 µg/dl (60 µmol/L) over baseline (Coleman et al, 1986). If neither lactate nor ammonia concentration increases during the test, the subject did not exercise strenuously and the test should be repeated.

An abnormal increase in the concentration of serum creatine kinase, with or without failure to generate increased serum concentrations of lactate or ammonia, is an indication for muscle biopsy. Biopsy is likely to lead to the diagnosis if histochemical and biochemical techniques can be applied. Patients with a normal lactate and ammonia response and a normal creatine kinase concentra-

tion are unlikely to have an abnormal muscle biopsy result, but these patients should have EMG. Muscle biopsy is indicated if EMG findings are abnormal or if the family has a history of cramps or muscle disease.

An elevated lactate concentration at rest suggests a mitochondrial myopathy. Failure to raise the serum lactate concentration more than 5 mg/dl (0.5 mmol/L) above baseline, coupled with a normal rise in ammonia concentration, is the basis for a diagnosis of glycogen storage disease. However, patients who lack debrancher enzyme in both liver and muscle may have serum lactate elevations of between 5 and 10 mg/dl (0.5 to 1 mmol/L); those with only liver debrancher deficiency have a normal response.

Failure to increase ammonia concentrations more than 100 µg/dl (60 µmol/L) above baseline,

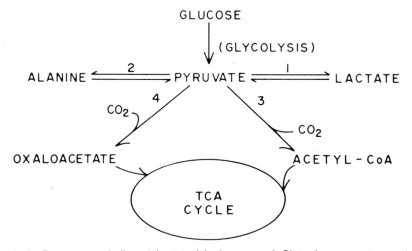

Figure 8–2 Pyruvate metabolism. *1,* Lactate dehydrogenase. *2,* Glutamic-pyruvate transaminase. *3,* Pyruvate dehydrogenase complex. *4,* Pyruvate carboxylase. (From Fenichel GM: Neonatal Neurology, 2nd edition. Churchill Livingstone, New York, 1985. By permission.)

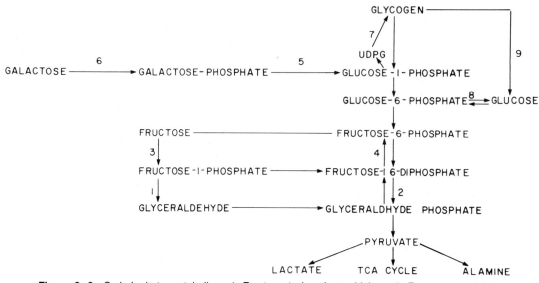

Figure 8–3   Carbohydrate metabolism. *1,* Fructose-1-phosphate aldolase. *2,* Fructose-1,6-diphosphate aldolase. *3,* Fructokinase. *4,* Fructose-1,6-diphosphatase. *5,* Galactose-1-phosphate uridyltransferase. *6,* Galactokinase. *7,* Glycogen synthase. *8,* Glucose-6-phosphatase. *9,* Acid maltase. (From Fenichel GM: Neonatal Neurology, 3rd edition. Churchill Livingstone, New York, 1990. By permission.)

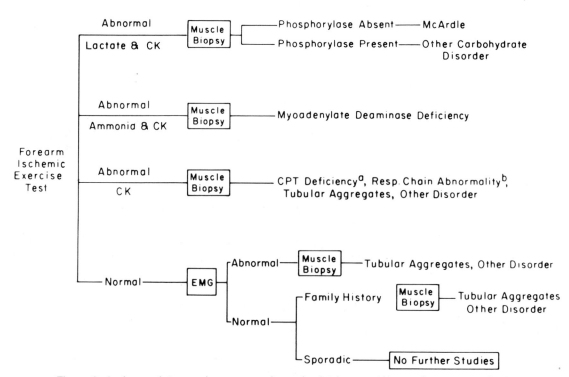

Figure 8–4   Approach to muscle cramps and exercise intolerance. [a]Abnormal response to fasting. [b]Elevated serum lactate.

Table 8–5 ◆ Forearm Ischemic Exercise Test

1. Explain the procedure to the patient.
2. The patient should rest for at least 30 minutes before the test.
3. Place the blood pressure cuff around the arm.
4. Insert the indwelling catheter in the antecubital vein and obtain blood samples for lactate, ammonia, and creatine kinase 10 minutes before exercise and immediately preceding it. Collect urine sample for myoglobin.
5. Inflate the cuff 20 mm Hg above systolic pressure and ask the patient to squeeze a hand dynamometer 40 times in 1 minute and then two times per second for 1 minute.
6. Release the pressure in the cuff at the end of the exercise.
7. Collect blood samples for lactate, ammonia, and creatine kinase determinations at 1, 3, 5, 10, and 20 minutes following release of the cuff.
8. Collect a second urine sample for myoglobin at completion of the blood collection.

coupled with a normal lactate response, suggests myoadenylate deaminase deficiency and is an indication for muscle biopsy (Sinkeler et al, 1986). However, this aspect of the test produces many false positive results.

CARNITINE PALMITOYL TRANSFERASE DEFICIENCY

Long-chain fatty acids are the principal lipid oxidized to produce acetyl-CoA. Carnitine palmitoyl transferase is an essential enzyme that allows long-chain fatty acids to pass through the inner mitochondrial membrane to the inner portion of the mitochondria, where oxidation to acetyl-CoA occurs. A 50% to 75% deficiency in the activity of carnitine palmitoyl transferase produces a characteristic syndrome of exercise intolerance. The disorder is transmitted by autosomal recessive inheritance. However, the clinical expression of the deficiency varies depending on the percentage of enzyme activity and the organs involved (Angelini et al, 1981; DiDonato et al, 1981). Carnitine palmitoyl transferase deficiency may affect several tissues other than muscle: leukocytes, platelets, fibroblasts, and liver. During periods of prolonged fasting, patients with a liver deficiency of carnitine palmitoyl transferase are slow to make ketones, and the concentration of long-chain fatty acids becomes elevated in the serum.

Clinical Features. The manifestations of muscle carnitine palmitoyl transferase deficiency usually begin during late childhood. No difficulty

is experienced in performing even heavy exercise of short duration; energy for this activity is provided by glycogen. However, pain, tenderness, and swelling of muscles develop when sustained aerobic exercise is attempted. Severe muscle cramps, as in myophosphorylase deficiency, do not occur. Associated with the pain may be actual muscle injury characterized by increased concentrations of serum creatine kinase and the appearance of myoglobin in the urine. Muscle injury may also accompany periods of prolonged fasting, especially in patients on low-carbohydrate, high-fat diets. Prolonged exercise and prolonged fasting produce generalized muscle weakness that may lead to respiratory disease and death.

In the interval between attacks, results of muscle examination, serum concentration of creatine kinase, and EMG are usually normal, but permanent myopathy develops in some children (Gieron and Korthals, 1987).

Diagnosis. The diagnosis is suggested by the demonstration of reduced or delayed production of ketone bodies in blood and urine when fasting. The fast should be ended by the administration of intravenous glucose at the first sign of clinical symptoms or the elevation of serum creatine kinase. Muscle biopsy may demonstrate an accumulation of lipid droplets within muscle fibers, but the results may also be normal. The definitive diagnosis requires measurement of carnitine palmitoyl transferase in platelets, fibroblasts, or muscle.

Treatment. Frequent carbohydrate feedings and the avoidance of prolonged aerobic activity minimize muscle destruction.

DEFECTS OF CARBOHYDRATE UTILIZATION
Myophosphorylase Deficiency (McArdle Disease)

Myophosphorylase deficiency is ordinarily transmitted by autosomal recessive inheritance, but transmission by autosomal dominant inheritance occurs as well. Phosphorylase activity is deficient only in muscle; the first step of glycogenolysis is prevented, and muscle glycogen is unavailable to produce glucose for energy. Liver phosphorylase concentrations are normal, and hypoglycemia does not occur.

Clinical Features. The severity of symptoms varies with the percentage of enzyme activity. Children with only mild deficiency states have few or no symptoms until adolescence. Aching becomes increasingly prominent and then, after an episode of vigorous exercise, severe cramps are noted in the exercised muscles. Myoglobinuria is sometimes present. The pain can last for hours. Thereafter, exercise leads to repeated bouts of cramps that cause a decline in the overall level of activity. Pain begins soon after vigorous exercise is initiated, and myoglobinuria is noted several hours later. Some patients exercise through the pain by slowing down just before the time of fatigue. Once they pass that point, exercise may continue unimpeded. This is probably due to an increase in cardiac output, the use of blood glucose and free fatty acids as a substrate for muscle metabolism, and the recruitment of more motor units (Braakhekke et al, 1986).

Examination is generally unrevealing. Muscle mass and strength and the tendon reflexes are normal. Weakness is detected only in adult patients, and even then the tendon reflexes are normal.

Myophosphorylase deficiency can also be manifested as slowly progressive proximal weakness that begins during childhood or adult life (Abarbanel et al, 1987). Affected individuals may never complain of cramps on exercise or of myoglobinuria. Tendon reflexes are preserved until late in the course of disease.

Diagnosis. The ischemic exercise test is the initial step to establish a defect in carbohydrate utilization. Patients with myophosphorylase deficiency develop cramps during the test and usually cannot complete the exercise, and the serum lactate concentration increases less than 5 mg/dl (0.05 mmol/L) above baseline. Normal individuals have lactate concentrations between 15 and 25 mg/dl (0.15 and 0.25 mmol/L) within 2 to 3 minutes, which rapidly decline to normal levels after 20 minutes. Cramps are not shown by EMG examination. The serum concentration of creatine kinase is elevated, and myoglobin may appear in the urine coincidentally with the cramps.

Salient features of muscle biopsy specimens are histochemical evidence of subsarcolemmal blebs containing glycogen and the absence of phosphorylase. Muscle fiber degeneration and regeneration are present immediately after an episode of cramps and myoglobinuria. Definitive diagnosis requires the biochemical demonstration of decreased myophosphorylase activity.

Treatment. A high-protein diet consisting of 20% to 30% protein, 30% to 35% fat, and 40% to 45% carbohydrate was found to increase exercise tolerance in one patient (Slonim and Goans, 1985). This observation has not been confirmed by others.

Other Disorders of Glucose Utilization

A syndrome identical to myophosphorylase deficiency—cramps on exercise and myoglobinuria—has also been described in four other enzyme deficiencies associated with the anaerobic glycolysis of carbohydrates (Figure 8–1). They are muscle phosphofructokinase deficiency (Agamanolis et al, 1980), muscle phosphoglycerate kinase deficiency (DiMauro et al, 1981), muscle phosphoglycerate mutase deficiency (DiMauro et al, 1982), and lactate dehydrogenase deficiency. Phosphofructokinase deficiency is the most common of this group and has also been described as a cause of infantile hypotonia (see Chapter 6).

The preceding disorders are transmitted by autosomal recessive inheritance. Myophosphorylase deficiency is usually suspected because of the clinical manifestations, elevation of serum creatine kinase concentrations during attacks, and failure to produce a normal rise in venous lactate after ischemic exercise. Muscle biopsy results demonstrate subsarcolemmal collections of glycogen, but the histochemical reaction for phosphorylase is normal. These disorders are correctly identified only by biochemical analysis. A high-protein diet should be tried in these patients.

MITOCHONDRIAL (RESPIRATORY CHAIN) MYOPATHIES

The respiratory chain, located in the inner mitochondrial membrane, consists of five protein complexes: complex I (NADH–coenzyme Q reductase); complex II (succinate–coenzyme Q reductase); complex III (reduced coenzyme Q–cytochrome c reductase); complex IV (cytochrome c oxidase); and complex V (ATP synthase) (Figure 8–5).

Coenzyme Q is a shuttle between complexes I and II and complex III. A defect of coenzyme Q has been recorded in only one patient, who had neonatal seizures, abnormal ocular movements, and lactic acidosis (Fischer et al, 1986).

The clinical syndromes associated with mitochondrial disorders are continually expanded and revised (Moraes et al, 1991). The organs affected are those highly dependent on aerobic metabolism: nervous system, skeletal muscle, heart, and kidney (Table 8–6). Exercise intolerance, either alone or in combination with symptoms of other organ failure, is a common feature of mitochondrial disorders. Although several clinical syndromes have been defined, they do not correspond exactly with any one of the respiratory complexes (Table 8–7).

Clinical Features. The age at which mitochondrial myopathies begin ranges from birth to adult life but is before 20 in 61% of patients. Half of patients have ptosis or ophthalmoplegia, one fourth have exertional complaints in the limbs, and one fourth have cerebral dysfunction. With time,

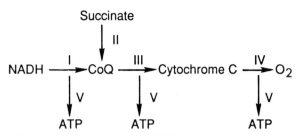

Figure 8–5 Respiratory complexes: complex I (NADH–coenzyme Q reductase); complex II (succinate–coenzyme Q reductase); complex III (reduced coenzyme Q–cytochrome *c* reductase; complex IV (cytochrome *c* oxidase); complex V (adenosine triphosphate synthase).

considerable overlap occurs among the three groups. Seventy-five percent eventually have ophthalmoplegia and 50% have exertional complaints. Pigmentary retinopathy occurs in 33% and neuropathy in 25% (Yiannikas et al, 1986).

Exercise intolerance usually develops by 10 years of age. With ordinary activity, active muscles become tight, weak, and painful, but cramps and myoglobinuria do not occur. One exception was two brothers with multiple deletions of mitochondrial DNA who had recurrent myoglobinuria and progressive weakness (Ohno et al, 1991). Nausea, headache, and breathlessness are sometimes associated features. During these episodes the serum concentration of lactate and creatine kinase may increase. Generalized weakness with ptosis and ophthalmoplegia may follow prolonged periods of activity or fasting. Such symptoms

may last for several days, but recovery is usually complete.

Diagnosis. A mitochondrial myopathy should be considered in all children with exercise intolerance and ptosis or ophthalmoplegia. This combination of symptoms may also suggest myasthenia gravis, which can be differentiated with edrophonium chloride (Tensilon).

Some children with mitochondrial myopathies have increased concentrations of serum lactate at rest but demonstrate lactic acidosis after exercise at 90% of predicted work rate (Nashef and Lane, 1989). Another test, easier to perform but not as sensitive as controlled exercise, is the glucose-lactate tolerance test. An ordinary oral glucose tolerance test is administered, and lactate and glucose determinations are made at the same time. In some children with mitochondrial disorders, lactic acidosis develops and glucose is slow to clear.

Muscle biopsy reveals a clumping of the mitochondria, which become red when the Gomori trichrome stain is applied (Figure 8–6). These muscle cells are referred to as ragged-red fibers.

Defects of specific respiratory complexes can be demonstrated only in specialized laboratories.

Treatment. One boy with a myopathy caused by complex I deficiency responded to treatment with riboflavin and carnitine (Bernsen et al, 1991). Attempts to treat other patients with high doses of thiamine, menadione, or coenzyme Q have not produced encouraging results (Morgan-Hughes et al, 1984).

MYOADENYLATE DEAMINASE DEFICIENCY

Deficiency of myoadenylate deaminase is clearly a familial trait, and the mode of inheritance is probably autosomal recessive (Sinkeler et al, 1988). This enzyme deficiency was discovered accidentally when muscle biopsy specimens from patients with several different clinical syndromes were surveyed for enzyme activity. The few biopsy

Table 8–6 ◆ Clinical Features of Mitochondrial Disease

Nervous System
1. Ataxia
2. Central apnea
3. Deafness
4. Dementia
5. Hypotonia
6. Mental retardation
7. Neuropathy
8. Ophthalmoplegia
9. Optic atrophy
10. Retinitis pigmentosa

Heart
1. Cardiomyopathy
2. Conduction defects

Kidney
1. Aminoaciduria
2. Hyperphosphaturia

Skeletal Muscle
1. Exercise intolerance
2. Myopathy

specimens that demonstrated myoadenylate deaminase deficiency were from patients with exercise intolerance. Myoadenylate deaminase deficiency has also been demonstrated in patients with infantile hypotonia, in patients with progressive myopathies beginning in childhood, and in asymptomatic individuals. Whether myoadenylate deaminase deficiency is responsible for familial syndromes of exercise intolerance is questionable. Most patients identified as having myoadenylate deaminase deficiency are asymptomatic.

Clinical Features.   The typical history is one of intermittent muscle pain and weakness with exercise (Ashwal and Peckham, 1985). The pain varies from a diffuse aching to a severe cramping type associated with muscle tenderness and swelling. Between attacks the children are normal. Symptoms last from 1 to 20 years with a mean of less than 9 years.

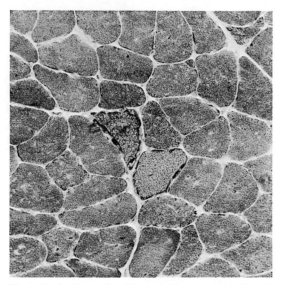

Figure 8–6   Ragged-red fibers (trichrome stain). The mitochondria are enlarged and stain intensely with hematoxylin.

Table 8–7 ◆ Mitochondrial Disorders

Complex I (NADH–Coenzyme Q Reductase)
1. Congenital lactic acidosis, hypotonia, seizures, and apnea
2. Exercise intolerance and myalgia
3. Kearns-Sayre syndrome (see Chapter 15)
4. Metabolic encephalopathy, lactic acidosis, and stroke (see Chapter 11)
5. Progressive infantile poliodystrophy (see Chapter 5)
6. Subacute necrotizing encephalomyelopathy (see Chapter 5)

Complex II (Succinate–Coenzyme Q Reductase)
1. Encephalomyopathy (?)

Complex III (Coenzyme QH₂–Cytochrome c Reductase)
1. Cardiomyopathy
2. Kearns-Sayre syndrome (see Chapter 15)
3. Myopathy and exercise intolerance with or without progressive external ophthalmoplegia

Complex IV (Cytochrome c Oxidase)
1. Fatal neonatal hypotonia (see Chapter 6)
2. Menkes syndrome (see Chapter 5)
3. Myoclonus epilepsy and ragged-red fibers
4. Progressive infantile poliodystrophy (see Chapter 5)
5. Subacute necrotizing encephalomyelopathy (see Chapter 5)
6. Transitory neonatal hypotonia (see Chapter 6)

Complex V (Adenosine Triphosphate Synthase)
1. Congenital myopathy
2. Neuropathy, retinopathy, ataxia, and dementia
3. Retinitis pigmentosa, ataxia, neuropathy, and dementia

Diagnosis.   During attacks the serum concentration of creatine kinase may be normal or markedly elevated. EMG and muscle histologic studies usually do not show abnormalities. The diagnosis is suggested by the ischemic exercise test (Figure 8–4). Patients with myoadenylate deaminase deficiency fail to generate ammonia but demonstrate normal elevations of lactate. However, ammonia levels may fail to rise even in normal individuals, and enzyme analysis of muscle is required for diagnosis.

Obligate heterozygotes have reduced concentrations of myoadenylate deaminase in muscle but are capable of normal ammonia production and are asymptomatic.

Treatment.   No treatment is available.

◆ Myopathic Stiffness and Cramps

This section discusses several conditions that are manifested as muscle stiffness or cramps, or both, in which the primary abnormality is thought to be in skeletal muscle.

BRODY DISEASE

Brody disease is caused by a deficiency of calcium-activated ATP in sarcoplasmic reticulum (Karpati et al, 1986). The disorder is clearly familial but occurs only in males, suggesting X-linked inheritance.

Clinical Features.   The major clinical manifestation is difficulty in relaxation after contraction. Myotonia is suspected but not supported by EMG. Symptoms of exercise-induced stiffness and cramping begin in the first decade and become progressively worse with age. Unlike myotonia, stiffness becomes worse rather than better with continued exercise. Exercise can be resumed after a period of rest. Muscle strength and tendon reflexes are normal.

Diagnosis.   Patients with Brody disease are thought to have myotonia, but the cramps are not shown by EMG, suggesting myophosphorylase deficiency. The ischemic exercise test results are normal. Muscle biopsy results reveal type II atrophy. Definitive diagnosis requires the demonstration of the biochemical defect.

Treatment.   Dantrolene and nifedipine have been tried without success.

CRAMPS AND TUBULAR AGGREGATES

Tubular aggregates are abnormal double-walled structures that originate from the sarcoplasmic reticulum and are located in a subsarcolemmal position (Figure 8–7). They are found in muscle biopsy specimens from patients with a variety of neuromuscular disorders but are most often present in patients with cramps or myalgia (Niakan et al, 1985; Rosenberg et al, 1985). Indeed, cramps or myalgia may be the only symptom of neuromuscular disease.

Most cases of cramps and tubular aggregates are sporadic and have a male predominance (Lazaro et al, 1980). A genetic form is transmitted by autosomal dominant inheritance (Pierobon-Bormioli et al, 1985).

Sporadic Cases

Clinical Features.   Onset is usually in the second or third decade. Cramps may occur at rest or are induced by exercise. Thigh and calf muscles are usually affected and become swollen, stiff, and tender. Cramping occurs more often in cold weather and may also occur at night, interfering with sleep. Myalgia is present between cramps.

Episodic stiffness of the mouth and tongue interferes with speech. Cramps are not associated with myoglobinuria. Muscle mass, strength, and tendon reflexes are normal.

Diagnosis.   The serum concentration of creatine kinase is normal. EMG results are normal except that in some patients the cramps are electrically silent. This suggests a disorder of carbohydrate metabolism. An ischemic tolerance test

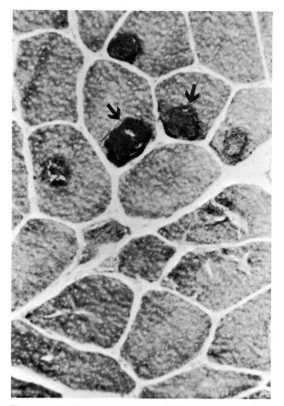

Figure 8–7   Tubular aggregates (ATPase reaction). Dark material is present beneath the sarcolemma in type I and type II fibers.

produces severe cramps, but there is normal generation of lactate with no elevation of the creatine kinase concentration.

Muscle biopsy results are the basis for a diagnosis. Light and electron microscopic examinations reveal tubular aggregates in type II fibers. No evidence of glycogen or lipid storage is present.

Treatment.   The cramps do not respond to medication.

Autosomal Dominant Cases

Clinical Features.   Muscle aches, cramps, and proximal weakness begin in the second decade (Ricker and Moxley, 1990). The cramps are exercise induced but also may occur at rest and during sleep. The legs are usually more severely affected than the arms, but the pattern of cramping varies from family to family. Weakness, when it occurs, is mild and progresses slowly.

Diagnosis.   The serum concentration of creatine kinase is moderately elevated. EMG suggests a myopathic process in some families and a neuropathic process in others. Muscle biopsy may show tubular aggregates in type I and type II fibers. Type I fiber predominance and type II hypertrophy are present in some patients.

Treatment.   No treatment is available for either the myopathy or the cramps.

FAMILIAL MYOEDEMA, MUSCULAR HYPERTROPHY, AND STIFFNESS

Myoedema, muscular hypertrophy, and stiffness constitute a rare disorder transmitted by autosomal dominant inheritance (Sadeh et al, 1990).

Clinical Features.   The onset of symptoms is usually in the second decade. Pain follows exercise and persists for several hours. Stiffness occurs during rest after the patient exercises or maintains a posture for a long period. Percussion of muscles causes local swelling, myoedema, that lasts 10 to 20 seconds. Muscle hypertrophy develops. Muscle strength, tone, and coordination, as well as tendon reflexes, are normal.

Diagnosis.   The serum creatine kinase concentration is mildly elevated, and muscle biopsy findings are normal. EMG of the muscle swelling after percussion does not show any electrical activity.

Treatment.   No treatment is available.

FAMILIAL X-LINKED MYALGIA AND CRAMPS

Familial X-linked myalgia and cramps is a new phenotype associated with a deletion in the dystrophin gene usually associated with Duchenne muscular dystrophy (see Chapter 7). It was described in nine males from one family (Gospe et al, 1989).

Clinical Features.   Symptoms begin in early childhood, frequently between 4 and 6 years of age. The children first have cramps with exercise and then cramps at rest. Usually the limb muscles are affected, but chest pain may occur as well. The cramping continues throughout life but is not associated with atrophy or weakness. Tendon reflexes are normal.

Diagnosis.   Affected family members have elevated concentrations of serum creatine kinase, especially after exercise. This disorder and the *McLeod phenotype* (acanthocytosis, elevated serum concentrations of creatine kinase, and absence of the Kell antigen) are probably allelic conditions. EMG and muscle biopsy show nonspecific myopathic changes.

DNA analysis indicates a deletion in the first third of the dystrophin gene. The dystrophin molecule is smaller than normal.

Treatment.   Phenytoin, carbamazepine, and nifedipine have not relieved the cramps. Exercise avoidance is the only way to avoid cramping.

MALIGNANT HYPERTHERMIA

Malignant hyperthermia is transmitted by autosomal dominant inheritance with variable penetrance. Attacks of muscular rigidity and necrosis in association with a rapid rise in body temperature are triggered by the administration of several inhalation anesthetics or by succinylcholine. Therefore the syndrome is seen almost exclusively in the operating suite.

Clinical Features.   The first symptoms are tachycardia, tachypnea, muscle fasciculations, and increasing muscle tone. Body temperature rises dramatically, as much as 2° C per hour. All muscles become rigid, and a progressive and severe metabolic acidosis develops. Seizures and death may occur if the patient is not treated promptly.

Diagnosis.   The diagnosis is based on the response to anesthesia or succinylcholine. Serum concentrations of creatine kinase rise to 10 times the upper limit of normal. No reliable test for identifying susceptible individuals is available.

Treatment.   Treatment includes termination of anesthesia, body cooling, treatment of metabolic acidosis, and intravenous injection of dantrolene, 1 to 2 mg/kg, which may be repeated every 5 to 10 minutes up to a total dose of 10 mg/kg (Gronert, 1980). When malignant hyperthermia is suspected in a child, pretreatment with dantrolene before anesthetics is used.

NEUROLEPTIC MALIGNANT SYNDROME

Clinical Features.   Several neuroleptic agents may induce an idiosyncratic response characterized by muscle rigidity, hyperthermia, altered states of consciousness, and autonomic dysfunction in susceptible individuals (Moore et al, 1986). Phenothiazines, butyrophenones, and thioxanthenes have been implicated. All ages have been affected, but young men predominantly. Symptoms develop over 1 to 3 days. The first symptoms are rigidity and akinesia, followed by fever, excessive sweating, urinary incontinence, and hypertension. Consciousness fluctuates, and the 20% mortality rate is due to respiratory failure.

Diagnosis.   The diagnosis is based primarily on clinical findings. The only helpful laboratory test results are an increased serum concentration of creatine kinase and a leukocytosis.

Treatment.   The offending neuroleptic agent must be promptly withdrawn and general supportive care provided. Bromocriptine reverses the syndrome completely.

RIGID SPINE SYNDROME

Rigid spine syndrome encompasses a heterogeneous group of disorders, usually sporadic, with a male predominance (Merlini et al, 1989). An autosomal dominant form has been described (Vanneste et al, 1988). Emery-Dreifuss muscular dystrophy (see Chapter 7) has similar features but is a distinct nosologic entity.

Clinical Features. Symptoms begin at any age from a few months until 13 years; the average is 5 years. The first manifestation may be stiffness, weakness, or both. Exercise intolerance is common. Stiffness is characterized by marked limitation of spinal flexion, especially in the cervical and dorsolumbar portions. Scoliosis is present, and flexion contractures develop at the elbows, limiting extension. The initial symptom of weakness is usually difficulty in climbing stairs or arising from the floor. Some children are toe-walkers and may be thought to have Duchenne dystrophy.

Examination reveals a pattern of scapuloperoneal or limb-girdle weakness in addition to spinal rigidity and scoliosis. Some patients have little subcutaneous fat. Tendon reflexes are diminished in weak muscles and sometimes in strong muscles as well.

The course is variable. In some children weakness and rigidity are only slowly progressive or remain stationary. Others experience severe, progressive scoliosis that compromises respiratory effort. Contractures may form at the hip, knee, and ankle in addition to the elbow and spine. Cardiomyopathy develops in some cases, which should probably be classified as Emery-Dreifuss muscular dystrophy (see Chapter 7).

Diagnosis. The serum concentration of creatine kinase is slightly elevated, and EMG is consistent with a myopathic process. Muscle biopsy usually reveals fibers undergoing degeneration with fatty replacement and fibrosis. Some patients have type I predominance, others have type II predominance, and one family had multicore fibers.

Treatment. No treatment is available for the myopathy, but scoliosis should be treated surgically to prevent respiratory distress. Patients with cardiomyopathy usually need a pacemaker.

TRILAMINAR MYOPATHY

A single case of trilaminar myopathy has been reported and is mentioned here because it was manifested as rigidity in the newborn (Ringel et al, 1978).

Clinical Features. A full-term newborn girl, the product of a normal pregnancy and delivery, had marked rigidity of the trunk and limbs immediately after birth that persisted during sleep. She had difficulty sucking and swallowing, with recurrent episodes of cyanosis and pneumonia. All skeletal muscles were firm when palpated, and the limbs resisted efforts to move them. Tendon reflexes were normal.

Diagnosis. EMG results were normal. No evidence of continuous motor unit activity or fasciculations was present. Muscle biopsy revealed fibers with three concentric zones: an innermost zone of densely packed myofibrils, a middle zone consisting of myofibrils, and an outer zone resembling a sarcoplasmic mass. The serum concentration of creatine kinase was elevated.

Treatment. No treatment is available, but the child improved spontaneously during infancy.

References

Abarbanel JM, Potashnik R, Frisher S, et al: Myophosphorylase deficiency: The course of an unusual congenital myopathy. Neurology 37:316, 1987.

Agamanolis DP, Askari AD, DiMauro S, et al: Muscle phosphofructokinase deficiency: Two cases with unusual polysaccharide accumulation and immunologically active enzyme protein. Muscle Nerve 3:456, 1980.

Angelini C, Freddo L, Battistella P, et al: Carnitine palmityltransferase deficiency: Clinical variability, carrier detection, and autosomal-recessive inheritance. Neurology 31:883, 1981.

Ashizawa T, Butler IJ, Harati Y, et al: A dominantly inherited syndrome with continuous motor neuron discharges. Ann Neurol 13:285, 1983.

Ashwal S, Peckham N: Myoadenylate deaminase deficiency in children. Pediatr Neurol 1:185, 1985.

Bernsen PLJA, Gabreels FJM, Ruitenbeek W, et al: Successful treatment of pure myopathy, associated with complex I deficiency, with riboflavin and carnitine. Arch Neurol 48:334, 1991.

Blum P, Jankovic J: Stiff-person syndrome: An autoimmune disease. Movement Dis 6:12, 1991.

Bonen A, McDermott JC, Hurber CA: Carbohydrate metabolism in skeletal muscle: An update of current concepts. Int J Sports Med 10:385, 1989.

Braakhekke JP, de Bruin MI, Stegeman DF, et al: The second wind phenomenon in McArdle's disease. Brain 109:1087, 1986.

Coleman RA, Stajich JM, Pact VW, et al: The ischemic exercise test in normal adults and in patients with weakness and cramps. Muscle Nerve 9:216, 1986.

DiDonato S, Castiglione A, Rimoldi A, et al: Heterogeneity of carnitine-palmityltransferase deficiency. J Neurol Sci 50:207, 1981.

DiMauro S, Dalakas M, Miranda AF: Phosphoglycerate kinase deficiency: A new cause of recurrent myoglobinuria [Abstract]. Ann Neurol 10:90, 1981.

DiMauro S, Miranda AF, Olarte M, et al: Muscle phosphoglycerate mutase deficiency. Neurology 32:584, 1982.

Fischer JC, Ruitenbeek W, Gabreels FJM, et al: A mitochondrial encephalomyopathy: The first case with an established defect at the level of coenzyme Q. Eur J Pediatr 144:441, 1986.

Gieron MA, Korthals JK: Carnitine palmityltransferase deficiency with permanent weakness. Pediatr Neurol 3:51, 1987.

Gospe SM, Lazaro RP, Lava NS, et al: Familial x-linked myalgia and cramps: A nonprogressive myopathy associated with a deletion in the dystrophin gene. Neurology 39:1277, 1989.

Gronert GA: Malignant hyperthermia. Anesthesiology 53:395, 1980.

Karpati G, Charuk J, Jablecki C, et al: Myopathy caused by a deficiency of Ca^{2+}-adenosine triphosphatase in sarcoplasmic reticulum (Brody's disease). Ann Neurol 20:38, 1986.

Kuhn E, Fiehn W, Seiler D, et al: The autosomal recessive (Becker) form of myotonia congenita. Muscle Nerve 2:109, 1979.

Layzer RB: Neuromuscular Manifestations of Systemic Disease. FA Davis, Philadelphia, 1985, p 16.

Lazaro RP, Fenichel GM, Kilroy AW, et al: Cramps, muscle pain, and tubular aggregates. Arch Neurol 37:715, 1980.

Lazaro RP, Rollinson RD, Fenichel GM: Familial cramps and muscle pain. Arch Neurol 38:22, 1981.

McEvoy KM: Stiff-man syndrome. Mayo Clin Proc 66:300, 1991.

McGuire SA, Tomosovic JJ, Ackerman N: Hereditary continuous muscle fiber activity. Arch Neurol 41:395, 1984.

Merlini L, Granata C, Ballestrazzi A, et al: Rigid spine syndrome and rigid spine sign in myopathies. J Child Neurol 4:274, 1989.

Moore A, O'Donohoe NV, Monagham H: Neuroleptic malignant syndrome. Arch Dis Child 61:793, 1986.

Moraes CT, Schon EA, DiMauro S: Mitochondrial diseases: Toward a rational classification. In Appel SH, ed: Current Neurology, vol 11. Mosby–Year Book, St Louis, 1991, p 83.

Morgan-Hughes JA, Hayes DJ, Clark JB, et al: Mitochondrial myopathies: Results of exploratory therapeutic trials. In Folkers K, Yamamura Y, eds: Biomedical and Clinical Aspects of Coenzyme Q, Elsevier Science Publishers, Amsterdam, 1984.

Nashef L, Lane RJM: Screening for mitochondrial cytopathies: The sub-anaerobic threshold exercise test (SATET). J Neurol Neurosurg Psychiatry 52:1090, 1989.

Neal CR, Resnikoff E, Unger AM: Treatment of dialysis-related muscle cramps with hypertonic dextrose. Arch Intern Med 141:171, 1981.

Niakan E, Harati Y, Danon MJ: Tubular aggregates: Their association with myalgia. J Neurol Neurosurg Psychiatry 48:882, 1985.

Nielsen VK: The peripheral nerve function in chronic renal failure. I. Clinical symptoms and signs. Acta Med Scand 190:105, 1986.

Ohno K, Tanakas M, Sahashi K, et al: Mitochondrial DNA deletions in inherited recurrent myoglobinuria. Ann Neurol 29:364, 1991.

Pascuzzi RM, Gratianne R, Azzarelli B, et al: Schwartz-Jampel syndrome with dominant inheritance. Muscle Nerve 13:1152, 1990.

Pierobon-Bormioli S, Armani M, Ringel SP, et al: Familial neuromuscular disease with tubular aggregates. Muscle Nerve 8:291, 1985.

Ricker K, Moxley RT: Autosomal dominant cramping disease. Arch Neurol 47:810, 1990.

Ringel SP, Neville E, Duster MC, et al: A new congenital neuromuscular disease with trilaminar muscle fibers. Neurology 28:282, 1978.

Rosenberg NL, Neville HE, Ringel SP: Tubular aggregates: Their association with neuromuscular diseases, including the syndrome of myalgias/cramps. Arch Neurol 42:973, 1985.

Sadeh M, Berg S, Sandbank U: Familial myoedema, muscular hypertrophy and stiffness. Acta Neurol Scand 81:201, 1990.

Shannon M: Clinical toxicity of cocaine adulterants. Ann Emerg Med 17:1243, 1988.

Sinkeler SP, Joosten MG, Wevers RA, et al: Myoadenylate deaminase deficiency: A clinical, genetic, and biochemical study in nine families. Muscle Nerve 11:312, 1988.

Sinkeler SP, Wevers RA, Joosten EM, et al: Improvement of screening in exertional myalgia with a standardized ischemic forearm test. Muscle Nerve 9:731, 1986.

Slonim AE, Goans PJ: Myopathy in McArdle's syndrome. N Engl J Med 312:355, 1985.

Tahmoush AJ, Alonso RJ, Tahmoush GP, et al: Cramp-fasciculation syndrome: A treatable hyperexcitable peripheral nerve disorder. Neurology 41:1021, 1991.

Teasley J, Garcia C, Malamut R, et al: Tocainide in pediatric patients with myotonia congenita [Abstract]. Neurology 40(suppl 1):205, 1990.

Trudell RG, Kaiser KK, Griggs RC: Acetazolamide-responsive myotonia congenita. Neurology 37:488, 1987.

Valli G, Barbieri S, Cappa S, et al: Syndromes of abnormal muscular activity: Overlap between continuous muscle fiber activity and the stiff man syndrome. J Neurol Neurosurg Psychiatry 46:241, 1983.

Vanneste JAL, Augustijn PB, Stam FC: The rigid spine syndrome in two sisters. J Neurol Neurosurg Psychiatry 51:131, 1988.

Yiannikas C, McLeod JG, Pollard JD, et al: Peripheral neuropathy associated with mitochondrial myopathy. Ann Neurol 20:249, 1986.

Sensory and Autonomic Disturbances

This chapter deals primarily with disturbed or lost sensation in the limbs and trunk. Autonomic disturbances are often associated with sensory loss but sometimes occur alone. Sensory disturbances of the face are considered in Chapter 17.

◆ Sensory Symptoms

The important symptoms of disturbed sensation are pain, dysesthesias, and loss of sensibility. Peripheral neuropathy is the most common cause of disturbed sensation at any age. Discomfort is more likely than numbness to bring a patient to medical attention. Several terms are used to describe sensory disturbances. Muscle aches, pains, and cramps are discussed in Chapter 8. Nerve root pain generally follows the course of a dermatome and is ordinarily described as deep and aching. The pain is more proximal than distal and may be constant or intermittent. When intermittent, the pain may radiate in a dermatomal distribution. The most common cause of root pain in adults is sciatica associated with lumbar disk disease. Disk disease also occurs in adolescents, usually because of trauma. In children root pain is more commonly due to radiculitis. Examples of radiculitis are the migratory aching of a limb preceding paralysis in the Guillain-Barré syndrome (see Chapter 7) and the radiating pain in a C-5 distribution that heralds an idiopathic brachial neuritis (see Chapter 13).

Polyneuropathy involving small nerve fibers produces dysesthetic pain. This pain differs from previously experienced discomfort and is described as pins and needles, tingling, or burning. It is often compared to the abnormal sensation felt when dental anesthesia is wearing off. The discomfort is superficial, distal, and usually symmetric. Dysesthetic pain is never a feature of hereditary neuropathies in children.

Loss of sensibility is the sole initial feature in children with sensory neuropathy. Diagnosis is often delayed because clumsiness is the first manifestation and strength is normal, as are tests of cerebellar function. Tendon reflexes are absent. The combination of areflexia and clumsiness should indicate a sensory neuropathy.

The pattern of sensory loss as a guide to the anatomic site of abnormality is summarized in Table 9–1.

◆ Brachial Neuritis

Three painful arm syndromes have been described: acute idiopathic brachial neuritis (neuralgic amyotrophy), familial recurrent brachial neuritis, and reflex sympathetic dystrophy. The first two are characterized by initial pain in the shoulder or arm, which then subsides and is followed by

Table 9–1 ◆ Patterns of Sensory Loss

Pattern	Site
Glove-and-stocking	Peripheral nerve
One leg	Plexus or spinal cord
One arm	Plexus
Both legs	Spinal cord or peripheral nerve
Legs and trunk	Spinal cord
All limbs	Spinal cord or peripheral nerve
Unilateral arm and leg	Brain or spinal cord

muscle atrophy. Weakness is the prominent feature, and these two syndromes are therefore discussed in Chapter 13. Although muscle atrophy also occurs in reflex sympathetic dystrophy, pain is the prominent feature, and this syndrome is discussed later in this chapter.

◆ Congenital Insensitivity (Indifference) to Pain

Most children with congenital insensitivity to pain have a hereditary sensory neuropathy. In many early reports of this condition, specific tests for sensory neuropathy and complete postmortem examinations were not performed. However, in some children and families with congenital universal insensitivity to pain, sensory neuropathy has been excluded (Landrieu et al, 1990). Many affected children are mentally retarded as well, and testing pain sensation is difficult. The Lesch-Nyhan syndrome is a specific disorder characterized by self-mutilation (presumably because of indifference to pain) and mental retardation without evidence of sensory neuropathy (see Chapter 5).

Clinical Features.   Children with congenital insensitivity to pain come to medical attention when they begin to move around the environment independently. Their parents then note that injuries do not produce crying and that the children fail to learn from experience the potential of injury. The result is repeated bruising, fractures, ulcerations of the fingers and toes, and mutilation of the tongue. Sunburn and frostbite are common.

Examination reveals absence of the corneal reflex and insensitivity to pain and temperature but relative preservation of touch and vibration sensations. Tendon reflexes are present.

Diagnosis.   Intelligence tests, electroencephalograms, and examination of the cerebrospinal fluid provide normal results.

Treatment.   No treatment is available for the underlying insensitivity, but supportive care is needed for the repeated injuries. Life is shortened by injuries and recurrent infections.

◆ Foramen Magnum Tumors

Extramedullary tumors in and around the foramen magnum are known for false localizing signs and for mimicking other disorders, especially syringomyelia and multiple sclerosis. In children, neurofibroma caused by neurofibromatosis is the only tumor found in this location (Yasuoka et al, 1978).

Clinical Features.   The most common initial symptom is unilateral or bilateral dysesthesias of the fingers. Half of patients experience suboccipital or neck pain. These two symptoms are often ignored early in the course. Numbness and tingling usually begin in one hand and then migrate to the other. Dysesthesias in the feet are a late occurrence. Gait disturbances, incoordination of the hands, and bladder disturbances generally follow sensory symptoms and are so alarming that they prompt medical consultation.

Many patients have café au lait spots, but few have evidence of subcutaneous neuromas. Weakness may be confined to one arm, one side, or both legs; 25% of patients have weakness in all limbs. Atrophy of the hands is uncommon. Sensory loss may involve only one segment or may have a "cape" distribution. Pain and temperature are usually diminished, and other sensory disturbances may be present. Tendon reflexes are brisk in the arms and legs.

Patients with neurofibromatosis may have multiple neurofibromas causing segmental abnormalities in several levels of the spinal cord.

Diagnosis.   Magnetic resonance imaging (MRI) is the best method for demonstrating abnormalities at the foramen magnum.

Treatment.   Symptoms can be relieved completely by surgical excision of neurofibroma of the C2 root.

◆ Hereditary Metabolic Neuropathies
ACUTE INTERMITTENT PORPHYRIA

Acute intermittent porphyria is transmitted by autosomal dominant inheritance. It is characterized by at least 50% deficiency in the activity of porphobilinogen deaminase. Individuals with similar degrees of enzyme deficiency may have considerable variation in phenotypic expression (Kappas et al, 1989).

Clinical Features.   Approximately 90% of individuals with acute intermittent porphyria never have clinical symptoms. The minority who do become symptomatic have no difficulty before puberty. Symptoms are periodic and occur at irregular intervals. The attacks are triggered by alterations in hormonal levels during a normal menstrual cycle or pregnancy and by exposure to certain drugs, especially barbiturates. Most attacks begin with abdominal pain, which is often followed by nausea and vomiting. Pain in the limbs is common, and muscle weakness often develops as well. The weakness is a result of a motor neuropathy that causes greater weakness in proximal than distal muscles and in the arms more than the legs. Tendon reflexes are usually decreased and may be absent in weak muscles. Approximately half of patients have symptoms of cerebral dysfunction; mental changes are particularly common, and seizures sometimes occur. Hypertension and tachycardia may accompany attacks. Chronic mental symptoms, such as depression and anxiety, sometimes continue even between attacks.

Diagnosis. Diagnosis is made by measuring porphobilinogen deaminase activity in red blood cells and urine.

Treatment. The most important aspect of managing symptomatic disease is to prevent acute attacks. This is done in part by avoiding known precipitating factors. During an attack, patients frequently need to be hospitalized because of severe pain. Carbohydrates are believed to reduce porphyrin synthesis and should be administered intravenously daily at a dose of 300 to 500 g as a 10% dextrose solution.

Intravenous infusion of hematin is in general use to prevent attacks and abort attacks in progress. It is given over 30 minutes or more in doses of 4 mg/kg every 12 hours during an acute attack and 200 mg weekly to prevent attacks.

HEREDITARY TYROSINEMIA

Hereditary tyrosinemia is transmitted by autosomal recessive inheritance and is caused by deficiency of the enzyme fumarylacetoacetate hydrolase (Mitchell et al, 1990).

Clinical Features. The major features are acute and chronic liver failure and a renal Fanconi syndrome. However, recurrent attacks of painful dysesthesias or paralysis are often the most prominent feature of the disease.

The attacks begin during infancy, usually at 1 year of age, and are preceded by an infection in half of cases. Perhaps because of the child's age, the pain is poorly localized to the legs and lower abdomen. Associated with the pain is axial hypertonicity ranging in severity from mild neck stiffness to opisthotonos. Generalized weakness occurs in 30% of attacks and may necessitate respiratory support. Less common features of attacks are seizures and self-mutilation. Between attacks the infants appear normal.

Diagnosis. The diagnosis of hereditary tyrosinemia is based on increased blood levels of tyrosine and demonstration of the enzyme deficiency. The crises are caused in part by an acute axonal neuropathy that can be demonstrated by electromyography. Succinylacetone, a metabolite of tyrosine, accumulates and inhibits porphyrin metabolism. Increased urinary excretion of gamma-aminolevulinic acid is present in both acute intermittent porphyria and hereditary tyrosinemia.

Treatment. Children with hereditary tyrosinemia are treated with a special diet similar to the one used for phenylketonuria (see Chapter 5). During a crisis, high-carbohydrate gavage without phenylalanine or tyrosine is used to provide adequate caloric intake. Narcotics may be needed to control pain.

◆ Hereditary Sensory and Autonomic Neuropathy

The classification of hereditary sensory and autonomic neuropathy provided in Table 9–2 is modified from the one suggested by Dyck (1984). This classification attempts to synthesize information based on natural history, mode of inheritance, and electrophysiologic characteristics. It is likely that each of these disorders is heterogeneous and that

Table 9–2 ◆ Disturbances of Sensation

Brachial Neuritis
1. Neuralgic amyotrophy (see Chapter 13)
2. Recurrent familial brachial neuropathy (see Chapter 13)

Congenital Insensitivity (Indifference) to Pain
1. Mental retardation
2. Lesch-Nyhan syndrome
3. With normal nervous system

Foramen Magnum Tumors

Hereditary Metabolic Neuropathies
1. Acute intermittent porphyria
2. Hereditary tyrosinemia

Hereditary Sensory and Autonomic Neuropathy (HSAN)
1. HSAN I (autosomal dominant)
2. HSAN II (autosomal recessive)
3. HSAN III (familial dysautonomia)
4. HSAN IV (with anhidrosis)
5. X-linked hereditary sensory neuropathy
6. HSAN with spastic paraplegia
7. Familial distal dysautonomia
8. Familial amyloid neuropathy

Lumbar Disk Herniation

Reflex Sympathetic Dystrophy

Syringomyelia

Thalamic Syndromes

several different genetic errors may produce a similar phenotype.

HEREDITARY SENSORY AND AUTONOMIC NEUROPATHY TYPE I

Hereditary sensory and autonomic neuropathy type I (HSAN I) appears in the literature under several names, most commonly "hereditary sensory radiculoneuropathy." Transmission is by autosomal dominant inheritance. As with other dominantly inherited neuropathies, variable expression is the rule. Therefore history alone is insufficient to determine whether parents are affected; physical examination and electrophysiologic studies are required.

Clinical Features.   Symptoms begin during the second decade or later (Ouvrier et al, 1990). The major clinical features are lancinating pains in the legs and ulcerations of the feet. However, initial symptoms are usually insidious and it is often difficult to date the onset. A callus develops on the sole of the foot, usually in the skin overlying a weight-bearing bony prominence. The callus blackens, becomes necrotic, and breaks down into an ulcer that is difficult to heal. The ulcer is preceded by sensory loss, but often it is the ulcer and not the sensory loss that brings the patient to medical attention. Although plantar ulcers are an important feature, they are not essential for diagnosis. Most patients with HSAN I do not have ulcers. When the proband in a kindred has typical features of plantar ulcers and lancinating pain, other family members may have sensory loss in the feet, mild pes cavus or peroneal atrophy, and loss of the Achilles tendon reflex.

Sensory loss in the feet is a constant feature, whereas sensory loss in the hands is variable. The hands are never affected as severely as the feet, and finger ulcers do not occur. The sensations of pain and temperature are lost before the sensations of touch and pressure. In some patients the dissociation of sensory loss is constant, whereas in others the dissociation is only a first stage before the development of global sensory loss. The Achilles tendon reflex is absent, and the quadriceps tendon reflex may also be absent. Tendon reflexes in the arms are preserved.

Foot ulcers are caused by trauma to the insensitive skin of the feet. They occur more often and are more difficult to heal in boys than in girls, in individuals who wear ill-fitting shoes, and in individuals who are on their feet much of the day. Lancinating pain is a late occurrence. It comes as recurring attacks usually affecting a single arm or leg. Other limbs may be affected on subsequent days. The intensity of pain varies.

Diagnosis.   Autosomal dominant inheritance and sensory loss in the feet are essential for the diagnosis. The presence of plantar ulcers and lancinating pain is helpful but is not critical for the diagnosis. HSAN I can be differentiated from familial amyloid polyneuropathy on clinical grounds. Urinary incontinence, impotence, and postural hypotension are frequent features of amyloidosis but do not occur in HSAN I.

Electrophysiologic studies demonstrate slowing of sensory nerve conduction velocity and reduced amplitude of sensory action potentials. Sural nerve biopsy reveals a marked decrease or absence of myelinated fibers and a mild to moderate reduction of small myelinated fibers.

Treatment.   No treatment is available for the neuropathy, but plantar ulcers can be prevented by good foot care. Tight shoes and activities that produce trauma to the feet should be avoided. Weight bearing must be discontinued at the first sign of a plantar ulcer. Much of the foot mutilation reported in previous years was due to secondary infection of the ulcers. This should be avoided by warm soaks, elevation, and antibiotics.

HEREDITARY SENSORY AND AUTONOMIC NEUROPATHY TYPE II

HSAN II probably includes several disorders transmitted by autosomal recessive inheritance. Many of the cases are sporadic, instances of parental consanguinity have been reported, and siblings are affected in some kindreds.

Clinical Features.   Symptoms probably begin during infancy and possibly at birth. Unlike HSAN I, which affects primarily the feet, HSAN II involves the arms and legs equally, as well as the trunk and forehead. The result is a diffuse loss of all sensation; touch and pressure are probably affected earlier and to a greater extent than temperature and pain. Affected infants and children are constantly hurting themselves without a painful response and are sometimes believed to have "congenital absence of pain" (Ouvrier et al, 1990). The absence of the protection pain provides against injury results in ulcerations and infections of the fingers and toes, stress fractures, and injuries to long bones. Loss of deep sensibility causes injury and swelling of joints, and loss of touch makes simple tasks, such as tying shoes, manipulating small objects, and buttoning buttons, difficult if not impossible. Tendon reflexes are absent throughout. Sweating is diminished in all areas of decreased sensibility, but no other symptoms or signs of autonomic dysfunction are present. Children with features of HSAN II and retinitis pigmentosa have been described (Landwirth, 1964), and one family has features of HSAN II and the early onset of cataracts (Donaghy et al, 1987). It is not clear whether such children represent separate genetic disorders or are part of the phenotypic spectrum of a single genetic disorder. Anhidrosis is also prominent in HSAN IV (discussed later), and the boundary between HSAN II and HSAN IV is difficult to delineate.

Diagnosis. The diagnosis relies primarily on the history and examination. Absence of sensory potentials confirms that the congenital absence of pain is due to peripheral neuropathy and not to a cerebral abnormality. Motor nerve conduction velocities are normal, as are the morphologic characteristics of motor unit potentials. Fibrillations are sometimes present. Sural nerve biopsy reveals an almost complete absence of myelinated fibers (Nukada et al, 1982).

Treatment. No treatment is available for the neuropathy. However, parents must be vigilant for painless injuries. Discoloration of the skin and swelling of joints or limbs should raise the possibility of fracture. Children must be taught to avoid activities that might cause injury and to examine themselves for signs of superficial infection.

HEREDITARY SENSORY AND AUTONOMIC NEUROPATHY TYPE III

HSAN III is ordinarily referred to as *familial dysautonomia* or the *Riley-Day syndrome*. This disorder is present at birth. Cardinal features are hypotonia, feeding difficulties, and poor control of autonomic function. Because neonatal hypotonia is prominent, the disorder is discussed in Chapter 6.

HEREDITARY SENSORY AND AUTONOMIC NEUROPATHY TYPE IV

HSAN IV is probably a heterogeneous group of disorders transmitted by autosomal recessive inheritance. The major features are congenital insensitivity to pain, anhidrosis, and mental retardation (Ouvrier et al, 1990). All the clinical abnormalities are present at birth, and although complications of the pain-free state are a continuous problem, the underlying disease may not be progressive.

Clinical Features. The initial symptoms may result from anhidrosis or insensitivity to pain. During infancy many affected children have repeated episodes of fever, sometimes associated with seizures. These episodes most commonly occur during the summer and are caused by the inability to sweat in response to exogenous heat. Sweat glands are present in the skin but lack sympathetic innervation. Most infants are hypotonic and areflexic. Developmental milestones are attained slowly, and

by 2 or 3 years of age the child has had several self-inflicted injuries caused by pain insensitivity. Injuries may include ulcers of the fingers and toes, stress fractures, self-mutilation of the tongue, and Charcot joints. Sensory examination reveals widespread absence of pain and temperature sensation. Touch, vibration, and stereognosis are intact in some patients. Mild to moderate retardation is present in almost every case.

Other features, present in some but not all patients, are blond hair and fair skin, Horner syndrome, and aplasia of dental enamel.

Diagnosis. Familial dysautonomia (HSAN III) and HSAN IV have many features in common and are easily confused. However, insensitivity to pain is not prominent in HSAN III and fungiform papillae of the tongue are present in HSAN IV. Anhidrotic ectodermal dysplasia is another hereditary disorder that shares many features with HSAN IV. Affected children also have unexplained fevers and abnormalities of tooth formation. However, children with ectodermal dysplasia are anhidrotic because sweat glands are absent. The nervous system is intact, and sensation to pain is present. Diagnosis of HSAN IV depends primarily on the clinical features but can be confirmed by demonstrating the absence of sensory evoked potentials, the absence of an axon reflex when histamine is injected into the skin, and the presence of sweat glands on skin biopsy specimens.

Treatment. No treatment is available for the underlying disease. However, constant vigilance is required to prevent injuries to the skin and bones with secondary infection.

X-LINKED HEREDITARY SENSORY NEUROPATHY

X-linked hereditary sensory neuropathy was described in five members of one family (Jestico et al, 1985).

Clinical Features. Painless deformities of the feet characterized by calcaneovalgus and loss of arch are noted between the ages of 3 and 13. Repeated trauma to the feet leads to painless ulcerations. Pain and touch sensations in the feet are reduced but not absent. The ankle tendon reflex is difficult to elicit but may be obtained with reinforcement. Other tendon reflexes are present. Autonomic function is preserved.

The rate of progression varies. Ulcers tend to enlarge and lead to osteomyelitis, which may necessitate amputation. The neuropathy remains limited to the feet.

Diagnosis. The only abnormality on EMG is reduction or absence of the sural nerve potential. Motor conduction velocities and motor unit potentials are normal. Sural nerve biopsy demonstrates selective loss of the small-diameter myelinated fibers.

Treatment. No treatment is available, but management requires the same concern for foot care as outlined for HSAN I.

HEREDITARY SENSORY AND AUTONOMIC NEUROPATHY WITH SPASTIC PARAPLEGIA

Hereditary sensory and autonomic neuropathy with spastic paraplegia may be caused by more than one genetic error. Some cases are sporadic, and others have occurred in siblings (Cavanagh et al, 1979). Autosomal recessive inheritance is suspected, but other modes of transmission cannot be excluded. Some patients with HSAN I or HSAN II have mild signs of corticospinal tract dysfunction, such as brisk reflexes and extensor plantar responses. Possibly cases with spastic paraplegia are variant phenotypes of HSAN I or HSAN II. However, it is reasonable to consider these cases separately at present.

Clinical Features. Progressive spastic paraplegia and sensory neuropathy are the major clinical features. The spasticity occurs first, or at least simultaneously with the sensory symptoms (see Chapter 12). A stiff-legged gait is noted during infancy or early childhood. Developmental motor milestones may be delayed. Tendon reflexes in the legs are increased, plantar responses are extensor, and sphincter control may not be attained. Either coinciding with the development of paraplegia or following it by several years, a relative insensitivity to pain is noticed by parents. This is characterized by repeated episodes of injury, ulcerations of the fingers and toes, and fractures. Pain and temperature sensations are much more severely affected than are the sensations of touch and vibration.

Intelligence is normal, and cranial nerves are unaffected. As the neuropathy becomes more profound, tendon reflexes, which initially were brisk, become depressed and are lost.

When the disease begins during infancy or early childhood, the course is relentlessly progressive and may lead to early death. Disease with onset in the second decade has a slower progression.

Diagnosis. A diagnosis cannot be established during early stages of the disease when spastic paraplegia is present but neuropathy is not. The development of insensitivity to pain and ulcers of the feet and fingers is essential for the diagnosis. Nerve conduction studies demonstrate prolonged sensory latencies and a reduced amplitude of action potentials. Motor conduction velocity may be nor-

mal. Sural nerve biopsy shows a profound loss of myelinated and unmyelinated fibers.

Treatment. No treatment for the underlying disease is available, but symptomatic care is needed to prevent injury to the hands and feet.

FAMILIAL DISTAL DYSAUTONOMIA

Familial distal dysautonomia is transmitted by autosomal dominant inheritance and was described in three generations of a single family (Robinson et al, 1989).

Clinical Features. Symptoms begin during childhood. Vasodilation is not induced by exercise, and burning pain occurs in the digits because of ischemia. Running causes swelling and reddening of the feet. The skin of the hands and feet is dry and cracks easily. Pedal pulses, tendon reflexes, and sensation are normal. The disorder does not shorten life expectancy.

Diagnosis. Warming of the hands or feet does not produce sweating. Motor and sensory nerve conduction is normal.

Treatment. Vasodilatory agents and sympathetic nerve block are not helpful. Symptoms are best managed by alterations in life-style.

FAMILIAL AMYLOID POLYNEUROPATHY

Familial amyloid polyneuropathy is a heterogeneous group of disorders, all transmitted by autosomal dominant inheritance, in which amyloid is deposited in the peripheral somatic and autonomic nervous systems. The abnormality is caused by a mutation in the gene for prealbumin located on chromosome 18 (Benson and Wallace, 1989). Other organs may be affected. The disorder has been described in several ethnic groups. Whether the genetic defect is the same among the different nationalities is not clear.

Clinical Features. Symptoms usually begin between the second and seventh decades, most often between the ages of 25 and 35. Dysesthesias are an early feature. Pain and temperature sensations are lost first, followed by touch, pressure, and vibration sensations. Lancinating pains and foot ulcers may be present, suggesting the diagnosis of HSAN I. However, autonomic dysfunction is much more profound and occurs earlier in the course of amyloid neuropathy than in HSAN I. Symptoms of autonomic dysfunction include impotence, constipation, diarrhea, fecal or urinary incontinence, and anhidrosis. Cardiac involvement is relatively common, as evidenced by bundle branch block, left ventricular hypertrophy, and atrioventricular dissociation. Postural hypotension occurs in approximately 10% of patients.

Motor involvement is a late feature; weakness and atrophy occur in both the hands and the feet. Tendon reflexes are depressed or absent in all limbs. Symptoms of other organ involvement tend to be mild. Vitreous opacities and perivascular amyloid deposition in retinal vessels are common. Some patients have proteinuria, but renal insufficiency is rare.

The course of disease is a steady progression, leading to cachexia and death within 15 years. Postmortem studies demonstrate amyloid deposition predominantly in peripheral nerves and blood vessels and to a lesser degree in cardiac muscle, smooth muscle, spleen, and kidneys.

Diagnosis. Clinical symptoms of a hereditary mixed motor sensory neuropathy with prominent autonomic dysfunction should suggest the diagnosis of familial amyloid polyneuropathy. Electrophysiologic findings are consistent with a mixed motor sensory neuropathy of the axonal type. Examination reveals amyloid deposition around the sural nerve causing compression within the endoneurium and in the walls of the vasa nervorum.

Treatment. No treatment is available for the underlying disease. Cardiac arrhythmias may necessitate a permanent cardiac pacemaker. For other manifestations of autonomic dysfunction, treatment is directed to the symptoms.

◆ Lumbar Disk Herniation

Lumbar disk herniation in children is usually caused by trauma. Almost all cases occur after age 10; they are more common in boys than in girls and are frequently sports related (Epstein et al, 1984; Kurihara and Kataoka, 1980). Because lumbar disk herniation is unusual in children, diagnosis may be delayed for months or years.

Clinical Features. Sciatica or back pain or both are the initial manifestations. Twenty percent of patients never have back pain, but all have sciatica at some time in the course. Almost half of patients report bilateral sciatica.

Physical findings may include diminished lumbar lordosis, vertebral muscle spasm, and scoliosis. The patient tries to hold the lumbar spine rigid. Point tenderness may be present over the involved disk space. Straight leg raising routinely provokes sciatica. Sensation to pinprick may be diminished in the distribution of the L-5 and S-1 dermatome, and the ankle tendon reflex is diminished or absent in more than half of patients.

Diagnosis. Radiographs of the lumbosacral spine reveal minor congenital anomalies (hemivertebrae, sacralization of the lumbar spine) in an unusually large number of cases. The diagnosis is confirmed by computed tomography of the spine or by myelography.

Treatment. Conservative treatment (bed rest and traction) provides immediate relief in the majority of patients, but surgery is often required for permanent relief of symptoms.

◆ Reflex Sympathetic Dystrophy

In the medical literature, reflex sympathetic dystrophy has several names, including causalgia, algodystrophy, neurovascular reflex dystrophy, posttraumatic sympathetic dystrophy, and Sudeck atrophy. The essential feature is sustained burning pain in a limb, combined with vasomotor and pseudomotor dysfunction, leading to atrophic changes in skin, muscle, and bone following trauma. The inciting trauma, which may be accidental or surgical, injures the nerves in a limb or the cervical spinal cord. The mechanism of reflex sympathetic dystrophy remains a debated issue, and several different central and peripheral mechanisms probably produce the same result (Janig et al, 1991).

Clinical Features. The mean age at onset in children is 11 years, and girls are affected more often than boys (Dietz et al, 1990). Reflex sympathetic dystrophy frequently follows trauma to one limb with or without fracture. The trauma may be relatively minor, and the clinical syndrome is so unusual that many affected individuals are first labeled "hysterical" or "malingering." Time until onset after injury is usually 1 or 2 months but may be longer. The first symptom is pain at the site of injury, which progresses either proximally or distally without regard for dermatomal distribution or anatomic landmarks. Generalized swelling and vasomotor disturbances of the limb follow in 80% of children. Pain is intense, is described as burning or aching, and is out of proportion to the injury. It may be maximally severe at onset or may become progressively worse for 3 to 6 months. Pain is exacerbated by movement or dependence, causing the arm to be held in a position of abduction and internal rotation as if it were swaddled to the body. The hand becomes swollen and hyperesthetic and feels warmer.

Children with reflex sympathetic dystrophy do better than adults: 42% have resolution in less than 12 weeks, 25% in less than 1 month, and the remainder within 6 months. Long-term pain is unusual, as are the trophic changes of the skin and bones that often occur in adults. Most children recover completely and do not have recurrences.

Diagnosis. The diagnosis is clinical and cannot be confirmed by laboratory tests. Because the syndrome follows accidental or surgical trauma, litigation is commonplace, and careful documentation of the examination is needed. One simple test is to immerse the affected hand in warm water. Wrinkling of the fingers requires an intact sympathetic innervation. The absence of wrinkling is evidence of a lesion in either the central or the peripheral sympathetic pathway (Braham et al, 1979).

Treatment. I have satisfactorily treated children with range of motion exercise and over-the-counter analgesics. Treatment of more severe syndromes, which almost always occur in adults, includes the oral administration of guanethidine, 20 to 30 mg/day, prednisone with or without stellate ganglion blockade, and sympathectomy.

◆ Syringomyelia

Syringomyelia is a generic term for disorders with cavitation in the spinal cord. The cavity varies in length and may extend into the brainstem. Such a cephalic extension is termed *syringobulbia*. The cavity, or syrinx, is centrally placed in the gray matter and may enlarge in all directions. The cervicothoracic region is a favorite site, but thoracolumbar syrinx also occurs, and occasionally a syrinx extends from the brainstem to the conus medullaris (Epstein and Epstein, 1981).

The mechanism of syrinx formation has been debated (Newman et al, 1981). Cavitation of the spinal cord sometimes follows trauma and infarction, but these are not important mechanisms of syringomyelia in children. In childhood, primary syringomyelia is generally regarded as either a congenital malformation or a cystic astrocytoma. In the past, congenital cysts could be distinguished from astrocytoma only by postmortem examination. Astrocytomas of the spinal cord, like those of the cerebellum, may have large cysts with only a nubbin of solid tumor. The development of MRI has greatly enhanced antemortem diagnosis of cystic astrocytoma by demonstrating small areas of increased signal intensity in one or more portions of the cyst. Cystic astrocytoma is more likely to produce symptoms during the first decade, whereas congenital syringomyelia is manifested in the second decade or later and is usually associated with the Chiari anomaly (Newman et al, 1981). Cystic astrocytoma of the spinal cord is considered further in Chapters 12 and 13; this section deals primarily with congenital syringomyelia.

Clinical Features. The initial symptoms of syringomyelia depend on the cyst's location. Because the cavity is near the central canal, crossing fibers subserving pain and temperature are often affected first. When the syrinx is in the cervical area, pain and temperature are typically lost in a "cape" or "vest" distribution. However, early involvement is often unilateral or at least asymmetric and sometimes involves the fingers before the shoulders. Touch and pressure are ordinarily preserved until the cyst enlarges into the posterior columns or the dorsal root entry zone. Loss of pain sensibility in the hands often leads to injury, ulceration, and infection as seen in hereditary sensory and autonomic neuropathies. Pain is not ordinarily a feature of syringomyelia, but lancinating limb pain is occasionally reported.

Scoliosis is common, and torticollis may be an initial sign in children with cervical cavities (Kiwak et al, 1983). As the cavity enlarges into the ventral horn, weakness and atrophy develop in the hands and may be associated with fasciculations; pressure on the lateral columns causes hyperreflexia and spasticity in the legs. Very long cavities may produce lower motor neuron signs in all four limbs. Sphincter control is sometimes impaired. The posterior columns are generally the last to be affected so that vibration sense and touch are preserved until relatively late in the course. The progress of symptoms is extremely slow and insidious. The spinal cord accommodates well to the slowly developing pressure within. Thus, at the time a physician is consulted, a long history of minor neurologic handicap such as clumsiness or difficulty running may be elicited.

Bulbar signs are relatively uncommon and usually asymmetric. They include hemiatrophy of the tongue with deviation on protrusion, facial weakness, dysphasia, and dysarthria. The descending pathway of the trigeminal nerve is frequently affected, causing loss of pain and temperature sensations on the same side of the face as the facial weakness and tongue hemiatrophy.

Diagnosis. MRI is the diagnostic test of choice. It not only allows visualization of the cavity (Figure 9–1) and the Chiari malformation, but also shows the presence of small foci of glioma.

Treatment. Several surgical approaches have been used in treating syringomyelia. Syringoperitoneal shunting has provided the most favorable results (Barbaro et al, 1984). Some degree of stabilization is achieved in most patients.

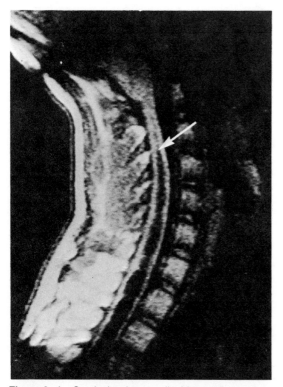

Figure 9–1 Cervical syringomyelia. Magnetic resonance image demonstrates a long cavity, beginning *(arrow)* just below the foramen magnum.

◆ Thalamic Pain

The thalamic pain syndrome of Déjérine and Roussy occurs almost exclusively in adults following infarction of the thalamus or of the white matter of the parietal lobe. Similar symptoms sometimes occur in patients with thalamic glioma. Such tumors more often produce hemiparesis than thalamic pain.

Clinical Features. Touching the affected limb or part of the body produces intense discomfort described as "sharp," "crushing," or "burning." Suffering is considerable, and the quality of pain is unfamiliar to the patient. Several different modes of stimulation, such as changes in ambient temperature, auditory stimulation, and even changes in emotional state, can accentuate the pain. Despite the severity of these dysesthesias, the affected limb is otherwise anesthetic to ordinary sensory testing.

Diagnosis. The presence of thalamic pain should prompt imaging studies to determine the presence of tumor, infarction, or demyelinating disease.

Treatment. The combination of levodopa and a peripheral decarboxylase inhibitor may be helpful for relieving pain (Plasencia et al, 1984). If this does not prove satisfactory, some combination of analgesic and tranquilizing medication should be administered.

References

Barbaro NM, Wilson CB, Gutin PH, et al: Surgical treatment of syringomyelia: Favorable results with syringoperitoneal shunting. J Neurosurg 61:531, 1984.

Benson MD, Wallace MR: Amyloidosis. In Scriver CR, Beaudet AL, Sly WS, et al, eds: The Metabolic Basis of Inherited Disease, 6th edition. McGraw-Hill, New York, 1989, p 2439.

Braham J, Sadeh M, Sarova-Pinhas I: Skin wrinkling on immersion of hands: A test of sympathetic function. Arch Neurol 36:113, 1979.

Cavanagh NPC, Eames RA, Galvin RJ, et al: Hereditary sensory neuropathy with spastic paraplegia. Brain 102:79, 1979.

Dietz FR, Mathews KD, Montgomery WJ: Reflex sympathetic dystrophy in children. Clin Orthop 258:225, 1990.

Donaghy M, Hakin RN, Bamford JM, et al: Hereditary sensory neuropathy with neurotrophic keratitis: Description of an autosomal recessive disorder with a selective reduction of small myelinated nerve fibres and a discussion of the classification of the hereditary sensory neuropathies. Brain 110:563, 1987.

Dyck PJ: Neuronal atrophy and degeneration predominantly affecting peripheral sensory and autonomic neurons. In Dyck PJ, Thomas PK, Lambert EH, Bunge R, eds: Peripheral Neuropathy. WB Saunders, Philadelphia, 1984, p 1557.

Epstein F, Epstein N: Surgical management of holocord intramedullary spinal cord astrocytomas in children: Report of three cases. J Neurosurg 54:829, 1981.

Epstein JA, Epstein NE, Marc J, et al: Lumbar intervertebral disk herniation in teenage children: Recognition and management of associated anomalies. Spine 9:427:1984.

Janig W, Blumberg H, Boas RA, et al: The reflex sympathetic dystrophy syndrome: Consensus statement and general recommendations for diagnosis and clinical research. In Bond MR, Charlton JE, Woolf CJ, eds: Proceedings of the VI World Congress On Pain. Elsevier Science, Amsterdam, 1991, p 373.

Jestico JV, Urry PA, Efphimiou J: An hereditary sensory and autonomic neuropathy transmitted as an X-linked recessive trait. J Neurol Neurosurg Psychiatry 48:1259, 1985.

Kappas A, Sassa S, Galbraith RA, et al: The porphyrias. In Scriver CR, Beaudet AL, Sly WS, et al, eds: The Metabolic Basis of Inherited Disease, 6th edition. McGraw-Hill, New York, 1989, p 1305.

Kiwak KJ, Deray MJ, Shields WD: Torticollis in three children with syringomyelia and spinal cord tumor. Neurology 33:946, 1983.

Kurihara A, Kataoka O: Lumbar disc herniation in children and adolescents: A review of 70 operated cases and their minimum 5-year follow-up studies. Spine 5:443, 1980.

Landrieu P, Said G, Allaire C: Dominantly transmitted congenital indifference to pain. Ann Neurol 27:574, 1990.

Landwirth J: Sensory radicular neuropathy and retinitis pigmentosa. Pediatrics 34:519, 1964.

Mitchell G, Larochelle J, Lambert M, et al: Neurologic crises in hereditary tyrosinemia. N Engl J Med 322:432, 1990.

Newman PK, Terenty TR, Foster JB: Some observations on the pathogenesis of syringomyelia. J Neurol Neurosurg Psychiatry 44:964, 1981.

Nukada H, Pollock M, Haas LF: The clinical spectrum and morphology of type II hereditary sensory neuropathy. Brain 105:647, 1982.

Ouvrier R, McLeod JG, Pollard J: Sensory neuropathies. In Peripheral Neuropathy in Childhood. International review of Child Neurology Series. Raven Press, New York, 1990, p 127.

Plasencia RJ, Gilroy J, Cullis P: Treatment of thalamic pain syndrome with levodopa. Neurology 34(suppl 1):137, 1984.

Robinson B, Johnson R, Abernathy D, et al: Familial distal dysautonomia. J Neurol Neurosurg Psychiatry 52:1281, 1989.

Yasuoka S, Okazaki H, Daube JR, et al: Foramen magnum tumors. J Neurosurg 49:828, 1978.

Ataxia

The term "ataxia" can be used for any disturbance in gait but is used here in a more restricted sense to denote disturbances of coordination rather than strength. Disturbances of coordination are typically caused by dysfunction of the cerebellum or its major input systems from the frontal lobes or the posterior columns of the spinal cord. An ataxic gait is wide based, lurching, and staggering, and in the observer it provokes fear that the patient is in danger of falling. The same gait is seen in people who are attempting to walk in a vehicle that has several directions of movement at once, such as a train. When an abnormality occurs in the vermis of the cerebellum, the child cannot sit still but constantly moves the body to and fro and bobs the head (titubation). In contrast, disturbances of the cerebellar hemispheres cause a tendency to veer in the direction of the affected hemisphere, with dysmetria and hypotonia in the ipsilateral limbs. Bifrontal lobe disease may produce symptoms and signs indistinguishable from cerebellar disease.

Loss of sensory input to the cerebellum, because of peripheral nerve or posterior column disease, necessitates constant looking at the feet to know their location in space. The gait is also wide based but is not so much lurching as careful. The foot is raised high with each step and slaps down heavily on the ground. Station and gait are considerably worse with the eyes closed, and the patient may actually fall to the floor (positive Romberg sign).

The differential diagnosis of a child with acute ataxia or recurrent attacks of ataxia (Table 10–1) is quite different from that of a child with chronic static or progressive ataxia (Table 10–2). Therefore these two presentations are discussed separately in the text. However, the reader must remember that a slowly progressive ataxia may be noticed "acutely" and that children with recurrent ataxia may never return to baseline after each attack and may have a progressive ataxia superimposed on the acute attacks.

Table 10–1 ◆ Acute or Recurrent Ataxia

Brain Tumor

Conversion Reaction

Drug Ingestion

Encephalitis (brainstem)

Genetic Disorders
1. Carnitine acetyltransferase deficiency
2. Dominant recurrent ataxia
3. Hartnup disease
4. Maple syrup urine disease
5. Paroxysmal ataxia and myokymia
6. Pyruvate decarboxylase deficiency

Migraine
1. Basilar
2. Benign paroxysmal vertigo

Postinfectious Immune
1. Acute postinfectious cerebellitis
2. Miller-Fisher syndrome
3. Myoclonic encephalopathy and neuroblastoma
4. Multiple sclerosis

Pseudoataxia (epileptic)

Trauma
1. Hematoma (Chapter 2)
2. Postconcussion
3. Vertebrobasilar occlusion

Vascular Disorders
1. Cerebellar hemorrhage
2. Kawasaki disease
3. Lupus erythematosus

Table 10–2 ◆ Chronic or Progressive Ataxia

Brain Tumors
1. Cerebellar astrocytoma
2. Cerebellar hemangioblastoma (von Hippel–Lindau disease)
3. Ependymoma
4. Medulloblastoma
5. Supratentorial tumors (see Chapter 4)

Congenital Malformations
1. Basilar impression
2. Cerebellar aplasias
   a. Cerebellar hemisphere aplasia
   b. Dandy-Walker malformation (see Chapter 18)
   c. Vermal aplasia
3. Chiari malformation

Hereditary Ataxias
1. Autosomal dominant inheritance
   a. Machado-Joseph disease
   b. Olivopontocerebellar degeneration
   c. Ramsay Hunt syndrome
      1. With pallidoluysian atrophy
      2. With mitochondrial myopathy
2. Autosomal recessive inheritance
   a. Abetalipoproteinemia
   b. Ataxia–ocular motor apraxia
   c. Ataxia-telangiectasia
   d. Ataxia with episodic dystonia
   e. Friedreich ataxia
   f. Harding ataxia
   g. Hartnup disease
   h. Hypobetalipoproteinemia
   i. Juvenile GM$_2$ gangliosidosis
   j. Juvenile sulfatide lipidoses
   k. Maple syrup urine disease
   l. Marinesco-Sjogren syndrome
   m. Pyruvate dysmetabolism (see Chapters 5, 7, and 8)
   n. Ramsay Hunt syndrome
   o. Refsum disease (HSMN IV) (see Chapter 7)
   p. Respiratory chain disorders (see Chapter 8)
   q. Sea-blue histiocytosis
3. X-linked inheritance
   a. Adrenoleukodystrophy (see Chapter 5)
   b. Leber optic neuropathy (see Chapter 16)
   c. With adult-onset dementia

◆ Acute or Recurrent Ataxia

The two most common causes of ataxia among children who were previously healthy and then suddenly have an ataxic gait are drug ingestion and acute postinfectious cerebellitis (Table 10–1). Migraine, brainstem encephalitis, and an underlying neuroblastoma are the next considerations. In preadolescent and adolescent girls a conversion reaction is always a possibility. Recurrent ataxia is uncommon and is usually caused by hereditary disorders; migraine is the most common cause, and disorders of pyruvate metabolism are second.

BRAIN TUMOR

Primary brain tumors ordinarily produce chronic progressive ataxia and are discussed later in the chapter. However, tumors may also be manifested as acute ataxia because of bleeding, sudden shifts in position that cause hydrocephalus, or growth. In addition, clumsiness may be overlooked until it becomes severe enough to cause an obvious gait disturbance. For this reason, brain imaging is recommended for all children with acute cerebellar ataxia (Figure 10–1).

CONVERSION REACTION

Clinical Features. Hysterical gait disturbances are common in children, especially girls between 10 and 15 years of age. The disturbance is involuntary, usually provides a secondary gain such as attention, and should be distinguished from malingering, which is a voluntary act. Hysterical gait disturbances are often extreme and if so are termed *astasia-abasia*. The child appears to sit without difficulty but when brought to standing immediately begins to sway from the waist. The child does not assume a wide-based stance to increase stability. Instead the child lurches, staggers, and otherwise travels across the room from object to object. The lurching maneuvers are often complex and require extraordinary balance. Strength, tone, sensation, and tendon reflexes are normal.

Diagnosis. Hysterical gait disturbances are usually diagnosed by observation; laboratory tests are not ordinarily required to exclude other possibilities.

Treatment. Determination of the precipitating stress is important. Conversion may represent a true call for help in a desperate situation such as child abuse. Such cases require referral to a multispecialty team able to deal with the whole family.

Most children with hysterical gait disturbances are responding to a more immediate and less serious difficulty. Symptoms can usually be treated by the use of suggestion and do not require psychiatric referral except when conversion is used repeatedly to handle stress.

DRUG INGESTION

The incidence of accidental drug ingestion is highest between 1 and 4 years of age.

Clinical Features. An overdose of most psy-

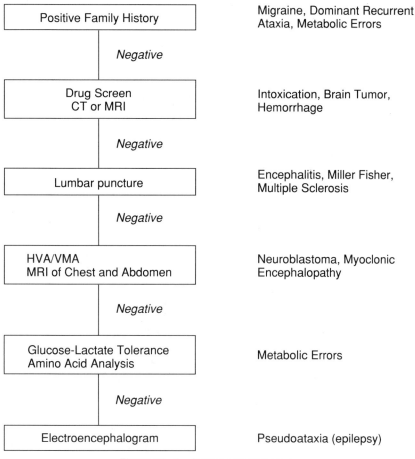

Positive Family History	Migraine, Dominant Recurrent Ataxia, Metabolic Errors
Negative	
Drug Screen CT or MRI	Intoxication, Brain Tumor, Hemorrhage
Negative	
Lumbar puncture	Encephalitis, Miller Fisher, Multiple Sclerosis
Negative	
HVA/VMA MRI of Chest and Abdomen	Neuroblastoma, Myoclonic Encephalopathy
Negative	
Glucose-Lactate Tolerance Amino Acid Analysis	Metabolic Errors
Negative	
Electroencephalogram	Pseudoataxia (epilepsy)

Figure 10–1   Acute cerebellar ataxia.

choactive drugs can produce ataxia, which is usually associated with some change in personality or sensorium. Toxic doses of anticonvulsant drugs, especially phenytoin, may produce marked ataxia without an alteration in sensorium. Nystagmus usually is present as well. Excessive use of antihistamines in the treatment of an infant or young child with allergy or an upper respiratory infection may produce ataxia. This is especially true in children with otitis media, who may have underlying unsteadiness because of middle ear infection.

Diagnosis.   The parents or care providers of every child with acute ataxia should be carefully questioned concerning drugs intentionally administered to the child and other drugs accessible in the home. It is worthwhile to inquire specifically if anyone in the family is using anticonvulsant or psychoactive drugs. Urine should be screened for drug metabolites, and blood should be sent for analysis when a specific drug is suspected.

Treatment.   Treatment depends on the specific drug ingested and its blood concentration. In most cases of ataxia caused by drug ingestion, the drug can be safely eliminated spontaneously if vital function is not compromised, if acid-base balance is not disturbed, and if liver and kidney function is normal. In life-threatening situations dialysis may be necessary while vital function is supported in an intensive care unit.

ENCEPHALITIS (BRAINSTEM)

Ataxia may be the initial feature of viral encephalitis affecting primarily the structures of the posterior fossa. Echoviruses, coxsackieviruses, and adenoviruses have been implicated as etiologic agents.

Clinical Features.   Cranial nerve dysfunction is often associated with the ataxia. A more diffuse encephalitis characterized by declining consciousness and seizures may develop later. Meningismus is sometimes present. The course is variable, and although most children recover completely, some are left with considerable neurologic impairment. Those who have only ataxia and cranial nerve palsies, with no disturbance of neocortical function, tend to recover best. Such cases cannot be distinguished from the Miller-Fisher syndrome on clinical grounds alone.

Diagnosis. Diagnosis requires the demonstration of a cellular response, primarily mononuclear leukocytes, in the cerebrospinal fluid, with or without some elevation of the protein content. Prolonged interpeak latencies of the brainstem auditory evoked response are evidence of an abnormality within the brainstem parenchyma and not the peripheral sensory input system. The electroencephalogram (EEG) is usually normal in children with brainstem encephalitis who have a normal sensorium. A mild increase in theta activity may be recorded as well.

Treatment. No specific treatment is available for viral infection.

GENETIC DISORDERS
Carnitine Acetyltransferase Deficiency

Carnitine acetyltransferase is a putative enzyme in the control of acetylcoenzymeA (acetyl-CoA) flux in mitochondria. Enzyme deficiency has been described in a single patient (DiDonato et al, 1979).

Clinical Features. A previously healthy girl had recurrent episodes of confusion, ataxia, and decreased states of consciousness beginning at 2 years of age. Hypotonia with reduced tendon reflexes and ophthalmoparesis accompanied episodes. Most functions recovered within 3 days, but mild ataxia and dysmetria persisted after several episodes. Episodes became progressively severe between ages 3 and 6. They were characterized by vomiting, delirium, ptosis, large or small pupils, and ataxia. The clinical syndrome suggests a disturbance in the pyruvate dehydrogenase complex, except that the liver is enlarged. Death occurred during one of the episodes.

Diagnosis. The EEG is normal between episodes and diffusely slow during an episode. Serum transaminase concentrations are normal at first and then become progressively elevated. Serum concentrations of lactate and pyruvate are normal. Definitive diagnosis requires demonstration of enzyme deficiency in liver or cultured fibroblasts.

Treatment. No treatment is available.

Dominant Recurrent Ataxia (Acetazolamide-Responsive)

Several families have been reported in whom episodic ataxia and vertigo are transmitted by autosomal dominant inheritance (Zasorin et al, 1983). The underlying metabolic defect has not been identified and may not be the same in all families. However, the clinical findings are sufficiently similar from family to family to suggest a uniform cause.

Clinical Features. The onset of symptoms is usually in childhood, often during the first 3 years, but may be delayed until adult life (Farris et al, 1986). The child first becomes unsteady and then is unable to maintain posture because of vertigo and ataxia. Vomiting is frequent and severe. Jerk nystagmus, sometimes with a rotary component, is observed during attacks. Young children have one to three attacks per month with symptoms lasting from 1 hour to 1 day. Attacks become milder and less frequent with age. Slowly progressive truncal ataxia and nystagmus may persist between attacks. In some patients, ataxia is the only symptom, others have only vertigo, and still others have only nystagmus (Baloh and Winder, 1991).

Most affected individuals are normal between attacks, but some demonstrate nystagmus and clumsiness (Farris et al, 1986).

Diagnosis. Diagnosis is based on the clinical features and a family history of the disorder. Selective atrophy of the cerebellar vermis has been documented by magnetic resonance imaging (MRI) (Vighetto et al, 1988). Basilar artery migraine and benign paroxysmal vertigo must be distinguished. In these conditions older family members have migraine but do not have recurrent ataxia. Attacks of benign paroxysmal vertigo rarely last more than a few minutes.

None of the other hereditary recurrent ataxias, other than migraine, are transmitted by autosomal dominant inheritance. Nevertheless, disorders of pyruvate metabolism, many of which produce intermittent ataxia, must be excluded.

Treatment. Daily oral acetazolamide prevents recurrence of attacks in almost every case. Its mechanism of action is unknown. The dose is generally 125 mg twice a day in young children and 250 mg twice a day in older children. Flunarizine, 5 to 10 mg/day, was effective in one patient and may serve as an alternative therapy when acetazolamide is not tolerated (Boel and Casaer, 1988). Anticonvulsant and antimigraine medications are without value.

Hartnup Disease

Hartnup disease is a rare disorder transmitted by autosomal recessive inheritance (Levy, 1989). The basic error is a defect of amino acid transport in cells of the proximal renal tubules and small intestine. The result is massive aminoaciduria and the retention of amino acids in the small intestine, where they are converted by bacteria into useless or toxic products that may be absorbed. Tryptophan is converted to nonessential indole products instead of nicotinamide.

Clinical Features.   Affected children are normal at birth but may be slow in attaining developmental milestones. Most achieve only borderline intelligence; others are normal. Affected individuals are photosensitive and have a severe, pellagra-like skin rash after exposure to sunlight. The rash is attributed to nicotinamide deficiency. Many patients have episodes of limb ataxia, sometimes associated with nystagmus. Mental changes, ranging from emotional instability to delirium, or states of decreased consciousness may occur. Tone is decreased, and the tendon reflexes are normal or exaggerated. The neurologic disturbances are triggered by stress or intercurrent infection and may be due to the intestinal absorption of toxic amino acid breakdown products.

Most patients have both rash and neurologic disturbances, but each can occur without the other. Neurologic symptoms progress over several days and last from a week to a month before recovery occurs.

Diagnosis.   The constant feature of Hartnup disease is massive aminoaciduria involving neutral monoaminomonocarboxylic amino acids. These include alanine, serine, threonine, asparagine, glutamine, valine, leucine, isoleucine, phenylalanine, tyrosine, tryptophan, histidine, and citrulline.

Treatment.   The rash can be prevented by daily oral administration of nicotinamide, 50 to 300 mg. Whether nicotinamide has a beneficial effect on the neurologic symptoms is not known.

Maple Syrup Urine Disease (Intermittent)

Maple syrup urine disease is a disorder of branched-chain amino acid metabolism caused by deficiency of the enzyme branched-chain ketoacid dehydrogenase. The defect is transmitted by autosomal recessive inheritance. Three phenotypes are associated with this enzyme deficiency. The *classic* form begins as seizures in the newborn (see Chapter 1), the *intermediate* form produces progressive mental retardation (see Chapter 5), and the *intermittent* form produces recurrent attacks of ataxia and encephalopathy (Danner and Elsas, 1989).

Clinical Features.   Affected individuals are normal during the first year. During the second year episodes of ataxia, irritability, and progressive lethargy are provoked by minor infections, vaccination, surgery, or a diet rich in protein. The length of an attack is variable; most children recover spontaneously, but some die of severe metabolic aci-

dosis. Psychomotor development remains normal in survivors.

Diagnosis.   The urine has a maple syrup odor during the attack, and the blood and urine have elevated concentrations of branched-chain amino acids and ketoacids. Between attacks the concentrations of branched-chain amino acids and ketoacids are normal in both blood and urine. Definitive diagnosis requires the demonstration of enzyme deficiency in cultured fibroblasts.

Treatment.   Children with intermittent maple syrup disease should be put on a protein-restricted diet. Some children have a thiamine-responsive enzyme defect and should have a trial of 1 g of thiamine a day for the acute attack (Pueschel et al, 1979). If this is successful, a maintenance dose of 100 mg/day is recommended. The major objective during an acute attack is to reverse ketoacidosis. Protein should not be given. Peritoneal dialysis may be helpful in life-threatening situations.

Paroxysmal Ataxia and Myokymia

Paroxysmal ataxia and myokymia is a syndrome related to autosomal dominant ataxia and also to paroxysmal choreoathetosis (see Chapter 1) (Ewout et al, 1990). The additional feature of continuous motor unit activity (see Chapter 8) suggests a defect in membrane stability affecting the central and peripheral nervous system.

Clinical Features.   The onset of attacks usually occurs between 5 and 7 years of age. The child has a sudden awareness that an attack is to begin by the sensation of spreading limpness or stiffness lasting a few seconds. Incoordination, trembling of the head or limbs, and often blurry vision then develop. A few children feel warm and perspire. Some can continue standing or walking, but most sit down. Attacks usually last less than 10 minutes, but some are as long as 6 hours. Attacks may begin spontaneously but more usually are brought on by sudden and unexpected movement (kinesiogenic). Startle and anxiety increase the potential for attacks. Myokymia of the hands is observed even between attacks.

Diagnosis.   The clinical diagnosis is based on the history of typical attacks and the family history. Electromyography confirms the diagnosis by the demonstration of continuous motor unit activity, most often in the hands but also in the proximal arm muscles and sometimes the face.

Treatment.   Acetazolamide reduces the frequency of attacks or completely stops them in about half of patients. The effect is noted within a few days. Anticonvulsants are not effective.

Pyruvate Decarboxylase Deficiency

Pyruvate decarboxylase is the first enzyme system in the pyruvate dehydrogenase complex. This complex is responsible for the oxidative decarboxylation of pyruvate to carbon dioxide and acetyl-CoA. Disorders of the complex are associated with several neurologic conditions, including subacute necrotizing encephalomyelopathy (Leigh syndrome), mitochondrial myopathies, and lactic acidosis.

An X-linked form of pyruvate decarboxylase deficiency is characterized by episodes of intermittent ataxia and lactic acidosis (Evans, 1984; Livingstone et al, 1984).

Clinical Features.   Most patients demonstrate mild developmental delay during early childhood. Episodes of ataxia, dysarthria, and sometimes lethargy usually begin after 3 years of age. In more severely affected patients episodes may begin during infancy and are associated with generalized weakness and states of decreased consciousness. Some attacks are spontaneous, but others are provoked by intercurrent infection, stress, or a high-carbohydrate meal. Attacks recur at irregular intervals and may last from 1 day to several weeks.

The severity of neurologic dysfunction in any individual probably reflects the level of residual enzyme activity. Those with generalized weakness are also areflexic and have nystagmus or other disturbances in ocular motility. Ataxia is the predominant symptom. Intention tremor and dysarthria may be present. Hyperventilation is common and may be caused by metabolic acidosis.

Patients with almost complete decarboxylase deficiency die of lactic acidosis and central hypoventilation during infancy.

Diagnosis.   Many patients have mild elevation in the concentration of blood lactate between attacks; all have elevated concentrations of blood lactate and pyruvate during attacks. Some have hyperalaninemia as well. The diagnosis of a pyruvate dysmetabolism state may be further verified by an oral glucose tolerance test. When oral glucose is administered, hyperglycemia is prolonged and blood concentrations of lactate are elevated. The test may provoke clinical symptoms. Definitive diagnosis requires analysis of enzyme activity in cultured fibroblasts, leukocytes, or muscle.

Treatment.   In patients with disorders of pyruvate metabolism, a high-fat (ketogenic) diet is useful to provide substrate that bypasses carbohydrate metabolism. In addition, oral acetazolamide, 125 mg twice a day in small children and 250 mg twice a day in older children, may significantly abort the attacks. Biotin and thiamine supplements have been used in several patients, but the value of vitamin supplementation has not been established.

MIGRAINE
Basilar Migraine

The term "basilar (artery) migraine" is used to characterize recurrent attacks of brainstem or cerebellar dysfunction that occur as a manifestation of migraine. Girls are affected more often than boys. The peak incidence is during adolescence, but attacks may occur at any age (Lapkin and Golden, 1978). Infant-onset cases are more likely to be manifested as benign paroxysmal vertigo.

Clinical Features.   Gait ataxia occurs in approximately 50% of patients. Other symptoms include visual loss, vertigo, tinnitus, alternating hemiparesis, and paresthesias of the fingers, toes, and corners of the mouth. An abrupt loss of consciousness, usually lasting only a few minutes, may be reported. Cardiac arrhythmia and brainstem stroke are rare life-threatening complications. Neurologic disturbances are usually followed by a severe, throbbing, occipital headache. Nausea and vomiting occur in less than one third of cases.

Several authors have stressed the association of seizures and occipital lobe spike discharges with attacks of basilar migraine. Such cases should be considered examples of benign occipital epilepsy and not migraine (see Chapter 1).

Children may have repeated basilar migraine attacks, but with time the episodes evolve into a pattern of classic migraine. Even during attacks of classic migraine the patient may continue to complain of vertigo and even ataxia.

Diagnosis.   The diagnosis of basilar migraine, like other forms of migraine, relies heavily on a family history of migraine. An EEG is informative, not only to eliminate the possibility of benign occipital epilepsy, but also because occipital intermittent rhythmic delta activity (Figure 10–2) may be present during and just after an attack.

Treatment.   Many authors have recommended the use of anticonvulsant drugs for basilar migraine. This is probably the result of confusing benign occipital epilepsy with basilar migraine. Prophylactic migraine therapy (see Chapter 3) is indicated in children with basilar migraine.

Benign Paroxysmal Vertigo

Benign paroxysmal vertigo is primarily a disorder of infants and preschool children but may occur in older children.

Clinical Features.   Episodes are characterized by the sudden onset of vertigo. True cerebellar

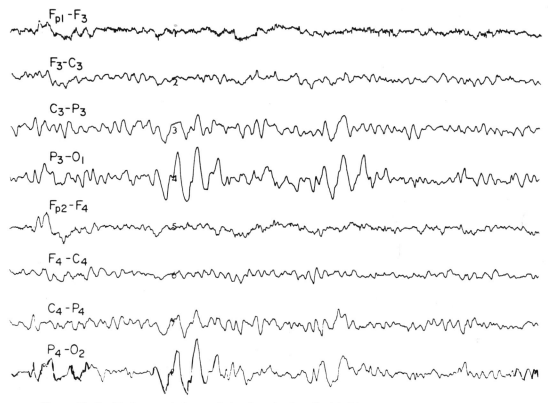

Figure 10–2 Electroencephalogram in basilar migraine. Occipital intermittent rhythmic delta waves are present shortly after an attack.

ataxia is not present, but vertigo is so profound that posture cannot be maintained. The child either lies motionless on the floor or indicates the need to be held by a parent. Consciousness is not altered, and headache is not reported. The predominant symptoms are pallor, nystagmus, and fright. Episodes last only minutes and may recur at irregular intervals. With time, attacks of paroxysmal vertigo are replaced by episodes of headache and vomiting that are more readily recognized as migraine (Fenichel, 1967).

Diagnosis. The diagnosis is primarily clinical, and laboratory tests are useful only to exclude other possibilities. A family history of migraine, although not necessarily paroxysmal vertigo, can be obtained in almost every case. Some parents indicate that they experience vertigo with their attacks of migraine. Only in rare cases does a parent have a history of benign paroxysmal vertigo.

Treatment. The attacks are so brief and harmless that treatment is seldom indicated. Standard migraine therapy can be employed when the child grows older and vertiginous episodes are replaced by headache and vomiting.

POSTINFECTIOUS IMMUNE DISORDERS

In many of the conditions discussed in this section an altered immune state is blamed for cerebellar dysfunction and sometimes for other neurologic deficits. Preceding viral infections are usually incriminated but are documented in only half of cases. Considering that children have an average of four to six viral infections a year, it is not surprising that 50% of any group of children have a history of a viral illness during the preceding 30 days. There is no evidence that acute cerebellar ataxia is caused by immunization.

Acute Cerebellar Ataxia

Acute cerebellar ataxia affects children between 1 and 5 years of age but may occur as late as 14 years. Males and females are affected equally, and the incidence among family members is not increased.

Clinical Features. The onset is explosive. A previously healthy infant awakens from a nap and cannot stand. Ataxia is maximal at onset. Some worsening may occur during the first hours, but a longer progression, or a waxing and waning course, makes the diagnosis unlikely. Ataxia varies from mild unsteadiness while walking to complete inability to stand or walk. Even when ataxia is severe, sensorium is clear and the child is otherwise normal. Tendon reflexes may be present or absent; their absence suggests Miller-Fisher syndrome. Nystagmus, when present, is usually mild. Chaotic movements of the eyes (opsoclonus) should suggest the myoclonic encephalopathy–neuroblastoma syndrome.

Symptoms may begin to remit after a few days, but complete recovery takes 3 weeks to 5 months. Patients with pure ataxia of the trunk or limbs and only mild nystagmus are likely to recover completely. Marked nystagmus or opsoclonus (myoclonic encephalopathy), tremors of the head and trunk, or moderate irritability is likely to be followed by persistent neurologic sequelae.

Diagnosis.   The diagnosis of acute postinfectious cerebellitis is one of exclusion. Every child should have drug screening and a brain imaging study. One possible exception is a child in whom ataxia develops during varicella infection. The association between the two is well established, and further diagnostic tests may not be needed. If cranial computed tomography (CT) or MRI findings are normal, lumbar puncture is indicated to exclude encephalitis (Figure 10–1).

Treatment.   Acute postinfectious cerebellitis is a self-limited disease. Treatment is not required.

Miller-Fisher Syndrome

The Miller-Fisher syndrome is characterized by ataxia, ophthalmoplegia, and areflexia. It is generally regarded as a variant of the Guillain-Barré syndrome (Asbury, 1981), although some believe that it may represent a brainstem encephalitis (Al-Din et al, 1982). The disorder is believed to be harmless, and recovery is expected.

Clinical Features.   A viral illness precedes the neurologic symptoms by 5 to 10 days in 50% of cases. Either ophthalmoparesis or ataxia may be the initial feature. Both are present early in the course. The most common ocular motor disturbance is paralysis of vertical gaze; upward gaze is more severely affected than downward gaze. The Bell phenomenon may be preserved despite paralysis of voluntary upward gaze, suggesting the possibility of a supranuclear palsy (Meienberg and Ryffel, 1983). Horizontal gaze is generally preserved, but dissociated nystagmus, most marked in the abducting eye, may be present. Ptosis occurs but is less severe than the vertical gaze palsy.

Ataxia is more prominent in the limbs than in the trunk and like the areflexia is probably caused by decreased peripheral sensory input. Weakness of the limbs may be noted. Unilateral or bilateral facial weakness occurs in a significant minority of children. The course is similar to that of Guillain-Barré syndrome. Recovery generally begins 2 to 4 weeks after symptoms become maximal and is complete within 6 months.

Diagnosis.   The clinical distinction between the Miller-Fisher syndrome and brainstem encephalitis can be difficult. Disturbances of sensorium, multiple cranial nerve palsies, an abnormal EEG, or prolongation of the interpeak latencies of the brainstem auditory evoked response should suggest a brainstem encephalitis. The cerebrospinal fluid profile in the Miller-Fisher syndrome parallels that of the Guillain-Barré syndrome. A cellular response is noted early in the course, and protein elevation occurs later.

Treatment.   Corticosteroids, adrenocorticotropic hormone (ACTH), and plasmapheresis have not shown benefit in treating the Miller-Fisher syndrome. The outcome in untreated children is excellent.

Multiple Sclerosis

Multiple sclerosis is usually a disease of young adults, but children as young as 24 months have been reported who fulfill the criteria for multiple sclerosis (Bejar and Ziegler, 1984). Whether the childhood forms of multiple sclerosis are etiologically distinct from the adult types has not been determined.

Clinical Features.   The female-to-male ratio varies from 2:1 to 4:1 (Bouton et al, 1988; Bye et al, 1985). Ataxia, concurrent with a febrile episode, is the most common initial feature in children. Encephalopathy, hemiparesis, or seizures are alternative initial manifestations. Intranuclear ophthalmoplegia that may be unilateral or bilateral develops in one third of patients (see Chapter 15).

Clinical features are sufficiently protean that a single prototype cannot be provided. The essential feature is repeated episodes of demyelination in noncontiguous areas of the central nervous system. Each episode is characterized by the rapid development of focal neurologic deficits that persist for weeks and months; afterward the child has partial or complete recovery. Recurrences are separated by months or years and are frequently associated with febrile illnesses. Lethargy, nausea, and vomiting sometimes accompany the attacks in children, but rarely in adults.

The child is usually irritable and demonstrates

truncal and limb ataxia. Tendon reflexes are generally brisk throughout. Long-term outcome is unpredictable.

Diagnosis. Multiple sclerosis may be suspected at the time of the first attack, but definitive diagnosis requires recurrence to establish a polyphasic course. Examination of the cerebrospinal fluid at the time of exacerbation reveals fewer than 25 lymphocytes/mm³, a normal or mildly elevated protein content, and sometimes the presence of oligoclonal bands.

Low-density lesions in the white matter can often be seen on a contrast-enhanced CT scan, but MRI is a considerably more powerful technique for imaging areas of demyelination (Figure 10–3). However, the extent and severity of lesions on MRI may not correlate with the clinical syndrome (Osborn et al, 1990). Visual evoked responses are useful to document prior or concurrent optic neuritis, and peroneal somatosensory evoked responses can be used to document myelitis.

Treatment. A course of ACTH or corticosteroids is recommended at the time of acute exacerbations. Prednisone is generally administered orally at a dosage of 2 mg/kg/day for 1 week and is then rapidly tapered and discontinued at the end of a month. Some believe that ACTH is superior to corticosteroids in adults with multiple sclerosis.

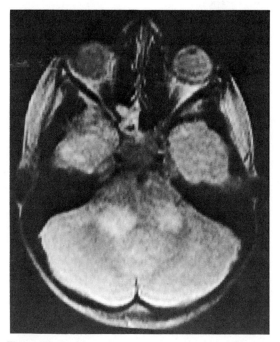

Figure 10–3 Magnetic resonance image in multiple sclerosis. Two areas of increased signal intensity are present in the cerebellum.

Aqueous ACTH, 80 units, is given intravenously over 8 hours in 5% dextrose and water each day for 3 days. Forty units of ACTH gel is then given intramuscularly every 12 hours for 7 days. Each injection is reduced by 5 units every 3 days. Improvement, when it occurs, is expected during the first 2 weeks.

Myoclonic Encephalopathy–Neuroblastoma Syndrome

Myoclonic encephalopathy is a syndrome characterized by chaotic eye movements (dancing eyes, opsoclonus), myoclonic ataxia, and encephalopathy. It may occur either as an idiopathic syndrome or as the result of an occult neuroblastoma. The common pathophysiologic mechanism is an altered immune state. The clinical presentation and the neurologic outcome are the same regardless of whether neuroblastoma is present (Bolthauser et al, 1979).

Clinical Features. The mean age at onset is 19 months with a range from 6 months to 6 years. Unlike acute postinfectious cerebellitis and the Miller-Fisher syndrome, in which neurologic symptoms are fully expressed within 1 to 2 days, the evolution of symptoms in myoclonic encephalopathy may take a week or longer.

Either ataxia or chaotic eye movements may bring the child to medical attention. Almost half of these children demonstrate personality change or irritability, suggesting the presence of a more diffuse encephalopathy. Some children are described as having a cerebellar ataxia, whereas others are said to be incoordinated because of myoclonus, constant rapid muscular contractions that have an irregular occurrence and a widespread distribution (see Chapter 14). Opsoclonus is a disorder of ocular muscles that is similar to myoclonus. It is characterized by spontaneous, conjugate, irregular jerking of the eyes in all directions. The movements are most prominent with attempts to change fixation and are then associated with blinking or eyelid flutter. Opsoclonus persists even in sleep and becomes more severe with agitation.

Diagnosis. The myoclonic encephalopathy syndrome can be diagnosed on clinical grounds, but laboratory investigation is required to determine the underlying cause (Figure 10–1). The presence of an occult neuroblastoma should be suspected in all children with recurrent ataxia or the myoclonic encephalopathy syndrome. Acute ataxia that progresses over several days or waxes and wanes is more likely to be caused by neuroblastoma than by acute cerebellitis.

In children with myoclonic encephalopathy

caused by occult neuroblastoma, the tumor is equally likely to be in the chest or the abdomen. In contrast, only 10% to 15% of neuroblastomas are in the chest when myoclonic encephalopathy is absent. The evaluation for neuroblastoma should include careful palpation of the abdomen, MRI of chest and abdomen (Figure 10–4), and measurement of the urinary excretion of homovanillic acid (HVA) and vanillylmandelic acid (VMA) and of serum metanephrine (Tuchman et al, 1985). I have found elevated excretion of VMA or HVA to be the most reliable indicator of tumor. Studies should be repeated until the tumor is found.

Treatment.   Partial or complete remission of the neurologic syndrome may occur regardless of whether neuroblastoma is present. In most patients the course is prolonged, with waxing and waning of neurologic dysfunction. Either ACTH or oral corticosteroids provide partial or complete relief of symptoms in 80% of patients, including those with neuroblastoma. Marked improvement usually occurs 1 to 4 weeks after initiation of therapy. Relapses occur when therapy is discontinued but may also occur while treatment is in progress.

Neuroblastoma, when present, must be removed. However, the long-term neurologic outcome is the same regardless of whether neuroblastoma is present or corticosteroids are used. Approximately half of affected children will have impaired motor ability, and one third will have some disturbance in intellectual function (Bolthauser et al, 1979).

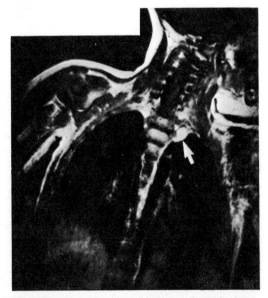

Figure 10–4 Apical neuroblastoma *(arrow)* demonstrated by magnetic resonance imaging in a child with normal radiographs and computed tomograms of chest.

Pseudoataxia (Epileptic)

Clinical Features.   Ataxia and other gait disturbances may be the only manifestation of epileptiform activity (Bennett et al, 1982). The child's epilepsy may not have been recognized before the onset of ataxia. Both gait and limb ataxia may be present. The gait disturbance may be blamed on overdose if the child is already taking anticonvulsant medication.

During the ataxic episode the child may appear inattentive or confused. Like other seizure manifestations, ataxia is sudden in onset and episodic.

Diagnosis.   The absence of nystagmus should suggest that ataxia is a seizure manifestation and is not caused by drug toxicity. Concurrent with the ataxia are prolonged, generalized, 2 to 3 Hz spike-wave complexes that have a frontal predominance. This is the typical EEG finding in the Lennox-Gastaut syndrome (see Chapter 1). Such discharges are ordinarily associated with myoclonic jerks or akinetic seizures. Either one occurring momentarily, but repeatedly, could interrupt smooth movement and produce ataxia.

Treatment.   Pseudoataxia usually responds to anticonvulsant drugs. Clonazepam and valproate are most often used for slow spike-wave discharges (see Chapter 1).

TRAUMA

Mild head injuries are common in children, especially toddlers. Recovery is always complete despite considerable parental concern. More serious head injuries, associated with loss of consciousness, seizures, and cerebral contusion, are less common but still account for several thousand deaths in children annually. Ataxia may follow head injuries, even mild ones. In most of these cases the ataxia is part of the so-called postconcussion syndrome, in which no structural derangement of the nervous system can be demonstrated. In others a cerebellar contusion or posterior fossa hematoma may be present (see Chapter 2).

Ataxia may also follow cervical injuries, especially during sports. These are usually caused by trauma to the vertebrobasilar artery.

Postconcussion Syndrome

Clinical Features.   Many adults complain of headache, dizziness, and mental changes following even a mild head injury. The frequency of such complaints is greater and the symptoms are more severe and long lasting when litigation is pending. Some of these symptoms also occur after head injury in children and probably represent a transitory derangement of cerebral function caused by the trauma. Even mild head trauma can produce structural disturbances in the brain, which may explain the persistence of symptoms.

In infants and small children the most prominent postconcussive symptom is ataxia. This is not necessarily a typical cerebellar ataxia but may be only an unsteady gait. No limb dysmetria is present, and the remainder of the neurologic findings are normal.

In older children with postconcussive syndromes, headache and dizziness are as common as ataxia. The headache is usually described as low grade and constant, sometimes made worse by movements of the head. Gait is less disturbed, possibly because an older child better compensates for dizziness, but the sensation of unsteadiness is still described.

Diagnosis. An imaging study is necessary in many children with postconcussive symptoms to exclude the possibility of subdural hematoma.

Treatment. Ataxia usually clears completely within 1 month and always within 6 months. Decreased activity during this time is recommended. Usually no further treatment is required.

Vertebrobasilar Occlusion

Trauma to the vertebrobasilar arteries is reported with chiropractic manipulation and sports injuries (Zimmerman et al, 1978). The vertebral arteries are encased in bony canals from C-2 to the foramen magnum. Sudden stretching of the arteries by hyperextension or hyperflexion of the neck causes endothelial injury and thrombosis.

Clinical Features. Symptoms are noted within minutes or hours of injury. Vertigo, nausea, and vomiting are the initial manifestations of brainstem ischemia. Occipital headache may be present as well. Ataxia is due to incoordination of the limbs on one side. It may be maximal at onset or progress over several days.

Examination demonstrates some combination of unilateral brainstem disturbances (diplopia, facial weakness) and ipsilateral cerebellar dysfunction.

Diagnosis. CT or MRI reveals a unilateral infarction in the cerebellar hemisphere. The lateral medulla may also be infarcted. The location of arterial thrombosis is visualized by arteriography.

Treatment. Many children recover completely in the months that follow injury. The value of anticoagulation has not been established.

VASCULAR DISORDERS
Cerebellar Hemorrhage

Spontaneous cerebellar hemorrhage in children, in the absence of a coagulopathy, is due to arteriovenous malformation, even though less than 10% of intracranial arteriovenous malformations in children are in the cerebellum. The two major features of cerebellar hemorrhage are ataxia and headache.

Lupus Erythematosus

Cerebellar disturbances occur in systemic lupus erythematosus (Sergent et al, 1975). The peak incidence of lupus erythematosus is in girls near the time of puberty.

Clinical Features. The major clinical features are fever, rash, arthritis or arthralgia, and cardiac abnormalities, including cardiomegaly, pericarditis, myocarditis, and congestive heart failure. Gastrointestinal bleeding, abnormal renal function, and cardiac disturbances indicate a poor prognosis for survival. Neurologic complications of lupus erythematosus ordinarily occur late in the course of disease, after the diagnosis is already established. The most common neurologic manifestations are seizures, personality changes, and chorea. However, cerebellar ataxia is sometimes noted as an isolated finding or in association with other neurologic manifestations.

Diagnosis. Systemic lupus erythematosus is an unlikely diagnosis in a previously healthy child with acute ataxia. When clinical symptoms and signs are compatible with the diagnosis, the demonstration of high concentrations of antinuclear antibody is confirmatory.

Treatment. Corticosteroids alone or in combination with cytotoxic agents are used to treat the underlying disease and its neurologic complications. Daily administration of high-dose corticosteroids is recommended, although their benefit has not been established.

Kawasaki Disease

Kawasaki disease is a systemic vasculitis that occurs predominantly in infants and children.

Clinical Features. Five of the following six criteria are required for diagnosis: fever, conjunctival congestion, reddening of the oropharynx and lips, indurative edema of the limbs, polymorphic exanthems, and lymphadenopathy. Arthralgia, carditis, and aseptic meningitis may be associated features. The disease is thought to be identical to childhood polyarteritis nodosa.

Multiple infarcts may occur in the brain. Acute ataxia, facial palsy, ocular motor palsies, and hemiplegia have been reported (Scully et al, 1986). Prognosis is guarded, partly because of the neurologic complications but mainly because of coronary artery disease.

Diagnosis. Clinical features of multisystem disease are essential for diagnosis. Abnormal laboratory findings include an increased sedimentation rate, a positive test for C-reactive protein, and increased serum complement and globulin levels. Typical changes of arteritis are demonstrated by skin biopsy.

Treatment. No effective method of treatment has been established. Aspirin is usually recommended. Corticosteroids are thought to increase coronary artery disease. Some studies suggest that intravenous high-dose gammaglobulin may be useful.

◆ Chronic or Progressive Ataxia

Brain tumor is always an initial consideration when progressive ataxia develops in children who were previously normal, especially if headache is present as well (Table 10–2). Congenital abnormalities that cause ataxia are frequently associated with some degree of mental deficiency. The onset of symptoms may occur during infancy or be delayed until adult life. With the exception of Friedreich ataxia, chronic ataxia is rarely hereditary. However, most cases are easily diagnosed and many are treatable. Failure to diagnose the underlying cause of chronic ataxia can have unfortunate consequences for the child.

BRAIN TUMORS

Neuroectodermal tumors are the second most common malignancy of childhood and the most common solid tumor. Posterior fossa tumors are more common than supratentorial tumors between the ages of 1 and 8 years and account for approximately 50% of brain tumors in children of all ages (Schulte, 1984). The four major tumors of the posterior fossa are cerebellar astrocytoma, brainstem glioma, ependymoma, and medulloblastoma. Ataxia is a late manifestation of brainstem glioma; the initial features are disturbances of cranial nerve function (see Chapter 15). Although this discussion is limited to tumors of the posterior fossa, it is important to remember that supratentorial brain tumors may also cause ataxia. Twenty-two percent of children with supratentorial brain tumors have gait disturbances at the time of their first hospitalization, and 17% have "cerebellar signs" (Gjerris, 1978). Gait disturbances occur with equal frequency whether supratentorial tumors are in the midline or the hemispheres, whereas cerebellar signs are more common with midline tumors.

Cerebellar Astrocytoma

Cerebellar astrocytomas constitute 16% to 20% of brain tumors in children. Less than 20% are malignant. The tumor may be in the hemisphere, in the vermis, or in both hemisphere and vermis or may occupy the fourth ventricle (Tomita, 1983).

Clinical Features. Both sexes are affected equally. The onset of symptoms is usually after 3 years of age but may be as early as infancy. Headache is the most common initial complaint in school-age children, whereas unsteadiness of gait and vomiting are the initial symptoms in preschool children. Headache can be insidious and intermittent; only rarely is there typical morning headache and vomiting. The first complaints of headache and nausea are usually attributed to a flulike illness. Only when symptoms persist is the possibility of increased intracranial pressure considered. In infants and small children symptoms of increased intracranial pressure are often relieved by the separation of cranial sutures. For this reason gait disturbances without headache or vomiting are the common initial sign of cerebellar astrocytoma in infants.

Papilledema is present in almost 83% of affected children at initial examination but is often absent in infants with separation of cranial sutures. Ataxia is present in 72%, dysmetria in 50%, and nystagmus in only 22% of these children.

Ataxia varies in severity from a wide-based lurching gait to a subtle alteration of gait observed only with tandem walking or quick turning. It is caused in part by the cerebellar location of the tumor and in part by hydrocephalus. When the tumor is in the cerebellar hemisphere, ipsilateral or bilateral dysmetria may be present. Other neurologic signs sometimes present in children with cerebellar astrocytoma include abducens palsy, multiple cranial nerve palsies, stiff neck, and head tilt.

Diagnosis. CT or MRI is suitable for diagnosis.

Treatment. Children with life-threatening hydrocephalus should undergo a shunting procedure as the first step in treatment. The shunt relieves many of the symptoms and signs, including ataxia (Hendrick, 1983).

Corticosteroids are sufficient to relieve pressure in many children with less severe hydrocephalus.

An astrocytoma in the cerebellar hemisphere can be surgically extirpated. Such tumors are usually cystic, and removal of the mural nodule is curative. Deeper tumors that involve the floor of the fourth ventricle are rarely removed in toto. Local recurrence is common after partial resection. Repeat surgery may be curative in some cases, but postoperative radiation therapy appears to offer a better prognosis following partial resection. In one series the overall disease-free survival rates following either surgery alone or surgery and radiation therapy were 92% at 5 years and 88% at 25 years (Garcia et al, 1989). Chemotherapy is not currently recommended for low-grade cerebellar astrocytomas regardless of the degree of surgical resection.

High-grade cerebellar astrocytoma (glioblastoma) has rarely been reported in children. More than 30% of childhood patients have dissemination of tumor through the neuraxis (spinal cord drop metastases). Examination of cerebrospinal fluid for cytologic features and complete myelography are recommended following surgical resection in all patients with glioblastoma. If either result is abnormal, whole-axis radiation therapy is indicated.

Cerebellar Hemangioblastoma (von Hippel–Lindau Disease)

Von Hippel–Lindau disease is a multisystem disorder transmitted by autosomal dominant inheritance (Neumann and Wiestler, 1991). The most prominent feature is hemangioblastomas of the cerebellum and retina (Maher et al, 1990). All children with cerebellar hemangioblastoma have von Hippel–Lindau disease. Among adults, 60% have isolated tumors and do not have the genetic defect. The expression of von Hippel–Lindau disease is variable even within a kindred. The most common manifestations are cerebellar and retinal hemangioblastoma (59%), renal carcinoma (28%), and pheochromocytoma (7%).

Clinical Features.   Mean age at onset of cerebellar hemangioblastoma in von Hippel–Lindau disease is 32 years; onset before 15 is unusual. The initial features are headache and ataxia. Retinal hemangioblastomas occur at a younger age and may cause visual impairment resulting from hemorrhage as early as the first decade. They may be multiple and bilateral and appear on ophthalmoscopic examination as a dilated artery leading from the disk to a peripheral tumor with an engorged vein.

Diagnosis.   The diagnosis of von Hippel–Lindau disease is based on the presence of any of the following: more than one hemangioblastoma of the central nervous system; an isolated hemangioblastoma associated with a visceral cyst or renal carcinoma; or any known manifestation with a family history of the disease.

Gadolinium-enhanced MRI is useful for detecting tumors in the central nervous system (Filling-Katz et al, 1991). Visceral manifestations can be identified by abdominal CT scan and ultrasound.

Treatment.   Children at risk for von Hippel–Lindau disease should be screened for retinal hemangioblastomas by indirect ophthalmoscopy every 5 years. Cryotherapy or photocoagulation of smaller lesions can lead to complete tumor regression without visual loss.

MRI should be performed in any child with ataxia and at 5-year intervals after 15 years of age in persons with genetic risk factors. Cerebellar hemangioblastoma should be treated surgically and can often be totally extirpated.

Visceral manifestations are uncommon in childhood, but adults must be screened with abdominal CT.

Ependymoma

Posterior fossa ependymoma is derived from the cells that line the roof and floor of the fourth ventricle. These tumors can extend into both lateral recesses and grow out to the cerebellopontine angle. They account for 10% of primary brain tumors in children.

Clinical Features.   Ependymoma is primarily a tumor of young children; 50% become symptomatic before three years of age (Choux, 1983). Both sexes are affected equally.

Symptoms evolve more slowly in children with ependymoma than in those with medulloblastoma. Symptoms are commonly present for several months before medical consultation is sought. Symptoms for increased intracranial pressure are the first manifestation in 90% of patients. Disturbances of gait and coordination, neck pain, or cranial nerve dysfunction is the initial symptom in the remainder. Fifty percent of patients have ataxia, usually of the vermal type, and 33% have nystagmus. Head tilt or neck stiffness is present in one third of children and indicates extension of tumor into the cervical canal.

Although steady deterioration is expected, some children have an intermittent course. Transient episodes of headache and vomiting, ataxia, and even nuchal rigidity lasting for days or weeks are followed by periods of well-being. These intermittent symptoms are caused by transitory obstruction of the fourth ventricle or aqueduct by the tumor acting in a ball-valve fashion.

Diagnosis.   CT and MRI are equally useful for

diagnosis. The ventricular system is almost always markedly dilated. MRI better demonstrates the tumor's location in the fourth ventricle and its extraventricular extensions.

Treatment.   The goals of surgical therapy are to relieve the hydrocephalus and to remove as much tumor as possible without damaging the fourth ventricle. Postoperative irradiation to the posterior fossa, but not the neuraxis, is usually indicated. A postoperative mortality rate of approximately 30% is noted in several series. Five-year survival rates vary from 33% to 70%.

High-grade ependymomas and ependymoblastomas are likely to seed the spinal subarachnoid space and require whole neuraxis irradiation. In addition, chemotherapeutic agents similar to those used for medulloblastoma should be administered.

Medulloblastoma

Medulloblastoma is a primitive neuroectodermal tumor with the capacity to differentiate into neuronal and glial tissue. Most tumors are in the vermis or fourth ventricle with or without extension into the cerebellar hemispheres. Approximately 10% are in the hemisphere alone (Tomita, 1983).

Clinical Features.   Most series indicate a male-to-female ratio of 3:2. Ninety percent of cases have their onset during the first decade and the remainder during the second decade. Medulloblastoma is the most common primary brain tumor with onset of symptoms during infancy.

The tumor grows rapidly, and the interval between onset of symptoms and medical consultation is generally brief: 2 weeks in 25% of cases and less than a month in 50%. Vomiting is an initial symptom in 58% of children, headache in 40%, an unsteady gait in 20%, and torticollis or stiff neck in 10%. The predominance of vomiting, with or without headache, as an early symptom is probably caused when the tumor irritates the floor of the fourth ventricle. Gait disturbances are more common in young children and are characterized by refusal to stand or walk rather than by ataxia.

Two thirds of children have papilledema at the time of initial examination. Truncal ataxia and limb ataxia are equally common, and both may be present. Only 22% of children have nystagmus. Tendon reflexes are hyperactive when hydrocephalus is present and hypoactive when the tumor is causing primarily cerebellar dysfunction.

Diagnosis.   Medulloblastoma is readily diagnosed with CT or MRI (Figure 10–5). The tumors are highly vascular and become enhanced when contrast medium is used.

Treatment.   The prognosis for children with

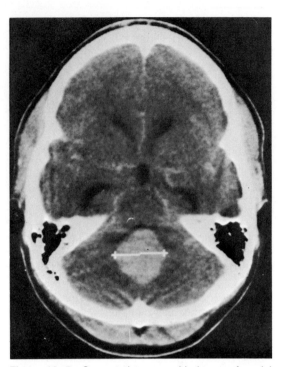

Figure 10–5   Computed tomographic image of medulloblastoma. The tumor is demonstrated as an enhancing mass in the vermis of the cerebellum.

medulloblastoma is greatly improved by the combined use of surgical extirpation, radiation therapy, and chemotherapy. The role of surgery is to provide histologic identification, debulk the tumor, and relieve obstruction of the fourth ventricle.

Children with medulloblastoma are divided into high- and low-risk groups for the purpose of designing therapy. The high-risk, or poor prognosis, group includes those with any evidence of tumor dissemination, more than 1.5 cm^2 of residual tumor following initial surgery, tumors invading two structures or completely filling the fourth ventricle, or tumor filling the fourth ventricle and extending to the third ventricle or the cervical cord. Radiation therapy is necessary for children in both the high- and low-risk groups. Medulloblastoma is more radiosensitive than is glioma, and a lower total dose of radiation can be used (Tomita and McLone, 1986). Before radiation is initiated, a complete myelogram must be obtained to determine whether drop metastases are present. Areas with visible metastatic disease receive a larger radiation dose.

Children in the high-risk group are treated with chemotherapy as well as radiation. This combination has improved 5-year survival rates by more than 10%. Experimental protocols are being tested, and children with medulloblastoma should be referred to specialized centers for chemotherapy (Packer, 1990).

When the combined approaches of surgery, irradiation, and chemotherapy are used, the 5-year survival rate is 50% to 70%.

CONGENITAL MALFORMATIONS
Basilar Impression

Basilar impression is a disorder of the craniovertebral junction in which the odontoid process is displaced posteriorly and compresses the spinal cord or brainstem.

Clinical Features.   The first symptoms are often head tilt, neck stiffness, and headache. The onset of symptoms is frequently precipitated by minor trauma to the head or neck. Examination reveals ataxia, nystagmus, and hyperreflexia (Teodori and Painter, 1984).

Diagnosis.   CT demonstrates invagination of the odontoid process into the foramen magnum. MRI may be useful to delineate an associated Chiari malformation or syringobulbia (Figure 10–6).

Treatment.   Surgical decompression of the foramen magnum usually relieves symptoms.

Cerebellar Malformations
Cerebellar Hemisphere Hypoplasia

Congenital hypoplasia of the cerebellum occurs in humans as an autosomal recessive disease and can be experimentally induced in immature animals by cytotoxic drugs, irradiation, or viral infection. The common histologic feature is the absence of granular cells with a relative preservation of Purkinje cells. In the human hereditary form, granular cell degeneration may continue postnatally and cause progressive cerebellar dysfunction during infancy. Most cases of human cerebellar hypoplasia are sporadic. Although the causes are diverse, the clinical features are relatively constant (Sarnat and Alcala, 1980).

Clinical Features.   Developmental delay and hypotonia are the first features suggesting a cerebral abnormality in the infant. Titubation of the head is a constant feature, and some combination of ataxia, dysmetria, and intention tremor is also noted. A jerky coarse nystagmus is usually present. Tendon reflexes may be increased or diminished. Those with hyperactive reflexes probably have congenital abnormalities of the corticospinal tract in addition to cerebellar hypoplasia. Seizures occur in some hereditary and some sporadic cases. Other neurologic signs and symptoms may be present, depending on associated malformations. Mental retardation is a constant feature but varies from mild to severe.

Diagnosis.   Cerebellar hypoplasia can be demonstrated by CT or MRI (Figure 10–6). The folial pattern of the cerebellum is prominent, and there is compensatory enlargement of the fourth ventricle, cisterna magna, and vallecula.

Treatment.   No treatment is available.

Vermal Aplasia

Aplasia of the vermis is relatively common and often associated with other cerebral malformations. All or part of the vermis may be missing, and when

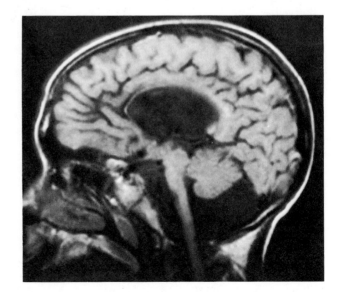

Figure 10–6   Aplasia of the cerebellum associated with thinnng of the corpus callosum.

the vermis is incomplete, the caudal portion is usually lacking.

Clinical Features. Partial agenesis of the cerebellar vermis may be asymptomatic. Three families with dominantly inherited aplasia of the anterior vermis have been reported; whether the pattern is autosomal or X-linked dominant is unknown (Fenichel and Phillips, 1989). Symptoms are nonprogressive and vary from only mild gait ataxia and upbeating nystagmus to severe ataxia.

Complete agenesis causes titubation of the head and truncal ataxia. Vermal agenesis is frequently associated with other cerebral malformations, producing a constellation of symptoms and signs referable to neurologic dysfunction. Two such examples are the Dandy-Walker malformation (see Chapter 18) and the *Joubert syndrome* (Appleton et al, 1989).

Cerebellar vermal agenesis is a constant feature of the Joubert syndrome, but several other cerebral malformations are usually present as well. More than one sibling in a family may be involved, but the parents are normal. The typical clinical manifestation in newborns and infants is periods of hyperpnea, usually about 120 breaths/min and lasting for up to 16 seconds, alternating with episodes of apnea lasting up to 12 seconds. Abnormal, conjugate jerking eye movements are observed in half of infants. Most infants are hypotonic. Tendon reflexes may be normal or exaggerated. All patients are mentally retarded, and some are microcephalic. Several affected children have died unexpectedly, possibly from respiratory failure.

Diagnosis. CT or MRI shows agenesis of the vermis of the cerebellum with enlargement of the cisterna magna. Other cerebral malformations, such as agenesis of the corpus callosum, may be observed as well.

Treatment. No treatment is available.

Chiari Malformation

The Chiari malformation is a displacement of the cerebellar tonsils into the upper cervical canal, sometimes accompanied by caudal dislocation of the hindbrain. Children with the Chiari malformation may have myelomeningocele as well (see Chapter 12). When the Chiari malformation is present without meningocele, the onset of symptoms is frequently delayed until adolescence or adult life.

Clinical Features. Major clinical features are headache, head tilt, pain in the neck and shoulders, ataxia, and lower cranial nerve dysfunction (Levy et al, 1983). Physical signs vary among patients. Features found in approximately half of cases include weakness of the arms, hyperactive tendon reflexes in the legs, nystagmus, and ataxia.

Diagnosis. MRI provides the best visualization of posterior fossa structures. The distortion of the cerebellum and hindbrain is precisely identified (Figure 10–7).

Treatment. Surgical decompression of the foramen magnum to at least the C3 vertebra is recommended (Park et al, 1983). More than half of patients are significantly improved by surgery.

HEREDITARY ATAXIA
Autosomal Dominant Inheritance

Several types of ataxia are transmitted by autosomal dominant inheritance. Some have been reported in only a single family (Farmer et al, 1989). Unfortunately, the dominantly inherited ataxias are difficult to differentiate on clinical grounds, and perhaps even on pathologic grounds, because the abnormal gene and the abnormal gene product(s) are unknown. Considerable phenotypic variability is seen even within a kindred. Two terms are used in the literature to describe progressive dominantly inherited ataxia: *olivopontocerebellar degeneration* and *Machado-Joseph disease*. The neuropathologic features of olivopontocerebellar atrophy have also been described as part of a multisystem disease that is transmitted by autosomal recessive inheritance and is manifested in newborns as hypotonia and arthrogryposis (see Chapter 6).

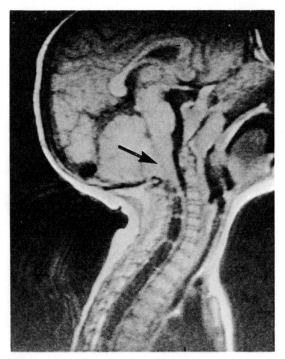

Figure 10–7 Chiari malformation. Magnetic resonance image demonstrates displacement of the cerebellar tonsils *(arrow)* into the foramen magnum.

Machado-Joseph Disease

In contrast to the olivopontocerebellar degenerations, Machado-Joseph disease is genetically homogeneous. It originated in Portuguese-Azorean populations and was transmitted worldwide by Portugese sailors during the age of exploration. The age at onset appears to be earlier with each generation (anticipation), and onset during adolescence is relatively common.

Clinical Features. Machado-Joseph disease is characterized by a degeneration of all motor systems: cerebellar, extrapyramidal, pyramidal, and motor unit. However, ataxia is usually the first symptom. Unsteadiness of gait is followed by dysmetria of the hands. Nystagmus is often present, and tendon reflexes may be diminished or brisk if the corticospinal tract is involved.

Within a family some members have predominantly a dystonic disorder, others have ataxia and pyramidal signs, and still others demonstrate amyotrophy (Fowler, 1984; Lima and Coutinho, 1980). Dystonia is somewhat more common than ataxia as the initial sign in children. Bulging eyes are a characteristic, but not constant, early feature of the disorder. Multimotor system degeneration eventually develops in all cases, with death occurring in middle to late adult life.

Diagnosis. Diagnosis depends on the clinical features and a family history of the disease. Neurodiagnostic studies do not add to the physical examination. In families with several affected members, individuals recognize the disease in themselves and may not seek medical attention.

Treatment. Treatment is not available for the underlying genetic defect, but Parkinson-like symptoms may be reversed by L-dopa and dystonia may respond to trihexyphenidyl.

Olivopontocerebellar Degeneration

The olivopontocerebellar degenerations have their onset between 15 and 35 years of age. They are broadly divided into two subgroups, one in which the genetic defect is linked to the HLA locus on the short arm of chromosome 6 and the other in which this linkage is not present (Nino et al, 1980). When the linkage is present, the onset is usually after 20 years of age but can be in childhood (Zoghbi et al, 1988).

Clinical Features. Cerebellar ataxia is invariably present and is frequently the initial manifestation. Gait ataxia, dysmetria, dysdiadochokinesia, finger-nose ataxia, and decomposition of movement are present. Patients with childhood onset often have mental retardation and seizures. Tendon reflexes are exaggerated, and the plantar response is usually extensor. Optic nerve atrophy is a constant finding in some families. Other variable features include nystagmus, dysarthria, decreased pupillary response, ptosis, and impaired position sense.

Diagnosis. Diagnosis depends on the clinical features and family history.

Treatment. No treatment is available.

Ramsay Hunt Variants

The Ramsay Hunt syndrome is discussed with genetic ataxias transmitted by autosomal recessive inheritance (see later discussion). However, the same complex of symptoms also occurs in two dominantly inherited disorders in which dentatorubral degeneration is associated with (1) progressive atrophy of the globus pallidus and subthalamic nucleus *(dentatorubral-pallidoluysian degeneration)* (Takahashi et al, 1988) or (2) a mitochondrial myopathy (Feit et al, 1983; Fitzsimons et al, 1981).

Clinical Features. In families with combined dentatorubral-pallidoluysian degeneration the onset of symptoms may be in childhood or adult life and a wide variety of clinical syndromes occur within a kindred. Patients with childhood onset usually have a progressive myoclonic epilepsy syndrome (see Chapter 1), whereas those with an adult onset have ataxia, dementia, and chorea as initial features. Dementia, dysarthria, and ataxia of gait and limbs eventually occur in all cases.

Patients with widespread mitochondrial disease have mental retardation and proximal weakness in addition to the cerebellar ataxia and myoclonus.

Diagnosis. Ramsay Hunt variants transmitted by autosomal dominant inheritance are easy to differentiate from sporadic cases by family history.

Treatment. Myoclonus and seizures should be treated with valproate. One patient with a mitochondrial disorder responded to oral doses of L-5-hydroxytryptophan and carbidopa.

Autosomal Recessive Inheritance
Abetalipoproteinemia

Abetalipoproteinemia is a disorder of lipid metabolism transmitted by autosomal recessive inheritance. Other terms for the disorder are *acanthocytosis* and the *Bassen-Kornzweig syndrome.* Apolipoprotein B, which is essential for the synthesis and structural integrity of low-density and very-low-density lipoproteins, is missing from the serum. The results are fat malabsorption and a progressive deficiency of vitamins A, E, and K.

Clinical Features. Fat malabsorption is present from birth, and most newborns come to medical attention because of failure to thrive, vomiting, and large volumes of loose stool. The correct diagnosis may be made at that time.

Psychomotor development during infancy is delayed. A cerebellar ataxia develops in one third of children during the first decade and in almost every child by the end of the second decade. The progression of symptoms may suggest Friedreich ataxia. Tendon reflexes are usually lost by 5 years of age. Progressive limb ataxia is characterized by gait disturbances, dysmetria, and difficulty with performing rapid alternating movements. Ataxia progresses until the third decade and then becomes stationary. Proprioceptive sensation is lost in the hands and feet, and pinprick and temperature sensations are mildly reduced. Sensory loss results from demyelination in the posterior columns of the spinal cord and the peripheral nerves (Wichman et al, 1985).

Retinitis pigmentosa is an almost constant feature of abetalipoproteinemia. The age at onset is variable but is usually during the first decade. The initial symptom is night blindness. Nystagmus is common and may be caused either by the cerebellar disturbance or by loss of central vision.

Diagnosis. The acanthocyte is the hallmark of abetalipoproteinemia and other lipoprotein deficiencies. It is an abnormal erythrocyte characterized by thorny projections from the cell surface that prevent normal rouleau formation and cause a very low erythrocyte sedimentation rate. Between 50% and 70% of peripheral erythrocytes undergo transformation to acanthocytes. Acanthocytes are also seen in association with other neurologic disorders in which lipoproteins are normal (see the discussions of McLeod syndrome and neuroacanthocytosis).

Severe anemia, with hemoglobin levels less than 8 g/dl (5 mmol/L), is common in young children but not in adults. The anemia may result from malabsorption and can be corrected with parenteral supplementation of iron or folate. Plasma cholesterol levels are less than 100 mg/dl (2.5 mmol/L), and triglyceride levels are less than 30 mg/dl (0.3 mmol/L). The diagnosis is confirmed by the absence of apolipoprotein B in plasma. Parents should be screened for apolipoprotein B as well. In abetalipoproteinemia the heterozygote is normal; if partial deficiency of apolipoprotein B is present, the diagnosis of familial hypobetalipoproteinemia is more likely.

Treatment. It is not clear how much of the neurologic abnormality is a direct effect of lipoprotein deficiency and how much is caused by de-

ficiency of fat-soluble vitamins. Steatorrhea in newborns responds to a restricted intake of triglycerides containing long-chain fatty acids. In addition to maintaining a low-fat diet, for the rest of their lives patients should take daily doses of vitamin E, 200 to 300 IU/kg, and vitamin A, 200 to 400 IU/kg. Evidence suggests that vitamin supplementation not only prevents or retards the development of neurologic sequelae, but also may reverse a neuropathy or myopathy already present (Hegele and Angel, 1985).

Ataxia–Ocular Motor Apraxia

Ataxia–ocular motor apraxia is believed to be transmitted as an autosomal recessive trait. It shares the neurologic features of ataxia-telangiectasia but lacks the disorder of immunity (Aicardi et al, 1988).

Clinical Features. Development is normal until 2 to 7 years of age. The first symptom, ataxia of gait, is followed by ataxia of the trunk and arms. The progression of neurologic deterioration is slow. All patients have choreic movements, and some have tremor as well. Abnormal movements of the head caused by ocular motor apraxia develop between the ages of 6 and 12 years. Oculomotor apraxia is a disturbance of voluntary gaze with intact following responses. Consequently, the head turns first and the eyes follow after. The apraxia of gaze is both vertical and horizontal. Tendon reflexes are normal in the arms but diminished or absent in the legs. Intellectual function is normal. The ultimate outcome has not been established.

Diagnosis. Ataxia–ocular motor apraxia is distinguished from ataxia-telangiectasia because the onset of ataxia is after the first year and only the nervous system is involved.

Treatment. No treatment is available.

Ataxia-Telangiectasia

Ataxia-telangiectasia is a multisystem disorder affecting primarily the nervous and immune systems. It is transmitted by autosomal recessive inheritance, and the genetic abnormality is on the long arm of chromosome 11. Ataxia-telangiectasia has worldwide distribution, occurs in all races, and occurs in an estimated 1 in 40,000 births (Gatti et al, 1991).

Clinical Features. The principal feature is a progressive truncal ataxia that begins during the first year. In some infants choreoathetosis develops instead of, or in addition to, ataxia. The ataxia begins as clumsiness and progresses so slowly that cerebral palsy is often the erroneous diagnosis. Oculomotor apraxia is present in 90% of patients but may be mild at first and overlooked (see Chapter 15). Many children are said to have a dull or expressionless face. Intellectual development is normal at first but often lags with time. One third of children ultimately function in the mildly retarded range.

Telangiectasia usually develops after 2 years of age and sometimes as late as age 10. It first appears on the bulbar conjunctivae, giving the eyes a bloodshot appearance. Similar telangiectasia appears on the upper half of the ears, on the flexor surfaces of the limbs, and in a butterfly distribution on the face. Telangiectasia may be exacerbated by exposure to sun or by irritation or friction.

Recurrent sinopulmonary infection is one of the more serious features of the disease and reflects an underlying immunodeficiency. The synthesis of antibodies and certain immunoglobulin subclasses is disturbed because of disorders in B cell and helper T cell function. Serum and salivary IgA is absent in 70% to 80% of children, and IgE is absent or diminished in 80% to 90%. The IgM concentration may be elevated in compensation for the IgA deficiency. The thymus has an embryonic appearance, and alpha-fetoprotein concentrations are elevated in the majority of patients (Waldmann et al, 1983).

Taken together, the many features of this disease suggest a generalized disorder of tissue differentiation and cellular repair. The result is an increased incidence of neoplasia, especially lymphoma and lymphocytic leukemia. Two thirds of patients are dead by 20 years of age. After infection, neoplastic disease is the most common cause of death.

Diagnosis. The diagnosis should be suspected in infants who have the combination of ataxia, chronic sinopulmonary infections, and oculomotor apraxia. As the child gets older, the addition of telangiectasia to the other clinical features makes the diagnosis a certainty. Complete studies of immunocompetence should be performed. Elevated concentrations of alpha-fetoprotein and carcinoembryonic antigen are the most constant laboratory markers. Ataxia–ocular motor apraxia without telangiectasia or abnormal immunity occurs as a genetic trait that is probably different from ataxia-telangiectasia.

Treatment. All infections must be treated vigorously. Intravenous antibiotics are sometimes required for what would be trivial sinusitis in a normal child. Patients with ataxia-telangiectasia are exquisitely sensitive to radiation, which produces cellular and chromosomal damage. Radia-

tion may be a precipitant in the development of neoplasia. Therefore, despite the frequency of sinopulmonary infections, radiologic studies must be minimized.

Ataxia with Episodic Dystonia

Families are described in which the combination of ataxia, brisk tendon reflexes, and episodic dystonia is transmitted by autosomal recessive inheritance (Graff-Radford, 1986). No underlying metabolic disturbance has been identified. The syndrome begins in the first decade with the onset of progressive ataxia, which is followed by episodes of dystonia that may be unilateral. The dystonia responds to anticonvulsant drugs. The syndrome shares many features with the syndrome of familial paroxysmal choreoathetosis, except for the pattern of inheritance and the progressive nature of the ataxia (see Chapter 1).

Friedreich Ataxia

The term "Friedreich ataxia" has been used in a generic sense to describe all spinocerebellar degenerations. This usage is not helpful. Strict clinical criteria for Friedreich ataxia define a more homogeneous group of patients who have a predictable course (Harding, 1981; Stumpf, 1985). These criteria include autosomal recessive inheritance, onset of ataxia or scoliosis before 20 years of age, rapid early progression, and absence of ophthalmoplegia and dementia.

Clinical Features. Clinical features are similar in members of the same family. Heterozygotes have no manifestations of disease, and the presence of abnormal signs, such as pes cavus or scoliosis, in parents should suggest a dominantly inherited ataxia or Charcot-Marie-Tooth disease (Harding, 1981).

In the majority of cases the onset occurs between 2 and 16 years of age, but occasionally the symptoms begin earlier or later. The initial manifestation is ataxia or clumsiness of gait in 95% of cases and scoliosis in 5%. The course is one of steady deterioration; most patients are confined to a wheelchair within 20 years of onset. Dysarthria develops in all patients. Disturbances of ocular motility occur in 32% of patients and deafness in 8%. Titubation of the head is present in only 4%. Symptoms of cerebellar dysfunction are more severe and more common in the arms than in the legs. Finger-nose ataxia and difficulty in performing rapid alternating movements develop in almost every patient. Only 28% of patients demonstrate the same symptoms in the legs, but spastic weakness is often present and may hide the cerebellar signs.

All tendon reflexes are absent in 75% of patients. In the other 25%, reflexes are obtained only at the biceps muscles. Children with a Friedreich-like syndrome but in whom tendon reflexes are retained at the arms and knees probably have a different genetic disorder (see discussion of Harding ataxia). Extensor plantar responses are present in 89%. Joint position sense and vibration sense are absent in the feet in 90% and in the hands in 27%. Light touch and pain sensations are impaired in less than 10% of patients.

Scoliosis develops in 79% and pes cavus in 55% of patients. The severity of the skeletal deformities varies and is usually mild. A cardiomyopathy characterized by dyspnea on exertion, palpitations, and angina develops in 40% of patients. Systolic ejection murmurs, heard best over the apex or left sternal edge, are relatively common.

Diabetes is present in 10% of patients and has its onset during the third decade. The diabetes tends to be severe, may be difficult to control with insulin, and can significantly contribute to death from the disease.

Diagnosis.   The diagnosis relies primarily on the clinical features. Motor nerve conduction velocities in the arms and legs are slightly slower than normal. In contrast, sensory action potentials are either absent or markedly reduced in amplitude. Spinal somatosensory evoked responses are usually absent.

Common changes on the electrocardiogram (EKG) are a reduced amplitude of T waves and left or right ventricular hypertrophy. Arrhythmias and conduction defects are uncommon.

Treatment.   The underlying disturbance is not curable, but symptomatic treatment is available. Severe scoliosis should be prevented by orthopedic intervention. The development of cardiomyopathy must be monitored by regular EKG and chest radiographs to determine heart size. Chest pain on exertion responds to propranolol, and congestive heart failure responds to digitalis. Patients should be checked for diabetes and should be given insulin when necessary.

Harding Ataxia (Early-Onset Cerebellar Ataxia with Retained Tendon Reflexes)

Harding ataxia is less common than Friedreich ataxia, with which it is often confused (Filla et al, 1990; Harding, 1981).

Clinical Features.   Onset is always before 20 years of age. Ataxia is usually the initial symptom and is soon followed by dysarthria and limb weakness, affecting legs more than arms. Tone in the weak limbs is increased; tendon reflexes may be decreased or increased but are not absent. The preservation of tendon reflexes distinguishes Harding ataxia from Friedreich ataxia. Other distinguishing features are a better prognosis and the absence of optic atrophy, cardiomyopathy, diabetes mellitus, and skeletal deformities.

Diagnosis.   Harding ataxia is a clinical diagnosis made more difficult by considerable phenotypic heterogeneity within a family. CT may show cerebellar atrophy. Nerve conduction velocities and evoked responses may be prolonged.

Treatment.   No treatment is available.

Hypobetalipoproteinemia

Clinical Features.   Reports have described several different disorders in which serum lipid profiles reveal hypocholesterolemia and reduced, but not absent, concentrations of apolipoprotein B and apolipoprotein A. Some patients have no neurologic symptoms; others have severe ataxia beginning in infancy (Agamanolis et al, 1986). Malabsorption does not occur, but the infant fails to thrive and has progressive fatty cirrhosis of the liver. Severe hypotonia and absence of tendon reflexes are noted in the first months. The course is characterized by inanition, slow development, and recurrent infection. Death occurs in the second year.

Diagnosis.   Total serum lipid content is normal, and the concentration of triglycerides is increased. Total high- and low-density lipoprotein cholesterol concentrations are reduced, as are levels of apolipoprotein B and apolipoprotein A_1.

Treatment.   No treatment is available.

Juvenile GM₂ Gangliosidosis

Several juvenile forms of both alpha- and beta-hexosaminidase A deficiency have been described (Johnson, 1981). All are transmitted by autosomal recessive inheritance. Some, like Tay-Sachs disease, are restricted to Ashkenazi Jews, whereas others occur in individuals of non-Jewish descent (see Chapter 5). In all of these conditions, GM_2 gangliosides are stored within the central nervous system.

Clinical Features.   Several different syndromes have been described; some resemble the Ramsay Hunt syndrome, and others mimic Friedreich ataxia or other spinocerebellar degenerations (Willner et al, 1981). Clumsiness of gait and ataxia are the usual early features. Onset is usually after 2 years of age but can be as late as adult life. Intention tremor is frequently an associated feature.

Affected children may be considered clumsy for several years before neurologic deterioration is evident. Although ataxia is a constant feature, other neurologic findings and the rate of progression vary from family to family but are relatively constant within a kindred. Associated neurologic disturbances may include spasticity, dysarthria, optic atrophy, athetoid posturing of the hands, and dementia. Many patients eventually enter a vegetative state. Other findings in some families include pes cavus, scoliosis, and visceromegaly.

Diagnosis. Any child with an apparent "spinocerebellar degeneration" may have juvenile GM_2 gangliosidosis. Diagnosis requires the measurement of alpha- and beta-hexosaminidase activity in fibroblasts or the demonstration of neuronal ganglioside storage by rectal biopsy.

Treatment. No treatment is available.

Juvenile Sulfatide Lipidosis

Sulfatide lipidosis (metachromatic leukodystrophy) is a disorder of central and peripheral myelin metabolism caused by deficient activity of the enzyme arylsulfatase A. The defect is transmitted by autosomal recessive inheritance. The late infantile form is discussed in Chapters 5 and 7. The juvenile form is genetically distinct and affects central myelin more than peripheral myelin.

Clinical Features. Onset usually takes place after 5 years of age but may be as early as infancy or as late as adult life. When onset is in infancy, the initial symptoms are developmental delay and clumsiness. School-age children have spasticity, progressive ataxia of the trunk and limbs, and generalized tonic-clonic convulsions (Haltia et al, 1980; MacFaul et al, 1982). Mental deterioration follows. Peripheral neuropathy is not a prominent clinical feature, but motor conduction velocities are usually prolonged late in the course. Protein concentration in the cerebrospinal fluid may be normal or only slightly elevated.

Once symptoms start, progression is relatively rapid. Most children deteriorate into a vegetative state and die within 10 years. The time from onset to death ranges from 3 to 17 years and cannot be predicted by age at onset.

Diagnosis. Among the many causes of progressive ataxia, this is the only one that demonstrates rapid and severe degeneration of multiple neurologic systems. It should be especially considered when the family has a history of similar illness. Nevertheless, many such families have gone for years without diagnosis. Physicians are frequently misled by normal motor conduction velocities early in the course. CT and MRI demonstrate widespread demyelination of the cerebral hemispheres. Patients with late-onset disease are often thought to have multiple sclerosis. Diagnosis requires the demonstration of markedly reduced or absent arylsulfatase A in peripheral leukocytes.

Treatment. No treatment is available.

Marinesco-Sjogren Syndrome

The Marinesco-Sjogren syndrome, characterized by cerebellar ataxia, congenital cataracts, and mental retardation, is transmitted by autosomal recessive inheritance. It is a rare disorder; by 1985 slightly more than 60 cases had been reported. The inherited abnormality is unknown, but electron microscopic studies suggest the possibility of a lysosomal storage disorder (Walker et al, 1985).

Clinical Features. A constant feature is cataracts, which may be congenital or develop during infancy. The type of cataract varies and is not specific. Cerebellar dysfunction during infancy is characterized by dysarthria, nystagmus, and ataxia of trunk and limbs. Strabismus and hypotonia are frequently present in childhood. Developmental delay is a constant feature but varies from mild to severe. Other features include short stature, delayed sexual development, pes valgus, and scoliosis.

Although the onset of symptoms is in infancy, the progress is slow or stationary. Ataxia leads to a wheelchair existence by the third or fourth decade, and the life span is significantly shortened.

Diagnosis. Diagnosis of the Marinesco-Sjogren syndrome relies primarily on the triad of bilateral cataracts, progressive cerebellar ataxia, and mental retardation. The underlying biochemical defect is unknown, and laboratory tests are not helpful.

Treatment. No treatment is available.

Ramsay Hunt Syndrome

Ramsay Hunt syndrome, also termed *dyssynergia cerebellaris myoclonica,* is a progressive degeneration of the dentate nucleus and superior cerebellar peduncle characterized by myoclonus, cerebellar ataxia, and infrequent seizures in the absence of dementia (Marsden et al, 1990). Many patients prove to have mitochondrial encephalomyopathies (see Chapter 5). Sporadic occurrence is common, and autosomal recessive inheritance is only presumed.

Clinical Features. Sporadic cases are not homogeneous, but a general clinical picture can be delineated. The initial symptom is clumsiness, usually noted during the first decade, which evolves into progressive ataxia. Intention tremor and dysarthria may follow. Myoclonus usually begins in the second decade. It is present at rest but is made worse by attempted movement. Myoclonus may be so severe as to throw the patient to the floor. The combination of ataxia and myoclonus is severely disabling. Generalized tonic-clonic convulsions develop late in the course and are not a constant feature. Tendon reflexes are depressed, and scoliosis may be present.

Diagnosis. The diagnosis of Ramsay Hunt syndrome is based on the combination of cerebellar ataxia and myoclonus. However, diagnosing the syndrome does not diagnose a disease. Variants with autosomal dominant inheritance, as well as other syndromes causing myoclonic epilepsy, must be considered (see Chapter 1). CT or MRI may reveal atrophy of the pons, cerebellar peduncles, and cerebellum. EEG frequently demonstrates epileptiform activity of the slow spike-wave type.

Treatment. Seizures usually respond to ordinary anticonvulsant drugs. Valproate has been found useful in reducing the severity and frequency of myoclonus (Somerville and Olanow, 1982).

Sea-Blue Histiocytoses

Sea-blue histiocytoses are a heterogeneous group of neurovisceral storage diseases, similar to Niemann-Pick disease, for which the enzymatic error has not been established. Sea-blue histiocytes are large macrophages 20 to 60 μm in diameter with a single eccentric nucleus and a prominent nucleolus. Wright-Giemsa staining reveals blue or blue-green granules in the cytoplasm that contain ceroid, lipofuscin, and sphingomyelin. The histiocytes are present in the bone marrow, liver, and lymph glands.

Clinical Features. Several clinical presentations have been described (Ashwal et al, 1984; Gartner et al, 1986). Hepatosplenomegaly is usually the first manifestation, but neurologic deterioration may precede the visceral dysfunction. Onset of symptoms can be as early as 2 months of age but more commonly occurs after 1 year and sometimes after ten years of age. Ataxia and spasticity are prominent features. The initial progress of neurologic dysfunction is so slow that the child is thought to have cerebral palsy. Involuntary movements and tremor may be present.

Neurologic deterioration accelerates as the child gets older. Later symptoms include dementia, seizures, speech disturbances, and supranuclear ophthalmoplegia. Severe bulbar palsy leads to aspiration and death.

Diagnosis. Sea-blue histiocytosis is a diag-

nosis of exclusion. When sea-blue histiocytes are present in the bone marrow or liver, an extensive search for a lysosomal enzyme defect must be made. Niemann-Pick disease type C should be especially suspect (see Chapter 5).

Treatment. No treatment is available. Liver transplantation was tried in one patient without success.

Other Metabolic Disorders

Hartnup disease and maple syrup urine disease were both described in the section on acute or recurrent ataxia. After an acute attack of these diseases some patients never return to baseline but instead have chronic progressive ataxia. Such patients should be screened for metabolic disorders (Table 10–3). Refsum disease is an inborn error of phytanic acid metabolism and is transmitted by autosomal recessive inheritance. The cardinal features are retinitis pigmentosa, chronic or recurrent polyneuropathy, and cerebellar ataxia. Affected individuals usually have night blindness or neuropathy (see Chapter 7).

Disorders of pyruvate metabolism and the respiratory chain enzymes produce widespread dis-

Table 10–3 ◆ Metabolic Screening in Progressive Ataxias

Disease	Abnormality
Blood	
Adrenoleukodystrophy	Very-long-chain fatty acids
Ataxia-telangiectasia	IgA, IgE, alpha-fetoprotein
Abetalipoproteinemia	Lipoproteins, cholesterol
Hypobetalipoproteinemia	Lipoproteins, cholesterol
Mitochondrial disorders	Lactate, glucose-lactate tolerance
Sulfatide lipidoses	Arylsulfatase A
Urine	
Hartnup disease	Amino acids
Maple syrup urine disease	Amino acids
Fibroblasts	
GM$_2$ gangliosidosis	Hexosaminidase
Refsum disease	Phytanic acid
Carnitine acetyltransferase deficiency	Carnitine acetyltransferase
Bone Marrow	
Neurovisceral storage	Sea-blue histiocytes

turbances in the nervous system and are described in Chapters 5, 7, and 8. The common features among the several disorders of mitochondrial metabolism include lactic acidosis, ataxia, hypotonia, ophthalmoplegia, mental retardation, and peripheral neuropathy. These disorders are suggested by a raised concentration of blood lactate or the production of lactic acidosis by administration of a standard glucose tolerance test. A deficiency of pyruvate decarboxylase may produce acute, recurrent, or chronic ataxia and is discussed in the section on acute or recurrent ataxia. Respiratory chain disorders produce a combination of ataxia, dementia, myoclonus, and seizures.

X-Linked Inheritance

The infantile form of adrenoleukodystrophy (see Chapter 5) and Leber optic neuropathy (see Chapter 16) may initially be manifested as ataxia. Adrenoleukodystrophy may more closely mimic a spinocerebellar degeneration and should be considered in any family with only males affected (Kobayashi et al, 1986). Leber optic neuropathy is readily distinguished from other cerebellar degenerations because other family members have characteristic ophthalmologic features.

Ataxia with Dementia

Clinical Features. Age at onset of ataxia with dementia is 2 to 3 years. The initial features are delayed developmental milestones, clumsiness, and intention tremor. Early school performance is acceptable. Progressive ataxia and spasticity develop in affected males during the second decade. Incoordination becomes progressively severe, leading to loss of ambulation. Progressive dementia begins in the third and fourth decades. Death usually occurs in the seventh decade (Farlow et al, 1987).

Cerebellar, corticospinal, and intellectual function are abnormal. Other neurologic systems are intact.

Diagnosis. CT or MRI shows cerebellar atrophy. No biochemical defect has been identified. Adrenoleukodystrophy is a major consideration, and plasma concentrations of very-long-chain fatty acids should be determined.

Treatment. No treatment is available.

References

Agamanolis DP, Potter JL, Naito HK, et al: Lipoprotein disorder, cirrhosis and olivopontocerebellar degeneration in two siblings. Neurology 36:674, 1986.

Aicardi J, Barbosa C, Andermann E, et al: Ataxia-ocular motor apraxia: A syndrome mimicking ataxia-telangiectasia. Ann Neurol 24:497, 1988.

Al-Din AN, Anderson M, Bickerstaff ER, et al: Brainstem encephalitis and the syndrome of Miller Fisher: A clinical study. Brain 105:481, 1982.

Appleton RE, Chitayat D, Jan JE, et al: Joubert's syndrome associated with congenital ocular fibrosis and histidinemia. Arch Neurol 46:579, 1989.

Asbury AK: Diagnostic considerations in Guillain Barré syndrome. Ann Neurol 9:1, 1981.

Ashwal S, Thrasher TV, Rice DR, et al: A new form of sea-blue histiocytosis associated with progressive anterior horn cell and axonal degeneration. Ann Neurol 16:184, 1984.

Baloh RW, Winder A: Acetazolamide-responsive vestibulocerebellar syndrome: Clinical and oculographic features. Neurology 41:429, 1991.

Bejar JM, Ziegler DK: Onset of multiple sclerosis in a 24-month-old child. Arch Neurol 41:881, 1984.

Bennett HS, Selman JE, Rapin I, et al: Nonconvulsive epileptiform activity appearing as ataxia. AJDC 136:30, 1982.

Boel M, Casaer P: Familial periodic ataxia responsive to flunarizine. Neuropediatrics 19:218, 1988.

Bolthauser E, Deonna A, Hirt HR: Myoclonic encephalopathy of infants or "dancing eyes syndrome." Helv Paediatr Acta 34:119, 1979.

Boutin B, Esquivel E, Mayer M, et al: Multiple sclerosis in children: Report of clinical and paraclinical features of 19 cases. Neuropediatrics 19:118, 1988.

Bye AME, Kendall B, Wilson J: Multiple sclerosis in childhood: A new look. Dev Med Child Neurol 27:215, 1985.

Choux M: Ependymomas in the posterior fossa of children. In Amador LV, ed: Brain Tumors in the Young. Charles C Thomas, Springfield, Ill, 1983, p 526.

Danner DJ, Elsas LJ: Disorders of branched chain amino acid metabolism. In Scriver CR, Beaudet AL, Sly WS, et al, eds: The Metabolic Basis of Metabolic Disorders, 6th edition. New York, McGraw-Hill, 1989, p 671.

DiDonato S, Rimoldi M, Moise A, et al: Fatal ataxic encephalopathy and carnitine acetyltransferase deficiency: A functional defect of pyruvate oxidation? Neurology 29:1578, 1979.

Evans OB: Episodic weakness in pyruvate decarboxylase deficiency. J Pediatr 105:961, 1984.

Ewout R, Brunt P, van Weerden TW: Familial paroxysmal kinesiogenic ataxia and continuous myokymia. Brain 113:1361, 1990.

Farlow MR, DeMyer W, Dlouhy SR, et al: X-linked recessive inheritance of ataxia and adult-onset dementia: Clinical features and preliminary linkage analysis. Neurology 37:602, 1987.

Farmer TW, Wingfield MS, Lynch SA, et al: Ataxia, chorea, seizures, and dementia. Arch Neurol 46:774, 1989.

Farris BK, Smith JL, Ayyar R: Neuro-ophthalmologic findings in vestibulocerebellar ataxia. Arch Neurol 43:1050, 1986.

Feit H, Kirkpatrick J, Van Woert MH, et al: Myoclonus, ataxia, and hypoventilation: Response to L-5-hydroxytryptophan. Neurology 33:109, 1983.

Fenichel GM: Migraine as a cause of benign paroxysmal vertigo in childhood. J Pediatr 71:114, 1967.

Fenichel GM, Phillips JA: Familial aplasia of the cerebellar vermis: Possible X-linked dominant inheritance. Arch Neurol 46:582, 1989.

Filla A, De Michele G, Cavalcanti F, et al: Clinical and genetic heterogeneity in early onset cerebellar ataxia with retained tendon reflexes. J Neurol Neurosurg Psychiatry 53:667, 1990.

Filling-Katz MR, Choyke PL, Oldfield E, et al: Central nervous system involvement in Von Hippel–Lindau disease. Neurology 41:41, 1991.

Fitzsimons RB, Clifton-Bligh P, Wolfenden WH: Mitochondrial myopathy and lactic acidemia with myoclonic epilepsy, ataxia and hypothalamic infertility: A variant of Ramsay-Hunt syndrome? J Neurol Neurosurg Psychiatry 44:79, 1981.

Fowler HL: Machado-Joseph-Azorean disease: A ten-year study. Arch Neurol 41:921, 1984.

Garcia DM, Latifi HR, Simpson JR, et al: Astrocytomas of the cerebellum in children. J Neurosurg 71:661, 1989.

Gartner JC, Bergman I, Malatack J, et al: Progression of neurovisceral storage disease with supranuclear ophthalmoplegia following orthotopic liver transplantation. Pediatrics 77:104, 1986.

Gatti RA, Boder E, Vinters HV, et al: Ataxia-telangiectasia: An interdisciplinary approach to pathogenesis. Medicine 70:99, 1991.

Gjerris F: Clinical aspects and long-term prognosis in supratentorial tumors of infancy and childhood. Acta Neurol Scand 57:445, 1978.

Graff-Radford NR: A recessively inherited ataxia with episodes of dystonia. J Neurol Neurosurg Psychiatry 49:591, 1986.

Haltia T, Palo J, Haltia M, et al: Juvenile metachromatic leukodystrophy: Clinical, biochemical, and neuropathologic studies in nine new cases. Arch Neurol 37:42, 1980.

Harding AE: Friedreich's ataxia: A clinical and genetic study of 90 families with an analysis of early diagnostic criteria and intrafamilial clustering of clinical features. Brain 104:589, 1981a.

Harding AE: Early onset cerebellar ataxia with retained tendon reflexes: Clinical and genetic study of a disorder distinct from Friedreich ataxia. J Neurol Neurosurg Psychiatry 44:503, 1981b.

Hegele RA, Angel A: Arrest of neuropathy and myopathy in abetalipoproteinemia with high-dose vitamin E therapy. Can Med Assoc J 132:41, 1985.

Hendrick EB: Medulloblastomas, astrocytomas, and sarcomas of the posterior fossa. In Amador LV, ed: Brain Tumors in the Young. Charles C Thomas, Springfield, Ill, 1983, p 498.

Johnson WG: The clinical spectrum of hexosaminidase deficiency diseases. Neurology 31:1453, 1981.

Kobayashi T, Noda S, Umezaki H, et al: Familial spinocerebellar degeneration as an expression of adrenoleukodystrophy. J Neurol Neurosurg Psychiatry 49:1438, 1986.

Lapkin ML, Golden GS: Basilar artery migraine. AJDC 132:278, 1978.

Levy HL: Hartnup disorder. In Scriver CR, Beaudet AL, Sly WS, et al, eds: The Metabolic Basis of Inherited Disease, 6th edition. McGraw-Hill, New York, 1989, p. 2515.

Levy WJ, Mason L, Hahn JF: Chiari malformation presenting in adults: A surgical experience in 127 cases. Neurosurgery 12:377, 1983.

Lima L, Coutinho P: Clinical criteria for diagnosis of Machado-Joseph disease: Report of a non-Azorean Portuguese family. Neurology 30:319, 1980.

Livingstone IR, Gardner-Medwin D, Pennington RJT: Familial intermittent ataxia with possible X-linked recessive inheritance. J Neurol Sci 64:89, 1984.

MacFaul R, Cavanagh N, Lake BD, et al: Metachromatic leucodystrophy: Review of 38 cases. Arch Dis Child 3:168, 1982.

Maher ER, Yates JRW, Harries R, et al: Clinical features and natural history of von Hippel–Lindau disease. Q J Med 77:1151, 1990.

Marsden CD, Harding AE, Obesio JA, et al: Progressive myoclonic ataxia (the Ramsay Hunt syndrome). Arch Neurol 47:1121, 1990.

Meienberg O, Ryffel R: Supranuclear eye movement disorders in Fisher's syndrome of ophthalmoplegia, ataxia, and areflexia: Report of a case and literature review. Arch Neurol 40:402, 1983.

Neumann HPH, Wiestler OT: Clustering of features of von Hippel–Lindau syndrome: Evidence for a complex genetic locus. Lancet 337:1052, 1991.

Nino HE, Noreen HJ, Dubey DP, et al: A family with hereditary ataxia: HLA typing. Neurology 30:12, 1980.

Osborn AG, Harnsberger HR, Smoker WRK, et al: Multiple sclerosis in adolescents: CT and MR findings. AJNR 11:489, 1990.

Packer RJ: Chemotherapy for medulloblastoma/primitive neuroectodermal tumors of the posterior fossa. Ann Neurol 28:823, 1990.

Park TS, Hoffman HJ, Hendrick EB, et al: Experience with surgical decompression of the Arnold-Chiari malformation in young infants with myelomeningocele. Neurosurgery 13:147, 1983.

Pueschel SM, Bresnan MJ, Shih VE, et al: Thiamine-responsive intermittent branched chain ketoaciduria. J Pediatr 94:629, 1979.

Sarnat HB, Alcala H: Human cerebellar hypoplasia: A syndrome of diverse causes. Arch Neurol 37:300, 1980.

Schulte FJ: Intracranial tumors in childhood—concepts of treatment and prognosis. Neuropediatrie 15:3, 1984.

Scully RE, Mark EJ, McNeely BU: Case records of the Massachusetts General Hospital. N Engl J Med 315:1143, 1986.

Sergent JS, Lockshin MD, Klempner MS, et al: Central nervous system disease in systemic lupus erythematosus. Am J Med 58:644, 1975.

Somerville ER, Olanow CW: Valproic acid: Treatment of myoclonus in dyssynergia cerebellaris myoclonica. Arch Neurol 39:527, 1982.

Stumpf DA: The inherited ataxias. Pediatr Neurol 1:129, 1985.

Takahashi H, Ohama E, Naito H, et al: Hereditary dentatorubral-pallidoluysian atrophy: Clinical and pathological variants in a family. Neurology 38:1065, 1988.

Teodori JB, Painter MJ: Basilar impression in children. Pediatrics 74:1097, 1984.

Tomita T: Statistical analysis of symptoms and signs in cerebellar astrocytoma and medulloblastoma. In Amador LV, ed: Brain Tumors in the Young, Charles C Thomas, Springfield, Ill, 1983, p 514.

Tomita T, McLone DG: Medulloblastoma in childhood: Results of radical resection and low-dose neuraxis radiation therapy. J Neurosurg 64:238, 1986.

Tuchman M, Morris CL, Ramnaraine ML, et al: Value of random urinary homovanillic acid and vanillylmandelic acid levels in diagnosis and management of patients with neuroblastoma. Pediatrics 75:324, 1985.

Vighetto A, Froment JC, Trillet M, et al: Magnetic resonance imaging in familial paroxysmal ataxia. Arch Neurol 45:547, 1988.

Waldmann TA, Misiti J, Nelson DL, et al: Ataxia-telangiectasia: A multisystem hereditary disease with immunodeficiency, impaired organ maturation, X-ray hypersensitivity, and a high incidence of neoplasia. Ann Intern Med 99:367, 1983.

Walker PD, Blitzer MG, Shapira E: Marinesco-Sjogren syndrome: Evidence for a lysosomal storage disorder. Neurology 35:415, 1985.

Wichman A, Buchthal F, Pezeshkpour GH, et al: Peripheral neuropathy in abetalipoproteinemia. Neurology 35:1279, 1985.

Willner JP, Grabowski GA, Gordon RE, et al: Chronic GM_2 gangliosidosis masquerading as atypical Friedreich ataxia: Clinical, morphologic, and biochemical studies of nine cases. Neurology 31:787, 1981.

Zasorin NL, Baloh RW, Myers LB: Acetazolamide-responsive episodic ataxia syndrome. Neurology 33:1212, 1983.

Zimmerman AW, Kumar AJ, Gadoth N, et al: Traumatic vertebrobasilar occlusive disease in childhood. Neurology 28:185, 1978.

Zoghbi HY, Pollack MS, Lyons LA, et al: Spinocerebellar ataxia: Variable age of onset and linkage to human leukocyte antigen in a large kindred. Ann Neurol 23:580, 1988.

Hemiplegia

The approach to children with hemiplegia must distinguish between acute hemiplegia, in which weakness develops within a few hours, and chronic progressive hemiplegia, in which weakness evolves over days, weeks, or months. The distinction between an acute and an insidious onset should be easy but sometimes poses a problem. In children with a slowly evolving hemiplegia, early weakness may be missed until an obvious level of functional disability is reached; then the hemiplegia seems new and acute.

A third form is found in infants who come to medical attention because they are slow in meeting motor milestones or are not using one hand; they are then found to have a hemiplegia. They have a static structural problem from birth *(hemiplegic cerebral palsy),* but the clinical features are not apparent until the child is old enough to use the affected limbs.

Magnetic resonance imaging (MRI) has become the diagnostic modality of choice for investigating acute and progressive hemiplegia, while computed tomography (CT) is generally satisfactory in children with hemiplegic cerebral palsy. Magnetic resonance arteriography (MRA) is a developing technique that will obviate the need for arteriography in many children (Wiznitzer and Masaryk, 1991).

◆ Hemiplegic Cerebral Palsy

The term "hemiplegic cerebral palsy" covers several pathologic entities that result in limb weakness on one side of the body. In premature infants the common causes are periventricular hemorrhagic infarction and periventricular leukomalacia (see Chapter 4). In full-term infants the underlying causes are more often cerebral malformations, cerebral infarction, and intracerebral hemorrhage.

Imaging studies of the brain are useful to sort out the underlying pathologic conditions (Wiklund and Uvebrant, 1991).

Infants with hemiplegia from birth are often brought for evaluation because crawling or walking is delayed, and attention is directed at the legs. An associated but seldom recognized abnormality is that hand dominance was established during the first year; this is not normal.

NEONATAL INFARCTION

Cerebral infarction from arterial occlusion occurs more often in full-term newborns than in premature newborns. Three patterns of infarction are seen with MRI (Smith and Baumann, 1991): (1) arterial border zone infarction is usually associated with resuscitation and probably is caused by hypotension; (2) multiartery infarction is less often associated with perinatal distress and may be caused by congenital heart disease, disseminated intravascular coagulation, and polycythemia; and (3) single artery infarction can be caused by injury to the cervical portion of the carotid artery during a difficult delivery owing to either misapplication of obstetric forceps or hyperextension and rotation of the neck with stretching of the artery over the lateral portion of the upper cervical vertebrae. However, trauma is probably a rare event and the cause of most single artery infarctions cannot be determined.

Clinical Features.   Single artery infarcts, usually frontal or parietal, occur in newborns without systemic disease or obvious risk factors (Fenichel et al, 1984). Subarachnoid hemorrhage is frequently an associated feature. Such newborns appear normal at birth, but repetitive, focal, or generalized seizures develop during the first 4 days post partum (Clancy et al, 1985; Levy et al, 1985).

Some recover fully, whereas others are left with hemiparesis. The face is usually spared when hemiplegia begins perinatally (Lenn and Freinkel, 1989).

Diagnosis. CT or MRI is necessary to demonstrate small infarcts, but large infarcts in the complete distribution of the middle cerebral artery can be detected by ultrasound. Follow-up imaging studies may show either unilateral enlargement of the lateral ventricle (Figure 11–1) or porencephaly in the distribution of the middle cerebral artery contralateral to the hemiparesis. Hemiatrophy of the pons contralateral to the abnormal hemisphere may be an associated feature.

Maternal use of cocaine during pregnancy can cause cerebral infarction and hemorrhage in the fetus. Cocaine can be detected in the newborn's urine during the first week post partum.

Treatment. Anticonvulsant drugs are usually effective for seizure control (see Chapter 1). Hemispherectomy or commissurotomy should be considered in children with intractable focal seizures (Goodman, 1986).

NEONATAL HEMORRHAGE

Small unilateral parietal or temporal hemorrhages occur almost exclusively in full-term new-

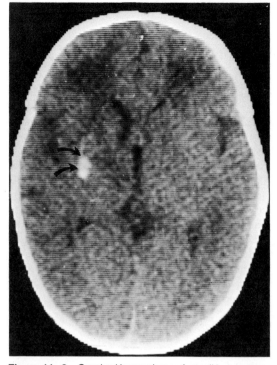

Figure 11–2 Cerebral hemorrhage. A small hemorrhage is indicated by the arrows.

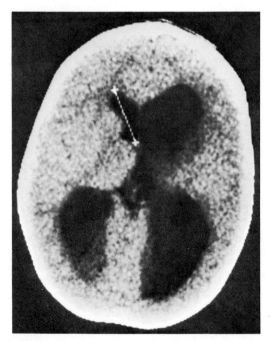

Figure 11–1 Cerebral hemiatrophy with ventricular enlargement. The lateral ventricle on the right side is considerably larger than on the left (marked) because of right hemispheric atrophy.

borns and are not associated with either trauma or asphyxia (Cartwright et al, 1979; Leblanc and O'Gorman, 1980). Larger hemorrhages into the temporal lobe are sometimes caused when excessive force is applied with obstetric forceps, but more often they are idiopathic (Bergman et al, 1985). Intraventricular hemorrhage may be an associated feature.

Clinical Features. Newborns with small hemorrhages are normal at birth and seem well until seizures begin, anytime during the first week. Larger hemorrhages may be manifested as apneic spells or seizures, or both. Seizures may be focal or generalized, and hemiplegia or hypotonia is present on examination. Some infants recover completely, whereas others are left with hemiplegia and mental retardation.

Diagnosis. Seizures and apneic spells usually prompt lumbar puncture to exclude the possibility of sepsis. The cerebrospinal fluid is grossly bloody. The initial CT demonstrates hemorrhage (Figure 11–2), and follow-up studies reveal focal encephalomalacia.

Treatment. Treatment is available for seizures, but not for hemorrhage.

◆ Acute Hemiplegia

The sudden onset of an acute, focal neurologic deficit suggests either a vascular or an epileptic mechanism (Table 11–1). Infants and children who have acute hemiplegia can be divided almost equally into two groups according to whether the hemiplegia was preceded by epilepsia partialis continua (Gastaut et al, 1979). Both groups may have seizures on the paretic side after hemiplegia is established. Cerebral infarction, usually in the distribution of the middle cerebral artery, accounts for 23% of cases in which seizures precede the hemiplegia and 57% of cases in which hemiplegia is the first manifestation. Whatever the cause, the probability of a permanent motor deficit is almost 100% when the initial manifestation is epilepsia partialis continua and about 50% when it is not (Solomon et al, 1970).

ALTERNATING HEMIPLEGIA

Alternating hemiplegia is a rare and poorly understood clinical syndrome, with hemiplegia as a cardinal feature. Its nosologic identity has been linked to migraine, epilepsy, and familial paroxysmal choreoathetosis (Aicardi, 1987).

Clinical Features.   Affected infants are developmentally normal before the attacks begin, which usually occurs before 18 months of age, but I have seen one child whose first attack was at 6 years. The attacks may be characterized by body stiffening and limb dyskinesia, hemiplegia, autonomic disturbances, or some combination of the three. Nystagmus and disturbances of ocular motility are often present during the attack. Episodes last for minutes to hours and become more frequent with time. Mental retardation develops in all children, and some have ataxia and choreoathetosis.

Diagnosis.   Results of electroencephalography (EEG), cerebral arteriography, and MRI are normal. The diagnosis relies entirely on the clinical features.

Table 11–1 ◆ Differential Diagnosis of
Acute Hemiplegia

1. Alternating hemiplegia
2. Asthmatic amyotrophy (see Chapter 13)
3. Cerebrovascular disease
4. Diabetes mellitus
5. Epilepsy
6. Hypoglycemia (see Chapter 2)
7. Kawasaki disease (see Chapter 10)
8. Migraine
9. Trauma
10. Tumor

Treatment.   Anticonvulsant and antimigraine medications have consistently failed to prevent attacks or prevent progression. Flunarizine, a calcium channel blocking agent, was found to reduce the frequency of attacks in one report (Casaer et al, 1987), but this has not been my experience.

CEREBROVASCULAR DISEASE

The annual incidence of stroke in children is 2.5:100,000, which is about half the incidence of brain tumors (Schoenberg et al, 1976). Some children with acute hemiplegia from stroke have a known predisposing condition, such as congenital heart disease or sickle cell anemia. In such children the index of suspicion for stroke is high whenever an acute neurologic disturbance occurs. Stroke may also occur in the absence of known risk factors (Table 11–2). In a previously healthy child, stroke is usually considered because of the sudden onset of a focal neurologic disturbance and is then confirmed by CT. Infarction is identified as an area of increased lucency that becomes enhanced with contrast material (Figure 11–3). As a rule the lucency cannot be visualized in the first 24 hours after stroke. Cerebral infarction is often superficial, affecting both gray and white matter, and is in the distribution of a single artery. Multiple infarcts suggest either embolism or vasculitis. Small, deep lesions of the internal capsule are rare but can occur in infants.

The evaluation of a child with cerebral infarction is summarized in Table 11–3. The usual line of investigation includes tests for blood dyscrasias, a search for cardiac sources of emboli, and cerebral arteriography to identify the site of vascular occlusion.

Children of all ages who are otherwise healthy may experience a single episode of cerebral infarction. Despite the most extensive evaluation, no underlying cause can be found. Clinical features vary with age and site of infarction. Hemiplegia, either immediately or as a late sequela, is one of the more common features.

Intracerebral hemorrhage is readily identified as an area of increased density on a non-contrast-enhanced CT (Figure 11–3). It is frequently surrounded by edema and may produce a mass effect with shift of midline structures.

Arteriovenous Malformations

Supratentorial malformations may cause acute or chronic, progressive hemiplegia. The acute form usually results from intraparenchymal hemorrhage.

Table 11–2 ◆ Causes of Stroke

Arteriovenous Malformation	**Hypercoagulable States** 1. Arterial thrombosis 2. Venous thrombosis
Cancer 1. Disseminated intravascular coagulation 2. Drug-induced thrombosis 3. Metastatic neuroblastoma	**Idiopathic Infarction** **Lipoprotein Disorders**
Carotid Disorders 1. Cervical infection 2. Fibromuscular dysplasia 3. Trauma	**Mitochondrial Encephalopathy, Lactic Acidosis, and Stroke (MELAS)** **Moyamoya Disease**
Cocaine Use	**Sickle Cell Anemia**
Heart Disease 1. Congenital 2. Mitral valve prolapse 3. Rheumatic	**Vasculopathies** 1. Hypersensitivity vasculitis 2. Kawasaki disease (see Chapter 10) 3. Systemic lupus erythematosus 4. Takayasu arteritis
Hemolytic-Uremic Syndrome (see Chapter 2)	
Homocystinuria (see Chapter 5)	

The major clinical manifestations of hemorrhage into a hemisphere are loss of consciousness, seizures, and hemiplegia. Large hematomas shift midline structures and increase intracranial pressure. Arteriovenous malformations are discussed fully in Chapter 4.

Brain Tumors

Acute hemiplegia from brain tumor is usually caused by hemorrhage into or around the tumor. The underlying tumor may be hidden by the hemorrhage on CT and is better appreciated by MRI (see Chapter 4).

Cancer

Cerebrovascular accidents occur in 4% of children with cancer (Packer et al, 1985). Two thirds occur in children with lymphoreticular cancers and the rest in children with solid tumors. Strokes are often caused by the vasculi thrombi that result from disseminated intravascular coagulation. This is especially true in children with leukemia, either as an initial manifestation or during therapy. Multiple infarctions and hemorrhages may be present. Hemiparesis and obtundation are major clinical features.

L-Asparaginase causes a coagulopathy that leads to acute arterial or sagittal sinus thrombosis in children with acute lymphocytic leukemia, and high-dose methotrexate produces infarction of unknown mechanism in children being treated for osteogenic sarcoma.

Neuroblastoma may metastasize to the sagittal sinus and produce increased intracranial pressure, obtundation, seizures, and alternating hemiplegia.

Carotid and Vertebral Artery Disorders
Cervical Infections

Unilateral and bilateral occlusions of the cervical portion of the internal carotid arteries may

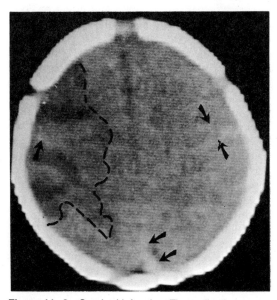

Figure 11–3 Cerebral infarction. The outlined area represents early changes caused by infarction in the middle cerebral artery distribution. Arrows indicate hemorrhage.

Table 11–3 ◆ Evaluation of Cerebral Infarction

Evaluation	Condition
Blood	
Complete blood cell count, erythrocyte sedimentation rate, culture, anti-DNA, lipid profile, lactic acid	Bacterial endocarditis Hyperlipidemia Leukemia Lupus erythematosus Mitochondrial encephalopathy, lactic acidosis, stroke (MELAS) Polycythemia Sickle cell anemia
Urine	
Cocaine Nitroprusside reaction Urinalysis	Cocaine abuse Homocystinuria Nephritis Nephrosis
Heart	
Echocardiography Electocardiography	Bacterial endocarditis Congenital heart disease Mitral valve prolapse Rheumatic heart disease
Brain	
Arteriography, magnetic resonance imaging	Arterial dissection Arterial thrombosis Arteriovenous malformation Fibromuscular hypoplasia Moyamoya disease Vasculitis

occur in children with a history of chronic tonsillitis and cervical lymphadenopathy (Tagawa et al, 1985). Whether this is cause and effect or coincidence is uncertain. It is speculated that tonsillitis produces carotid arteritis.

Unilateral cerebral infarction may occur in the course of cat scratch disease (see Chapter 2) and mycoplasmal pneumonia (Parker et al, 1981). In both diseases the presence of submandibular lymph node involvement is associated with arteritis of the adjacent carotid artery.

Necrotizing fasciitis is a serious cause of inflammatory arteritis with subsequent occlusion of one or both carotid arteries (Bush et al, 1984). The source of parapharyngeal space infection is usually chronic dental infection. Mixed aerobic and anaerobic organisms are isolated on culture.

Clinical Features. The usual sequence in cervical arteritis is fever and neck tenderness followed by sudden hemiplegia. Bilateral hemiplegia may occur when both sides are infected.

Diagnosis. The offending organism or organisms must be identified by culture of the throat or lymph node specimens. Carotid occlusion is identified by arteriography.

Treatment. Aggressive therapy with antibiotics, especially for necrotizing fasciitis, is indicated. The outcome is variable, and recovery may be partial or complete.

Fibromuscular Dysplasia

Fibromuscular dysplasia is an idiopathic segmental nonatheromatous disorder of the internal carotid artery. The cervical portion of the artery is most often affected.

Clinical Features. Transient ischemic attacks and stroke are the only clinical features. Fibromuscular dysplasia occurs most often in women over 50 years of age but also has been reported in children (Llorens-Terol et al, 1983).

Diagnosis. Arteriography reveals an irregular contour of the internal carotid artery in the neck, resembling a string of beads. Concomitant fibromuscular dysplasia of the renal arteries should be suspected if hypertension is present.

Treatment. The occlusion may be treated by operative transluminal balloon angioplasty (Smith et al, 1985) or by carotid endarterectomy. The long-term prognosis in children is unknown.

Trauma to Carotid Artery

Older children may experience carotid thrombosis and dissection from trivial injuries sustained in child abuse (grabbing and shaking the neck) or during exercise and sports. The carotid artery may be injured in the tonsillar fossa during a tonsillectomy or when a child falls with a blunt object (e.g., pencil, lollipop) in the mouth.

Clinical Features. The onset of symptoms is usually delayed for several hours and sometimes days (Yamada et al, 1967). The delay probably represents the time needed for thrombus formation within the artery. Clinical features usually include hemiparesis, hemianesthesia, hemianopia, and aphasia when the dominant hemisphere is affected. Deficits may be transitory or permanent, but some recovery always occurs. Seizures are uncommon.

Diagnosis. Carotid occlusions in the neck may be demonstrated by ultrasonic imaging, but arteriography is essential for diagnosis.

Treatment. Neither anticoagulation nor surgical repair has proved useful in reversing hemiplegia.

Trauma to Vertebral Artery

Vertebral artery thrombosis or dissection may follow minor neck trauma, especially rapid neck rotation (Katirji et al, 1985).

Clinical Features. The usual features of vertebral artery injury are headache and brainstem dysfunction. Repeated episodes of hemiparesis associated with bitemporal throbbing headache and vomiting are reported as well (Lewis and Berman, 1986). Episodes are provoked by exercise, last up to 4 hours, and are readily misdiagnosed as basilar artery migraine.

Diagnosis. The clue to diagnosis is the presence of one or more areas of infarction on CT or MRI. This should raise the possibility of stroke and lead to arteriography. Occlusion of the basilar artery is then visualized.

Treatment. Aspirin, 300 mg twice daily, was found effective in preventing further attacks in one patient (Lewis and Berman, 1986).

Cocaine Use

Cocaine is a potent vasoconstrictor that causes infarction in several organs. Stroke occurs mainly in young adults and may follow any route of administration but takes place more often when "crack" is smoked (Levine et al, 1991). The interval from administration to stroke is unknown in most cases but may be minutes to hours. Intracerebral and subarachnoid hemorrhage are more common than cerebral infarction and often occur in people with underlying aneurysms or arteriovenous malformations. Infarction may be due to vasospasm or vasculitis.

Heart Disease
Congenital Heart Disease

Cerebrovascular complications of congenital heart disease are most likely in children with cyanotic disorders. The usual complications are venous sinus thrombosis in infants and embolic arterial occlusion in children. Emboli may occur from valvular vegetations or bacterial endocarditis. In either case the development of cerebral abscess is a major concern. Cerebral abscess of embolic origin is exceedingly uncommon in children younger than 2 years with congenital heart disease and occurs only as a complication of meningitis or surgery.

Clinical Features. Venous thrombosis occurs most often in infants with cyanotic heart disease who are dehydrated and polycythemic. One or more sinuses may become occluded. Failure of venous drainage always increases intracranial pressure. Hemiparesis is a major clinical feature and may occur on first one side and then the other when the sagittal sinus is obstructed. Seizures and decreased consciousness are almost always associated features. The mortality rate is high in infants with thrombosis of major venous sinuses, and most survivors have neurologic morbidity.

Children with cyanotic heart disease are at risk for arterial embolism when vegetations are present within the heart or if right-to-left shunt allows peripheral emboli to bypass the lungs and reach the brain. This can occur spontaneously or at the time of cardiac surgery. The potential for cerebral abscess formation increases in children with right-to-left shunt because decreased arterial oxygen saturation lowers cerebral resistance to infection.

The initial feature is sudden onset of hemiparesis associated with headache, seizures, and loss of consciousness. Seizures may at first be focal and recurrent but then become generalized.

Diagnosis. MRI is the preferred procedure for the detection of venous thrombosis and emboli. A pattern of hemorrhagic infarction is seen adjacent to the site of venous thrombosis, and multiple areas of infarction are associated with embolization.

The CT appearance may be normal during the first 12 to 24 hours following embolization. By the next day a low-intensity lesion can be observed with contrast enhancement. Although the sequence is consistent with a sterile embolus, the possibility of subsequent abscess formation must be considered (Kurlan and Griggs, 1983). Enhanced CT or MRI should be repeated within 1 week to search for ring enhancement as a sign of abscess development.

Treatment.   Treatment for venous thrombosis is primarily supportive and directed toward correcting dehydration and controlling increased intracranial pressure. Dexamethasone can be used to decrease cerebral volume, but osmotic diuretics are contraindicated and may cause further thrombosis. The infarction is usually hemorrhagic, and anticoagulants are contraindicated. Whether a thrombosis is septic or sterile is impossible to determine, and all infants should be treated with antibiotics.

Children with arterial emboli, but without evidence of hemorrhagic infarction, should undergo anticoagulation to prevent further embolization. If the infarction is associated with cerebral edema and a mass effect, dexamethasone should be administered as well. All such children should be given antibiotic therapy to prevent cerebral abscess formation. If an abscess does not form, antibiotics can be stopped after 1 week. If an abscess forms, therapy must be continued for 6 to 8 weeks.

Mitral Valve Prolapse

Mitral valve prolapse is a familial disorder present in 5% of children (Greenwood, 1984). It is almost always asymptomatic but is estimated to cause recurrent attacks of cerebral ischemia in 1 per 6000 cases each year (Cheng, 1989). The attacks are attributed to sterile emboli from thrombus originating either from the prolapsing leaflet or at its junction with the atrial wall.

Clinical Features.   The initial manifestation is usually a transitory ischemic attack in the distribution of the carotid circulation producing partial or complete hemiparesis. Weakness usually clears within 24 hours, but recurrent episodes, not necessarily in the same arterial distribution, are the rule. Basilar insufficiency is less common and usually results in visual field defects. The interval between recurrences varies from weeks to years. Fewer than 20% of individuals are left with permanent neurologic deficits.

Diagnosis.   Only 25% of patients have late systolic murmurs or a midsystolic click. In the remainder a cardiac examination shows no abnormality. Two-dimensional echocardiography is required to establish the diagnosis.

Treatment.   No treatment is needed for asymptomatic children with auscultatory or electrocardiographic abnormalities, nor is there specific treatment for a transient ischemic attack. However,

once a child has suffered a transient ischemic attack, daily aspirin should be administered to reduce the likelihood of further thrombus formation in the heart.

Rheumatic Heart Disease

The frequency and severity of rheumatic fever and rheumatic heart disease in North America had been decreasing for several decades. Unfortunately, the incidence of acute rheumatic fever is now increasing. Rheumatic heart disease involves the mitral valve in 85% of patients, the aortic valve in 54%, and the tricuspid and pulmonary valves in less than 5% (Kaplan, 1983).

Clinical Features.   The cardinal features of mitral valve disease are cardiac failure and arrhythmia. Aortic valve disease is often asymptomatic. Neurologic manifestations are due to bacterial endocarditis or embolism from a valvular vegetation during surgery. Symptoms are much the same as in congenital heart disease except that cerebral abscess is less common.

Diagnosis.   Children are known to have rheumatic heart disease long before their first stroke. The onset of neurologic abnormalities, except in the period following cardiac surgery, should suggest bacterial endocarditis as the underlying cause. Embolization is a more likely explanation in the postoperative period. Multiple blood cultures may be needed to identify the organism and select the best drug for intravenous antibiotic therapy.

Treatment.   Bacterial endocarditis must be treated vigorously with intravenous antibiotics.

Hypercoagulable States

Venous thrombosis in children is usually due to a hypercoagulable state, polycythemia, or dehydration. Congenital heart disease and cancer, two of the leading causes, are discussed in previous sections. Partial thrombosis of the sagittal sinus may also occur in young women taking oral contraceptives and during pregnancy (Imai et al, 1982).

Clinical Features.   The typical clinical presentation is headache and obtundation caused by increased intracranial pressure, seizures, and successive hemiplegia on each side.

Diagnosis.   Venous thrombosis should be suspected when hemiplegia and increased intracranial pressure suddenly develop. Sagittal sinus thromboses can be suspected when parasagittal hemorrhage or infarction is present on CT. Definitive diagnosis requires cerebral arteriography.

Treatment.   Treatment is directed at decreasing intracranial pressure and rehydrating the patient without increasing cerebral edema.

Idiopathic Infarction
Capsular Stroke

Small, deep infarcts involving the internal capsule are usually seen in adults with hypertensive angiopathy. They also occur, but rarely, in infants and young children (Aram et al, 1983; Young et al, 1983). The onset of weakness is sudden and may occur during sleep or wakefulness.

Clinical Features.   The face and limbs are involved, and a typical hemiplegic posture and gait develop. Hypalgesia and decreased position sense are difficult to demonstrate in infants but can be observed in older children. Larger infarcts affecting the striatum and the internal capsule of the dominant hemisphere produce speech disturbances. At the onset of hemiplegia the child is mute and lethargic. As speech returns, evidence of dysarthria and aphasia develops. Eventually speech becomes normal. Hemiplegia may clear completely in the following year, but some children have residual weakness of the hand.

Diagnosis.   Capsular infarcts are demonstrated by CT or MRI. A cause is rarely determined despite extensive study (Table 11–3).

Treatment.   No treatment is available.

Cerebral Artery Infarction

Acute infantile hemiplegia may result from infarction in the distribution of the middle cerebral artery or one of its branches, the posterior cerebral artery, or the anterior cerebral artery.

Clinical Features.   Sudden hemiplegia is the typical clinical manifestation. Hemianesthesia, hemianopia, and aphasia (with dominant hemisphere infarction) are present as well. Some children are lethargic at the onset of symptoms, but consciousness is seldom lost completely.

In approximately one third of cases epilepsia partialis continua precedes the hemiplegia (Gastaut et al, 1979). In such cases permanent hemiplegia is a constant feature, and epilepsy is common. When hemiplegia occurs without seizures, half of patients recover completely and the remainder are left with partial paralysis.

Diagnosis.   Complete occlusion of the middle cerebral artery produces a large area of lucency on CT involving the cortex, underlying white matter, basal ganglia, and internal capsule. Occlusion of superficial branches of the middle cerebral artery produces a wedge-shaped area of lucency extending from the cortex into the subjacent white matter.

Treatment.   Seizures should be treated with anticonvulsant drugs (see Chapter 1). When seizures are intractable, hemispherectomy or commissurotomy should be considered (Goodman, 1986; Goodman et al, 1985).

Lipoprotein Disorders

Familial lipid and lipoprotein abnormalities may cause premature cerebrovascular disease in infants and children (Glueck et al, 1982). These disorders are transmitted by autosomal dominant inheritance.

Clinical Features.   Ischemic episodes produce transitory or permanent hemiplegia, sometimes associated with hemianopia, hemianesthesia, and aphasia. The family has a history of cerebrovascular and coronary artery disease developing at an early age.

Diagnosis.   Most children have low plasma concentrations of high-density lipoprotein (HDL) cholesterol, others have high plasma concentrations of triglycerides, and some have both. The mechanism of arteriosclerosis is lipoprotein-mediated endothelial damage with secondary thrombus formation.

Treatment.   Dietary treatment and daily aspirin administration are indicated.

Mitochondrial Encephalopathy, Lactic Acidosis, and Stroke

Approximately one third of patients with mitochondrial encephalopathy, lactic acidosis, and stroke (MELAS) have a biochemical defect that involves complex I (NADH–coenzyme Q reductase). Maternal transmission occurs in this disorder as well as several other mitochondrial disorders (Koga et al, 1988; Montagna et al, 1988).

Clinical Features.   Affected children are normal at birth and may develop normally. Mental deterioration, when present, occurs anytime during childhood. Growth retardation is common, and progressive deafness may be an associated feature. The cardinal neurologic features are recurrent attacks of prolonged migrainelike headaches and vomiting, seizures (myoclonic, focal, generalized) that often progress to status epilepticus, the sudden onset of focal neurologic defects (hemiplegia, hemianopia, aphasia), and encephalopathy. Neurologic abnormalities are initially intermittent and then become progressive, leading to coma and death.

Diagnosis. T_2-weighted MRI shows multifocal areas of hyperintense signal in the cerebral and cerebellar cortices and in the immediate adjacent white matter with sparing of deep structures (Matthews et al, 1991). The concentration of lactate in the blood and cerebrospinal fluid is elevated. Ragged-red fibers are noted on muscle biopsy (see Figure 7–6).

Treatment.   No treatment is available.

Moyamoya Disease

Moyamoya disease is a slowly progressive, bilateral occlusion of the internal carotid arteries starting at the carotid siphon. The basilar artery is sometimes occluded as well. Because the occlusion is slowly progressive, multiple anastomoses have time to form between the internal and external carotid arteries. The result is a new vascular network at the base of the brain composed of collaterals from the anterior or posterior choroidal arteries, the basilar artery, and the meningeal arteries. These telangiectasias produce a hazy appearance on angiography from which the Japanese word *moyamoya* ("puff of smoke") is derived (Figure 11–4). The disorder is worldwide in distribution with a female-to-male bias of 3:2. The underlying cause or causes have not been identified, but an arteritis is suspected.

Clinical Features.   The initial symptoms vary from recurrent headache to abrupt hemiparesis. Infants and young children tend to have an explosive onset characterized by the sudden development of complete hemiplegia affecting face and limbs. The child is at least lethargic and sometimes comatose.

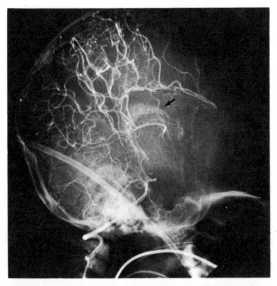

Figure 11–4 Moyamoya disease. Arteriography demonstrates occlusion of the carotid artery at the siphon and new anastomotic vessel formation *(arrow)*.

When the child is sufficiently alert to be examined, hemianopia, hemianesthesia, and aphasia may be found. Some children have chorea of the face and all limbs that may be worse on one side (Watanabe et al, 1990). Recovery follows, but before it is complete, new episodes of focal neurologic dysfunction occur on either the same or the opposite side. These episodes include hemiparesis, hemianesthesia, or aphasia, alone or in combination. The outcome is generally poor. Most children are left with chronic weakness of one or both sides, epilepsy, and mental retardation. Some have died.

Recurrent transient ischemic attacks are an alternative manifestation (Fukuyama and Umezu, 1985). These are characterized by episodic hemiparesis and dysesthesias lasting minutes or hours. Consciousness is retained. Attacks are frequently triggered by hyperpnea or excitement and may recur daily. After 4 or 5 years the attacks cease, but the child may be left with residual deficits.

Repeated episodes of monoparesis or symptoms of subarachnoid hemorrhage are other possible features of moyamoya disease. Monoparesis generally occurs after infancy and subarachnoid hemorrhage after sixteen years of age.

Diagnosis.   CT is likely to be the first diagnostic test performed on a child with acute hemiplegia. A large infarction is usually demonstrated because of stenosis in the internal carotid artery. Definitive diagnosis requires arteriographic demonstration of bilateral stenosis in the distal internal carotid arteries and the development of collaterals in the basal ganglia and meninges.

Treatment.   Intravenous verapamil was reported to be effective early in the course to provide return of function and radiographic evidence of increased perfusion (McLean et al, 1985). Temporal muscle graft, in which temporal muscle is placed over the arachnoid, has been attempted and found useful in providing better circulation to the superficial cortex (Takeuchi et al, 1983). However, this approach seems unlikely to add substantially to the natural development of arterial anastomoses.

Sickle Cell Anemia

Sickle cell anemia is a genetic disorder of black children that is transmitted by autosomal recessive inheritance. Neurologic manifestations occur in up to 25% of homozygotes and may occur at times of stress, such as surgery, in heterozygotes. The abnormal erythrocytes clog large and small vessels, decreasing total, hemispheric, or regional blood flow. Cerebral infarction usually occurs in the region of arterial border zones (Pavlakis et al, 1988).

Clinical Features. The major systemic manifestations are jaundice, pallor, weakness, and fatigability from chronic hemolytic anemia. Half of homozygotes show symptoms by 1 year, and all have symptoms by 5 years of age.

Strokes occur at the time of a thrombotic, vasoocclusive crisis. Such crises are frequently precipitated by dehydration or anoxia and are characterized by fever and pain in the abdomen and chest. Focal or generalized seizures are the initial neurologic manifestation in 70% of patients. After the seizures have ended, hemiplegia and other focal neurologic deficits are noted. Some recovery follows, but there is a tendency for recurrent strokes, epilepsy, and mental retardation. Strokes affecting both hemispheres produce a pseudobulbar palsy with brainstem dysfunction.

The worst case is a child who is in a coma and has meningismus. Such a case is usually caused by a diffuse decrease in cerebral blood flow associated with subarachnoid or intracerebral hemorrhage (Van Hoff et al, 1985). The mortality rate is high.

Diagnosis. The abnormal hemoglobin can be diagnosed at birth with acid agar gel electrophoresis or microcolumn chromatography. In most affected children sickle cell anemia is diagnosed long before their first stroke. The extent of cerebral infarction and hemorrhage during a cerebral vasoocclusive crisis can be documented by CT. After several such crises, cortical atrophy may be present.

Cerebral arteriography should be avoided, since it offers little additional information and carries the risk of increasing ischemia.

Treatment. A vasoocclusive crisis requires prompt hydration, oxygen administration, and transfusions of packed red blood cells. Hydration should not reach the point of increasing cerebral edema. Recurrent strokes may be prevented by a regimen of regular transfusions designed to keep the level of hemoglobin A above 60% (Russell et al, 1976).

Vasculopathies
Hypersensitivity Vasculitis

The term "hypersensitivity vasculitis" covers several disorders that have a known underlying cause (drugs, infection) and are characterized by purpura of the legs and venulitis. Neurologic manifestations occur only in *Henoch-Schonlein purpura,* for which the cause has not been established but is thought to be an antecedent infection.

Clinical Features. The systemic features of Henoch-Schonlein purpura are fever, a purpuric rash on the extensor surfaces of the limbs, and abdominal pain with nausea and vomiting. Joint and renal disturbances may be present. Almost half of affected children have headache and abnormalities on the EEG (Ostergaard and Storm, 1991). Focal neurologic deficits occur in one third of patients, with hemiplegia accounting for half of these cases (Belman et al, 1985). Hemiplegia may be preceded by a seizure and may be associated with hemianesthesia, hemianopia, and aphasia. These deficits may be permanent.

Diagnosis. Infarction or hemorrhage, or both, may be demonstrated by CT.

Treatment. Corticosteroids are used to treat the underlying disease.

Systemic Lupus Erythematosus

Several collagen vascular disorders can cause neurologic disturbances in adults, but systemic lupus erythematosus is the only major cause in children.

Clinical Features. Lupus is a systemic disorder, and 90% of children who have it have fever, 88% have joint complaints, and 74% have skin rash at the time of diagnosis (Meislin and Rothfield, 1968). Neurologic dysfunction is present in one fourth of children at the time of diagnosis and, unlike systemic complaints, is likely to progress or develop anew even after treatment is initiated. Neurologic dysfunction develops in 38% of children during the course of disease. Seizures, cranial neuropathies, and mental disorders are common features. Hemiplegia usually follows a seizure and may be caused by cerebral infarction or hemorrhage.

Diagnosis. The diagnosis of lupus requires a compatible clinical syndrome and the detection of antinuclear antibody. CT or MRI of the head is useful to determine the presence of hemorrhage or infarction. Results of cerebral arteriography may be normal.

Treatment. Large doses of corticosteroids are the mainstay of therapy, but the mortality rate is higher in children than in adults.

Takayasu Arteritis

Takayasu arteritis, a disorder of unknown cause, involves the aorta and its major branches.

Clinical Features. Onset usually occurs between 15 and 20 years of age but may occur as early as infancy (Kohrman and Huttenlocher, 1986). Ninety percent of patients are female. The most common manifestations are hypertension, absent pulses, and vascular bruits. Stroke occurs in only 5% to 10% of patients and is characterized by focal seizures and sudden hemiplegia.

Diagnosis. CT reveals a focal hypodense area, indicating infarction. Arteriography demonstrates involvement of the ascending aorta and its major branches. Cardiac catheterization is necessary to define the full extent of arteritis. Some vessels have a beaded appearance; others terminate abruptly and have prestenotic dilation.

Treatment. Aggressive immunosuppressive therapy with prednisone, 2 mg/kg/day, and azathioprine, 1 mg/kg/day, is indicated. If the disease is left untreated, the mortality rate is 75%. Early diagnosis and treatment can lead to full recovery.

DIABETES MELLITUS

Acute but transitory attacks of hemiparesis occur in children with insulin-dependent diabetes mellitus (MacDonald and Brown, 1979). Complicated migraine is a suggested mechanism (Korobkin, 1980), but the pathophysiology remains unknown.

Clinical Features. Attacks frequently occur during sleep in a child with a respiratory illness. Hemiparesis is present on awakening; the face and arm are more affected than the leg. Sensation is intact, but aphasia is present if the dominant hemisphere is affected. Tendon reflexes may be depressed or brisk in the affected arm, and an extensor plantar response is usually present. Headache is a constant feature and may be unilateral or generalized. Some patients are nauseated. The family does not have a history of migraine.

Attacks last for 3 to 24 hours, and recovery is complete. Recurrences are common.

Diagnosis. Stroke is not a complication of juvenile insulin-dependent diabetes except during episodes of ketoacidosis (see Chapter 2). Head CT in children with transitory hemiplegia does not demonstrate infarction. EEG reveals a focus of polymorphic delta activity that returns to normal after several days.

Treatment. Although some children have further attacks, no way of preventing recurrences has been found. Prophylactic phenobarbital was useful in one child.

EPILEPSY
Absence Status

Absence attacks in children are characterized by brief episodes of staring or eye blinking associated with 3 Hz generalized spike-wave complexes on the EEG (see Chapter 1). Prolonged absence at-

tacks are characterized by confusion and automatisms similar to complex partial seizures. In addition, a variant form of absence status with hemiparesis as the primary feature has been described (Niedermeyer et al, 1979).

Clinical Features. Some patients have a history of generalized tonic-clonic seizures but are not known to have a history of absence. The patient seems confused, has poor motor performance, and is unable to carry on a conversation. Transient hemiparesis or face-hand weakness is noted, and aphasia may be present. The attack ends spontaneously or with the intravenous administration of diazepam.

Diagnosis. EEG is essential for diagnosis. Several different epileptiform patterns may be seen. Most constant are 3 Hz spike-wave complexes from the frontal region during an attack. These complexes are often generalized but always have a unilateral predominance.

Treatment. Standard anticonvulsant drugs provide seizure control. However, the appropriate class of drugs to use in any individual is difficult to determine. Some respond to phenytoin or carbamazepine, whereas others respond to ethosuximide, valproate, or clonazepam.

Hemiconvulsions-Hemiplegia Syndrome

Explosive and intractable focal motor seizures followed by hemiplegia in an infant or child without a history of epilepsy is sometimes caused by infarction and is described in the previous section on cerebrovascular disease. An additional small percentage are caused by focal "inflammatory disease" (Rasmussen, 1978) or viral infections such as herpes. No cause can be identified in the majority of cases.

Clinical Features. Jerking in part of the face or in a limb develops in an infant or young child who was previously healthy. At onset the movements may be infrequent and of low amplitude, but they become continuous and involve the eyes, face, and both limbs within hours or days. Anticonvulsant therapy may stop the seizures temporarily or permanently. Afterward the affected limbs are hemiparetic. Hemianopia develops in some children. Permanent hemiplegia and mental retardation can be expected in every case, and most patients continue to have epilepsy.

Diagnosis. EEG demonstrates a continuous spike discharge on a background of polymorphic slowing in the hemisphere contralateral to the hemiparesis. Occasional spike discharges may be seen in the other hemisphere as well. Contrast-enhanced CT or MRI is indicated to search for infarction, hemorrhage, or arteriovenous malformation. The initial CT results are usually normal, but a year later CT demonstrates atrophy of the hemisphere with dilation of the ipsilateral ventricle.

The cerebrospinal fluid is usually normal, although a few monocytes may be present as a result of the prolonged seizure. In one patient the cerebrospinal fluid contained oligoclonal bands and an elevated IgG concentration (Andrews et al, 1990). Subsequent pathologic study of the affected hemisphere showed a vasculitis and immune complex disease.

Treatment.   An intravenous load of phenytoin or phenobarbital should be administered first and may stop, or at least decrease, the frequency of seizures. Unfortunately, most cases are refractory and complete control is not the rule. Several standard anticonvulsant drugs (see Chapter 1), alone or in combination, may be tried before acceptable control is established.

Uncontrolled focal seizures may evolve into intractable tonic-clonic seizures. In such cases interhemispheric commissurotomy can be considered (Goodman et al, 1985). This procedure prevents the development of a mirror focus and progression to generalized tonic-clonic seizures and allows easier management of focal seizures with anticonvulsant drugs.

Hemiparetic Seizures

Todd paralysis is a term used to describe hemiparesis that lasts minutes or days and follows a focal or generalized seizure. It most often occurs when seizures are prolonged or caused by an underlying structural abnormality. An ischemic mechanism has been suggested, and radioisotope studies demonstrate focal uptake in the contralateral hemisphere during the paralysis in support of that suggestion (Yarnell, 1975).

Hemiparesis may be a seizure manifestation as well as a postictal event. The seizures are called "hemiparetic" or "focal inhibitory" (Hanson and Chodos, 1978). Todd paralysis may be difficult to distinguish from hemiparetic seizures because it is not always clear whether a seizure preceded the hemiparesis or whether the hemiparesis is ictal or postictal.

Clinical Features.   The initial manifestation may be a brief focal seizure followed by flaccid hemiparesis or the abrupt onset of flaccid monoparesis or hemiparesis. Consciousness is not impaired, and the child seems well otherwise. The severity and distribution of weakness fluctuate, affecting one limb more than the other, and sometimes the face. Tendon reflexes are normal in the hemiparetic limbs, but the plantar response may be extensor.

Diagnosis.   EEG reveals recurrent spike and slow-wave discharges in the contralateral hemisphere. A radioisotope scan demonstrates increased focal uptake in the affected hemisphere. Results of CT and cerebral arteriography are normal.

Treatment.   Seizures respond to standard anticonvulsant drugs (see Chapter 1).

INFECTIONS

Hemiplegia occurs during the course of bacterial meningitis, resulting from vasculitis or venous thromboses, and during the course of viral encephalitis, especially herpes simplex, resulting from parenchymal necrosis. In both bacterial and viral infections, hemiplegia is usually preceded by prolonged or repetitive focal seizures.

Brain abscess may cause hemiplegia, but its evolution is usually slowly progressive rather than acute.

MIGRAINE

Migraine is a hereditary disorder associated with paroxysmal alterations in cerebral blood flow. Transitory neurologic abnormalities may accompany the attack, but these are believed to reflect a primary neuronal disturbance rather than cerebral ischemia. However, cerebral infarction may occur in adolescents during a prolonged attack of classic migraine (Bogousslavsky et al, 1988; Rothrock et al, 1988).

The occurrence of focal motor deficits, usually hemiplegia or ophthalmoplegia (see Chapter 15), during an occasional migraine attack is called *complicated migraine*. In some families hemiplegic migraine is a familial trait. This condition is called *familial hemiplegic migraine*.

Complicated Migraine

Clinical Features.   The family has a history of migraine, but other family members have not experienced hemiplegia during an attack. The evolution of symptoms is variable but usually incudes scintillating or simple scotomas, unilateral dysesthesias of the hand and mouth, and unilateral weakness of the arm and face. The leg is usually spared. Occurring concurrently with hemiparesis is a throbbing frontotemporal headache contralateral to the affected hemisphere (Heyck, 1973). Nausea and vomiting follow. The patient falls asleep and has usually recovered on awakening. Hemiparesis lasts less than 24 hours.

Diagnosis. Migraine is a clinical diagnosis that relies heavily on a family history of the disorder. During an attack of hemiplegic migraine an EEG focus of polymorphic delta activity is present in the hemisphere contralateral to weakness. Arteriography is contraindicated and may prolong the attack.

Treatment. The management of migraine is summarized in Chapter 3.

Familial Hemiplegic Migraine

Familial hemiplegic migraine differs from complicated migraine because other family members with migraine have at least one hemiplegic attack. The trait is transmitted by autosomal dominant inheritance.

Clinical Features. Attacks are stereotyped, occur primarily in childhood or adolescence, are precipitated by trivial head trauma, and rarely occur more often than once a year (Glista et al, 1975). The hemiplegia, although usually more severe in the face and arm, affects the leg too. Hemianesthesia of the hemiplegic side is a prominent feature. Aphasia is present when the dominant hemisphere is affected. Confusion, stupor, or psychosis may be present during an attack. The psychosis includes both auditory and visual hallucinations, as well as delusions (Feely et al, 1982). Occasionally patients have fever and a stiff neck.

Symptoms last for 2 or 3 days. When the attack is over, the neurologic deficits usually resolve completely, but permanent sequelae are possible. Recurrent hemiplegic attacks may occur on either the same or the opposite side.

Diagnosis. A family history of hemiplegic migraine is essential for diagnosis.

Treatment. There has been theoretical concern that propranolol may increase the chance of stroke in people with complicated migraine. This has not been substantiated, and I continue to recommended propranolol therapy in familial hemiplegic migraine (see Chapter 3).

TRAUMA

Trauma accounts for half of all deaths in children. Approximately 10% of traumatic injuries in children are not accidental. Head injury is the leading cause of death from child abuse, and half of survivors are left with permanent neurologic handicaps (McClelland et al, 1980).

Epidural hematoma, subdural hematoma, cerebral laceration, and intracerebral hemorrhage can produce focal signs such as hemiplegia. However, brain swelling is such a prominent feature of even trivial head injury in children (Snoek et al, 1984) that diminished consciousness and seizures are the typical clinical manifestations (see Chapter 2).

TUMORS

Primary tumors of the cerebral hemispheres are more likely to be manifested as chronic progressive hemiplegia than as acute hemiplegia and are discussed in Chapter 4. However, tumors may cause acute hemiplegia when they bleed or provoke seizures and must be considered in the evaluation of acute hemiplegia.

◆ Chronic Progressive Hemiplegia

The important causes of chronic progressive hemiplegia are brain tumor, brain abscess, and arteriovenous malformations. All three frequently are manifested by symptoms of increased intracranial pressure and are discussed in Chapter 4. Less often, progressive hemiplegia is an initial feature of demyelinating diseases, which are discussed in Chapters 5 and 10 (Table 11–4).

STURGE-WEBER SYNDROME

The Sturge-Weber syndrome is a sporadic neurocutaneous disorder characterized by unilateral venous angioma of the pia mater and an ipsilateral port-wine stain of the face (Aicardi and Arzimanoglou, 1991).

Clinical Features. The cutaneous angioma is flat and variable in size but usually involves the upper lid. The size of the cutaneous angioma does not predict the size of the intracranial angioma.

Seizures occur in 75% to 90% of children with Sturge-Weber syndrome. Onset is generally within the first year, and the seizure type is usually focal motor, sometimes leading to partial or generalized status epilepticus (see Chapter 1). Mental retardation is a common concurrent feature in children with seizures.

Table 11–4 ◆ Causes of Progressive Hemiplegia

1. Arteriovenous malformation (see Chapter 4)
2. Brain abscess (see Chapter 4)
3. Cerebral hemisphere tumor (see Chapter 4)
4. Demyelinating diseases
   a. Adrenoleukodystrophy (see Chapter 5)
   b. Late-onset globoid leukodystrophy (see Chapter 5)
   c. Multiple sclerosis (see Chapter 10)
5. Sturge-Weber syndrome

Hemiplegia, contralateral to the facial angioma, occurs in up to 50% of children. It is often noted initially after a focal-onset seizure and progresses in severity after subsequent seizures. Transient episodes of hemiplegia that cannot be related to clinical or EEG evidence of seizure activity may occur. Some episodes are associated with migraine-like headache. Others occur in the absence of other symptoms and may be caused by transitory ischemia.

Diagnosis. The association of neurologic abnormalities and a port-wine stain of the face should suggest the syndrome. The eyelid and the skin above the eye should be examined for angioma in any child with focal motor seizures. The pial angioma is best visualized by contrast-enhanced MRI and only rarely by angiography.

Treatment. The seizures are often difficult to control with anticonvulsant medications. Hemispherectomy is recommended when seizures are refractory and disabling.

References

Aicardi J: Alternating hemiplegia of childhood. Int Pediatr 2:115, 1987.

Aicardi J, Arzimanoglou A: Sturge-Weber syndrome. Int Pediatr 6:129, 1991.

Andrews JM, Thompson JA, Pysher TJ, et al: Chronic encephalitis, epilepsy, and cerebrovascular immune complex deposits. Ann Neurol 28:88, 1990.

Aram DM, Rose DF, Rekate HL, et al: Acquired capsular/striatal aphasia in childhood. Arch Neurol 40:614, 1983.

Belman AL, Leicher CR, Moshe SL, et al: Neurologic manifestations of Schoenlein-Henoch purpura: Report of three cases and review of the literature. Pediatrics 75:687, 1985.

Bergman I, Bauer RE, Barmada MA, et al: Intracerebral hemorrhage in the fullterm neonatal infant. Pediatrics 75:488, 1985.

Bogousslavsky J, Regli F, Van Melle G, et al: Migraine stroke. Neurology 38:223, 1988.

Bush JK, Giunere LB, Whitaker S, et al: Necrotizing fasciitis of the parapharyngeal space with carotid artery occlusion and acute hemiplegia. Pediatrics 73:343, 1984.

Cartwright GW, Culbertson K, Schreiner RL, et al: Changes in clinical presentation of term infants with intracranial hemorrhage. Dev Med Child Neurol 21:730, 1979.

Casaer P, Aicardi J, Curatolo P, et al: Flunarizine in alternating hemiplegia in childhood: An international study in 12 children. Neuropediatrics 18:191, 1987.

Cheng TO: Mitral valve prolapse. Annu Rev Med 40:201, 1989.

Clancy R, Malin S, Laraque D, et al: Focal motor seizures heralding stroke in full-term neonates. AJDC 139:601, 1985.

Feely MP, O'Hara J, Veale D, et al: Episodes of acute confusion or psychosis in familial hemiplegic migraine. Acta Neurol Scand 65:369, 1982.

Fenichel GM, Webster DL, Wong WKT: Intracranial hemorrhage in the term newborn. Arch Neurol 41:30, 1984.

Fukuyama Y, Umezu R: Clinical and cerebral angiographic evolutions of idiopathic progressive occlusive disease of the circle of Willis ("moyamoya" disease) in children. Brain Dev 7:21, 1985.

Gastaut H, Pinsard N, Gaustaut JL, et al: Acute hemiplegia in children. In Goldstein M, ed: Advances in Neurology. Raven Press, New York, 1979, p 329.

Glista GG, Mellinger JF, Rooke ED: Familial hemiplegic migraine. Mayo Clin Proc 50:307, 1975.

Glueck CJ, Daniels SR, Bates S, et al: Pediatric victims of unexplained stroke and their families: Familial lipid and lipoprotein abnormalities. Pediatrics 69:308, 1982.

Goodman R: Hemispherectomy and its alternatives in the treatment of intractable epilepsy in in patients with infantile hemiplegia. Dev Med Child Neurol 28:251, 1986.

Goodman RN, Williamson PD, Reeves AG, et al: Interhemispheric commissurotomy for congenital hemiplegics with intractable epilepsy. Neurology 35:1351, 1985.

Greenwood RD: Mitral valve prolapse: Incidence and clinical course in a pediatric population. Clin Pediatr 23:318, 1984.

Hanson PA, Chodos R: Hemiparetic seizures. Neurology 28:920, 1978.

Heyck H: Varieties of hemiplegic migraine. Headache 12:135, 1973.

Imai WK, Everhart FR, Sanders JM: Cerebral venous sinus thrombosis: Report of a case and review of the literature. Pediatrics 70:965, 1982.

Kaplan S: Chronic rheumatic heart disease. In Adams FH, Emmanoullides GC, eds: Heart Disease in Infants, Children, and Adolescents. Williams & Wilkins, Baltimore, 1983, p 552.

Katirji MB, Reinmuth OM, Latchaw RE: Stroke due to vertebral artery injury. Arch Neurol 42:242, 1985.

Kelly JJ, Mellinger JF, Sundt TM: Intracranial arteriovenous malformations in childhood. Ann Neurol 3:338, 1978.

Koga Y, Nonaka I, Kobayashi M, et al: Findings in muscle in complex I (NADH coenzyme Q reductase) deficiency. Ann Neurol 24:749, 1988.

Kohrman MH, Huttenlocher PR: Takayasu arteritis: A treatable cause of stroke in infancy. Pediatr Neurol 2:154, 1986.

Korobkin R: Active hemiparesis in juvenile insulin-dependent diabetes mellitus (JIDDM). Neurology 30:220, 1980.

Kurlan R, Griggs RC: Cyanotic congenital heart disease with suspected stroke: Should all patients receive antibiotics? Arch Neurol 40:209, 1983.

Leblanc R, O'Gorman AM: Neonatal intracranial hemorrhage: A clinical and serial computerized tomographic study. J Neurosurg 53:642, 1980.

Lenn NJ, Freinkel AJ: Facial sparing as a feature of prenatal-onset hemiparesis. Pediatr Neurol 5:291, 1989.

Levine SR, Brust JCM, Futrell N, et al: A comparative study of the cerebrovascular complications of cocaine: Alkaloidal versus hydrochloride—a review. Neurology 41:1173, 1991.

Levy SR, Abroms IF, Marshall PC, et al: Seizures and cerebral infarction in the full-term newborn. Ann Neurol 17:366, 1985.

Lewis DW, Berman PH: Vertebral artery dissection and alternating hemiparesis in an adolescent. Pediatrics 78:610, 1986.

Llorens-Terol J, Sole-Llenas J, Tura A: Stroke due to fibromuscular hyperplasia of the internal carotid artery. Acta Paediatr Scand 72:299, 1983.

MacDonald JT, Brown DR: Acute hemiparesis in juvenile insulin-dependent diabetes mellitus (JIDDM). Neurology 29:893, 1979.

Matthews PM, Tampieri D, Bervokic SF, et al: Magnetic resonance imaging shows specific abnormalities in the MELAS syndrome. Neurology 41:1043, 1991.

McClelland CQ, Rekate H, Kaufman B, et al: Cerebral injury in child abuse: A changing profile. Child Brain 7:225, 1980.

McLean MJ, Gebarski SS, Van Der Spek AFL, et al: Response of moyamoya disease to verapamil. Lancet 1:163, 1985.

Meislin AG, Rothfield N: Systemic lupus erythematosus in childhood: Analysis of 42 cases, with comparative data on 200 adult cases followed concurrently. Pediatrics 42:37, 1968.

Montagna P, Gallassi R, Medori R, et al: MELAS syndrome: Characteristic migrainous and epileptic features and maternal transmission. Neurology 38:751, 1988.

Niedermeyer E, Fineyre F, Riley T, et al: Absence status (petit mal status) with focal characteristics. Arch Neurol 36:417, 1979.

Ostergaard JR, Storm K: Neurologic manifestations of Schonlein-Henoch purpura. Acta Paediatr Scand 80:339, 1991.

Packer RJ, Rorke LB, Lange BJ, et al: Cerebrovascular accidents in children with cancer. Pediatrics 76:194, 1985.

Parker P, Puck J, Fernandez F: Cerebral infarction associated with *Mycoplasma* pneumonia. Pediatrics 67:373, 1981.

Pavlakis SG, Bello J, Prohovnik I, et al: Brain infarction in sickle cell anemia: Magnetic resonance imaging correlates. Ann Neurol 23:125, 1988.

Rasmussen T: Further observations on the syndrome of chronic encephalitis and epilepsy. Appl Neurophysiol 41:1, 1978.

Rothrock JF, Walicke P, Swenson WR, et al: Migrainous stroke. Arch Neurol 45:63, 1988.

Russell MO, Goldberg HI, Reis L, et al: Transfusion therapy for cerebrovascular abnormalities in sickle cell disease. J Pediatr 88:382, 1976.

Schoenberg BS, Mellinger JF, Schoenberg DG: Cerebrovascular disease in infants and children: A study of incidence, clinical features and survivial. Neurology 26:358, 1976.

Smith CD, Baumann RJ: Clinical features and magnetic resonance imaging in congenital and childhood stroke. J Child Neurol 6:263, 1991.

Smith DC, Smith LL, Hesso AN: Fibromuscular dysplasia of the internal carotid artery treated by operative transluminal balloon angioplasty. Radiology 155:645, 1985.

Snoek JW, Minderhoud JM, Wilmink JT: Delayed deterioration following mild head injury in children. Brain 107:15, 1984.

Solomon GE, Hilal SK, Gold AP, et al: Natural history of acute hemiplegia of childhood. Brain 93:107, 1970.

Tagawa T, Mimaki T, Yabuuchi H, et al: Bilateral occlusions in the cervical portion of the internal carotid arteries in a child. Stroke 6:896, 1985.

Takeuchi S, Tsuchida T, Kobayashi K, et al: Treatment of moyamoya disease by temporal muscle graft "encephalo-myosynangiosis." Child Brain 10:1, 1983.

Van Hoff J, Ritchey K, Shaywitz BA: Intracranial hemorrhage in children with sickle cell disease. AJDC 139:1120, 1985.

Watanabe K, Negoro T, Maehara M, et al: Moyamoya disease presenting with chorea. Pediatr Neurol 6:40, 1990.

Wiklund L-M, Uvebrant P: Hemiplegic cerebral palsy: Correlation between CT morphology and clinical findings. Dev Med Child Neurol 33:512, 1991.

Wiznitzer M, Masaryk TJ: Cerebrovascular abnormalities in pediatric stroke: Assessment using parenchymal and angiographic magnetic resonance imaging. Ann Neurol 29:585, 1991.

Yamada S, Kindt GD, Youmans JR: Carotid artery occlusion due to non-penetrating injury. J Trauma 7:333, 1967.

Yarnell PR: Todd's paralysis: A cerebrovascular phenomenon? Stroke 6:301, 1975.

Young RSK, Coulter DL, Allen RJ: Capsular stroke as a cause of hemiplegia in infancy. Neurology 33:1044, 1983.

Paraplegia and Quadriplegia

The term "paraplegia" is used in this text to denote partial or complete weakness of both legs, therefore obviating need for the term "paraparesis." Many conditions described fully in this chapter are abnormalities of the spinal cord. The same spinal abnormality can cause paraplegia or quadriplegia, depending on the location of injury. Therefore the two are discussed together in this chapter. The term "quadriplegia" is used to denote partial or complete weakness of all limbs, and the term "quadriparesis" is not used.

◆ Approach to Paraplegia

Weakness of both legs, without any involvement of the arms, suggests an abnormality of either the spinal cord or the peripheral nerves. Ordinarily peripheral neuropathies are readily identified by the pattern of distal weakness and sensory loss, atrophy, and loss of tendon reflexes (see Chapters 7 and 9). In contrast, spinal paraplegia causes spasticity, exaggerated tendon reflexes, and a dermatomal level of sensory loss. Disturbances in the conus medullaris and cauda equina, especially congenital malformation, may produce a complex of signs in which spinal cord or peripheral nerve localization is difficult. Indeed, both may be involved. Spinal paraplegia may be asymmetric at first, and then the initial feature is monoplegia (see Chapter 13). When anatomic localization between the spinal cord and peripheral nerves is difficult, electromyography (EMG) and nerve conduction studies are useful in making the distinction.

Paraplegia is sometimes caused by cerebral abnormalities. In such a case the child's arms as well as the legs are usually weak. However, leg weakness is so much greater than arm weakness that paraplegia is the chief complaint. It is important to remember that both the brain and the spinal cord may be abnormal and that the abnormalities can be in continuity (syringomyelia) or separated (Chiari malformation and myelomeningocele).

◆ Spinal Paraplegia and Quadriplegia

The conditions that cause acute, chronic, or progressive spinal paraplegia are listed in Table 12–1. In the absence of trauma the acute onset or rapid progression of paraplegia is caused by either spinal cord compression or myelitis. Spinal cord compression from any cause is a medical emergency requiring rapid diagnosis and therapy to avoid permanent paraplegia. Corticosteroids have the same dehydrating effect on the spinal cord as on the brain and provide transitory decompression before surgery.

Several techniques are available to visualize the spinal cord. The advantages and disadvantages of each are summarized in Table 12–2. Each has its place, and sometimes more than one technique must be used to achieve a comprehensive picture of the disease process. However, as resolution is increased and scan time decreased by newer magnetic resonance imaging (MRI) instruments, MRI is becoming the procedure of choice.

SYMPTOMS AND SIGNS

Clumsiness of gait, refusal to stand or walk, and loss of bladder or bowel control are the common complaints of spinal paraplegia. Clumsiness of gait is the usual feature of slowly progressive disorders. The decline in function can be sufficiently insidious to be overlooked for years. Refusal to stand or walk is a symptom of an acute process. When a young

Table 12–1 ◆ Spinal Paraplegia

Congenital Malformations
1. Arachnoid cyst
2. Arteriovenous malformations
3. Atlantoaxial dislocation
4. Caudal regression syndrome
5. Dysraphic states
   a. Chiari malformation
   b. Myelomeningocele
   c. Tethered spinal cord
6. Syringomyelia (see Chapter 9)

Familial Spastic Paraplegia
1. Autosomal dominant
2. Autosomal recessive
3. X-linked recessive

Infections
1. Asthmatic amyotrophy (see Chapter 13)
2. Diskitis
3. Epidural abscess
4. Herpes zoster myelitis
5. Polyradiculoneuropathy (see Chapter 7)
6. Tuberculous osteomyelitis

Neonatal Cord Infarction

Transverse Myelitis
1. Devic disease
2. Encephalomyelitis
3. Idiopathic

Trauma
1. Concussion
2. Epidural hematoma
3. Fracture dislocation
4. Neonatal cord trauma (see Chapter 6)

Tumors
1. Astrocytoma
2. Ependymoma
3. Neuroblastoma
4. Other

child refuses to support weight, the underlying cause may be weakness or pain. Sometimes both are present.

Scoliosis is a feature of many spinal cord disorders. It is seen with neural tube defects (McMaster, 1984; Park et al, 1985), spinal cord tumors (Citron et al, 1984; McMaster, 1984), and several degenerative disorders. The presence of scoliosis, in females before puberty and in males of all ages, should strongly suggest either a spinal cord disorder or a neuromuscular disease (see Chapters 6 and 7).

Abnormalities in the skin overlying the spine, such as an abnormal tuft of hair, pigmentation, a sinus opening, or a mass, may indicate an underlying dysraphic state. Spina bifida is almost always an associated feature.

Foot deformities and especially stunted growth of a limb are signs of lower spinal cord dysfunction. The usual deformity is foreshortening of the foot,

Table 12–2 ◆ Imaging the Spinal Cord

Imaging Method	Advantages	Disadvantages
Myelography	Allows visualization of entire spinal cord at one time; demonstrates blockage of cerebrospinal fluid flow	Invasive; requires use of contrast media (metrizamide), which may cause allergic reactions or seizures; two-dimensional; does not allow reconstruction in other planes
Computed tomography	Noninvasive; allows reconstruction in many planes; demonstrates bone–spinal cord relationship	Allows only limited portion of spinal cord to be visualized at one time
Magnetic resonance imaging	Noninvasive; no exposure to radiation; allows good cerebrospinal fluid–cord contrast; ease of multiplanar imaging; improved discrimination of extramedullary and intramedullary masses; better definition of cavities	Does not show bone

pes cavus. In such cases disturbances of bladder control are often an associated feature.

Spinal myoclonus is often misdiagnosed as seizure activity or fasciculations. It is characterized by brief, irregular contractions of small groups of muscles and persists in sleep. Myoclonus is caused by irritation to pools of motor neurons and interneurons, usually be an intramedullary tumor or syrinx. The dermatomal distribution of the myoclonus localizes the site of irritation within the spinal cord.

CONGENITAL MALFORMATIONS

Some congenital malformations, such as caudal regression syndrome and myelomeningocele, are obvious at birth. Many others do not cause symptoms until the teens or later. Congenital malformations must always be considered when progressive paraplegia appears in childhood.

Arachnoid Cysts

Arachnoid cysts of the spinal cord, like those of the brain (see Chapter 4), are usually asymptomatic and discovered incidentally on imaging studies. Familial cases should suggest neurofibromatosis type 2 (see Chapter 5).

Clinical Features. Arachnoid cysts may be single or multiple and are usually thoracic (Richaud, 1988). Symptomatic arachnoid cysts are unusual in children and are most often encountered in adolescents and young adults. The features are back or radicular pain and paraplegia. Symptoms are intensified when the child is standing and intermittent when the child changes position. They tend to become more severe with time.

Diagnosis. MRI is the diagnostic modality of choice.

Treatment. Shunting of the cyst is curative but should not be undertaken unless the cyst is known to be symptomatic. It is a common mistake to blame a subarachnoid cyst for symptoms that have another cause.

Arteriovenous Malformations

Arteriovenous malformations of the spinal cord are uncommon in childhood. The youngest patient reported was 1 year old, and only 14% of childhood cases begin before age 5 (Scarff and Reigel, 1979).

Clinical Features. The progression of symptoms is usually insidious. The average time from onset to diagnosis is approximately 5 years. Subacute or chronic pain is the initial feature in 38% of patients and subarachnoid hemorrhage in 26%. Paraplegia is an early feature in only 34%, but

monoplegia or paraplegia is present in 92% of children at the time of diagnosis. Most patients have a slowly progressive spastic paraplegia with loss of bladder control.

When subarachnoid hemorrhage is the initial manifestation, the malformation is more likely to be in the cervical portion of the spinal cord. Blunt trauma to the spine may be a precipitating factor. The onset of paraplegia or quadriplegia is acute and is associated with back pain.

Back pain and episodic weakness that improves completely or in part may be initial features in some children. Impairment is progressive. This type of presentation is misleading, and diagnosis may be delayed for several years.

Diagnosis. MRI has replaced myelography as the first step in diagnosis (Doppman et al, 1987). It distinguishes intramedullary from dural and extramedullary locations of the malformation and even allows recognition of thrombus formation (DiChiro et al, 1985). Arteriography is still necessary to demonstrate the intramedullary extent of the malformation and all of the feeding vessels.

Treatment. The potential approaches to therapy for intraspinal and intracranial malformations are similar (see Chapter 4).

Atlantoaxial Dislocation

The odontoid process is the major factor preventing dislocation of C-1 onto C-2. Aplasia of the odontoid process can occur alone or as part of Morquio syndrome, other mucopolysaccharidoses, Klippel-Feil syndrome, several types of genetic chondrodysplasia, and some chromosomal abnormalities (Roach et al, 1984; Skeletal Dysplasia Group, 1989). Asymptomatic atlantoaxial subluxation is thought to occur in 20% of children with Down syndrome as a result of congenital hypoplasia of the articulation of C-1 and C-2 (Chaudhry et al, 1987); symptomatic dislocation is much less common.

Clinical Features. Congenital atlantoaxial dislocation produces an acute or slowly progressive quadriplegia that may begin anytime from the neonatal period to adult life. When the onset is in a newborn, the clinical features resemble an acute infantile spinal muscular atrophy (see Chapter 6). The infant has generalized hypotonia with preservation of facial expression and extraocular movement. The tendon reflexes are absent at first but then become hyperactive.

Dislocations during childhood frequently follow a fall or head injury. In such cases symptoms may begin suddenly and include not only those of myelopathy but also those related to vertebral artery occlusion (Bhatnagar et al, 1991; Phillips et al, 1988).

Morquio syndrome is primarily a disease of the skeleton with only secondary abnormalities of the spinal cord. Beginning in the second year or thereafter, affected children have development of prominent ribs and sternum, knock-knees, progressive shortening of the neck, and dwarfism. The odontoid process is aplastic or absent. Acute, subacute, or chronic cervical myelopathy develops, sometimes precipitated by a fall. An insidious onset is characterized by loss of endurance, fainting attacks, and a "pins and needles" sensation in the arms.

The essential feature of the *Klippel-Feil syndrome* is a reduced number and abnormal fusion of cervical vertebrae. As in Morquio syndrome, the head appears to rest directly on the shoulders, the posterior hairline is low, and movement in all directions is limited (Nagib et al, 1985). Elevation of the scapulae and deformity of the ribs (Sprengel deformity) are frequently present. Weakness and atrophy of the arm muscles and mirror movements of the hands are associated with the paraplegia. Associated abnormalities may be present in several organ systems.

Symptomatic atlantoaxial dislocation in children with Down syndrome may occur anytime from infancy to the twenties. Females are affected more often than males. Symptoms include neck pain, torticollis, and an abnormal gait. Spinal cord compression is progressive and leads to quadriplegia and urinary incontinence.

Diagnosis.   Lateral radiographs of the cervical portion of the spine in extension and flexion may demonstrate atlantoaxial instability, but computed tomography (CT) of the cervical vertebrae provide better documentation of the instability and of the spinal cord compression. When Morquio syndrome is suspected, the urine should be checked for keratan sulfate.

Treatment.   Surgical stabilization of the atlantoaxial junction must be undertaken in any child with evidence of spinal cord compression. The choice of surgical procedure depends on the mechanism of compression.

Caudal Regression Syndrome

The term "caudal regression syndrome" covers several malformations of the caudal spine that range from sacral agenesis to sirenomelia, in which only one leg is present (Towfighi and Housman, 1991). The mechanism of caudal regression is poorly understood. Although the name implies that the cord was formed properly and then regressed,

defects in neural tube closure are often associated features. The risk of caudal regression is greater among infants of diabetic mothers.

The clinical spectrum varies from absence of the lumbrosacral spinal cord, resulting in small paralyzed legs, to a single malformed leg associated with malformations of the rectum and genitourinary tract.

Chiari Malformation

The type I Chiari malformation is elongation of the cerebellar vermis with herniation of its caudal end through the foramen magnum. The type II malformation combines the cerebellar herniation with distortion and dysplasia of the medulla and occurs in more than 50% of children with lumbar myelomeningocele (Azimullah et al, 1991). The herniated portion may become ischemic and necrotic and can cause compression of the brainstem and upper cervical spinal cord.

Clinical Features.   The onset of a type I malformation is often insidious (Dyste and Menezes, 1988). Headache and neck pain are the first features in 38% of children and weakness in 56%. Eighty percent demonstrate motor deficits on examination, usually atrophy and hyporeflexia in the arms and spasticity and hyperreflexia in the legs. Sensory loss and scoliosis are each present in 50% of cases.

The type II malformation should be suspected in every child with myelomeningocele. In most the cerebellar displacement is asymptomatic. Hydrocephalus may result from aqueductal stenosis or obstruction of the outflow of cerebrospinal fluid from the fourth ventricle, resulting from herniation. Respiratory distress is the most important feature of the Chiari malformation and the usual cause of death (Papasozomenos and Roessmann, 1981). Rapid respirations, episodes of apnea, and Cheyne-Stokes respirations may be observed. Other evidence of brainstem compression includes poor feeding, vomiting, dysphagia, and paralysis of the tongue. Sudden cardiorespiratory failure is the usual cause of death.

Diagnosis.   The malformation is best visualized by MRI of the posterior fossa and cervical cord, but recognition of bony abnormalities of the cervical cord may require CT or plain radiographs.

Treatment.   Newborns with myelomeningocele and respiratory distress caused by the Chiari malformation are often treated with posterior fossa decompression. Unfortunately, the results have not been encouraging. Posterior fossa decompression is usually successful in relieving symptoms of cord compression in older children without myelomeningocele. Ventriculoperitoneal shunt may be required as well.

Myelomeningocele

Dysraphia comprises all defects in the closure of the neural tube and its coverings. Closure occurs during the third and fourth weeks of gestation. The mesoderm surrounding the neural tube gives rise to dura, skull, and vertebrae, but not to the skin. Therefore defects in the final closure of the neural tube and its mesodermal case do not preclude the presence of a dermal covering.

Despite extensive epidemiologic studies the cause of myelomeningocele remains unknown. Causes are likely to be multifactorial, including both genetic and environmental factors. Because women who have previously had a child with dysraphia have an approximately 2% risk of recurrence, prenatal diagnosis can be offered to prevent repetition.

Alpha fetoprotein is the principal plasma protein of the fetus and is present in amniotic fluid. When the fetus has a defect of the skin that allows the exudation of plasma proteins, the concentration of alpha fetoprotein in the amniotic fluid increases. Prenatal diagnosis is possible in every case by the combination of measuring the maternal serum concentration of alpha fetoprotein and performing an ultrasound examination of the fetus (Nadel et al, 1990).

The incidence of dysraphic defects has been declining in the United States (Adams et al, 1985) and the United Kingdom (Carstairs and Cole, 1984). This decline cannot be explained by antenatal screening alone and may be due in part to changes in critical environmental factors.

The ingestion of folic acid supplements during early pregnancy reduces the incidence of neural tube defects (Milunsky et al, 1989). Women who have had a pregnancy resulting in an infant with a neural tube defect are advised to start folic acid supplementation, 4 mg/day, from at least 4 weeks before conception through the first 3 months of pregnancy (MRC Vitamin Study Research Group, 1991).

Clinical Features. *Spina bifida cystica,* the protrusion of a cystic mass through the defect, is an obvious deformity of the newborn's spine. More than 90% are thoracolumbar. Among newborns with spina bifida cystica the protruding sac is a meningocele without neural elements in 10% to 20% and is a myelomeningocele in the rest. Meningoceles tend to have a partial dermal covering and are often pedunculated, with a narrow base connecting the sac to the underlying spinal cord.

Myelomeningoceles usually have a broad base, are poorly epithelialized, and ooze a combination of cerebrospinal fluid and serum. Remnants of the spinal cord are fused to the exposed portion of the dome.

In newborns with spina bifida cystica it is important to determine the extent of neurologic dysfunction caused by the myelopathy, the potential for the development of hydrocephalus, and the presence of other malformations in the nervous system and in other organs. When myelomeningocele is the only deformity, the newborn is alert and responsive and has no difficulty in feeding. Diminished consciousness or responsiveness and difficulty in feeding should suggest perinatal asphyxia or cerebral malformations such as hydrocephalus. Cyanosis, pallor, or dyspnea may be due to associated malformations in the cardiovascular system. Multiple major defects are present in 27% of cases (Adams et al, 1985).

Location of the myelomeningocele with reference to the ribs and iliac crest provides reasonably accurate information concerning the spinal segments involved. Several patterns of motor dysfunction may be observed, depending on the cyst's location. Motor dysfunction results from interruption of the corticospinal tracts and from dysgenesis of the segmental innervation. At birth the legs are flaccid and the hips are dislocated. Spastic paraplegia, a spastic bladder, and sensory loss develop in infants with a thoracic lesion. Segmental withdrawal reflexes below the level of the lesion, which indicate the presence of an intact but isolated spinal cord segment below the cyst, can be demonstrated in 50% of patients. Infants with deformities of the conus medullaris maintain a flaccid paraplegia, have lumbosacral sensory loss, lack a withdrawal response in the legs, and have a distended bladder with overflow incontinence.

Only 15% of newborns with myelomeningocele have clinical evidence of hydrocephalus at birth, but hydrocephalus can be detected in 60% of affected newborns by ultrasound (Adams et al, 1985). Hydrocephalus eventually develops in 80% of these newborns. The first clinical manifestation frequently follows the repair of the myelomeningocele, but the two are not related. In 73% of newborns with myelomeningocele, hydrocephalus is caused by aqueductal stenosis.

Diagnosis. The diagnosis of spina bifida cystica is made by examination alone. Electromyography (EMG) may be useful to clarify the distribution of segmental dysfunction. Cranial ultrasound should be performed on every newborn to look for hydrocephalus. CT or MRI is useful to define malformations of the brain, especially the Chiari malformation (see Figure 10–7). This information may be needed in making therapeutic decisions. Even when hydrocephalus is not present at birth, ultrasound should be repeated in 2 to 4 weeks to evaluate ventricular size.

Treatment. The chance of surviving the first year is poor unless the back is closed (Adams et al, 1985; Charney et al, 1985). However, closure is not a surgical emergency and can be delayed for a week or longer without having an impact on survival rate (Charney et al, 1985). Other factors associated with an increased mortality are a high spinal location of the defect and clinical hydrocephalus at birth.

During the 1960s an aggressive approach to the treatment of myelomeningocele was pursued in the United Kingdom. The results were not encouraging; only 2% of patients were free of any handicap and 80% were severely impaired (Lorber, 1971). Better results have been reported from the United States (Reigel and McLone, 1988). Of 358 newborns with myelomeningocele who were transferred to one medical center between 1978 and 1986, 80% underwent closure of the back defect within 24 hours. Hydrocephalus requiring a shunt developed in 89%, of whom 18% developed ventriculitis. Eighty-four percent were not confined to a wheelchair, and seven patients with thoracic and upper lumbar level lesions were able to walk without braces.

The difference between the experience in the United States and that in the United Kingdom probably has several reasons, not the least of which is two decades of improvement in medical and surgical care. In the United States survival rates were higher in the last half of the 1970s than in the first half.

Tethered Spinal Cord

The conus medullaris is sometimes anchored to the base of the vertebrae by a thickened filum terminale, a lipoma, a dermal sinus, or a diastematomyelia. Spina bifida occulta is usually an associated feature, and for this reason these anomalies are considered part of the spectrum of dysraphia (Anderson, 1975). As the child grows, the tether causes the spinal cord to stretch and the lumbosacral segments to become ischemic. The mitochondrial oxidative metabolism of neurons is impaired, and neurologic dysfunction follows (Yamada et al, 1981).

Dermal sinus is a midline opening of the skin usually marked by a tuft of hair or port-wine stain. It is caused by an abnormal invagination of ecto-derm into the posterior closure site of the neural tube. Most sinuses terminate subcutaneously as a blind pouch or dermoid cyst. Others extend through a spina bifida to the developing neuraxis, at which point they attach to the dura or the spinal cord as a fibrous band or dermoid cyst. Such sinuses tether the spinal cord and may also serve as a route for bacteria from the skin to reach the subarachnoid space and cause meningitis.

Diastematomyelia consists of a bifid spinal cord (also diplomyelia) that is normal in the cervical and upper thoracic region and then divides into lateral halves (Figure 12–1). Two types of diastematomyelia occur with equal frequency. In one type each half of the cord is surrounded by its own dural sheath and the two halves are separated by a fibrous or bony septum. Once the cord separates, it never rejoins. In the other type the two halves are surrounded by a single dural sheath, no septum is present, and the two halves rejoin after one or two segments. Therefore splitting of the spinal cord is not caused by the presence of a septum but is instead a primary disturbance in the formation of luminal borders caused by faulty closure of the neural tube. It is usually associated with other dysraphic disturbances such as spina bifida occulta or cystica (Dryden, 1980).

Clinical Features. The initial manifestations of a tethered spinal cord occur at any age from infancy to young adulthood. The clinical features vary with age. External signs of spinal dysraphism (tuft of hair, subcutaneous lipoma, dermal sinus) are present in more than half of patients, and spina bifida occulta or sacral deformity is present in almost 90% (Anderson, 1975; Fitz and Harwood-Nash, 1975).

Infants and young children are most likely to demonstrate clumsiness of gait, stunted growth or deformity of one foot or leg, and disturbances in bladder function. These symptoms may occur alone or in combination. Consequently the first specialist consulted may be an orthopedic surgeon, a urologist, a neurologist, or a neurosurgeon. The progression of symptoms and signs is insidious, and at first most children are believed to have a static problem. Children with only a clumsy gait or disturbances in urinary control tend to have normal or exaggerated tendon reflexes and a Babinski sign. In some children the ankle tendon reflex is diminished or absent on one or both sides. Children with foot deformity usually have pes cavus and stunted growth of the entire leg. The other leg may appear normal or have a milder deformity without a growth disturbance. The tendon reflexes in the deformed foot are more likely to be diminished than increased.

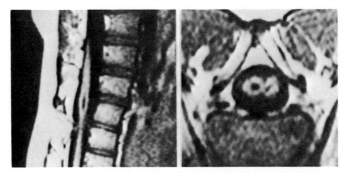

Figure 12–1 Diplomyelia. Magnetic resonance image shows two cords with two central canals. An enlarged segment with a cystic center is seen on longitudinal section.

The initial manifestation of tethered spinal cord in older children and adolescents is either clumsiness of gait or scoliosis. Bilateral, but mild, foot deformities are sometimes present, and urinary incontinence and constipation may be reported. Tendon reflexes in the legs are usually exaggerated at the knees and ankles, and the Babinski sign is frequently present.

Diagnosis. EMG is not useful as a screening procedure, since the results are almost always normal. Radiographs of the spine may demonstrate spina bifida, but a more definitive imaging procedure is needed in every case.

MRI is the appropriate diagnostic test and is particularly useful in the detection of lumbosacral lipoma (Brophy et al, 1989). The essential feature of a tethered spinal cord is a low-lying conus medullaris. At 28 weeks' gestational age the tip of the conus is at the L-3 vertebral level. It generally rises one L-2 level by 40 weeks' gestation (Fitz and Harwood-Nash, 1975). A conus tip below the L-2 to L-3 interspace in children 5 years and older is always abnormal.

Treatment. Surgical relief of the tethering prevents further deterioration of neurologic function. However, improvement of preexisting deficits occurs in only 25% of patients with lipoma and 50% of patients with a thickened filum terminale (James et al, 1984; Linder et al, 1982).

FAMILIAL SPASTIC PARAPLEGIA

Familial spastic paraplegia is a heterogeneous group of genetic disorders in which the prominent clinical manifestation is a progressive spastic paraplegia. Degeneration occurs in the lateral and posterior columns of the spinal cord, and for this reason these disorders are classified in the broader category of spinocerebellar degenerations. Some families have pure spastic paraplegia without clinical evidence of degeneration in the posterior columns or cerebellar pathways. Familial spastic paraplegia is usually transmitted by autosomal dominant (70%) or autosomal recessive (30%) inheritance. Genetic heterogeneity exists even within the dominant and recessive forms. An X-linked form has been reported in only 14 families (Ülkü et al, 1991).

Autosomal Dominant Inheritance

Two types of familial spastic paraplegia transmitted by autosomal dominant inheritance have been identified: type I designates cases with onset in childhood, and type II comprises cases with onset in adult life (Harding, 1981). Only type I is discussed here.

Clinical Features. As a rule, dominantly inherited spastic diplegia is not associated with other neurologic or nonneurologic features (Appleton et al, 1991). The mean age at onset is 11 years in boys and 16 years in girls. Onset may be as early as infancy. Such infants demonstrate toe-walking, and their condition is frequently misdiagnosed as cerebral palsy, especially if the affected parent is asymptomatic or has only a mildly stiff gait. Increased tone is more prominent than weakness. Tone increases slowly for 10 years and then stabilizes. At this point the child may have minimal stiffness of gait or be unable to stand or walk.

Tendon reflexes are usually increased in the legs and arms, and ankle clonus may be present. Occasionally tendon reflexes at the ankle are diminished or absent. Increased reflexes are usually the only sign of involvement of the arms, but almost 20% of patients have mild arm ataxia as well. One third of patients have urinary symptoms, usually in the form of frequency and urgency, and one third have a pes cavus deformity.

Diagnosis. This disorder is difficult to diagnose in the absence of a family history of the defect. It should be suspected in any child with very slowly progressive spastic paraplegia. Laboratory studies are not helpful except to exclude other conditions such as spinal cord compression and adrenoleukodystrophy.

Treatment.   No treatment is available.

Autosomal Recessive Inheritance

Autosomal recessive inheritance of hereditary spastic paraplegia is characterized by involvement of other neurologic systems (Appleton et al, 1991). The associated features vary from family to family, suggesting genetic heterogeneity.

Clinical Features.   Spastic paraplegia may begin during infancy but can be delayed until the teens. Involvement of other neurologic systems follows the establishment of spastic paraplegia. The common associated features are cerebellar dysfunction, pseudobulbar palsy, sensory neuropathy, and pes cavus. These features may be present in any combination.

Children with sensory neuropathy lose the tendon reflexes in the legs that had once been hyperactive. Some have delayed development and never achieve bladder control. When sensory loss is progressive, the symptoms resemble those of familial sensory neuropathies described in Chapter 9. The outcome varies from mild disability to wheelchair confinement.

Diagnosis.   The onset of paraplegia in infancy, in the absence of a family history of the disease, is likely to suggest cerebral palsy until the progressive nature of the spasticity is recognized. Sensory neuropathy with mutilation of digits may lead to the erroneous diagnosis of syringomyelia. Laboratory tests are useful only to exclude other diagnoses.

Treatment.   No treatment is available for the underlying defect, but supportive care for the sensory neuropathy is needed (see Chapter 9).

INFECTIONS
Diskitis

Diskitis is a relatively common disorder of childhood in which one disk space is inflamed; adjacent vertebral bodies may be affected as well. The cause is uncertain, but bacterial infection, viral infection, and trauma have been suspected. *Staphylococcus aureus* is the organism most often grown on cultures of disk material removed by needle biopsy and is probably the major cause (Wenger et al, 1978). The same organism is sometimes isolated on cultures of the blood.

Clinical Features.   The initial manifestation is either difficulty walking or pain. Difficulty walking occurs almost exclusively in children less than 3 years of age. The typical child has a low-grade fever, is observed to be limping, and refuses to stand or walk. This symptom complex evolves over 24 to 48 hours. Affected children prefer to lie on their sides rather than to rest supine, resist being brought to standing, and then seem uncomfortable and walk with a shuffling gait. Examination reveals loss of lumbar lordosis. The hips or back is sometimes tender.

Pain as an initial feature occurs more often after 3 years of age. The pain may be abdominal or vertebral. When abdominal, the pain generally increases in intensity and may radiate from the epigastrium to the umbilicus or pelvis. Abdominal pain in association with low-grade fever and an elevated peripheral white blood cell count invariably suggests the possibility of appendicitis or other intraabdominal disease. Fortunately, abdominal pain is the least common manifestation.

Back pain is the most common complaint. Older children may indicate a specific area of pain and tenderness. Younger children may have only an abnormal posture intended to splint the painful area. Back pain usually leads to prompt diagnosis because attention is immediately directed to the spine. Examination reveals point tenderness, loss of lumbar lordosis, and decreased movement of the spine.

Diagnosis.   Diskitis should be considered in all children who have a sudden back pain or refuse to walk and in whom neurologic findings are normal. Strength, tone, and tendon reflexes in the legs are normal. Radiographs of the spine reveal narrowing of the affected intervertebral space, most often in the lumbar region but sometimes as high as the C-5 to C-6 positions. The inflammation within the disk is best demonstrated by MRI, which shows osteomyelitis of the surrounding vertebrae as well as of the disk space (Figure 12–2).

Treatment.   Whether antibiotics are effective is a matter of controversy. However, a course of treatment directed at *S. aureus* seems reasonable, even if the organism cannot be grown on culture. Immobilization is important, as much to reduce pain as to encourage healing. Bed rest is sufficient immobilization for most children.

EPIDURAL ABSCESS

Most epidural abscesses result from hematogenous spread of bacteria, most often hemolytic *S. aureus,* rather than direct extension from vertebral osteomyelitis. The abscess is usually located on the

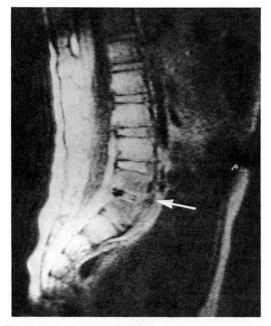

Figure 12–2 Diskitis. Magnetic resonance image reveals collapse of the disk space *(arrow)* and demineralization of the adjoining vertebral bodies.

dorsal surface of the midthoracic or lower lumbar spine, at which point the epidural space is large. The source of infection may be cutaneous or intraabdominal, and often no source can be identified. Despite occasional reports of epidural abscess in infancy, it rarely occurs in children less than 10 years of age.

Clinical Features. A bacterial infection or trauma to the back is described as an antecedent event in some children. The initial manifestation is usually back pain, which increases in severity and localizes at the site of the abscess. An effort is made to splint the trunk in extension; flexion and coughing intensify the pain. Fever is often present at the onset of pain but may be delayed for days. Headache, vomiting, and stiff neck often develop and suggest the diagnosis of meningitis. At this stage, examination reveals a rigid spine with tenderness to percussion over the involved area (Bell and McCormick, 1981).

Symptoms of root irritation and spinal cord compression develop 3 to 6 days after localized back pain begins. Because the abscess is usually thoracic, root irritation is characterized by radiating pain around the chest or into the groin. Spinal cord compression is characterized by progressive paraplegia and bladder dysfunction. Back pain intensifies and is more severe than the pain associated with spinal cord compression by tumor. Fever also suggests abscess.

Epidural abscess in the thoracic region may produce flaccid or spastic paraplegia with hyperreflexia in the legs. An abscess in the lumbar region produces flaccid paraplegia and diminished tendon reflexes.

Diagnosis. Most children with spinal epidural abscess undergo lumbar puncture because meningitis is suspected. If the abscess is lumbar and is pierced by the spinal needle, meningitis will follow. The cerebrospinal fluid is usually sterile, with an increased concentration of protein and a mixed pleocytosis in which lymphocytes predominate. The concentration of glucose is normal. Definitive diagnosis requires MRI of the painful area.

Treatment. Intravenous antibiotics directed against *S. aureus* should be started immediately when spinal epidural abscess is suspected. As with other causes of spinal cord compression, early surgical decompression is essential. The likelihood of recovery is diminished with each day that paraplegia is allowed to persist.

Herpes Zoster Myelitis

Immunosuppressed individuals may experience reactivation of the varicella-zoster virus that had been latent in sensory ganglia following primary chicken-pox infection (Devinsky et al, 1991).

Clinical Features. The spinal cord becomes involved within 3 weeks after a truncal rash appears. The myelopathy usually progresses for 3 weeks, but progression may last as long as 6 months in people with acquired immunodeficiency syndrome (AIDS). Cord involvement is bilateral in 80% of cases.

Diagnosis. Diagnosis depends on recognition of the characteristic herpetic rash at the dermatomal level of the myelitis. The spine should be imaged to exclude other causes. The cerebrospinal fluid shows a pleocytosis and protein elevation that is greatest at the time of maximal neurologic deficit.

Treatment. Corticosteroids and acyclovir are recommended for treatment, although their benefit is uncertain.

Tuberculous Osteomyelitis

Vertebral infection is due to hematogenous dissemination. Any level of the vertebral column may be affected. The infection usually begins in one vertebral body and spreads to adjacent vertebrae and the surrounding soft tissue. Less than 20% of patients with tuberculous osteomyelitis have symptoms of spinal cord dysfunction. The pathophysiologic mechanisms include epidural abscess, arteritis, and vertebral collapse. In addition, tuberculous granuloma of the spine may occur in the absence of vertebral disease.

Clinical Features.   Tuberculosis of the vertebrae and spine is primarily a disease of children and young adults. Young children with vertebral osteomyelitis not extending to the spinal cord may refuse to walk because of pain, and their symptoms may mimic paraplegia. The prominent features are fever, anorexia, and back pain. In children less than 10 years of age, infection is generally diffuse, affecting several vertebrae and adjacent tissues (Hsu and Leong, 1984). Older children tend to have localized infection, but with a higher incidence of spinal cord compression.

The symptoms and signs of spinal cord compression from tuberculosis are similar to those described for epidural abscess, except that progression is slower.

Diagnosis.   The cerebrospinal fluid is usually under pressure and demonstrates a pleocytosis with polymorphonuclear leukocytes predominating early in the course and lymphocytes predominating in the later stages. The total cell count rarely exceeds 500 cells/mm^3. Protein concentrations are elevated, and glucose concentrations are depressed. Acid-fast organisms can be seen on stained smear and can be isolated on cultures of the cerebrospinal fluid.

Early stages of vertebral osteomyelitis can be demonstrated by technetium bone scan or plain radiographs. As the disease progresses, radiographs reveal collapse of adjacent vertebrae and gibbus formation.

Treatment.   Tuberculous osteomyelitis and meningitis should be treated in a similar fashion. The recommended drug combinations are oral isoniazid, 20 mg/kg/day (up to 500 mg/day); intramuscular streptomycin, 20/mg/kg/day (up to 1 g/day); and oral rifampin, 15 mg/kg/day (up to 15 mg/kg). Streptomycin and rifampin are continued for 8 weeks following clinical improvement, and isoniazid is continued for 2 years (Bell and McCormick, 1981).

NEONATAL CORD INFARCTION

Infarction of the spinal cord is a hazard in newborns undergoing umbilical artery catheterization (Haldeman et al, 1983). The artery of Adamkiewicz arises from the aorta at the level of T-10 to T-12 and is the major segmental artery to the thoracolumbar spinal cord. Embolization of the artery may occur if the catheter tip is placed between levels T-8 and T-11. The result is acute and sometimes irreversible paraplegia. A similar syndrome can occur in premature or small-for-dates newborns who have not been catheterized (Singer et al, 1991). The mechanism is not understood but probably is caused by hypotension to the cord.

TRANSVERSE MYELITIS

Transverse myelitis is an acute demyelinating disorder of the spinal cord that evolves in hours or days. It may occur alone or in combination with demyelination in other portions of the nervous system. The association of transverse myelitis and optic neuritis is called *Devic disease;* acute demyelination throughout the neuraxis is called *diffuse encephalomyelitis.* These terms are descriptive and do not suggest an underlying cause.

Multiple sclerosis is usually suspected in adults with transverse myelitis, although only 15% eventually have other demyelinating lesions disseminated in time (Ropper and Poskanzer, 1978). Multiple sclerosis is exceedingly uncommon in childhood, and it is usually manifested as ataxia when it occurs (see Chapter 10).

Transverse myelitis, and especially encephalomyelitis, in children is frequently attributed to a preceding viral infection or immunization. No evidence supports such a notion. School-age children average four to six "viral" episodes annually. Therefore half of children with any illness may give a history of a viral infection within the preceding 30 days. Similarly, despite several case reports there is no epidemiologic evidence supporting a cause-and-effect relationship between licensed vaccines and demyelinating disorders of the central nervous system.

Clinical Features.   Mean age at onset is 9 years. Symptoms progress rapidly, and maximal deficit is attained within 2 days (Adams and Armstrong, 1990). The level of myelitis is usually thoracic and demarcated by the sensory loss. Asymmetric leg weakness is common. The bladder fills and does not empty voluntarily. Tendon reflexes may be increased or reduced. Recovery begins after 6 days but may be incomplete (Dunne et al, 1986). Fifty percent of patients make a full recovery, 10% have no recovery, and 40% recover incompletely. Most resume walking, but many continue to have sensory disturbances.

Diagnosis.   MRI of the spine should be performed to exclude acute cord compression, and it sometimes shows swelling at the level of myelitis. Cranial MRI is indicated to exclude more widespread disease. Vision should be checked daily because of the possibility of Devic disease.

Treatment.   Prednisone is generally used despite the absence of controlled studies.

Devic Disease (Neuromyelitis Optica)

A temporal association between pulmonary tuberculosis and Devic disease has been observed in adolescents and adults (Silber et al, 1990). In these cases the neurologic disease appears to be an immune reaction to tuberculosis and not caused by antituberculous therapy. No cause can be determined in most children.

Clinical Features.   A history of anorexia or a flulike syndrome a few days or a week before the first neurologic symptoms is common. The anorexia may be part of the acute demyelinating illness rather than a viral infection. Myelitis precedes optic neuritis in 13% of patients and follows it in 76%, myelitis and neuritis occur simultaneously in 10% (Whitham and Brey, 1985). Optic neuritis and transverse myelitis generally occur within 1 week of each other. The child remains irritable while the neurologic symptoms are evolving.

Bilateral optic neuritis occurs in 80% of patients (see Chapter 16). Both eyes may be affected at onset, or one eye may become affected before the other. Loss of vision is acute and accompanied by pain. Blindness is often complete within hours. The initial opthalmoscopic examination may have normal results but more often shows swelling of the disk. The pupils are dilated, and response to light is sluggish.

Myelitis is heralded by back pain and discomfort in the legs. The legs become weak, and the patient has difficulty standing and walking. Paraplegia becomes complete; it is first flaccid and then becomes spastic. Tendon reflexes may be diminished at first but later become exaggerated and are associated with extensor plantar responses. The bladder is spastic, and the patient has overflow incontinence. In some patients a sensory level may be detected, but more often the sensory deficit is patchy and difficult to delineate in an irritable child.

The course of Devic disease varies. Approximately one fourth of cases evolve into encephalomyelitis (see "Diffuse Encephalomyelitis"), another one fourth remain stationary, and the remaining half demonstrate some recovery that is usually incomplete (Cloys and Netsky, 1970).

Diagnosis.   Any child with acute transverse myelitis may also have a spinal cord compression syndrome. A space-occupying mass of the spine must be excluded by MRI. If none is found, MRI of the head should be performed to delineate the extent of demyelination.

Adrenoleukodystrophy should be considered in boys with Devic disease or diffuse encephalomyelitis. Carrier females may have paraplegia alone (Moser et al, 1984). This disorder may be explosive in onset and simulate an acute, acquired demyelinating disease (see Chapter 5). An adrenocorticotropic hormone (ACTH) stimulation test is useful for screening, but definitive diagnosis requires measuring the serum concentration of very-long-chain fatty acids.

The cerebrospinal fluid in children with Devic disease is usually abnormal. The protein content is mild to moderately elevated, and a mixed pleocytosis of neutrophils and mononuclear cells is present.

Treatment.   A course of corticosteroids is usually suggested for children with Devic disease. Although the value of corticosteroids has never been established, most physicians believe they are beneficial. The regimen is the same as for diffuse encephalomyelitis. Bladder care with intermittent catheterization is imperative, as are measures to prevent bed sores and infection. The child and the family often need psychologic counseling.

Diffuse Encephalomyelitis

Diffuse encephalomyelitis is discussed in the section on Devic disease and in Chapter 2. The major clinical difference from Devic disease is that the cerebral hemispheres are affected as well as the spinal cord. Cerebral demyelination may precede, follow, or occur concurrently with the myelitis.

Clinical Features.   In addition to the myelitis, an encephalopathy characterized by decreased consciousness, irritability, and spastic quadriplegia occur. If the brainstem is affected, dysphagia, fever, cranial nerve palsies, and irregular respiration are present.

Diagnosis.   The full extent of demyelination can be appreciated only with MRI (Perdue et al, 1985). Multiple white matter lesions that become confluent are noted in the cerebral hemispheres (see Figure 2–4), cerebellum, and brainstem. Adrenoleukodystrophy must be excluded by measuring very-long-chain fatty acids.

Treatment.   Most authorities agree that corticosteroids should be administered (Pasternak et al, 1980). Prednisone, 2 mg/kg/day (not to exceed 100 mg), or its equivalent in a parenteral form is the initial dose, which is then tapered over a 4-week period depending on the response. The benefit of such a course of therapy is not established, but some patients become corticosteroid dependent and have a relapse when prednisone is discontinued. Such children require long-term alternate day therapy.

TRAUMA

Spinal cord injuries are relatively rare before adolescence. The major cause is motor vehicle accidents, followed by sports-related injuries (Zabramski et al, 1986). The injuries affect the cervical spinal cord in 65% of cases before 15 years of age and 71% of cases before 9 years of age. Fifteen percent of patients have injuries at multiple levels. Neurologic function that is intact immediately after the injury remains intact afterward. Even those with incomplete function are likely to recover completely. Evidence of complete transection on initial examination indicates that paralysis is permanent.

Spinal Cord Concussion

A direct blow on the back may produce a transitory disturbance in spinal cord function (Zwimpfer and Bernstein, 1990). The dysfunction is caused by edema (spinal shock); the spinal cord is intact.

Clinical Features.   Most injuries occur at the level of the cervical cord or the thoracolumbar juncture. The major clinical features are flaccid paraplegia or quadriplegia, a sensory level at the site of injury, loss of tendon reflexes, and urinary retention. Recovery begins within a few hours and is complete within a week.

Diagnosis.   At the onset of weakness a spinal cord compression syndrome such as epidural hematoma cannot be excluded, and an imaging study of the spine is necessary.

Treatment.   Children with spinal cord concussion should be treated with methylprednisolone as outlined in the section on spinal cord transection.

Compressed Vertebral Body Fractures

Clinical Features.   Compression fractures of the thoracolumbar region occur when a child jumps or falls from a height greater than 10 feet and lands in a standing or sitting position. The spinal cord itself is not transected, but spinal cord concussion may cause paraplegia. Back pain at the fracture site is immediate and intense. Nerve roots are compressed, causing pain that radiates into the groin and legs.

Diagnosis.   Thoracolumbar radiographs reveal the fracture, but when paraplegia is present, a spinal cord imaging study is usually performed as well, and the results prove to be normal.

Treatment.   Immobilization relieves the back pain and promotes healing of the fracture.

Fracture Dislocation and Spinal Cord Transection

Transection of the spinal cord from fracture dislocation is the most serious vertebral injury and is usually caused by a motor vehicle accident. A forceful flexion of the spine fractures the articular facets and allows the vertebral body to move forward or laterally, with consequent contusion or transection of the spinal cord. The common sites of traumatic transection are the levels C-1 to C-2, C-5 to C-7, and T-12 to L-2.

Clinical Features.   Neurologic deficits at and below the level of spinal cord contusion or transection are immediate and profound. Many children with fracture dislocations sustained head injuries at the time of trauma and are unconscious.

Immediately after the injury the child has flaccid weakness of the limbs below the level of the lesion associated with loss of tendon and cutaneous reflexes (spinal shock). In high cervical spinal cord lesions, the knee and ankle tendon reflexes, anal reflex, and plantar response may be elicited during the initial period of spinal shock. Spinal shock lasts for approximately 1 week in infants and young children and up to 6 weeks in adolescents.

First the superficial reflexes return, then the plantar response becomes one of extension, and finally massive withdrawal reflexes (mass reflex) appear. The mass reflex is triggered by trivial stimulation of the foot or leg, usually in a specific zone unique to the patient. The response at first is dorsiflexion of the foot, flexion at the knees, and flexion and adduction at the thighs. Later, there are also contraction of the abdomen, sweating, piloerection, and emptying of the bladder and bowel. During this time of heightened reflex activity the tendon reflexes return and become exaggerated.

Below the level of injury, sensation is lost to a variable degree, depending on the completeness of the transection. When the injury is incomplete, sensation begins to return within weeks and may continue to improve for up to 2 years. Patients with partial or complete transections may complain of pain and tingling below the level of injury.

In addition to the development of a small spastic bladder, autonomic dysfunction includes constipation, lack of sweating, orthostatic hypotension, and disturbed temperature regulation.

Diagnosis.   Fracture dislocation is readily identified by radiographs of the vertebrae. Imaging of the spinal cord produces further information on the presence of compressive hematomas and the structural integrity of the spinal cord (Figure 12–3). The presence of a complete block on myelography indicates a poor prognosis for return of function.

Treatment.   The immediate treatment of fracture dislocation is to reduce the dislocation and prevent further damage to the cord. This is accomplished by corticosteroids, surgery, and immobilization. An intravenous infusion of methylprednisolone, 30 mg/kg within the first 8 hours after injury, followed by 4 mg/kg/hr for 23 hours, significantly reduces neurologic morbidity (Bracken et al, 1992). Long-term management of spinal cord injuries is beyond the scope of this text but is best accomplished at specialized centers.

Spinal Epidural Hematoma

Spinal epidural hematoma usually results from direct vertebral trauma and is especially common in children with an underlying bleeding tendency. The hematoma causes symptoms by progressive compression of the cord and is manifested like any other extradural mass lesion. Diagnosis is usually based on MRI. Treatment is surgical evacuation.

TUMORS OF THE SPINAL CORD

Astrocytoma, ependymoma, and neuroblastoma are the common spinal cord tumors of childhood. Sarcomas are next in frequency, followed by neu-

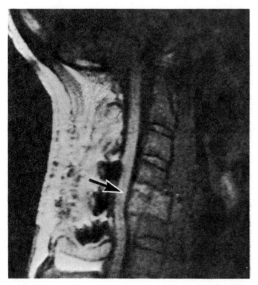

Figure 12–3 Fracture dislocation. C-4 is dislocated on C-5, causing compression *(arrow)* of the cord.

rofibroma and then by several different secondary tumors such as teratoma, dermoid, and chondroma. Motor deficits, usually paraplegia, are an early feature in 86% of spinal cord tumors, and back pain in 63%.

Astrocytoma

The problem of differentiating cystic astrocytoma of the spinal cord from syringomyelia is discussed in Chapter 9 (see "Syringomyelia").

Clinical Features.   Astrocytomas are usually long and may extend from the lower brainstem to the conus medullaris. Two distinct syndromes are associated with holocord astrocytoma (Epstein and Epstein, 1982). The first is characterized primarily by weakness of one arm as the initial manifestation. Pain in the neck may be an associated symptom, but bowel and bladder function are normal. Examination reveals mild spastic weakness of the legs. The solid portion of the tumor is in the neck, and its caudal extension is cystic.

The second syndrome is characterized by progressive spastic paraplegia, sometimes associated with thoracic pain. Scoliosis may be present. In these patients the solid portion of the tumor is in the thoracic or lumbar region. When solid tumor extends into the conus medullaris, tendon reflexes in the legs may be diminished or absent and bowel and bladder function is impaired.

Intraaxial tumors of the cervicomedullary junction may cause cranial nerve dysfunction or spinal cord compression (Epstein and Wisoff, 1987). Cranial nerve dysfunction is manifested by difficulty in swallowing and nasal speech (see Chapter 17).

Diagnosis.   MRI is the definitive diagnostic procedure. It allows visualization of both the solid and cystic portions of the tumor (Figure 12–4).

Treatment.   Complete resection should be attempted whenever possible. A laminectomy is performed over the solid portion of the tumor. With microsurgical technique the solid portion is removed and the cystic portion is aspirated. MRI should be repeated 1, 6, and 12 months after surgery. The benefits of radiation therapy, either after resection or at the time of recurrence, have not been determined (Rossitch et al, 1990).

Ependymoma

Ependymomas are composed primarily of ependymal cells and arise from the lining of the ventricular system or central canal. They are more often intracranial than intraspinal in children. When intraspinal, they tend to be located in the

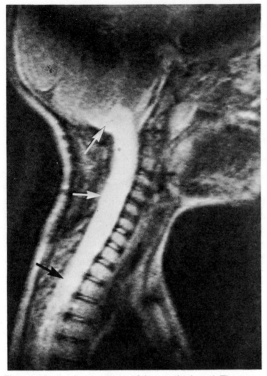

Figure 12–4   Astrocytoma of the cervical cord. The tumor demonstrates an intense signal *(arrow)* on T_2-weighted images.

lumbar region or in the cauda equina but may occur anywhere along the neuraxis (Dohrmann et al, 1976; Fischer and Mansuy, 1980).

Clinical Features.   Clinical features vary with the location of the tumor. The initial manifestation may be scoliosis, pain in the legs or back, paresthesia, or weakness in one or both legs. Diagnosis may be delayed for years when scoliosis is the only sign. Eventually all children have difficulty walking, and this is the symptom that usually leads to appropriate diagnostic testing.

Cervical ependymoma is manifested by stiff neck and cervical pain that is worse at night. Tumors of the cauda equina may sometimes rupture and produce meningismus, fever, and pleocytosis mimicking bacterial meningitis.

Spastic paraplegia is the usual finding on examination. Cervical tumors cause weakness of one arm as well. Tumors of the cauda equina produce flaccid weakness and atrophy of leg muscles associated with loss of tendon reflexes.

Diagnosis.   MRI is the primary modality for demonstrating tumors of the spinal cord. Lumbar puncture is rarely indicated but shows an elevated protein content of the cerebrospinal fluid.

Treatment.   Microsurgical techniques make possible the complete removal of intramedullary ependymoma (Fischer and Mansuy, 1980). The role of postoperative local radiation therapy for treating benign tumors is uncertain. Malignant ependymomas of the spinal cord are unusual in children but require total neuraxis irradiation when present.

Neuroblastoma

Neuroblastoma is the most common extracranial solid tumor of infancy and childhood. It produces neurologic dysfunction by direct invasion, by metastasis, and by distant "humoral" effects (see Chapter 10). Half of cases occur before 2 years of age, and 60% occur before 1 year (Jaffe, 1976). Neuroblastoma is derived from cells of the sympathetic chain and cranial ganglia. Tumors in a paraspinal location may extend through a neural foramen and compress the spinal cord.

Clinical Features.   Paraplegia is the initial manifestation of neuroblastoma extending into the epidural space from a paravertebral origin. Since most affected children are infants, the first symptom is usually refusal to stand or walk. Mild weakness may progress to complete paraplegia within hours or days. Examination generally reveals a flaccid paraplegia, a distended bladder, and exaggerated tendon reflexes in the legs. Sensation may be difficult to test.

Diagnosis.   Radiographs of the chest usually show the extravertebral portion of the tumor, and the extent of spinal compression is delineated with MRI.

Treatment.   In children with an acute spinal cord compression, some relief can be provided by high-dose corticosteroids before surgical extirpation and radiation therapy. The survival rate in infants with neuroblastoma confined to a single organ is greater than 60%.

Other Tumors

Other spinal cord tumors of infancy and childhood include sarcoma, neurofibroma, dermoid, teratoma, and epidermoid. Meningioma almost never occurs before the third decade.

The clinical features of the various spinal cord tumors are much alike. Paraplegia and back pain are prominent. Sensory deficits and sphincter disturbances are less common and depend on tumor location. Some combination of the studies listed in Table 12–2 leads to the diagnosis, and excision of the tumor is ordinarily the first step in treatment.

◆ Cerebral Paraplegia and Quadriplegia

Almost all progressive disorders of the brain that result in quadriplegia also have dementia as an initial or prominent feature (see Chapter 5). Pure paraplegia of cerebral origin is unusual. At the very least the patient has impairment of fine finger movements and increased tendon reflex activity in the arms. Pure paraplegia should always direct attention to the spinal cord.

CEREBRAL PALSY

Cerebral palsy is a chronic disability of cerebral origin characterized by aberrant control of movement or posture, onset of neurologic disturbance in the neonatal period, and absence of progressive disease.

Many slowly progressive disorders are mistakenly diagnosed as cerebral palsy (Table 12–3). Perinatal asphyxia is a known cause of cerebral palsy but accounts for only a minority of cases (Naeye et al, 1989). Most cerebral palsy is due to prenatal factors that are difficult to identify with precision in an individual patient.

Cerebral palsy is not always a permanent condition. Many infants with only mild motor impairments improve and achieve normal motor function in childhood (Nelson and Ellenberg, 1982).

Table 12–3 ◆ Slowly Progressive Disorders Sometimes Misdiagnosed as Cerebral Palsy

Condition	Chapter
Polyneuropathy	
1. GM$_1$ gangliosidosis type II	5
2. Hereditary motor and sensory neuropathies	7
3. Infantile neuroaxonal dystrophy	5
4. Metachromatic leukodystrophy	5
Ataxia	
1. Abetalipoproteinemia	10
2. Ataxia-telangiectasia	10
3. Friedreich ataxia	10
Spasticity-Chorea	
1. Familial spastic paraplegia	12
2. Lesch-Nyhan syndrome	5
3. Niemann-Pick disease, type C	5
4. Pelizaeus-Merzbacher disease	5
5. Rett syndrome	5

Unfortunately, up to 25% of such children will be retarded or will have some behavioral or cognitive disturbance.

Traditionally the cerebral palsies have been classified by the pattern of motor impairment. The spastic types are paraplegia or diplegia, quadriplegia, and hemiplegia (see Chapter 11). The hypotonic types are ataxic (see Chapter 10) and athetoid (see Chapter 14).

Spastic Diplegia (Paraplegia)

Diplegia means that all four limbs are affected but that the legs are affected more severely than the arms. The motor impairment in the arms may be limited to increased responses of tendon reflexes; such children are classified as paraplegic.

Clinical Features. Many children with spastic diplegia have normal tone, or even hypotonia, during the first 4 months. The onset of spasticity in the legs is insidious and slowly progressive during the first year. Four-point creeping is impossible because of leg extension, and early ambulation is usually achieved by either rolling or crawling on the floor with the belly on the ground, using the arms to pull the body forward.

Sitting up alone is delayed or never achieved. From the supine position the infant pulls to standing rather than to sitting. Sitting is later made possible by bending forward at the waist, to compensate for the lack of flexion at the hip and knee, and placing one hand on the floor for balance. Most children with spastic diplegia stand on their toes, with flexion at the knees and an increased lumbar lordosis. Walking is difficult because of the stiffness in the legs and can be accomplished only by throwing the body forward or side to side to transfer weight.

Examination reveals spasticity of the legs and lesser spasticity of the arms. The tendon reflexes are exaggerated in all limbs. Reflex sensitivity and responsiveness are increased; percussion at the knee causes a crossed adductor response. Ankle clonus and a Babinski sign are usually present. When the infant is suspended vertically, strong contractions of the adductor muscles cause the legs to cross at the thigh *(scissoring)*.

Subluxation or dislocation of the hips is relatively common in children with severe spasticity; this is caused in part by the constant adduction of the thighs and also by insufficient development of the hip joint resulting from delayed standing or inability to stand.

Diagnosis. Spastic diplegia is a clinical diagnosis. The important consideration is to be certain that the child does not have a progressive disease of the brain or cervical portion of the spine. Features that suggest a progressive disease are a family history of "cerebral palsy," deterioration of mental function, loss of motor skills previously obtained, atrophy of muscles, and sensory loss.

Treatment. There are probably as many "methods" to manage spastic diplegia and quadriplegia as there are children with cerebral palsy. In general, a multidisciplinary approach including infant stimulation, physical therapy, and occupational therapy is used to help the child achieve an adequate functional status. Controlled clinical trials are rarely accomplished, and one such trial concluded that physical therapy offered no short-term advantage (Palmer et al, 1988). Drugs to relieve spasticity generally have no value unless doses that produce unacceptable sedation are used.

Selective posterior rhizotomy has emerged as a useful procedure for the treatment of spasticity (Park and Owen, 1992). The best results are obtained in children younger than 8 years of age. Surgery is also useful to relieve contractures but should be carefully planned so that it is performed only once. Surgery is followed by a program of physical therapy that maintains the desired range of motion.

Spastic Quadriplegia

The whole body is affected in spastic quadriplegia, but one side is usually worse than the other and the arms are affected more than the legs. For this reason the condition is sometimes called *double hemiplegia*. If asymmetry is considerable, the child may be thought to have a hemiplegia.

Clinical Features. Developmental delay is profound, and the infant is quickly identified as neurologically abnormal. Failure to meet motor milestones and abnormal posturing of the head and limbs are the common reasons for neurologic evaluation.

In severely affected children the supine posture is characteristic. The head and neck are retracted, the arms are flexed at the elbows with the hands clenched, and the legs are held in extension. Infantile reflexes (Moro and tonic-neck) are obligatory and stereotyped and persist after 6 months of age. Microcephaly is frequently an associated feature.

Because both hemispheres are damaged, supranuclear bulbar palsy (dysphagia and dysarthria) is common. Disturbances in vision and ocular motility are frequently associated features, and seizures occur in 50% of affected children.

Diagnosis. Diagnosis is based on clinical findings. Laboratory studies are useful when the underlying cause is not obvious or the possibility of a genetically transmitted defect exists.

Treatment. Treatment is the same as described in the section on spastic diplegia.

References

Adams C, Armstong D: Acute transverse myelopathy in children. Can J Neurol Sci 17:40, 1990.

Adams MM, Greenberg F, Khoury MJ, et al: Trends in clinical characteristics of infants with spina bifida—Atlanta, 1972-1979. AJDC 139:514, 1985.

Anderson FM: Occult spinal dysraphism: A series of 73 cases. Pediatrics 55:826, 1975.

Appleton RE, Farrell K, Dunn HG: "Pure" and complicated forms of hereditary spastic paraplegia presenting in childhood. Dev Med Child Neurol 33:304, 1991.

Arens LJ, Peacock WJ, Peter J: Selective rhizotomy: A long-term follow-up study. Child Nerv Syst 5:148, 1989.

Azimullah PC, Smit LME, Rietveld-Knol E, et al: Malformations of the spinal cord in 53 patients with spina bifida studied by magnetic resonance imaging. Child Nerv Syst 7:63, 1991.

Bell WE, McCormick WF: Neurologic infections in children. In Markowitz M, ed: Major Problems in Clinical Pediatrics, vol 12. Saunders, Philadelphia, 1981, p 244.

Bhatnagar M, Sponseller PD, Carroll C IV, et al: Pediatric atlantoaxial instability presenting as cerebral and cerebellar infarcts. J Pediatr Orthop 11:103, 1991.

Bracken MB, Shepard MJ, Collins WF, et al: Methylprednisolone or naloxone treatment after acute spinal-cord injury: 1-year follow-up data. Results of the second National Acute Spinal Cord Injury Study. J Neurosurg 76:23, 1992.

Brophy JD, Sutton LN, Zimmerman RA, et al: Magnetic resonance imaging of lipomyelomeningocele and tethered cord. Neurosurgery 25:336, 1989.

Carstairs V, Cole S: Spina bifida and anencephaly in Scotland. Br Med J 289:1182, 1984.

Charney EB, Weller SC, Sutton LN, et al: Management of the newborn with myelomeningocele: Time for a decision-making process. Pediatrics 75:58, 1985.

Chaudhry V, Sturgeon C, Gates AJ, et al: Symptomatic atlantoaxial dislocation in Down's syndrome. Ann Neurol 21:606, 1987.

Citron N, Edgar MA, Sheeny J, et al: Intramedullary spinal cord tumors presenting as scoliosis. J Bone Joint Surg 66:513, 1984.

Cloys DE, Netsky MG: Neuromyelitis optica. In Vinken PJ, Brun GW, eds. Handbook of Clinical Neurology, vol 9. North Holland Publishing Co, Amsterdam, 1970, p 426.

Devinksy O, Eun-Sook C, Petito CK, et al: Herpes zoster myelitis. Brain 114:1181, 1991.

DiChiro G, Doppman JL, Dwyer AJ, et al: Tumors and arteriovenous malformations of the spinal cord: Assessment using MR. Radiology 156:689, 1985.

Dohrmann GJ, Farwell JR, Flannery JT: Ependymomas and ependymoblastomas in children. J Neurosurg 45:273, 1976.

Doppman JL, DiChiro G, Dwyer AJ, et al: Magnetic resonance imaging of spinal arteriovenous malformations. J Neurosurg 66:830, 1987.

Dryden RJ: Duplication of the spinal cord: A discussion of the possible embryogenesis of diplomyelia. Dev Med Child Neurol 22:234, 1980.

Dunne K, Hopkins IJ, Shield LK: Acute transverse myelopathy in childhood. Dev Med Child Neurol 28:198, 1986.

Dyste GN, Menezes AH: Presentation and management of pediatric Chiari malformations without myelodysplasia. Neurosurgery 23:589, 1988.

Epstein F, Epstein N: Surgical treatment of spinal cord astrocytomas of childhood: A series of 19 patients. J Neurosurg 57:685, 1982.

Epstein F, Wisoff J: Intra-axial tumors of the cervicomedullary junction. J Neurosurg 67:483, 1987.

Fischer G, Mansuy L: Total removal of intramedullary ependymomas: Follow-up study of 16 cases. Surg Neurol 14:243, 1980.

Fitz CR, Harwood-Nash DC: The tethered conus. AJR 125:515, 1975.

Haldeman S, Fowler GW, Ashwal S: Acute flaccid neonatal paraplegia: A case report. Neurology 33:93, 1983.

Harding AE: Hereditary "pure" spastic paraplegia: A clinical and genetic study of 22 families. J Neurol Neurosurg Psychiatry 44:871, 1981.

Hsu LC, Leong JC: Tuberculosis of the lower cervical spine (C2 to C7): A report of 40 cases. J Bone Joint Surg 66:1, 1984.

Jaffe N: Neuroblastoma: Review of the literature and an examination of factors contributing to its enigmatic character. Cancer Treat Rev 3:61, 1976.

James HE, Williams J, Brock W, et al: Radical removal of lipomas of the conus and cauda equina with laser microneurosurgery. Neurosurgery 15:340, 1984.

Linder M, Rosenstein J, Sklar FH: Functional improvement after spinal surgery for the dysraphic malformations. Neurosurgery 11:622, 1982.

Lorber J: Results of treatment of myelomeningocele: An analysis of 524 unselected cases with special reference to possible selection for treatment. Dev Med Child Neurol 13:279, 1971.

McMaster MJ: Occult intraspinal anomalies and congenital scoliosis. J Bone Joint Surg 66:588, 1984.

Milunsky A, Jick H, Jick SS, et al: Multivitamin/folic acid supplementation in early pregnancy reduces the prevalence of neural tube defects. JAMA 262:2847, 1989.

Moser HW, Moser AE, Singh I, et al: Adrenoleukodystrophy: Survey of 303 cases; Biochemistry, diagnosis, and therapy. Ann Neurol 16:628, 1984.

MRC Vitamin Study Research Group: Prevention of neural tube defects: Results Of The Medical Research Council Vitamin Study. Lancet 338:131, 1991.

Nadel AS, Green JK, Holmes LB, et al: Absence of need for amniocentesis in patients with elevated levels of maternal serum alpha-fetoprotein in normal ultrasonographic examinations. N Engl J Med 323:557, 1990.

Naeye RL, Peters EC, Bartholomew M, et al: Origins of cerebral palsy. AJDC 143:1154, 1989.

Nagib MG, Maxwell RE, Chou SN: Klippel-Feil syndrome in children: Clinical features and management. Child Nerv Syst 1:255, 1985.

Nelson KB, Ellenberg JH: Children who "outgrew" cerebral palsy. Pediatrics 69:529, 1982.

Palmer FB, Shapiro BK, Wachtel RC, et al: The effects of physical therapy on cerebral palsy: A controlled trial in spastic diplegia. N Engl J Med 318:803, 1988.

Papasozomenos S, Roessmann U: Respiratory distress in Arnold-Chiari malformation. Neurology 31:97, 1981.

Park TS, Cail WS, Maggio WM, et al: Progressive spasticity and scoliosis in children with myelomeningocele: Radiological investigation and surgical treatment. J Neurosurg 62:367, 1985.

Park TS, Owen JH: Surgical management of spastic diplegia in cerebral palsy. N Engl J Med 326:745, 1992.

Pasternak JF, DeVivo DC, Prensky AL: Steroid-responsive encephalomyelitis in childhood. Neurology 30:481, 1980.

Perdue Z, Bale JF, Dunn VD, et al: Magnetic resonance imaging in childhood disseminated encephalomyelitis. Pediatr Neurol 1:370, 1985.

Phillips PC, Lorentsen KJ, Shropshire LC, et al: Congenital odontoid aplasia and posterior circulation stroke in childhood. Ann Neurol 23:410, 1988.

Reigel DH, McLone DG: Myelomeningocele: Operative treatment and results—1987. Concepts Pediatr Neurosurg 8:41, 1988.

Richaud J: Spinal meningeal malformations in children (without meningoceles or meningomyeloceles). Child Nerv Syst 4:79, 1988.

Roach JW, Duncan D, Wenger DR, et al: Atlanto-axial instability and spinal cord compression in children—diagnosis by computerized tomography. J Bone Joint Surg 66:708, 1984.

Ropper AH, Poskanzer DC: The prognosis of acute and subacute transverse myelopathy based on early signs and symptoms. Ann Neurol 4:51, 1978.

Rossitch E Jr, Zeidman SM, Burger PC, et al: Clinical and pathological analysis of spinal cord astrocytomas in children. Neurosurgery 27:193, 1990.

Scarff TB, Reigel DH: Arteriovenous malformations of the spinal cord in children. Child Brain 5:341, 1979.

Silber MH, Willcox PA, Bowen RM, et al: Neuromyelitis optica (Devic's syndrome) and pulmonary tuberculosis. Neurology 40:934, 1990.

Singer R, Joseph K, Gilai AN, et al: Nontraumatic, acute neonatal paraplegia. J Pediatr Orthop 11:588, 1991.

Skeletal Dysplasia Group: Instability of the upper cervical spine. Arch Dis Child 64:283, 1989.

Towfighi J, Housman C: Spinal cord abnormalities in caudal regression syndrome. Acta Neuropathol 81:458, 1991.

Ülkü A, Karasoy H, Karatepe A, et al: X-linked spastic paraplegia. Arch Neurol Scand 83:403, 1991.

Wenger DR, Bobechko WP, Gilday DL: The spectrum of intervertebral disc-space infection in children. J Bone Joint Surg 60:100, 1978.

Whitham RH, Brey RL: Neuromyelitis optica: Two new cases and review of the literature. J Clin Neuroophthalmol 5:263, 1985.

Yamada S, Zinke DE, Sanders D: Pathophysiology of "tethered cord syndrome." J Neurosurg 54:494, 1981.

Zabramski JM, Hadley MN, Browner CM, et al: Pediatric spinal and vertebral column injuries. Barrow Neurol Inst Q 2:11, 1986.

Zwimpfer TJ, Bernstein M: Spinal cord concussion. J Neurosurg 72:894, 1990.

Monoplegia

Flaccid weakness of one limb is usually caused by abnormalities of the spine or proximal portion of the nerves. Many conditions that result in paraplegia or quadriplegia may begin as monoplegia. Therefore the differential diagnosis of spinal paraplegia provided in Table 12–1 must also be consulted for monoplegia. In addition, several cerebral disorders that cause hemiplegia may initially be manifested as monoplegia, so the tables in Chapter 11 must be consulted as well.

◆ Approach to Monoplegia

If a child refuses to use a limb, the problem may be caused by either pain or weakness. Painful limbs are usually caused by injury, but they may also be caused by arthritis, infection, or tumor. A trivial pull of the arm may dislocate the radial head in some infants and cause an apparent monoplegia. Pain and weakness together are a feature of plexitis.

The differential diagnosis of acute monoplegia is summarized in Table 13–1. Plexopathies and neuropathies are the leading cause of pure monoplegia. Stroke often affects one limb, usually the arm more than the leg. The presentation suggests monoplegia, but careful examination often reveals increased tendon reflexes and an extensor plantar response in the seemingly unaffected leg. Any suggestion of hemiplegia, rather than monoplegia, or increased tendon reflexes in the paretic limb should focus attention on the brain and cervical cord as the pathologic site.

Chronic progressive brachial monoplegia is uncommon. When it occurs, syringomyelia and tumors of the cervical cord or brachial plexus should be suspected. Chronic progressive weakness of one leg suggests a congenital malformation or tumor of the spinal cord.

A monomelic form of spinal muscular atrophy, affecting only one leg or one arm, has been reported repeatedly from Asia but is uncommon in Europe and the United States. However, childhood-onset spinal muscular atrophies may be asymmetric at onset and be manifested as monoplegia.

◆ Plexopathies
ACUTE IDIOPATHIC PLEXITIS

Acute plexitis is a demyelinating disorder of the brachial or lumbar plexus thought to be immune mediated. Brachial plexitis is far more common than lumbar plexitis and occurs with an annual incidence of 1.64:100,000 (Beghi et al, 1985).

Brachial Plexitis

Brachial plexitis (brachial neuritis, neuralgic amyotrophy) occurs from infancy to adult life (Charles and Jayam-Trouth, 1980; Tsairis et al, 1972). An antecedent infectious disease is recorded in 25% of patients; this is not a significant association. However, a 10% to 20% prior immunization with tetanus toxoid may be significant. The site of immunization does not correlate with the arm involved.

Clinical Features. The onset of symptoms is usually explosive. Pain is the initial manifestation in 95% of patients. Pain is frequently localized to the shoulder but may be more diffuse or limited to the lower arm. It is severe, may awaken the patient, and is described as sharp, stabbing, throbbing, or aching. The duration of pain, which is frequently constant, varies from several hours to 3 weeks. As the pain subsides, weakness appears. Weakness is in the distribution of the upper plexus in 56% of patients, the lower plexus in 6%, and the entire plexus in 38%. Although the initial pain has abated, paresthesias may accompany the weakness.

Table 13–1 ◆ Differential Diagnosis of
Acute Monoplegia

Complicated Migraine (see Chapter 11)

Dislocation of the Radial Head

"Hemiparetic" Seizures (see Chapter 11)

Plexopathy and Neuropathy
1. Acute neuritis
   a. Asthmatic plexitis
   b. Idiopathic plexitis
   c. Osteomyelitis plexitis
   d. Poliomyelitis (see Chapter 7)
   e. Tetanus toxoid (?) plexitis
2. Hereditary
   a. Hereditary brachial neuritis
   b. Hereditary recurrent pressure palsy
3. Injury
   a. Lacerations
   b. Pressure injuries
   c. Traction injuries

Stroke (see Table 11–2)

Two thirds of patients report improved strength during the month after onset. Upper plexus palsies improve faster than do lower plexus palsies. Among all patients, 36% recover within 1 year, 75% by 2 years, and 89% by 3 years. The rest may continue to show improvement after 3 years, but many are left with permanent residua. Recurrences are unusual and less severe than the initial episode.

Diagnosis. Pain and weakness in one arm are also symptoms of spinal cord compression, and an imaging study of the spinal cord is often needed. However, when the onset is characteristic of brachial plexus neuritis, the diagnosis can be established on clinical grounds and diagnostic tests can be deferred.

The cerebrospinal fluid is usually normal. A slight lymphocytosis and mild elevation in protein content are sometimes noted.

Electromyography (EMG) and nerve conduction studies are helpful in demonstrating the extent of plexopathy. Electrical evidence of bilateral involvement is often present in patients with unilateral symptoms.

Treatment. Corticosteroids have not been demonstrated to affect outcome. Range of motion exercises are recommended.

Lumbar Plexitis

Lumbar plexitis occurs at all ages and is similar to brachial plexitis, except that the leg is affected instead of the arm. An immune mechanism is sus-

pected, but no association with antecedent viral infection or immunization has been established.

Clinical Features. Fever is often the first symptom and is followed, after 3 to 8 days, by pain in one or both legs (Awerbuch et al, 1989). The pain has an abrupt onset and may occur in a femoral or sciatic distribution. Sciatica, when present, suggests disk disease. Young children refuse to stand or walk, and older children begin to limp.

Weakness may develop concurrent with pain or may be delayed for as long as 3 weeks. The onset of weakness is insidious and often difficult to date, but usually it begins 8 days after the onset of pain. Weakness progresses for a week and then stabilizes. Tendon reflexes are absent in the affected leg but are present in other limbs.

Recovery is characterized first by abatement of pain and then by increasing strength. The average time from onset of pain to maximal recovery is 18 weeks, with a range of 8 weeks to several years. Functional recovery is almost universal, but mild weakness may persist.

Diagnosis. The sudden onset of pain and weakness of one leg suggests spinal cord or disk disease. Magnetic resonance imaging (MRI) of the spine is a means of excluding other disorders; the results are invariably normal in lumbar plexitis. The cerebrospinal fluid is normal except for a mild elevation of protein concentration. EMG performed 3 weeks after onset demonstrates patchy denervation.

Treatment. Corticosteroids have not been demonstrated to affect outcome. Range of motion exercises are recommended.

OSTEOMYELITIS-NEURITIS

Apparent limb weakness that is due to pain is a well-recognized phenomenon. However, a true brachial neuritis may occur in response to osteomyelitis of the shoulder (Clay, 1982). The mechanism is thought to be ischemic nerve damage caused by vasculitis.

Clinical Features. Osteomyelitis-neuritis occurs predominantly during infancy. The initial manifestation is a flaccid arm without pain or tenderness. Body temperature may be normal at first but soon becomes elevated. Pain develops on movement of the shoulder, and tenderness to palpation follows. No swelling is present. The biceps and triceps reflexes may be depressed or absent.

Diagnosis. Osteomyelitis of the proximal humerus should be suspected when brachial plexitis develops during infancy. Radiographs of the humerus do not show abnormalities until the end of the first week, when they reveal destruction of the lateral margin of the humerus. A radioisotope bone scan demonstrates a focal area of uptake in the proximal humerus, the scapula, or both shortly after onset. After 3 weeks EMG demonstrates patchy denervation in the muscles innervated by the upper plexus. The EMG results support the idea that this is a true plexitis and not just a painful limb.

The organism can be identified in aspirate from the shoulder joint or by blood cultures. Group B *Streptococcus* is often isolated in specimens from young infants, and other species of bacteria are found in older children.

Treatment.   Intravenous antibiotics, usually penicillin, must be administered for 3 to 4 weeks. Recovery of arm strength may be incomplete.

ASTHMATIC AMYOTROPHY

Sudden flaccid paralysis of one or more limbs, resembling poliomyelitis, may occur during recovery from an asthmatic attack *(Hopkins syndrome)*. All affected children had been immunized against poliomyelitis. The syndrome is believed to be caused by anterior horn cell infection by a neurotropic virus other than poliovirus (Shahar et al, 1991). Adenovirus, echovirus, and coxsackievirus have been isolated from stool, throat, or cerebrospinal fluid in some cases.

Clinical Features.   Age at onset is from 1 to 11 years, and the male-to-female ratio is 7:4. The interval between the asthmatic attack and the paralysis is 1 to 11 days with an average of 5 days. Among 22 reported cases, monoplegia occurred in 18, the arm was involved in 12 children and the leg in 6, and hemiplegia was present in 2 and diplegia in 2. Meningeal irritation is not present, but muscle pain in the paralyzed limb is noted in half of cases. Recovery is incomplete, and all affected children have been left with some degree of permanent paralysis.

Diagnosis.   Asthmatic amyotrophy is primarily a clinical diagnosis based on the sequence of events. It must be distinguished from paralytic poliomyelitis and idiopathic brachial neuritis. The distinction from paralytic poliomyelitis is made on the basis of normal cerebrospinal fluid in asthmatic amyotrophy. A few white blood cells may be present in the cerebrospinal fluid but never to the extent encountered in poliomyelitis, and the protein concentration is normal.

EMG during the acute phase demonstrates active denervation of the paralyzed limb, but the pattern of denervation does not follow the radicular distribution expected in a brachial neuritis.

Treatment.   Treatment is directed to the symptoms and includes analgesics for pain and physical therapy.

HEREDITARY BRACHIAL PLEXOPATHY

Focal familial recurrent neuropathy has two major phenotypes: hereditary brachial plexopathy (Bradley et al, 1975; Dunn et al, 1978; Geiger et al, 1974) and hereditary recurrent pressure palsy (see later discussion of mononeuropathies). The phenotypes are genetically distinct but can be confused because isolated nerve palsies may occur in hereditary brachial plexopathy and brachial plexopathy is reported in patients with hereditary recurrent pressure palsy. Both disorders are transmitted by autosomal dominant inheritance.

Clinical Features.   Hereditary brachial plexopathy may be difficult to distinguish from idiopathic brachial plexitis in the absence of a family history or a patient's history of similar episodes.

Events that have been reported to trigger an attack in genetically predisposed individuals include infection, emotional stress, strenuous use of the affected limb, and childbirth. Immunization has not been implicated.

The initial attack usually occurs during the second or third decade but may appear in childhood. When brachial plexus palsy is present at birth, it is generally misinterpreted as traumatic even if the family history of the disease is known. Weakness resolves completely, only to recur later in childhood.

Attacks are characterized by severe arm pain that may be exacerbated by movement. Weakness follows in days to weeks; it is usually maximal within a few days and always by 1 month. The entire plexus may be involved, but most often the upper trunk is affected alone or most severely. Examination demonstrates proximal arm weakness and sometimes distal weakness. Tendon reflexes cannot be elicited from affected muscles. Weakness persists for weeks to months, during which time atrophy and fasciculations are observed. Pain, which is frequently the only sensory finding, subsides after the first week.

Recovery begins weeks to months after maximal weakness is attained. Return of function is usually complete, although some residual weakness may persist after repeated attacks. The frequency of attacks is variable; several attacks may occur within a single year, but two or three attacks per decade is more usual.

Occasional patients have an episode of lumbar plexopathy, which is characterized by pain in the thigh and by proximal weakness. Brachial and lumbar plexopathies are never concurrent, although bilateral brachial plexopathy is a relatively common event. Isolated cranial nerve palsies are reported in families with hereditary brachial plexopathy. The vagus nerve is most often affected, causing hoarseness and difficulty in swallowing. Transitory facial palsies and unilateral hearing loss are reported as well.

Diagnosis. The family history, early age at onset, unique triggering events, recurrences, and involvement of other nerves differentiate hereditary brachial plexopathy from idiopathic brachial neuritis. EMG demonstrates a diffuse axonopathy in the affected arm and some evidence of denervation in the asymptomatic arm. Asymptomatic legs are electrically normal.

Treatment. Corticosteroids have not shown benefit. Analgesics may be needed at the onset of an attack. Range of motion exercises are recommended.

NEONATAL BRACHIAL NEUROPATHY

The incidence of brachial plexus injuries in children born between 1959 and 1965 was 0.7 per 1,000 live births (Painter and Bergman, 1973). This was a decline from prior studies. Improved obstetric practices have probably resulted in a continued decline.

Brachial plexus injuries in the newborn are caused by excessive traction. Upper plexus injuries occur when the head is suddenly pulled away from the arm, which may occur in several scenarios. In vertex position the head may be forcefully pulled to deliver the after-coming shoulder or the head and neck may be forced downward by normal contractions, while the shoulder is caught by the pelvis. Injuries in breech position occur when the arm is pulled downward to free the after-coming head or when the head is rotated to occipitoanterior but the shoulder is fixed. Lower plexus injuries occur during vertex deliveries when traction is exerted on a prolapsed arm and in breech deliveries when the trunk is pulled downward but an aftercoming arm is fixed.

Clinical Features. Most neonatal brachial plexus injuries occur in large full-term newborns of primiparous mothers, especially when the fetus is malpositioned and the delivery is long and difficult. Although brachial plexus injuries are traditionally divided into those involving the upper roots (named for Erb and Duchenne) and those involving the lower roots (named for Klumpke), solitary lower root injuries do not occur. The fifth and sixth cervical roots are constantly affected, the seventh cervical root is additionally affected in 50% of injuries, and all roots from the fifth cervical to the first thoracic in 10% (Eng, 1971; Hardy, 1981). Bilateral, but not necessarily symmetric, involvement occurs in up to 23% of cases.

Because the upper plexus is always involved, the posture of the arm is typical and reflects weakness in the proximal muscles. The arm is abducted and internally rotated at the shoulder and is extended and pronated at the elbow, so that the partially flexed fingers face backward. When the seventh cervical segment is also involved, extension of the wrist is lost and fisting of the fingers is more prominent. The biceps and triceps reflexes are absent. Injuries that extend higher than the fourth cervical segment result in ipsilateral diaphragmatic paralysis.

Newborns with a complete brachial plexus palsy have a flaccid, dry limb with neither proximal nor distal movement. A Horner syndrome is sometimes associated. Sensory loss to pinprick is present with partial or complete palsies but may not conform to the segmental pattern of weakness.

Diagnosis. Brachial plexus palsy is easily recognized by the typical posture of the arm and by failure of movement when the Moro reflex is tested. Because the injury often takes place during a long and difficult delivery, asphyxia may be present. In such cases focal arm weakness may be missed because of generalized hypotonia. Approximately 10% of newborns with brachial plexus injuries have facial nerve palsy and fractures of the clavicle or humerus.

EMG may be useful for determining precise segmental localization of injury and for prognosis (Eng, 1971). Reinnervation can be predicted by the appearance of small polyphasic motor units, which precede clinical evidence of recovery by 1 month.

Treatment. Spontaneous recovery rates are good, and the only goal of therapy is to prevent the development of contractures. This is accomplished by range of motion exercises; splinting or other forms of immobilization should be avoided.

Complete recovery is reported in 70% to 95% of cases. Significant recovery occurs throughout the first year, only minor improvement occurs in the second year, and the deficit is fixed after the second year.

POSTNATAL INJURIES
Brachial Plexus

Traction and pressure injuries of the brachial plexus are relatively common because of its superficial position. Motor vehicle and sports accidents account for the majority of severe injuries. However, mild injuries can occur when an adult suddenly yanks a child's arm, either protectively or to force movement; by a blow to the shoulder, such as in a football scrimmage or from the recoil of a rifle (Wanamaker, 1974); because of prolonged wearing of a heavy knapsack; when the arm is kept hyperextended during surgery; and by pressure in the axilla from poorly positioned crutches.

Clinical Features.   Mild injuries do not affect all portions of the plexus equally. Diffuse weakness is uncommon. Pain may be an important initial feature, and sensory loss is uncommon. Recovery begins within days or weeks and is complete. Atrophy does not occur.

More severe injuries are usually associated with fractures of the clavicle and scapula and dislocation of the humerus. The upper plexus is generally affected more severely than is the lower plexus, but complete paralysis may be present at the onset. Sensory loss is less marked than weakness, and the two may not correspond in distribution. Pain is common, not only from the plexopathy but also from the bone and soft tissue injuries. The most painful injuries are those associated with root avulsion (Wynn-Parry, 1980).

Tendon reflexes are absent, and atrophy develops in denervated muscle. Recovery progresses proximal to distal and can be plotted by the Tinel sign: tingling in the distal part of a limb caused by tapping over the regenerating segment of a nerve. Complete reinnervation, when it occurs, may take several months or years. The completeness of recovery depends on the severity and nature of the injury. Pressure and traction injuries in which anatomic integrity is not disturbed recover best, whereas injuries that tear the nerve or avulse the root do not recover at all.

Diagnosis.   EMG is useful in identifying the pattern of nerve injury and providing information on prognosis (Trojaborg, 1977). Even with mild traction injuries the amplitude of motor and sensory action potentials is attenuated and motor and sensory conduction is slowed.

Treatment.   Mild injuries do not require treatment other than range of motion exercises. For more severe traction injuries, resting of the limb for the first month is usually necessary. During that time, analgesia is needed for pain and the muscles can be stimulated electrically, away from the site of injury, to maintain tone. Range of motion exercises should be started after the pain subsides.

Fractures and dislocations causing pressure on the brachial plexus must be corrected promptly. Where nerves have been lacerated, anatomic integrity must be restored surgically.

Lumbar Plexus

The lumbar plexus is much less likely to be injured than is the brachial plexus because the former is surrounded by the pelvis and the very heavy muscles of the proximal leg.

Clinical Features.   Lumbar plexus injuries are almost always associated with fracture-dislocation of the pelvis. Motor vehicle accidents or falls from considerable height are required to produce sufficient force to fracture the pelvis. Therefore the patient usually has multiple injuries and the lumbar plexus injury may not be identified early.

Lumbar plexus injuries produce a patchy weakness that is difficult to differentiate from mononeuritis multiplex.

Diagnosis.   EMG is critical in making the distinction between plexus injuries and nerve injuries.

Treatment.   Fracture-dislocations must be treated to relieve pressure on the plexus. As with brachial plexus injuries, the completeness of recovery depends on the anatomic integrity of the nerves.

PLEXUS TUMORS

Brachial plexus tumors in childhood are rare; when they do occur, they are likely to be malignant. The important primary tumor is a malignant schwannoma, and the important secondary tumors are neuroblastoma and other primitive neuroectodermal tumors arising in the chest.

◆ Mononeuropathies
RADIAL NEUROPATHY

The radial nerve is most often injured in the spinal groove of the humerus, just below the takeoff of the motor branch to the triceps muscle. Injury may occur with fractures of the humerus or by external pressure. Such pressure usually results when a sleeping or sedated patient is in a position that compresses the nerve between the humerus and a hard surface, such as an operating table or chair.

Clinical Features.   Radial nerve injuries in the spinal groove are characterized by wristdrop and fingerdrop. The brachioradialis muscle may be weak and its tendon reflex lost. Sensory disturbances are restricted to the back of the hand near the base of the thumb. With the wrist dropped, a fist is mechanically difficult to make but the finger flexors are not weak.

Diagnosis.   Electrophysiologic studies are useful for locating the site of injury and assessing the anatomic integrity of the nerve and the prognosis for recovery (Trojaborg, 1977).

Treatment.   Pressure injuries recover completely in 6 to 8 weeks. During that time a splint is useful for placing the wrist in extension so that the patient can flex the fingers.

ULNAR NEUROPATHY

The most common site of ulnar injury is the elbow. This type of injury can result from external pressure, recurrent dislocation of the nerve from its groove, and fracture of the distal humerus.

Clinical Features. Paresthesias are noted on the ulnar side of the hand, the little finger, and the ring finger. Tapping the ulnar groove increases the discomfort. Hand strength is lost, and the intrinsic muscles become wasted. Sensation over the little finger and the adjacent side of the ring finger is diminished or absent.

Diagnosis. The injury's precise location along the course of the nerve is readily determined by electrophysiologic techniques.

Treatment. Minor pressure injuries do not require treatment, and recovery is complete within a few weeks. For injuries to the elbow that cause fracture or nerve dislocation, surgical intervention is frequently needed.

PERONEAL NEUROPATHY

The peroneal nerve lies in a superficial position adjacent to the fibula and is readily compressed against the bone by external force. This most often occurs in people who have undergone significant weight loss (Jones, 1986; Sotaniemi, 1984). Such individuals may have a mild dietary polyneuropathy, and the peroneal nerve is selectively injured by the pressure of crossing the legs while sitting.

Clinical Features. The prominent feature is a painless footdrop. Both dorsiflexion and eversion of the foot are weak. Sensation is usually intact, but sometimes there is numbness over the lower lateral leg and dorsum of the foot. When only the deep branch of the peroneal nerve is involved, sensory loss is restricted to a small triangle between the first two toes.

Diagnosis. Electrodiagnosis is useful in discriminating peroneal nerve lesions from disturbances of the fifth lumbar root.

Treatment. A footdrop brace is a useful aid in walking until recovery is complete.

HEREDITARY RECURRENT PRESSURE PALSY

Transmitted by autosomal dominant inheritance, hereditary recurrent pressure palsy is characterized by the development of a mononeuropathy following trivial trauma (Attal et al, 1975; Roos and Thygesen, 1972). In some cases the brachial plexus is affected (Bosch et al, 1980).

Clinical Features. The first episode usually occurs during the second or third decade. Typical precipitating factors include sleeping on a limb, body contact in sports, constrictive clothing, or positioning during surgery. Individuals quickly learn to avoid activities that provoke episodes. Superficial nerves (radial, ulnar, median, peroneal) are the ones most commonly affected. The resulting mononeuropathy is painless and affects both motor and sensory fibers. Tendon reflexes are lost. Recovery is complete within days to weeks.

Diagnosis. Except for the family history, the first episode might suggest an ordinary pressure palsy, although the trivial nature of the trauma should alert the physician to the underlying neuropathy.

Electrophysiologic studies demonstrate slow conduction time, not only in the affected limb but in all limbs. Generalized slowing of conduction can be demonstrated in other family members between attacks.

Treatment. No treatment is available for the underlying neuropathy. Life-style may need to be altered to avoid pressure palsies. Acute episodes should be treated with physical therapy. In some patients a generalized motor and sensory neuropathy eventually develops.

◆ Monomelic Spinal Muscular Atrophy

Spinal muscular atrophies are genetic disorders characterized by progressive degeneration of anterior horn cells (see Chapter 7). Focal and generalized forms are worldwide in distribution, but 80% of monomelic cases have been reported from Asia (de Visser et al, 1988; Peiris et al, 1989).

Clinical Features. Monomelic spinal muscular atrophy is usually sporadic in occurrence and has a male bias of 10 to 1. There is a single report of a segmental spinal muscular atrophy affecting one hand and then the other in male identical twins (Tandan et al, 1990).

Age at onset is between 10 and 25 years but generally after 15 years. The progression of weakness and wasting is insidious. The arm is affected more often than the leg, and the distribution of weakness may be only proximal, be only distal, or involve the entire limb. The initial weakness and wasting are often unilateral and involve muscles innervated by C-7, C-8, and T-1. Bilateral weakness is usually present within 2 years. Tremor of one or both hands is often associated with the wasting. Fasciculations are then noted in the proximal muscles, and their appearance heralds weakness and wasting. Progression is slow, and spontaneous arrest within 5 years is the rule. However, another limb may become affected after a gap of 15 years.

Diagnosis. Monomelic spinal muscular atrophy is a rare disorder, and other causes of monoplegia must be excluded. Fasciculations are present in the affected muscles. EMG and muscle biopsy findings are consistent with denervation, but nerve conduction velocities are normal. MRI of the spinal cord shows no abnormalities.

Treatment. Treatment is supportive and includes physical and occupational therapy.

References

Attal C, Robain O, Chaouis G: Familial nerve trunk paralyses. Dev Med Child Neurol 17:787, 1975.

Awerbuch GI, Nigro MA, Dabrowski E, et al: Childhood lumbosacral plexus neuropathy. Pediatr Neurol 5:314, 1989.

Beghi E, Kurland LT, Mulder DW, et al: Brachial plexus neuropathy in the population of Rochester, Minnesota, 1970-1981. Ann Neurol 18:320, 1985.

Bosch EP, Chui HC, Martin MA, et al: Brachial plexus involvement in familial pressure-sensitive neuropathies: Electrophysiological and morphological findings. Ann Neurol 8:620, 1980.

Bradley WG, Madrid R, Thrush DC, et al: Recurrent brachial plexus neuropathy. Brain 98:381, 1975.

Charles LM, Jayam-Trouth A: Brachial plexus neuropathy: Three cases in children. AJDC 134:299, 1980.

Clay SA: Osteomyelitis as a cause of brachial plexus neuropathy. AJDC 136:1054, 1982.

de Visser M, de Visser BWO, Verbeeten B Jr: Electromyographic and computed tomographic findings in five patients with monomelic spinal muscular atrophy. Eur Neurol 28:135, 1988.

Dunn HG, Daube JR, Gomez MR: Heredofamilial brachial plexus neuropathy (hereditary neuralgic amyotrophy with brachial predilection) in childhood. Dev Med Child Neurol 20:28, 1978.

Eng GD: Brachial plexus palsy in newborn infants. Pediatrics 48:18, 1971.

Geiger LR, Mancall EL, Penn AS, et al: Familial neuralgic amyotrophy—report of three families with review of the literature. Brain 97:87, 1974.

Hardy AE: Birth injuries of the brachial plexus: Incidence and prognosis. J Bone Joint Surg 63B:98, 1981.

Jones HR: Compressive neuropathy in childhood: A report of 14 cases. Muscle Nerve 9:720, 1986.

Painter MJ, Bergman I: Obstetrical trauma to the neonatal central and peripheral nervous system. Semin Perinatol 6:89, 1973.

Peiris JB, Seneviratne KN, Wickremasinghe HR, et al: Non familial juvenile distal spinal muscular atrophy of upper extremity. J Neurol Neurosurg Psychiatry 52:314, 1989.

Roos D, Thygesen P: Familial recurrent polyneuropathy. Brain 95:235, 1972.

Shahar EM, Hwang PA, Niesen CE, et al: Poliomyelitis-like paralysis during recovery from acute bronchial asthma: Possible etiology and risk factors. Pediatrics 88:276, 1991.

Sotaniemi KA: Slimmer's paralysis—peroneal neuropathy during weight reduction. J Neurol Neurosurg Psychiatry 47:564, 1984.

Tandan R, Sharma KR, Bradley WG, et al: Chronic segmental spinal muscular atrophy of upper extremities in identical twins. Neurology 40:236, 1990.

Trojaborg W: Rate of recovery in motor and sensory fibers of the radial nerve: Clinical and electrophysiological aspects. J Neurol Neurosurg Psychiatry 33:625, 1970.

Trojaborg W: Electrophysiological findings in pressure palsy of the brachial plexus. J Neurol Neurosurg Psychiatry 40:1160, 1977.

Tsairis P, Dyck PJ, Mulder DW: Natural history of brachial plexus neuropathy: Report on 99 patients. Arch Neurol 27:109, 1972.

Wanamaker WM: Firearm recoil palsy. Arch Neurol 31:208, 1974.

Wynn-Parry CB: Pain in avulsion lesions of the brachial plexus. Pain 9:41, 1980.

Movement Disorders

Involuntary movements are usually associated with abnormalities of the basal ganglia and their connections and may occur in a variety of neurologic conditions. Abnormal movements can be the major or first feature of disease, or they can occur as a late manifestation. The former type is discussed in this chapter, and the latter is discussed in other chapters.

◆ Approach to the Patient

Movement disorders cannot be adequately described; they must be seen. If abnormal movements are not present at the time of examination, the parents should be instructed to videotape the movements at home. Some relatively common movements are recognizable by description, but the rich variety of abnormal movements and postures that may occur defies classification. The most experienced observer will at times mistake one movement for another or will have difficulty conceptualizing the nature of an abnormal movement.

Many abnormal movements are paroxysmal or at least intermittent. Some are induced by movement, startle, or emotional upset. The physician should always inquire what makes the movement worse. If the movements are action induced, the child should be asked to perform the action during the examination. Paroxysmal movements raise the question of epilepsy. Indeed, many neurologic disorders of childhood are characterized by the concurrent presence of seizures and involuntary movements. The clinical and conceptual distinction between spinal myoclonus and spinal seizures remains a gray area. No absolute rules distinguish involuntary movements from seizures, but in general the following guidelines apply: involuntary movements, with the exception of spinal myoclonus, abate or disappear during sleep and seizures

persist or worsen; involuntary movements have a more stereotyped appearance and are more persistent than seizures; seizures are often characterized by loss of consciousness or awareness, and involuntary movements are not; seizures are usually accompanied by epileptiform activity on electroencephalogram (EEG), and involuntary movements are not.

Involuntary contraction of a muscle that does not move a joint may be a fasciculation, a focal seizure, or myoclonus. Low-amplitude jerking movements that move a joint or muscles may be focal seizures, chorea, myoclonus, tics, or hemifacial spasms. High-amplitude jerking movements that move a limb or limbs may be seizures, ballismus, or myoclonus. Slow, writhing movements and abnormal posturing may be due to athetosis, dystonia, continuous motor unit activity, or seizures. Rhythmic movements may be caused by tremors, seizures, or myoclonus.

◆ Chorea and Athetosis

Chorea is a rapid jerk affecting any part of the body and may be incorporated into a voluntary movement to hide the jerk. The movements are repetitive but neither rhythmic nor stereotyped, and they migrate from side to side and limb to limb. Because the involuntary movement flows into a voluntary movement, it gives the appearance of constant movement ("restlessness"). Depending on the condition, chorea may be unilateral or bilateral and may affect the face and trunk as well as the limbs.

Chorea is more readily observed when separated from the superimposed voluntary movement that follows. This is achieved by asking the child to raise both hands upward beside the head with palms facing each other. Low-amplitude jerking movements that turn the arm into pronation are observed. When the child is asked to grip the examiner's fingers lightly, the grip alternately tightens and loosens, as if the patient is "milking" the examiner's hands. Hypotonia is common in many conditions causing chorea. Tendon reflexes may be normoreactive, but at times a choreic jerk occurs during the patellar response, producing an extra kick.

Athetosis is a slow, writhing movement of the limbs that may occur alone but is often associated with chorea (choreoathetosis). Athetosis without chorea is almost always due to perinatal brain injury. Kernicterus was the major cause, but perinatal asphyxia is now predominant. Many children with athetosis have atonic cerebral palsy, and others have spastic diplegia.

Ballismus is a high-amplitude, violent flinging of a limb from the shoulder or pelvis. It is considered an extreme form of chorea. In adults it may occur in limbs contralateral to a vascular lesion in the subthalamic nucleus; in children it is almost always associated with chorea and is seen in Sydenham chorea and lupus erythematosus (Dewey and Jankovic, 1989).

Tardive dyskinesia is a complex syndrome characterized by buccolingual masticatory movements that include tongue protrusion, lip smacking, puckering, and chewing. It is uncommon in children. Psychotropic drugs are the usual cause of tardive dyskinesia. It may be considered a subtype of chorea, or at least a related disorder, and is sometimes associated with choreic movements of the limbs.

The differential diagnosis of chorea and choreoathetosis is summarized in Tables 14–1 and 14–2. Chorea is a cardinal feature of the conditions listed in Table 14–1. Nevertheless, many are de-

tailed elsewhere in the text because concurrent features are more prominent. Although abnormal movements are the only manifestation, familial paroxysmal choreoathetosis is described in Chapter 1 because it is more likely to be confused with epilepsy than with other causes of chorea.

Table 14–2 contains a partial list of conditions in which chorea and choreoathetosis may occur but in which they are either late manifestations or at least not prominent early in the course. Movement disorders are relatively common in many progressive cerebral degenerations and are an expected part of the devastating illness. In contrast, chorea may be misinterpreted as seizures when it develops during acute illnesses such as bacterial meningitis (Burnstein and Breningstall, 1986), metabolic encephalopathies, or encephalitis. At times the movement disorder is due to the underlying brain disorder and at times to drugs used in treatment.

GENETIC DISORDERS

Abetalipoproteinemia and ataxia-telangiectasia ordinarily are first manifested by cerebellar ataxia. Chorea may be present in both conditions, but only in ataxia-telangiectasia does chorea occur without ataxia. Huntington disease is an important cause of chorea and dystonia and is described in most texts as a movement disorder. However, since the first sign of the childhood form of Huntington disease is usually declining school performance, it is discussed in Chapter 5.

Benign Familial Chorea

Benign familial chorea is a rare disorder transmitted by autosomal dominant inheritance (Sleigh

---

Table 14–1 ◆ Differential Diagnosis of Chorea as Initial or Prominent Symptom

Genetic Disorders
 1. Abetalipoproteinemia (see Chapter 10)
 2. Ataxia-telangiectasia (see Chapter 10)
 3. Benign familial chorea
 4. Fahr disease
 5. Familial paroxysmal choreoathetosis (see Chapter 1)
 6. Glutaric aciduria
 7. Hallervorden-Spatz disease
 8. Hepatolenticular degeneration (Wilson disease)
 9. Huntington disease (see Chapter 5)
10. Infantile bilateral striatal necrosis
11. Lesch-Nyhan syndrome (see Chapter 5)
12. Machado-Joseph disease (see Chapter 5)
13. Neuroacanthocytosis

Drug-Induced Movement Disorders
 1. Anticonvulsants
 2. Antiemetics
 3. Oral contraceptives
 4. Psychotropic agents
 5. Stimulants
 6. Theophylline

Systemic Conditions
 1. Hyperthyroidism
 2. Lupus erythematosus
 3. Pregnancy (chorea gravidarum)
 4. Sydenham (rheumatic) chorea

Tumors of Cerebral Hemisphere (see Chapter 4)

Table 14–2 ◆ Conditions That May Include Choreoathetosis

Alternating Hemiplegia (see Chapter 11)

Cerebral Palsy
1. Congenital malformations (see Chapters 5 and 18)
2. Kernicterus (see Chapter 1)
3. Perinatal asphyxia (see Chapter 1)
4. Unknown causes

Genetic Disorders
1. Ceroid lipofuscinosis (see Chapter 5)
2. Idiopathic torsion dystonia
3. Incontinentia pigmenti (see Chapter 1)
4. Pelizaeus-Merzbacher disease (see Chapter 5)
5. Phenylketonuria (see Chapter 5)
6. Porphyria (see Chapter 7)
7. Rett syndrome (see Chapter 5)

Infectious Diseases
1. Bacterial meningitis (see Chapter 4)
2. Viral encephalitis (see Chapter 2)

Metabolic Encephalopathies (see Chapter 2)
1. Addison disease
2. Burn encephalopathy
3. Hypernatremia
4. Hypocalcemia
5. Hypoparathyroidism
6. Vitamin B_{12} deficiency

Vascular
1. Moyamoya disease (see Chapter 11)
2. Poststroke (see Chapter 11)

and Lindenbaum, 1981). Benign familial chorea and familial paroxysmal choreoathetosis (see Chapter 1) may be genetically related disorders (Nardocci et al, 1989).

Clinical Features. The onset of chorea is always in early childhood. In some children motor development is delayed; other symptoms may include intention tremor, dysarthria, hypotonia, and athetosis. Most children have only chorea, which becomes less pronounced by adolescence. Adults may be asymptomatic or may have mild hypotonia and ataxia.

Diagnosis. Benign familial chorea may be difficult to distinguish from other causes of chorea in children, especially familial paroxysmal chorea. A family history of the disorder is critical to diagnosis but can be overlooked because of incomplete expression in parents. Chorea is continuous and not episodic or paroxysmal. Computed tomography (CT) and EEG results are normal.

Treatment. Tetrabenazine or haloperidol should be tried and are beneficial in some individuals (Table 14–3).

Fahr Disease

The combination of encephalopathy and progressive calcification of the basal ganglia is called Fahr disease. It may be familial or sporadic. Familial cases are transmitted by autosomal recessive or autosomal dominant inheritance (Smits et al, 1983). Those with dominant inheritance are associated with hypoparathyroidism or pseudohypoparathyroidism. Some sporadic cases probably represent autosomal recessive inheritance and others are a result of systemic disease. The common fea-

tures of diseases with basal ganglia calcification are thought to be defective iron transport and free radical production (Beall et al, 1989).

Clinical Features. Onset may be anytime from childhood to adulthood but is consistent within a family. Disorders occurring before 10 years of age are likely to be different from those that occur in adulthood. Affected children may have a Cockayne syndrome phenotype (see Chapter

Table 14–3 ◆ Generic and Brand Names of Drugs

Generic Name	Brand Name (Manufacturer)
Benztropine	Cogentin (Merck, Sharp & Dohme)
Carbamazepine	Tegretol (Geigy)
Clonazepam	Klonipin (Roche)
Clonidine	Catapres (Boehringer Ingelheim)
Dextroamphetamine	Dexedrine (Smith, Kline & French)
Diazepam	Valium (Roche)
Haloperidol	Haldol (McNeil)
Methylphenidate	Ritalin (CIBA)
Metoclopramide	Reglan (Robins)
Phenothiazines	
Chlorpromazine	Chlorpromazine
Fluphenazine	Permitil (Schering)
	Prolixin (Squibb)
Thioridazine	Mellaril (Sandoz)
Pimozide	Orap (McNeil)
Primidone	Mysoline (Ayerst)
Tetrabenazine	Nitoman (Roche)*
Trihexyphenidyl	Artane (Lederle)
Valproate	Depakene (Abbott)

*Not available in the United States.

16): dwarfism, senile appearance, and retinitis pigmentosa. Mental deterioration and choreoathetosis are constant features. Ataxia, dysarthria, spasticity, and seizures are variable. Progressive neurologic deterioration results in early disability and death.

Diagnosis. Plain radiographs of the skull demonstrate bilateral calcification in the region of the basal ganglia that can be localized more precisely by CT. Calcification appears first in the dentate nuclei and pons, then in the basal ganglia, and finally in the corpus callosum.

Parathyroid function must be assessed in every child with basal ganglia calcification to exclude the possibility of either hyperparathyroidism or pseudohypoparathyroidism.

Treatment. No treatment is available for the underlying condition except in cases of parathyroid dysfunction. The symptoms of chorea can be treated.

Hallervorden-Spatz Disease

Hallervorden-Spatz disease is a rare disorder of iron metabolism that is presumed to be transmitted by autosomal recessive inheritance (Swaiman, 1991).

Clinical Features. Symptoms begin between 2 and 10 years of age in more than half of patients but may appear as late as the third decade. The prominent features are choreoathetosis, dystonia, rigidity, and dysarthria. Dystonia may be more prominent than chorea. Retinitis pigmentosa and seizures each occur in 20% to 25% of cases. Mental deterioration and spasticity follow, with progression to spastic immobility and death within 5 to 10 years.

Diagnosis. Antemortem diagnosis is based primarily on the clinical presentation and is difficult to establish in the absence of a family history of the disorder. Cranial CT and EEG findings are normal early in the course. At onset, Hallervorden-Spatz disease may be difficult to distinguish from idiopathic torsion dystonia, but the later development of mental deterioration and retinitis pigmentosa suggests Hallervorden-Spatz disease and is not expected in idiopathic torsion dystonia.

Postmortem examination reveals degeneration of the pallidum and substantia nigra with deposition of iron-containing material.

Treatment. Levodopa reduces symptoms in some patients but not in others. In two siblings, benztropine, 2 mg twice daily, was found to produce a dramatic remission that persisted during 2 years of observation (Torch and Humphreys, 1986). Agents that chelate iron have not proved effective.

Infantile Bilateral Striatal Necrosis

The term "infantile bilateral striatal necrosis" has been applied to several clinical disorders, many genetic, that share pathologic features: bilateral, symmetric, spongy degeneration of the corpus striatum with variable degeneration of the globus pallidus (Leuzzi et al, 1988). These disorders may appear in infancy or early childhood, and the familial cases are thought to be transmitted by autosomal recessive inheritance (Mito et al, 1986).

Clinical Features. Three clinical syndromes are described: acute infantile, gradual infantile, and childhood. Probably most of the acute infantile cases are caused by subacute necrotizing encephalomyelopathy (see Chapter 5). In the gradual infant form, neurologic symptoms, including nystagmus, choreoathetosis, and seizures, often follow a febrile illness with nausea and vomiting. Optic atrophy is an associated feature in some families (Leuzzi et al, 1992). The course is marked by developmental delay, progressive spasticity, a decline to a vegetative state, and death.

When the onset is after 3 years of age, other family members are usually not affected and the disorder may not be genetic. Some cases are suspected to be "postinfectious," but a cause-and-effect relationship with a toxic or infectious cause has not been established.

Diagnosis. Diagnosis is suggested by showing progressive striatal necrosis on serial MRI examinations. Postmortem examination reveals diffuse but patchy neuronal loss and marked gliosis in the striatum and globus pallidus.

Treatment. No treatment is available.

Neuroacanthocytosis

Familial and nonfamilial cases of a progressive neurologic disorder have been described in which chorea is a prominent feature, associated with acanthocytosis and normal lipoproteins (Hardie et al, 1991). The acanthocyte is an abnormal erythrocyte that has thorny projections from the cell surface (see "Abetalipoproteinemia").

Clinical Features. Age at onset is usually in adulthood but may be as early as the first decade. Chorea or dystonia of the limbs and face occurs in all cases. Tics, oromandibular dyskinesia, and dystonia may be associated features. Self-mutilation of the lips may occur. Phenotypic variability is considerable and may include axonal neuropathy, loss of tendon reflexes, dementia, seizures, and neurosis.

Diagnosis. The association of acanthocytosis

or echinocytes (cells with rounded projections) and neurologic disease in the absence of lipoprotein abnormality is required for diagnosis. Erythrocyte deformity is enhanced by incubating the cells in saline solution for 5 minutes (Feinberg et al, 1991). McLeod syndrome is excluded by testing for the Kell antigen (see Chapter 8).

Treatment. Only the symptoms can be treated. Death occurs 10 to 20 years after onset.

DRUG-INDUCED CHOREA

Choreiform movements and akathisia (restlessness) or dystonic posturing may occur as effects of drugs. Chorea and akathisia are more likely to be dose-related effects, whereas dystonia is usually an idiosyncratic reaction (see "Dystonia"). Phenytoin and ethosuximide may induce chorea as a toxic or idiosyncratic manifestation. Phenothiazines and haloperidol are associated with idiosyncratic dystonic reactions and tardive dyskinesia, and stimulant drugs (dextroamphetamine and methylphenidate) are associated with chorea, akathisia, and tic (see "Tic and Tourette Syndrome").

Tardive Dyskinesia

The term "tardive dyskinesia" denotes drug-induced choreiform movements. These movements are often limited to the lingual, facial, and buccal muscles and appear late ("tardive") in the course of drug therapy. In my experience drug-induced buccolingual dyskinesia is unusual in children.

Tardive dyskinesias are most often associated with drugs used to modify behavior (neuroleptics), such as phenothiazines or haloperidol, and antiemetics, such as metoclopramide and prochlorperazine; they also occur in children with asthma treated with theophylline (Pranzatelli et al, 1991). The incidence of tardive dyskinesia in children taking neuroleptic drugs is estimated at 1% (Silverstein and Johnston, 1985).

Clinical Features. Tardive dyskinesia is a complex of stereotyped movements. It usually affects the mouth and face, resembles chewing, and includes tongue protrusion and lip smacking; the trunk may be involved in rocking movements and the fingers in alternating flexion and extension resembling piano playing. Limb chorea, dystonia, myoclonus, tics, and facial grimacing may be associated features. These movements are exacerbated by stress and relieved by sleep.

Symptoms appear months to years after the initiation of therapy and are not related to changes in dosage. In children the movements usually cease when the drug is discontinued, but they may remain unchanged in adults.

Diagnosis. Drug-induced dyskinesia should be suspected in any child who shows abnormal movements of the face or limbs while taking neuroleptic drugs. It is important to distinguish tardive dyskinesia from facial tics in children with Tourette syndrome and from facial mannerisms in children with schizophrenia.

Treatment. The risk of tardive dyskinesia in children may be reduced by intermittent interruption of therapy or scheduled exchange of drugs (Singer, 1986). All neuroleptic drugs should be discontinued as quickly as possible after symptoms of dyskinesia develop. This may not be possible when drugs are needed to treat psychosis. In such circumstances the movements sometimes respond to reserpine or diazepam.

Emergent Withdrawal Syndrome

Chorea and myoclonus may appear for the first time after neuroleptic drugs are abruptly discontinued or greatly reduced in dosage (Gualtieri et al, 1984). Lingual-facial-buccal dyskinesia may be present as well. The symptoms are self-limited and cease in weeks to months.

PAROXYSMAL CHOREOATHETOSIS

Paroxysmal choreoathetosis occurs in children who are otherwise normal and in children with an obvious underlying static encephalopathy. The former have a genetic disease, *familial paroxysmal choreoathetosis* (see Chapter 1), and the latter may have one of several nongenetic disorders (Erickson and Chun, 1987). The mechanism of both is unknown.

Acquired paroxysmal choreoathetosis occurs most often in children with cerebral palsy. Either hemiplegia or diplegia may be present, and the involuntary movements affect only the paretic limbs. The onset of the movement disorder often occurs 10 or more years after the acute encephalopathy.

SYSTEMIC CONDITIONS
Hyperthyroidism

The ocular manifestations of thyrotoxicosis are discussed in Chapter 15. Tremor is the most common associated movement disorder. Chorea is unusual, but when present it may affect the face, limbs, and trunk (Swanson et al, 1981). The movements cease when the child becomes euthyroid.

Lupus Erythematosus

Clinical Features.   Lupus-associated chorea is uncommon but may be the first manifestation of disease (Groothuis et al, 1977). The chorea begins from 7 years before to 3 years after the appearance of systemic features. It is indistinguishable from Sydenham chorea in appearance. Average duration is 12 weeks, but one fourth of patients suffer recurrence. Additional neurologic manifestations of lupus (ataxia, psychosis, seizures) are common in children who manifest chorea but occur only after the appearance of systemic symptoms. Therefore chorea may be a solitary manifestation of disease.

Diagnosis.   The diagnosis is clear in children with known lupus erythematosus. When chorea is an initial manifestation of lupus, it must be differentiated from Sydenham chorea. An elevated erythrocyte sedimentation rate may be present in both conditions and is not a distinguishing feature. The presence of elevated concentrations of antinuclear antibodies is critical to diagnosis.

Treatment.   Children with neurologic manifestations of lupus erythematosus should be treated with high doses of corticosteroids. The overall outcome is poor.

Pregnancy (Chorea Gravidarum)

Chorea should not be accepted as a complication of pregnancy. More likely pregnancy has added one more stress to an underlying condition. The major considerations are an initial attack or recurrence of Sydenham chorea and lupus erythematosus.

Sydenham (Rheumatic) Chorea

In the past, Sydenham chorea was the most common form of acquired chorea in children. Its incidence in the United States greatly diminished but has begun to increase again. Sydenham chorea is a cardinal manifestation of rheumatic fever and occurs primarily in populations with untreated streptococcal infections.

Clinical Features.   The onset is frequently insidious, and diagnosis is often delayed. Chorea, emotional lability, and hypotonia are cardinal features. Difficulty in school may bring the child to medical attention. Chorea causes the child to be restless, and discipline by the teacher results in emotional excess. The behavioral change is often thought to be a sign of mental illness.

Examination reveals a fidgeting child with migratory chorea of limbs and face. The limbs of only one side may be affected initially, but the chorea eventually becomes generalized in most patients. Efforts to conceal chorea with voluntary movement only add to the appearance of restlessness.

Gradual improvement occurs over several months. Most patients recover completely, but some have persistent behavioral disturbances (Bird et al, 1976). Rheumatic valvular heart disease develops in one third of untreated persons (Aron et al, 1965).

Diagnosis.   The diagnosis is clinical and cannot be confirmed by laboratory tests. The differential diagnosis is mainly between Sydenham chorea and lupus-associated chorea. They are difficult to distinguish on clinical grounds alone. Blood should be examined for lupus antinuclear antibodies and for thyroid function. The onset of Sydenham chorea is usually 4 months after the provocative streptococcal infection, and by that time the antistreptolysin O titer is back to normal or only slightly increased.

Treatment.   Pimozide usually controls the acute neurologic symptoms without producing sedation (Shannon and Fenichel, 1990). If pimozide does not relieve the symptoms, benzodiazepines, phenothiazines, or haloperidol should be tried. All children with Sydenham chorea must be treated as if they had acute rheumatic fever: penicillin in high doses for 10 days to eradicate active streptococcal infection and prophylactic penicillin therapy until age 21.

◆ Dystonia

Dystonia is a disturbance of posture caused by simultaneous contracture of agonist and antagonist muscles. The posturing is initiated by involuntary movement in the limbs, face, or trunk; the movement has a writhing quality. The overall appearance is not of an involuntary movement disorder, but rather of an abnormal posture of the limbs or trunk and grimacing of the face. Involvement may be of a single body part (*focal dystonia*), two or more contiguous body parts (*segmental dystonia*), the arm and leg on one side of the body (*hemidystonia*), or one or both legs and the contiguous trunk and any other body part (*generalized dystonia*).

The differential diagnosis of abnormal posturing is summarized in Table 14–4. Continuous motor unit activity (see Chapter 8) may be difficult to distinguish from dystonia by clinical inspection alone, especially when only one or two limbs are affected. The two disorders are differentiated by electromyography, which is recommended in most cases.

Table 14–4 ◆ Differential Diagnosis of Abnormal Posturing

1. Dystonia
2. Hysteria
3. Muscular dystrophy
4. Myotonia
5. Neuromyotonia
6. Rigidity
7. Spasticity
8. Stiffman syndrome

Persistent focal dystonias are relatively common in adults but are unusual in children except when drug induced. Most dystonias in children that begin focally eventually become generalized. Children with focal, stereotyped movements of the eyelids, face, or neck are much more likely to have a tic than focal dystonia. Only childhood forms of focal dystonia are listed in Table 14–5.

Generalized dystonia usually begins in one limb. The patient has difficulty performing an act rather than a movement, so that the foot becomes dystonic when walking forward but not when sitting, standing, or running.

FOCAL DYSTONIAS
Blepharospasm

Blepharospasm is an involuntary spasmodic closure of the eyes (Jankovic et al, 1982). The differential diagnosis for children is summarized in Table 14–6. Essential blepharospasm, an incapacitating focal dystonia, is a disorder of middle or late adult life and never begins in childhood. Tic accounts for almost all cases of involuntary eye closure in children. Eye fluttering occurs during absence seizures (see Chapter 1) but is not confused with dystonia. Focal dystonia involving eye closure in children is almost always drug induced.

Blepharospasm and orofacial dystonia in adult patients may be helped by treatment with baclofen, clonazepam, trihexyphenidyl, tetrabenazine with lithium, and subcutaneous injections of botulinum A toxin (Jankovic and Brin, 1991).

Drug-Induced Dystonia
Acute Reactions

Focal or generalized dystonia may occur as an acute idiosyncratic reaction following a first dose of phenothiazine or haloperidol. Possible reactions include trismus, opisthotonos, torticollis, and oculogyric crisis. Difficulty with swallowing and speaking may occur. The highest frequency of drug-induced generalized dystonia and oculogyric crisis is in children less than 15 years of age (Knight and Roberts, 1986).

Metoclopramide, a nonphenothiazine antiemetic that blocks postsynaptic dopamine receptors, may produce acute and delayed (tardive) dystonia. The acute reactions are usually self-limited or respond to treatment with benztropine, but they

Table 14–5 ◆ Differential Diagnosis of Dystonia in Childhood

Focal Dystonia
1. Blepharospasm
2. Drug-induced dystonia
3. Torticollis
4. Writer's cramp

Generalized Dystonia
1. Genetic disorders
   a. Ataxia with episodic dystonia (see Chapter 10)
   b. Ceroid lipofuscinosis (see Chapter 5)
   c. Cytochrome *b* deficiency
   d. Dopa-responsive dystonia
   e. Familial paroxysmal choreoathetosis (see Chapter 1)
   f. Glutaric acidemia
   g. Hallervorden-Spatz disease (see "Chorea")
   h. Hepatolenticular degeneration (Wilson disease)
   i. Huntington disease (see Chapter 5)
   j. Idiopathic torsion dystonia
   k. Leber disease (see Chapter 16)
   l. Machado-Joseph disease (see Chapter 10)
   m. Transient paroxysmal dystonia of infancy (see Chapter 1)
2. Symptomatic dystonia
   a. Perinatal cerebral injury (see Chapter 1)
   b. Postinfectious
   c. Poststroke
   d. Posttraumatic
   e. Toxin-induced
   f. Tumor-induced

Table 14–6 ◆ Differential Diagnosis of Blepharospasm in Childhood

1. Continuous motor unit activity
2. Drug-induced
3. Encephalitis
4. Hemifacial spasm
5. Hepatolenticular degeneration (Wilson disease)
6. Huntington disease
7. Hysteria
8. Myokymia
9. Myotonia
10. Schwartz-Jampel syndrome
11. Seizures

may be prolonged and resistant to therapy (Leopold, 1984).

Tardive Dystonia

Dystonia may occur 3 to 11 days after treatment with neuroleptic drugs is initiated. The dystonia is usually generalized in children but may be focal in adults (Burke et al, 1982). Spontaneous remissions are unusual. Tetrabenazine is helpful in 68% of patients, and anticholinergics offer relief in 39%.

Torticollis

The differential diagnoses of torticollis and head tilt are summarized in Table 14–7. The first step in diagnosis is to distinguish fixed from nonfixed torticollis. In fixed torticollis the neck cannot be readily moved back to the neutral position. This may be due to structural disturbance of cervical vertebrae, but more often the patient experiences pain and resists movement.

If evidence of dystonia in the face or limbs is also present, further evaluation should be directed at underlying causes of dystonia. Torticollis associated with hyperactive tendon reflexes, ankle clonus, or extensor plantar responses suggests a cervical spinal cord disturbance and is an indication for magnetic resonance imaging (MRI) of the cervical portion of the spine (see Figure 10–7). Symptoms of increased intracranial pressure indicate a posterior fossa tumor with early herniation. When torticollis is the only abnormal feature, the underlying causes are focal dystonia, injuries to the neck muscles, and juvenile rheumatoid arthritis.

Nonfixed torticollis that occurs in attacks suggests benign paroxysmal torticollis or familial paroxysmal choreoathetosis. The combination of head

Table 14–7 ◆ Differential Diagnosis of Torticollis and Head Tilt

1. Benign paroxysmal torticollis
2. Cervical cord syringomyelia (see Chapter 12)
3. Cervical cord tumors (see Chapter 12)
4. Cervicomedullary malformations (see Chapters 10 and 18)
5. Diplopia (see Chapter 15)
6. Dystonia
7. Familial paroxysmal choreoathetosis (see Chapter 1)
8. Juvenile rheumatoid arthritis
9. Posterior fossa tumors (see Chapter 10)
10. Sandifer syndrome
11. Spasmus nutans (see Chapter 15)
12. Sternocleidomastoid injuries
13. Tic and Tourette syndrome

tilt and nystagmus is termed "spasmus nutans" (see Chapter 15). Tic produces head turning but is so spasmodic that it should not be confused with torticollis.

Benign Paroxysmal Torticollis

Benign paroxysmal torticollis is a migraine variant occuring in infants and small children (Deonna and Martin, 1981). It is closely related to benign paroxysmal vertigo (see Chapter 10).

Clinical Features. Onset is always in the first year and is characterized by episodes in which the head is tilted to one side (not always the same side) and may be slightly rotated. The child may resist efforts to return the head to a neutral position, but this can be overcome. Some children have no other symptoms, whereas others have pallor, irritability, malaise, and vomiting. Attacks last for minutes to days, end spontaneously, and tend to recur monthly. Children old enough to stand and walk become ataxic during attacks.

With time the attacks may evolve into episodes characteristic of benign paroxysmal vertigo or classic migraine, or may simply cease without further symptoms. The disorder has been described in siblings, but more often the family history is only of migraine.

Diagnosis. The disorder should be suspected in any infant with attacks of torticollis that remit spontaneously. A family history of migraine is critical to the diagnosis. Familial paroxysmal choreoathetosis and familial paroxysmal dystonia do not begin during early infancy. *Sandifer syndrome,* intermittent torticollis associated with hiatal hernia, is an alternative consideration.

Treatment. No treatment is available or needed for the acute attacks.

Writer's Cramp

Writer's cramp is a focal dystonia that may occur only when writing, when performing other specific manual tasks such as typing or playing the piano *(occupational cramp),* or with nonspecific use of the hands (Sheehy and Marsden, 1982). The cramp is most often isolated but may be associated with other focal dystonias, such as torticollis, or with generalized dystonia.

Clinical Features. Onset is almost always after 20 years of age but may be in the second decade. Initial features are any of the following: aching in the hand when writing, loss of handwriting neatness or speed, and difficulty in holding a writing implement. All three symptoms are eventually present. Dystonic postures occur when the patient attempts to write. The hand and arm lift from the paper, and the fingers extend. An attempt is made to overcome forced finger extension by forced grasping. Writing with the affected hand becomes impossible, and the patient learns to write with the nondominant hand.

Symptoms are at first intermittent and are especially severe when others observe the writing. Later the cramp occurs with each attempt at writing. Some patients have lifelong difficulty with using the dominant hand for writing and may have difficulty with other manual tasks as well. Other experience remissions and exacerbations, and in a minority of patients generalized dystonia develops.

Diagnosis. Unfortunately, most people with writer's or occupational cramp are thought to have psychiatric illness despite the lack of associated psychopathologic features. Early diagnosis can save considerable expense and concern. Isolated focal dystonia must be distinguished from generalized dystonia with focal onset. Family history should be explored thoroughly and examination repeated to determine the presence of dystonia in other body parts.

Treatment. The same medications used to treat generalized dystonia should be used in patients with focal dystonia (see "Idiopathic Torsion Dystonia").

GENERALIZED DYSTONIAS
Genetic Dystonias
Cytochrome b Deficiency

Mitochondrial disorders cause widespread dysfunction of the central and peripheral nervous system (see Chapters 5, 8, and 11). Partial cytochrome *b* deficiency was identified in an 18-year-old girl in whom clinical features of idiopathic torsion dystonia developed at 2 years of age (Nigro et al, 1990). The possibility of mitochondrial dysfunction was suggested by an increased concentration of lactate and pyruvate in venous blood and by CT evidence of bilateral hypodensities in the putamen. Ragged-red fibers were present on muscle biopsy (see Chapter 8), and the cytochrome *b* deficiency was demonstrated in the muscle specimen.

Dopa-Responsive Dystonia

Dopa-responsive dystonia is also called the *dystonia-parkinsonism syndrome, dystonia with diurnal variation,* and *Segawa disease* (Nygaard et al, 1990). Dopa-responsive dystonia is probably inherited as an autosomal dominant trait with a 31% penetrance rate. Most cases of "juvenile parkin-

sonism" probably belong to this group (Nygaard et al, 1991).

Clinical Features. Age at onset is usually between 4 and 8 years but may be as early as infancy. Early-onset cases are often misdiagnosed as cerebral palsy. The initial feature is nearly always a gait disturbance caused by leg dystonia. Flexion at the hip and knee and plantar flexion of the foot cause toe-walking. Both flexor and extensor posturing of the arms develops, and finally parkinsonian features appear: cogwheel rigidity, masklike facies, and bradykinesia. The disease reaches a plateau in adolescence. Postural or intention tremor occurs in almost half of patients, but typical parkinsonian tremor is unusual.

Diurnal fluctuation in symptoms occurs in more than half of patients. Symptoms are considerably improved on awakening and become worse later in the day. Movement and exercise exacerbate dystonia in some patients. Whether other disorders with exercise-induced dystonia as the major or solitary feature are expressions of the same genetic error is unknown (Plant et al, 1984).

Diagnosis. Dopa-responsive dystonia may be difficult to differentiate from other genetic disorders with dystonia because of phenotypic variation among family members. The neurologist should examine as many close relatives as possible. Important clues to diagnosis are features of parkinsonism without other neurologic signs, diurnal variation in severity of symptoms, exacerbation of symptoms with exercise, and response to levodopa.

Treatment. A small dose of levodopa provides immediate and complete relief in most patients, even when treatment is initiated long after symptoms begin. No other dystonia responds so well. The daily dosage of levodopa when given as carbidopa-levodopa (Sinemet), 10 mg/kg, is 50 to 200 mg. Long-term therapy is beneficial and required; symptoms return when the drug is discontinued.

Trihexyphenidyl, in doses lower than ordinarily needed to treat idiopathic torsion dystonia, and bromocriptine are also effective.

Glutaric Acidemia

Glutaric acidemia is a rare inborn error in the catabolism of lysine, hydroxylysine, and tryptophan. It is transmitted by autosomal recessive inheritance and caused by deficiency of glutaryl–coenzyme-A dehydrogenase (Bergman et al, 1989).

Clinical Features. Megaloencephaly is usually present at birth (Iafolla and Kahler, 1989). Neurologic findings may be otherwise normal. Two patterns have been described in affected infants. One is characterized by hypotonia and developmental delay, and the other by dystonia, chorea, athetosis, and dysmetria. Infants have an acute encephalitis-like illness characterized by somnolence, irritability, and excessive sweating. Seizures sometimes occur. Afterward there are developmental regression, progressive choreoathetosis, and dystonia. The dystonic form may have an acute onset suggesting a drug reaction.

Diagnosis.   Metabolic acidosis may be present. Abnormal amounts of glutaric, 3-hydroxyglutaric, 3-hydroxybutyric, and acetoacetic acids are found in the urine. Definitive diagnosis requires demonstration of the enzyme deficiency in cultured fibroblasts. CT often shows diffuse attenuation of cerebral white matter and cerebral atrophy, most marked in the frontal and temporal lobes.

Treatment.   The course of disease may be improved by protein restriction and riboflavin supplementation.

Hepatolenticular Degeneration (Wilson Disease)

Hepatolenticular degeneration is transmitted by autosomal recessive inheritance. The disorder may be caused by a disturbance in the biliary excretion of copper and its incorporation into ceruloplasmin. The defective gene is located on chromosome 13 (Bowcock et al, 1988). Symptoms result from the accumulation of copper in liver, brain, and cornea.

Clinical Features.   Hepatic failure is the prominent clinical feature in children less than 10 years of age, usually without neurologic symptoms or signs. Neurologic manifestations with only minimal symptoms of liver disease are more likely when the onset of symptoms is in the second decade. A single symptom, such as a disturbance of gait or speech, is often the initial feature and may remain unchanged for years (Sternlieb et al, 1987). Eventually the initial symptom worsens and new features develop: dysarthria (97%), dystonia (65%), dysdiadochokinesia (58%), rigidity (52%), gait and postural abnormalities (42%), tremor (32%), and drooling (23%) (Starosta-Rubinstein et al, 1987).

Dystonia of bulbar muscles is responsible for three prominent features of the disease: dysarthria, a fixed pseudosmile (risus sardonicus), and a high-pitched whining noise on inspiration.

Psychiatric disturbances precede the neurologic abnormalities in 20% of cases. They range from behavioral disturbances to paranoid psychoses. Dementia is not an early feature of disease.

The Kayser-Fleischer ring, a yellow-brown granular deposit at the limbus of the cornea, is a certain indicator of the disease. It is caused by copper deposition in the Descemet membrane and is present in all patients with neurologic manifestations, although it may be absent in children with liver disease alone.

Diagnosis.   Hepatolenticular degeneration should be considered in any child with dysarthria and dystonia. The further association of chronic liver disease increases the probability of hepatolenticular degeneration. The diagnosis is confirmed by demonstrating an increased copper content by liver biopsy or by the demonstration of a Kayser-Fleischer ring by slitlamp examination. Ninety-six percent of patients have a serum ceruloplasmin concentration of less than 20 mg/dl, corresponding to less than 56 μg/dl of ceruloplasmin copper (Sternlieb et al, 1987).

MRI demonstrates increased signal intensity and decreased size of the caudate, putamen, subcortical white matter, midbrain, and pons. MRI findings do not correlate well with clinical features (Prayer et al, 1990).

Treatment.   The treatment of choice is the oral administration of D-penicillamine, 250 mg four times a day for children more than 10 years of age and half as much for children less than 10. Penicillamine must always be given on an empty stomach together with a daily dose of 25 mg pyridoxine. Twenty-four-hour urinary copper secretion is then monitored, and the dose is adjusted to produce urinary excretion of copper at a rate of 2 mg/day during the first year. Later an excretion of 1 mg/day is considered satisfactory. Improvement is slow, and recovery of neurologic function frequently takes several months. Symptoms may worsen during the first months of therapy, but this should not be a cause for alarm. When treatment is started early, the results are quite satisfactory without excess morbidity and mortality.

Discontinuation of penicillamine results in rapid clinical deterioration, which may prove fatal (Scheinberg et al, 1987). The replacement of penicillamine with trientine, a chelating agent, prevents the adverse course associated with penicillamine withdrawal.

Siblings of patients with Wilson disease should be carefully screened for disease and treated as early as possible (Strickland and Leu, 1975).

Idiopathic Torsion Dystonia

Idiopathic torsion dystonia encompasses several genetic disorders characterized by generalized dystonia without other symptoms of neurologic deterioration. *Dystonia musculorum deformans* is an older name for the same disorders. Most familial forms are transmitted by autosomal dominant inheritance with the abnormal gene located on chromosome 9 at the q32-34 site (Kramer et al, 1990). The frequency of idiopathic torsion dystonia in Ashkenazi Jews is five to ten times greater than in other groups. Nonfamilial cases probably represent autosomal dominant inheritance with incomplete penetrance. The penetrance rate is 40%, and the expression is highly variable (Fletcher et al, 1990).

Clinical Features. Dystonia often begins between 6 and 14 years of age but may begin anytime after infancy. The limbs are usually affected before the trunk.

Forty-three percent of patients initially have dystonia of the hands or arm, and 36% have gait abnormalities (Marsden and Harrison, 1974). Leg involvement as an initial feature is more common in children that adults. Despite the focal features at onset, dystonia always becomes generalized in children, affecting the limbs and trunk. Spontaneous stabilization is the rule, but remission is unusual. The eventual outcome varies from complete disability to functional independence (Angelini et al, 1989).

Other clinical features include dysarthria, orofacial movements, dysphagia, postural tremor, and blepharospasm. Mental deterioration does not occur, but as a group, patients with familial disease have a lower IQ than those with sporadic cases.

Diagnosis. Diagnosis depends on the clinical features of dystonic movements and postures, normal perinatal history, no exposure to drugs, no evidence of intellectual or corticospinal deterioration, and no demonstrable biochemical disorder.

Treatment. Trihexyphenidyl is effective in the treatment of idiopathic torsion dystonia. High dosages are required, usually 30 mg/day in three divided doses. Daily doses as high at 80 mg/day are sometimes necessary. Children can tolerate such high dosages if built up slowly, but adults rarely can. The response cannot be predicted from measurement of plasma concentration (Burke and Fahn, 1985).

If trihexyphenidyl is not effective, diazepam should be added at low dosages and slowly increased as tolerated. If a patient does not respond to this combination, tetrabenazine (Jankovic and Orman, 1988) or some combination of carbamazepine, levodopa, benztropine, pimozide, or bromocriptine may be tried (Gautier and Awada, 1983).

Symptomatic Dystonia

Dystonia may be caused by an underlying tumor, active encephalopathy (hypoxic, infectious, or metabolic), or prior brain damage resulting from encephalopathy, trauma, or stroke.

Clinical Features. The onset of dystonia may be at the time of an acute encephalopathy, after the acute phase is over, or several years later when the encephalopathy is thought to be static (Burke et al, 1980). Delayed-onset chorea and dystonia in children with perinatal disturbances such as asphyxia or kernicterus usually begin by 2 or 3 years of age but may be delayed for 17 years (Saint Hilaire et al, 1991). After involuntary movements appear, they tend to become progressively severe, but intellectual decline is not an associated feature. Delayed-onset dystonia is usually generalized.

Hemidystonia most often occurs after stroke or head injury but may be a symptom of neuronal storage diseases or tumors of the basal ganglia (Narbona et al, 1984; Pettigrew and Jankovic, 1985). The dystonic limbs are contralateral to the damaged basal ganglia.

Diagnosis. Children with a known cause for the development of dystonia or chorea need not be studied extensively. The new symptoms are discouraging for patients and families who have adjusted to a fixed neurologic deficit. They may be assured that this is not evidence of new degeneration in the brain, but only the appearance of new symptoms from old lesions. This sequence is most likely when injury is perinatal and brain maturation is required to manifest involuntary movements.

The appearance of hemidystonia, even when the predisposing event is known, necessitates MRI or CT to look for localized changes that may require treatment, such as an expanding cyst. The possibility of tumor must be considered in children who had been neurologically intact before hemidystonia appeared.

Treatment. The drugs used to treat symptomatic dystonia are no different from those used for genetic dystonia, but the results may not be as favorable.

◆ Hemifacial Spasm

Hemifacial spasm is characterized by involuntary, irregular contraction of the muscles innervated by one facial nerve. It is rare in children (Ronen et al, 1986). The spasms may develop because of aberrant regeneration following facial nerve injury, as a result of posterior fossa tumor, or without apparent cause.

Clinical Features. Spasms are embarrassing and disturbing but not painful. The orbicularis oculi muscles are affected first and most commonly, causing forced closure of the eye. As all facial muscles on one side become affected, the mouth is pulled to one side. Spasms may occur several times a minute, especially during times of stress. The subsequent course depends on the underlying cause.

Diagnosis. Hemifacial spasm in children may be mistaken for a focal seizure. The stereotyped appearance of the spasm and a concurrent normal EEG should differentiate them. Posterior fossa tumor must be suspected in every child with hemifacial spasm. MRI is indicated unless symptoms can be explained by a known history of facial nerve injury.

Treatment. Some patients respond to treatment with carbamazepine at anticonvulsant doses (see Chapter 1), but most have no response to medical therapy. Surgical procedures to relieve pressure on the facial nerve from adjacent vessels are of questionable value.

◆ Mirror Movements

Mirror movements are defined as involuntary movements of one side of the body, usually the hands, that occur as mirror reversals of an intended movement on the other side of the body (Cohen et al, 1991). They are normal during infancy and tend to disappear before 10 years of age, coincident with myelination of the corpus callosum. Persistence of mirror movements may be a familial trait caused by ipsilateral and contralateral organization of the corticospinal pathways. Obligatory mirror movements are abnormal even in infants and suggest a congenital abnormality at the cervicomedullary junction.

◆ Myoclonus

The term "myoclonus" encompasses several involuntary movements characterized by rapid muscle jerks. They are less frequent and severe during sleep but may not disappear. Myoclonus may be rhythmic or nonrhythmic; focal, multifocal, or generalized; or spontaneous or activated by movement (action myoclonus) or sensory stimulation (reflex myoclonus).

Nonepileptic myoclonus must be distinguished from tic, chorea, tremor, and seizures. Tics are usually more complex and stereotyped movements than myoclonus and can be briefly suppressed by voluntary effort; myoclonus cannot be suppressed. Chorea is more random than myoclonus and tends to be incorporated into voluntary movement; myoclonus is never part of a larger movement. Rhythmic myoclonus and tremor look alike and are distinguished with certainty only by special studies. Tremor is a continuous to-and-fro movement, whereas rhythmic myoclonus has a pause between movements.

Marsden and associates (1982) proposed an etiologic classification of myoclonus that has proved useful and is summarized in Table 14–8. Physiologic myoclonus occurs in normal people when falling asleep, during sleep (nocturnal myoclonus), when waking up, and during times of anxiety. Nocturnal myoclonus is a rhythmic jerking of the legs

Table 14–8 ◆ Etiologic Classification of Myoclonus

Physiologic
1. Anxiety-induced
2. Exercise-induced
3. Sleep jerks and nocturnal myoclonus

Essential
1. Familial
2. Sporadic

Epileptic (see Chapter 1)

Symptomatic
1. After-central nervous system injury
   a. Hypoxia (see Chapter 2)
   b. Trauma (see Chapter 2)
   c. Stroke (see Chapter 11)
2. Basal ganglia degenerations
   a. Idiopathic torsion dystonia
   b. Hallervorden-Spatz disease
   c. Hepatolenticular degeneration (Wilson disease)
   d. Huntington disease (see Chapter 5)
3. Drug-induced
   a. L-Dopa
   b. Tricyclic antidepressants
4. Lysosomal storage diseases (see Chapter 5)
5. Metabolic encephalopathies (see Chapter 2)
   a. Dialysis syndromes
   b. Disorders of osmolality
   c. Hepatic failure
   d. Renal failure
6. Myoclonic encephalopathy (see Chapter 10)
   a. Idiopathic
   b. Neuroblastoma
7. Spinal cord tumor (see Chapter 12)
8. Spinocerebellar degenerations (see Chapter 10)
9. Toxic encephalopathies (see Chapter 2)
10. Viral encephalitis

during sleep and is classified as an essential myoclonus by Marsden and associates (1982). I believe it is normal in children and have classified it as a physiologic myoclonus. Essential myoclonus is abnormal, but it occurs in people who have no other neurologic abnormality. Epileptic myoclonus is associated with epileptiform activity on the EEG (see Chapter 1). Symptomatic myoclonus is caused by drugs, follows a cerebral injury, or is part of a generalized and usually progressive encephalopathy.

ESSENTIAL MYOCLONUS

Essential myoclonus may be sporadic or familial. The familial form is transmitted by autosomal dominant inheritance.

Clinical Features. Onset is in the first or second decade. Males and females are affected equally. The movements are predominantly in the face, trunk, and proximal muscles. They are usually generalized but may be restricted to one side of the body. No other neurologic disturbances develop, and life span is not affected. Essential tremor may be present in the same family.

Diagnosis. A family history of isolated myoclonus limits the differential diagnosis. Unfortunately, sporadic cases are more common than familial cases. Symptomatic and epileptic myoclonus must be eliminated by careful neurologic examination, EEG, and brain imaging study. Even then, a period of observation and repeat laboratory investigations may be necessary to eliminate other causes.

Treatment. Mild essential myoclonus may not require treatment. Carbamazepine, clonazepam, tetrabenazine, and valproate have been found useful in symptomatic myoclonus and may have an effect in generalized myoclonus as well. Benztropine relieved symptoms completely in one family (Chokroverty et al, 1987).

SYMPTOMATIC MYOCLONUS

Myoclonus is often a symptom of an underlying neurologic disease. It tends to be generalized when caused by diffuse, progressive encephalopathies (such as lysosomal storage diseases) and segmental when there is a focal lesion of the brainstem or spinal cord.

Posthypoxic Myoclonus (Lance-Adams Syndrome)

Posthypoxic myoclonus is a form of action myoclonus in patients who have suffered an episode of hypoxia. It does not follow hypoxic-ischemic encephalopathy of the newborn. Single or repetitive myoclonic jerks occur when voluntary movement is attempted. Facial and pharyngeal muscles may be affected, interfering with speech and swallowing. Cerebellar disturbances are usually associated findings.

Myoclonus usually begins during recovery from anoxic encephalopathy and is lifelong. It may respond to valproate (Rollinson and Gilligan, 1979), 5-hydroxytryptophan, or clonazepam (Chadwick et al, 1977).

Segmental (Focal) Myoclonus

Segmental myoclonus is an involuntary contraction of contiguous muscles innervated by the brainstem or spinal cord. It may be rhythmic or nonrhythmic. Rhythmic segmental myoclonus looks like a focal seizure. The underlying causes in children are limited mainly to demyelinating diseases and intrinsic tumors.

Palatal myoclonus is the most common segmental myoclonus of brainstem origin. Cystic astrocytoma of the spinal cord is the major cause of spinal myoclonus and may be a presenting feature (see Chapter 12).

Palatal myoclonus is a unilateral or bilateral rhythmic contraction of the palate (80 to 180 per minute) that usually persists during sleep. It may be associated with rhythmic contractions of the eyes, larynx, neck, diaphragm, trunk, and limbs and results from lesions in the central tegmental tract or dentato-olivary pathways, which produce a denervation hypersensitivity and hypertrophy of the contralateral inferior olivary nucleus (Matsuo and Ajax, 1979). The median interval between the precipitating cause and the onset of palatal myoclonus is 10 to 11 months.

Clonazepam and tetrabenazine are the most useful drugs in the treatment of segmental myoclonus (Jankovic and Pardo, 1986).

◆ Tic and Tourette Syndrome

Tics or *habit spasms* are complex, stereotyped movements (motor tic) or utterances (verbal tic) that are sudden, brief, and purposeless. They may be confused with chorea but can be readily distinguished by their stereotyped appearance. Tic is more readily suppressed by voluntary effort than is chorea, and no effort is made to incorporate tic into voluntary movement. Tic and chorea are both exacerbated by stress and disappear during sleep.

Tourette syndrome is any combination of verbal and motor tics. It should not be considered a separate disease, but rather part of a phenotypic spectrum that includes simple motor tic, attention deficit disorder, and obsessive-compulsive behavior (Kurlan, 1989). It is believed to be transmitted as a highly penetrant, autosomal dominant trait in which tics and attention deficit disorder are more commonly expressed in males and obsessive-compulsive disease in females.

Clinical Features.   Affected children are not mentally disturbed before symptoms begin. Although the frequency of behavioral disturbances is increased in children with Tourette syndrome, the movement disorder and the behavioral disturbances should each be considered an expression of the same underlying genetic defect; one does not cause the other.

Onset is anytime from 2 to 15 years of age with the mean between 6 and 7 years. Neck muscles are often affected first, causing a head movement in which the child appears to be tossing hair back from the face. A haircut is frequently the first unsuccessful intervention. New motor tics develop either in place of or in addition to existing tics. They usually affect the head, eyes, or face. Common tics include eye blinking, grimacing, lip smacking, and shrugging in one or both shoulders.

The initial verbal tics are usually a clearing of the throat, a snorting or sniffing noise, and a cough-like noise. Many children who make sniffing or coughing noises undergo an extensive evaluation for allergy and are found to be allergic. Desensitization is then the next unsuccessful intervention. Grunting and hissing are other verbal tics. Coprolalia is a rare symptom in children. The profanity is quickly suppressed and replaced by barking or coughing noises.

Symptoms wax and wane spontaneously and in response to stress. Tics usually become less frequent when children are out of school. Most children outgrow their tics, but some have lifelong difficulty and others have prolonged remissions with recurrence in middle age or later (Klawans and Barr, 1985).

Among children with tic, attention deficit disorder is present in 54% and obsessive-compulsive disease in 33% (Comings and Comings, 1985). Attention deficit disorder is characterized by hyperactivity, short attention span, restlessness, poor concentration, and impaired impulse control. This syndrome is often treated with dextroamphetamine or methylphenidate, drugs that have the potential to accentuate tics in genetically predisposed children (Erenberg et al, 1985).

Obsessive-compulsive disease is characterized by ritualistic actions and thoughts, which may include touching things repeatedly, placing objects in a certain place, washing and rewashing hands, obsessive thoughts about sex or violence, and counting objects.

Diagnosis.   Tic and Tourette syndrome are diagnosed by history and observation. Laboratory tests are not helpful and need not be done in obvious cases. EEG, CT, and psychologic test results are normal (Lees et al, 1984).

Tics do not ordinarily occur in degenerative diseases of the nervous system or as an adverse reaction to drugs. Drug-induced tics should be considered the potentiation of Tourette syndrome in a genetically predisposed child. Carbamazepine, as well as amphetamine and methylphenidate, may trigger the disorder (Neglia et al, 1984). Withdrawal of the potentiating drug does not always stop the tics (Singer et al, 1986).

A degenerative disorder that begins as a spinal muscular atrophy during childhood has been described in two brothers of consanguineous parents. Tourette syndrome develops in adult life and is replaced by parkinsonism (Spitz et al, 1985). Acanthocytosis is an associated feature. This is the only degenerative disease that includes Tourette syndrome; tics are not present in childhood.

Treatment.   Most children with tics and Tourette syndrome do not require drug treatment. The decision to prescribe medication depends on whether the tics bother the child. Drugs should not be used if the tics bother the parents but do not disturb the child's life. The parents must be told that tics are not a sign of progressive neurologic or mental illness, are made worse by stress, and will diminish in frequency if ignored.

Drug treatment is often difficult to evaluate because the disorder's natural history is one of exacerbation and remission. Haloperidol is widely used and provides some improvement in 80% of cases. It is started as a single dose of 0.5 mg at night and is slowly increased by 0.5 mg each week until tics are reasonably controlled or adverse reactions are noted. The usual maintenance dosage is 1 to 3 mg/day in two divided doses. The major toxic effects are sedation, irritability, and depression of appetite. Dystonia and akathisia are idiosyncratic reactions.

I prefer pimozide, which is equally effective and has a lower incidence of adverse effects (Regeur et al, 1986). The dosage is initially 2 mg/day in two divided doses and is increased 2 mg each week as needed. The maintenance dosage is 0.2 mg/kg/day or 10 mg/day whichever is less.

Other recommended drugs are fluphenazine (Goetz et al, 1984; Singer et al, 1986) and clonidine

(Leckman et al, 1985). Fluphenazine is started at 1 mg/day and increased 1 mg each week. The usual maintenance dosage is 2 to 6 mg/day. Adverse reactions are the same as with haloperidol but occur less frequently. Clonidine is started at a dosage of 0.05 mg/day and is increased 0.05 mg each week. The usual maintenance dosage is 0.1 to 0.6 mg/day.

Any of the aforementioned drugs may lose their efficacy after prolonged use, but effectiveness may return after an interval of withholding the drug. Interrupted therapy with one drug or alternating between two drugs is reasonable.

Clomipramine may be useful for obsessive-compulsive disorders when they occur as part of the Tourette phenotype.

◆ Tremor

Tremor is an involuntary oscillating movement with a fixed frequency. The product of tremor frequency and amplitude is constant; since frequency decreases with age, amplitude increases. Shuddering, cerebellar ataxia or dysmetria, and asterixis are not tremors because they lack rhythm. Myoclonus may be rhythmic but is interrupted between oscillations.

All normal people have a low-amplitude *physiologic tremor* inherent to movement that is not ordinarily observed without instrumentation. Physiologic tremor may be enhanced to a clinically detectable level by situations (anxiety, excitement, exercise, fatigue, stress) and drugs (adrenergic agonists, nicotine, prednisone, thyroid hormone, xanthines). Hyperthyroidism is routinely associated with enhanced physiologic tremor.

Parkinsonism is a major cause of pathologic tremors in adults, but it does not occur in children except when drug induced or as part of a complex degenerative disorder. Typical parkinsonian tremor is seldom present in these situations. Essential (familial) tremor is the major cause of tremor in children.

ESSENTIAL (FAMILIAL) TREMOR

Essential (familial) tremor is a monosymptomatic condition probably transmitted as an autosomal dominant trait. Sporadic cases are called essential tremor, and familial cases are called familial tremor. Probably they are the same condition with subclinical penetrance in the affected parent. Tremor may coexist with other movement disorders, especially in adult-onset cases (Lou and Jankovic, 1991). However, no evidence has shown that essential tremor in childhood is part of a larger neurologic disturbance.

Shuddering attacks in young children may be a form of essential tremor and occur in families where other members have essential tremor (Barron and Younkin, 1992).

Clinical Features. Essential tremor occurs only in a limb being used (action tremor). The head, face, and neck are sometimes affected. Neck tremor gives the appearance of torticollis. The frequency of essential tremor is typically between 4 and 8 Hz (Findley and Koller, 1987).

Childhood-onset tremor usually appears in the second decade but can begin as early as 2 years of age. Essential tremor may impair function, especially schoolwork, and therefore disturbs the patient. In young children the tremor has the appearance of restlessness or clumsiness. Later its nature as an action tremor is appreciated.

Tremor is enhanced by greater precision of movement and therefore appears first and most prominently in the hands. It is further enhanced by anxiety, concentrated effort to stop the tremor, and fatigue. In such cases the worsening of tremor may be due to enhanced physiologic tremor rather than enhanced essential tremor. The distinction is important in considering treatment options.

Essential tremor is generally lifelong.

Diagnosis. Essential tremor in children is often mistaken for cerebellar dysfunction because it occurs with action (intention). The two can be easily differentiated because essential tremor is rhythmic and not dysmetric (does not become worse at the endpoint) and because it is not associated with other signs of cerebellar dysfunction.

The distinction between essential tremor and enhanced physiologic tremor may be more difficult because the two are often concurrent. Enhanced physiologic tremor is always circumstantial, whereas essential tremor remains even when the patient is alone and relaxed.

Treatment. Not all patients with essential tremor require treatment. Medication should be reserved for situations in which tremor impairs function. Propranolol (1 to 2 mg/kg/day) and primidone (2 to 10 mg/kg/day) are each effective drugs to control tremor in approximately 70% of cases (Koller and Vetere-Overfield, 1989; Lou and Jankovic, 1991). Propranolol has fewer side effects and should be the first drug chosen.

PAROXYSMAL DYSTONIC HEAD TREMOR

Clinical Features. Paroxysmal dystonic head tremor is an uncommon, nonfamilial syndrome of unknown cause (Hughes et al, 1991). The major feature is attacks of horizontal head tremor (frequency 5 to 8 Hz), as if the person were saying no. Onset occurs in adolescence, and two reported patients as well as my two patients were male. The attacks vary from 1 to 30 minutes, are not provoked by any single stimulus, and cannot be suppressed. My patients also had a head tilt that had predated the onset of tremor by 5 to 10 years. The attacks are reported to continue for more than 10 years but do not progress to other neurologic symptoms. Results of the examination are otherwise normal.

Diagnosis.   Imaging studies of the brain show no abnormalities. In an infant the combination of head nodding and head tilt would be diagnosed as spasmus nutans even in the absence of nystagmus (see Chapter 15), and perhaps the underlying mechanism is similar.

Treatment.   Daily clonazepam reduces the frequency and severity of attacks.

References

Angelini L, Nardocci N, Rumi V, et al: Idiopathic dystonia with onset in childhood. J Neurol 236:319, 1989.

Aron AM, Freeman JM, Carter S: The natural history of Sydenham's chorea: Review of the literature and long-term evaluation with emphasis on cardiac sequelae. Am J Med 38:83, 1965.

Barron TF, Younkin DP: Propanolol therapy for shuddering attacks. Neurology 42:258, 1992.

Beall SS, Patten BM, Mallette L, et al: Abnormal systemic metabolism of iron, porphyrin, and calcium in Fahr's syndrome. Ann Neurol 26:569, 1989.

Bergman I, Finegold D, Gartner JC Jr, et al: Acute profound dystonia in infants with glutaric acidemia. Pediatrics 83:228, 1989.

Bird MT, Palkes H, Prensky AL: A follow-up study of Sydenham's chorea. Neurology 26:601, 1976.

Bowcock AM, Farrer LA, Hebert JM, et al: Eight closely linked loci place the Wilson disease locus within 13q14q21. Am J Hum Genet 43:554, 1988.

Burke RE, Fahn S: Pharmacokinetics of trihexyphenidyl after short-term and long-term administration to dystonic patients. Ann Neurol 18:35, 1985.

Burke RE, Fahn S, Gold AP: Delayed-onset dystonia in patients with "static" encephalopathy. J Neurol Neurosurg Psychiatry 43:789, 1980.

Burke RE, Fahn S, Jankovic J, et al: Tardive dystonia: Late-onset and persistent dystonia caused by antipsychotic drugs. Neurology 32:1335, 1982.

Burnstein L, Breningstall GN: Movement disorders in bacterial meningitis. J Pediatr 109:260, 1986.

Chadwick D, Hallett M, Harris R, et al: Clinical, biochemical and physiological factors distinguishing myoclonus responsive to 5-hydroxytryptophan, tryptophan plus a monoamine oxidase inhibitor and clonazepam. Brain 100:455, 1977.

Chokroverty S, Manocha M, Duvoisin RC: A physiologic and pharmacologic study in anticholinergic-responsive essential myoclonus. Neurology 37:608, 1987.

Cohen LG, Meer J, Tarkka I, et al: Congenital mirror movements: Abnormal organization of motor pathways in two patients. Brain 114:381, 1991.

Comings DE, Comings BG: Tourette syndrome: Clinical and psychological aspects of 250 cases. Am J Hum Genet 37:435, 1985.

Deonna T, Martin D: Benign paroxysmal torticollis in infancy. Arch Dis Child 56:956, 1981.

Dewey RB Jr, Jankovic J: Hemiballismus-hemichorea: Clinical and pharmacologic findings in 21 patients. Arch Neurol 46:862, 1989.

Erenberg C, Cruse RP, Rothner AD: Gilles de la Tourette's syndrome: Effect of stimulant drugs. Neurology 35:1436, 1985.

Erickson GR, Chun RWM: Acquired paroxysmal movement disorders. Pediatr Neurol 3:226, 1987.

Feinberg TE, Cianci CD, Morroe JS, et al: Diagnostic tests for choreoacanthocytosis. Neurology 41:1000, 1991.

Findley LJ, Koller WC: Essential tremor: A review. Neurology 37:1194, 1987.

Fletcher NA, Harding AE, Marsden CD: A genetic study of idiopathic torsion dystonia in the United Kingdom. Brain 113:379, 1990.

Gautier JC, Awada A: Dystonia musculorum deformans improved by bromocriptine. Rev Neurol 139:449, 1983.

Goetz CG, Tanner CM, Klawans HL: Fluphenazine and multifocal tic disorder. Arch Neurol 41:271, 1984.

Groothuis JR, Groothuis DR, Mukhopadhyay D, et al: Lupus-associated chorea in children. AJDC 131:1131, 1977.

Gualtieri CT, Quade D, Hicks RE, et al: Tardive dyskinesia and other clinical consequences of neuroleptic treatment in children and adolescence. Am J Psychiatry 141:20, 1984.

Hardie RJ, Pullon HWH, Harding AE, et al: Neuroacanthocytosis: A clinical, haematological and pathological study of 19 cases. Brain 114:13, 1991.

Hughes AJ, Lees AJ, Marsden CD: Paroxysmal dystonic head tremor. Movement Dis 6:85, 1991.

Iafolla AK, Kahler SG: Megalencephaly in the neonatal period as the initial manifestation of glutaric aciduria type I. J Pediatr 114:1004, 1989.

Jankovic J, Brin MF: Therapeutic uses of botulinum toxin. N Engl J Med 324:1186, 1991.

Jankovic J, Havins WE, Wilkins RB: Blinking and blepharospasm: Mechanism, diagnosis, and management. JAMA 248:3160, 1982.

Jankovic J, Orman J: Tetrabenazine therapy of dystonia, chorea, tics, and other dyskinesias. Neurology 38:391, 1988.

Jankovic J, Pardo R: Segmental myoclonus: Clinical and pharmacologic study. Arch Neurol 43:1025, 1986.

Klawans HL, Barr A: Recurrence of childhood multiple tic in late life. Arch Neurol 42:1079, 1985.

Knight ME, Roberts RJ: Phenothiazine and butyrophenone intoxication in children. Pediatr Clin North Am 33:299, 1986.

Koller WC, Vetere-Overfield B: Acute and chronic effects of propranolol and primidone in essential tremor. Neurology 39:1587, 1989.

Kramer PL, de Leon D, Ozelius L, et al: Dystonia gene in Ashkenazi Jewish population is located on chromosome 9q32-34. Neurology 27:114, 1990.

Kurlan R: Tourette's syndrome: Current concepts. Neurology 39:1625, 1989.

Leckman JF, Detlor J, Harcherik DF, et al: Short- and long-term treatment of Tourette syndrome with clonidine: A clinical perspective. Neurology 35:343, 1985.

Lees AJ, Robertson M, Trimble MR, et al: A clinical study of Gilles de la Tourette syndrome in the United Kingdom. J Neurol Neurosurg Psychiatry 47:1, 1984.

Leopold NA: Prolonged metoclopramide-induced dyskinetic reaction. Neurology 34:238, 1984.

Leuzzi V, Bertini E, De Negri AM, et al: Bilateral striatal necrosis, dystonia and optic atrophy in two siblings. J Neurol Neurosurg Psychiatry 55:16, 1992.

Leuzzi V, Favata I, Seri S: Bilateral striatal lesions. Dev Med Child Neurol 30:252, 1988.

Lou J-S, Jankovic J: Essential tremor: Clinical correlates in 350 patients. Neurology 41:234, 1991.

Marsden CD, Harrison MJG: Idiopathic torsion dystonia (dystonia musculorum deformans): A review of forty-two patients. Brain 97:793, 1974.

Marsden CD, Hallett M, Fahn S: The nosology and pathophysiology of myoclonus. In Marsden CD, Fahn S, eds: Movement Disorders. Butterworth's International Medical Reviews: Neurology, Vol 2. Butterworth, London, 1982, p 196.

Matsuo F, Ajax E: Palatal myoclonus and denervation supersensitivity in the central nervous system. Ann Neurol 5:72, 1979.

Mito T, Tanaka T, Becker LE, et al: Infantile bilateral striatal necrosis: Clinicopathologic classification. Arch Neurol 43:677, 1986.

Narbona J, Obeso JA, Martinez-Lage, et al: Hemi-dystonia secondary to localized basal ganglia tumor. J Neurol Neurosurg Psychiatry 47:704, 1984.

Nardocci N, Lamperti E, Rumi V, et al: Typical and atypical forms of paroxysmal choreoathetosis. Dev Med Child Neurol 31:670, 1989.

Neglia JP, Glaze DG, Zion TE: Tics and vocalizations in children treated with carbamazepine. Pediatrics 73:841, 1984.

Nigro MA, Martens ME, Awerbuch GI, et al: Partial cytochrome b deficiency and generalized dystonia. Pediatr Neurol 6:407, 1990.

Nygaard TG, Marsden CD, Fahn S: Dopa-responsive dystonia: Long-term treatment response and prognosis. Neurology 41:174, 1991.

Nygaard TG, Trugman JM, de Yebenes JG, et al: Dopa-responsive dystonia: The spectrum of clinical manifestations in a large North American family. Neurology 40:66, 1990.

Pettigrew LC, Jankovic J: Hemidystonia: A report of 22 patients and a review of the literature. J Neurol Neurosurg Psychiatry 48:650, 1985.

Plant GT, Williams AC, Earl CJ, et al: Familial paroxysmal dystonia induced by exercise. J Neurol Neurosurg Psychiatry 47:275, 1984.

Pranzatelli MR, Albin RL, Cohen BH: Acute dyskinesias in young asthmatics treated with theophylline. Pediatr Neurol 7:216, 1991.

Prayer L, Wimberger D, Kramer J, et al: Cranial MRI in Wilson's disease. Neuroradiology 32:211, 1990.

Regeur L, Pakkenberg B, Fog R, et al: Clinical features and long-term treatment with pimozide in 65 patients with Gilles de la Tourette's syndrome. J Neurol Neurosurg Psychiatry 49:791, 1986.

Rollinson RD, Gilligan BS: Postanoxic action myoclonus (Lance-Adams syndrome) responding to valproate. Arch Neurol 36:44, 1979.

Ronen G, Donat JR, Hill A: Hemifacial spasm in children. Can J Neurol Sci 13:342, 1986.

Saint Hilaire M-H, Burke RE, Bressman SB, et al: Delayed-onset dystonia due to perinatal or early childhood asphyxia. Neurology 41:216, 1991.

Scheinberg IH, Jaffe ME, Sternlieb I: The use of trientine in preventing the effects of interrupting penicillamine therapy in Wilson's disease. N Engl J Med 317:209, 1987.

Shannon KM, Fenichel GM: Pimozide treatment of Sydenham's chorea. Neurology 40:186, 1990.

Sheehy MP, Marsden CD: Writer's cramp—a focal dystonia. Brain 105:461, 1982.

Silverstein F, Johnston MV: Risks of neuroleptic drugs in children with neurological disorders. Ann Neurol 18:392, 1985.

Singer HS: Tardive dyskinesia: A concern for the pediatrician. Pediatrics 77:553, 1986.

Singer HS, Gammon K, Quaskey S: Haloperidol, fluphenazine and clonidine in Tourette syndrome: Controversies in treatment. Pediatr Neurosci 12:71, 1986.

Sleigh G, Lindenbaum RH: Benign (non-paroxysmal) familial chorea: Pediatric perspectives. Arch Dis Child 56:616, 1981.

Smits MG, Gabeels FJM, Thijssen HOM, et al: Progressive idiopathic strio-pallido-dentate calcinosis (Fahr's disease) with autosomal recessive inheritance: Report of three siblings. Eur Neurol 22:58, 1983.

Spitz MC, Jankovic J, Killian JM: Familial tic disorder, parkinsonism, motor neuron disease, and acanthocytosis: A new syndrome. Neurology 35:366, 1985.

Starosta-Rubinstein S, Young AB, Kluin K, et al: Clinical assessment of 31 patients with Wilson's disease: Correlations with structural changes on magnetic resonance imaging. Arch Neurol 44:365, 1987.

Sternlieb I, Giblin DR, Scheinberg IH: Wilson's disease. In Marsden CD, Fahn S, eds: Movement Disorders 2. Butterworth's International Medical Reviews. Neurology, Vol 7, Butterworth, London, 1987, p 288.

Strickland GT, Leu M-L: Wilson's disease: Clinical and laboratory manifestations in 40 patients. Medicine 54:113, 1975.

Swaiman KF: Hallervorden-Spatz syndrome and brain iron metabolism. Arch Neurol 48:1285, 1991.

Swanson JW, Kelly Jr JJ, McConahey WM: Neurologic aspects of thyroid dysfunction. Mayo Clin Proc 56:504, 1981.

Torch WC, Humphreys HK: Pharmacological therapy of Hallervorden-Spatz syndrome: Two cases responsive to benztropine. Ann Neurol 20:445, 1986.

Disorders of Ocular Motility

The maintenance of binocular vision by conjugate movement of the eyes is perhaps the most delicate feat of muscular coordination achieved by the nervous system. Disorders of the visual sensory system, ocular muscles, ocular motor nerves, neuromuscular transmission, or gaze centers of the central nervous system may disturb ocular motility. This chapter deals with nonparalytic strabismus, paralytic strabismus (ophthalmoplegia), gaze palsies (supranuclear palsies), ptosis, and nystagmus. Visual disorders and disorders of the pupil are discussed in Chapter 16.

◆ Nonparalytic Strabismus

Strabismus (squint), or abnormal ocular alignment, affects 3% to 4% of preschool children (Nelson, 1983). Most individuals have a latent tendency for ocular misalignment, *heterophoria,* which becomes apparent only under stress or fatigue. During periods of misalignment the child may have diplopia or headache. Constant ocular misalignment is called *heterotropia.* Children with heterotropia suppress the image in one eye to avoid diplopia. If only one eye is used for fixation, visual acuity may be permanently lost in the other (developmental amblyopia).

In nonparalytic strabismus the amount of deviation in different directions of gaze is relatively constant (comitant). Each eye moves through a normal range when tested separately (ductions), but the eyes are disconjugate when used together (versions). Many children with chronic brain damage syndromes, such as malformations or perinatal asphyxia, have nonparalytic strabismus. This is due to faulty fusion or control of conjugate gaze mechanisms by the abnormal brain. In neurologically normal children the most common cause of nonparalytic strabismus is either a genetic influence or

an intraocular disorder. Ocular alignment in the newborn is usually poor, with transitory shifts of alignment from convergence to divergence. Constant ocular alignment usually begins after 3 months of age. Approximately 2% of newborns exhibit chronic downward deviation of the eyes during the waking state. The eyes assume a normal position during sleep and are able to move upward reflexively (Hoyt et al, 1980).

ESOTROPIA

Esotropia is an inward deviation (convergence) of the eyes. Early-onset or infantile esotropia is noted between 3 and 6 months of age, and accommodative esotropia is noted after 6 months of age.

Clinical Features. Children with infantile esotropia often alternate fixation between eyes and may cross-fixate, that is, look to the left with the right eye and to the right with the left eye. The misalignment is sufficient to be noticed by family members. Some children fixate almost entirely with one eye and are at risk for permanent loss of visual acuity, *amblyopia,* in the other.

Accommodative esotropia occurs when accommodation is used to correct hyperopia. Accommodation causes the blurred hyperopic image to be more sharply focused. Because accommodation is accompanied by convergence, the eyes turn inward. Some children with accommodative esotropia cross-fixate so that both eyes are used. However, if one eye is more hyperopic than the other, the better eye may be used exclusively for fixation and the unused eye has a considerable potential for amblyopia.

Diagnosis. The eyes should be retinoscoped to determine whether hyperopia is present.

Treatment. Hyperopic errors should be corrected with eyeglasses. Early-onset esotropia in which only one eye is used for fixation is treated with alternate patching of the eyes. Early corrective surgery is required for persistent esotropia. A recently introduced alternative to surgery is chemodenervation of overactive muscles by injection of botulinum toxin. The technique has proved effective in research trials but is not yet approved for regular use (Magoon and Scott, 1987).

EXOTROPIA

Exotropia is an outward deviation of the eyes. It may be intermittent or constant.

Clinical Features. Intermittent exotropia is a relatively common condition that usually begins before 4 years of age. It is most often evident when the child is fatigued and fixating on a far object. The natural history of the condition is unknown.

Constant exotropia may be congenital but can also be caused by poor vision in the outward turning eye.

Diagnosis. The eyes must be examined for intraocular disease.

Treatment. In children with intermittent exotropia the decision to perform corrective surgery depends on the frequency and degree of the abnormality. When exotropia is constant, treatment depends on the underlying cause of visual loss.

◆ Ophthalmoplegia (Paralytic Strabismus)

Ophthalmoplegia can be due to disorders of the ocular motor nerves, the ocular muscles, or neuromuscular transmission. The muscles, the nerves, and their functions are summarized in Table 15–1. The eye appears to deviate in the direction opposite the field of action of the paralyzed ocular muscle, and diplopia occurs. Strabismus and diplopia are made worse when the child gazes in the direction of action of the paralyzed muscle.

CONGENITAL OPHTHALMOPLEGIA

Ophthalmoplegia in the newborn is often missed because eye movements are infrequently tested. It is common for strabismus to remain unnoticed for several months and then to be discounted as transient esotropia. Therefore congenital ophthalmoplegia should be considered even when there is no history of ophthalmoplegia at birth.

Oculomotor Nerve Palsy

Clinical Features. Congenital oculomotor nerve palsy usually is unilateral and complete. Involvement of the pupillary reflex varies (Victor, 1976). The palsy is observed at birth in only half of cases. An occasional case is familial or due to trauma of the orbit at birth, but most are idiopathic. The affected eye is exotropic and usually amblyopic. Aberrant regeneration may be evidenced by lid retraction on attempted adduction or downward gaze.

Diagnosis. Magnetic resonance imaging (MRI) is indicated to exclude the possibility of an intracranial mass compressing the nerve. Exophthalmos should suggest a tumor of the orbit. The presence of a dilated pupil excludes the possibility of myasthenia gravis, but an edrophonium chloride (Tensilon) test is indicated if the pupil is normal.

Treatment. Extraocular muscle surgery may improve the cosmetic appearance but does not improve ocular motility or visual function.

Trochlear Nerve Palsy

Clinical Features. Congenital superior oblique palsy is unilateral in 94% of cases (von Noorden et al, 1986). Birth trauma is often suspected but is rarely established. Most congenital cases are idiopathic.

Diplopia is not a common complaint and may be relieved by a compensatory head tilt away from the paralyzed side. The major features on examination include: noncomitant hypertropia, greatest in the nasal field of the involved eye; underaction of the paretic superior oblique and overaction of the inferior oblique muscle; and increased hypertropia when the head is tilted to the paralyzed side (positive Bielschowsky test).

Diagnosis. Many children have head tilt or torticollis (see Chapter 14). Once a superior

Table 15–1 ◆ Extraocular Muscles

Ocular Muscle	Innervation	Functions
Lateral rectus	Abducens	Abduction
Medial rectus	Oculomotor	Adduction
Superior rectus	Oculomotor	Elevation, intorsion, adduction
Inferior rectus	Oculomotor	Depression, extorsion, adduction
Inferior oblique	Oculomotor	Extorsion, elevation, abduction
Superior oblique	Trochlear	Intorsion, depression, abduction

oblique palsy is confirmed by examination, important etiologic considerations other than congenital ones include trauma, myasthenia gravis, and brainstem glioma.

Treatment. Most patients require surgery. Several procedures are available to restore balance between the superior and inferior oblique muscles.

Abducens Nerve Palsy

Clinical Features. Congenital abducens nerve palsy may be unilateral or bilateral and is sometimes associated with other cranial nerve palsies. Lateral movement of the affected eye(s) is limited, partially or completely. Most infants use cross-fixation and thereby retain vision in both eyes. In the few reported cases with pathologic correlation the abducens nerve is absent and its nucleus is hypoplastic (Hickey and Wagoner, 1983). *Möbius syndrome* is the association of congenital facial diplegia and bilateral abducens nerve palsies (see Chapter 17). *Duane syndrome* is characterized by a lateral rectus palsy, some limitation of adduction, and narrowing of the palpebral fissure because of globe retraction on attempted adduction. Other ocular, ear, and systemic malformations may be present (Tachibana et al, 1984).

Diagnosis. MRI is indicated to exclude the possibility of an intracranial mass lesion. Hearing should be tested, and if there is facial weakness, electromyography (EMG) may be useful to determine facial nerve function.

Treatment. Surgical procedures may be useful for cosmetic purposes and to provide binocular vision, but they do not restore ocular motility.

Brown Syndrome

Brown syndrome consists of mechanical limitation of elevation in adduction as a result of congenital shortening of the superior oblique muscle or tendon (Wang et al, 1984).

Clinical Features. Elevation is limited in adduction but normal in abduction. Passive elevation (forced duction) is also restricted. Other features include widening of the palpebral fissure on adduction and backward head tilt.

Diagnosis. Congenital Brown syndrome must be differentiated from shortening of the superior oblique muscle caused by juvenile rheumatoid arthritis, trauma, and inflammatory processes affecting the top of the orbit (see "Orbital Pseudotumor" later in this chapter).

Treatment. Surgical procedures that extend the superior oblique muscle can be useful in congenital cases.

Congenital Myasthenia Gravis

Several different syndromes of myasthenia gravis in the newborn have been described (see Chapter 6). Congenital myasthenia gravis is the only one with ophthalmoplegia as the primary clinical feature. It is probably transmitted by autosomal recessive inheritance and may be caused by several underlying defects, including abnormal acetylcholine resynthesis or immobilization, reduced endplate acetylcholinesterase, and impaired function of the acetylcholine receptor (Misulis and Fenichel, 1989).

Clinical Features. Although the disorder is transmitted by autosomal recessive inheritance, a male-to-female bias of 2:1 exists. Symmetric ptosis and ophthalmoplegia are noted at birth or shortly thereafter. Mild facial weakness may be present but is not severe enough to impair feeding. If partial at birth, the ophthalmoplegia becomes complete during infancy or childhood. Generalized weakness sometimes develops.

Diagnosis. The diagnosis should be suspected in any newborn with bilateral ptosis or limitation of eye movement. Intramuscular injection of Tensilon produces a transitory improvement in ocular motility. Repetitive nerve stimulation of the limbs at a frequency of 3 Hz may evoke a decremental response, reversible with Tensilon. This suggests that the underlying defect, although producing symptoms only in the eyes, is already generalized at birth.

Treatment. There is no evidence for an immunopathy or a rational basis for immunosuppressive therapy. Thymectomy and corticosteroids have been found ineffective. Anticholinesterases may decrease facial paralysis, but they have little or no effect on ophthalmoplegia. 3, 4-Diaminopyridine, an agent that releases acetylcholine, is beneficial in some children (Palace et al, 1991).

Congenital Ptosis

Clinical Features. Congenital drooping of one or both lids is relatively common, and the drooping is unilateral in 70%. The cause is unknown, but the condition is rarely familial. Congenital ptosis is often unnoticed until early childhood or even adult life and then is thought to be an "acquired" ptosis. Miosis is sometimes an associated feature and suggests the possibility of a Horner syndrome, except that the pupil responds normally to pharmacologic agents. Some patients have a synkinesis between the oculomotor and the trigeminal nerves, so that jaw movements produce opening of the eye (Marcus Gunn phenomenon).

Diagnosis. The differential diagnosis of ptosis is listed in Table 15–2. Distinguishing congenital from acquired ptosis is essential. This is best accomplished by examining baby pictures. If miosis is present, the eye must be tested with pharmacologic agents to determine whether sympathetic hypersensitivity is present. Concurrent paralysis of extraocular motility is evidence against congenital ptosis.

Treatment. Corrective surgery is useful in elevating the lid to improve appearance or when ptosis impairs vision.

Fibrosis of Extraocular Muscles

Fibrosis of extraocular muscles is an ill-defined entity with partial (Prakash et al, 1985) or complete (Apt and Axelrod, 1978) paralysis of ocular motility at birth. It is caused by maldevelopment of the ocular muscles, which are represented as fibrous bands. In some cases the underlying cause may be hypoplasia of the ocular motor nerves.

Clinical Features. The only clinical feature is restricted ocular motility, which is usually bilateral although unilateral occurrence has been reported. Ptosis is almost always present.

Diagnosis. Other causes of congenital ophthalmoplegia must be excluded. MRI shows the fibrotic muscles, but biopsy provides the more definitive diagnosis.

Treatment. Surgery may offer cosmetic benefit and relieve ptosis but does not correct the disturbed motility.

Acute Unilateral Ophthalmoplegia

The causes of acquired ophthalmoplegia are summarized in Table 15–3. Many of the conditions are discussed in other chapters.

Table 15–2 ◆ Causes of Ptosis

Congenital
1. Fibrosis of extraocular muscles
2. Horner syndrome
3. Myasthenia
4. Oculomotor nerve palsy

Acquired
1. Lid inflammation
2. Mitochondrial myopathies (see Chapter 8)
3. Myasthenia gravis
4. Oculomotor nerve palsy
5. Oculopharyngeal dystrophy (see Chapter 17)
6. Ophthalmoplegic migraine
7. Orbital cellulitis

Acute ophthalmoplegia reaches maximum intensity within 1 week of onset and may be partial or complete (Table 15–4). Generalized increased intracranial pressure is always an important consideration in patients with unilateral or bilateral abducens palsy (see Chapter 4).

Aneurysm

Arterial aneurysms are discussed fully in Chapter 4 because the important clinical feature in children is hemorrhage rather than nerve compression. This section deals only with possible ophthalmoplegic features.

Clinical Features. Aneurysms at the junction of the internal carotid and posterior communicating arteries are an important cause of unilateral oculomotor palsy. The palsy is attributed to hemorrhage within the sac to which the nerve adheres or to hemorrhage into the nerve. Intense pain in and around the eye is frequently experienced at the time of hemorrhage. Because the parasympathetic fibers are at the periphery of the nerve, mydriasis is an almost constant feature of ophthalmoplegia caused by aneurysms of the posterior communicating artery. However, pupillary involvement may develop several days after onset of an incomplete ophthalmoplegia (Kissel et al, 1983). A normal pupil with complete ophthalmoplegia effectively excludes the possibility of aneurysm.

The superior branch of the oculomotor nerve is sometimes affected earlier and more severely than the inferior branch. Ptosis may precede the development of other signs by hours or days.

Diagnosis. Many aneurysms can be identified by contrast-enhanced MRI, but arteriography provides better visualization.

Treatment. Surgical resection is the treatment of choice whenever technically feasible. Oculomotor function often returns to normal after the aneurysm is removed.

Brainstem Glioma

Clinical Features. Symptoms begin between 2 and 13 years of age with a peak at age 6 (Langmoen et al, 1991). Cranial nerve palsies, usually abducens and facial, are the initial features in most cases. Later, contralateral hemiplegia and ataxia, dysphagia, and hoarseness develop. Hemiplegia at onset is associated with a more rapid course. With time, cranial nerve and corticospinal tract involvement may become bilateral. Increased intracranial pressure is not an early feature, but vomiting may be caused by direct irritation of the brainstem emetic center. Intractable hiccough, facial spasm,

Table 15–3 ◆ Causes of Acquired Ophthalmoplegia

Brainstem	**Nerve** *continued*
1. Brainstem encephalitis (see Chapter 10)	5. Postinfectious
2. Intoxication	a. Idiopathic (postviral)
3. Multiple sclerosis (see Chapter 10)	b. Miller-Fisher syndrome (see Chapter 10)
4. Subacute necrotizing encephalopathy (see Chapter 10)	c. Polyradiculoneuropathy (see Chapter 7)
5. Tumor	6. Trauma
a. Brainstem glioma	a. Head
b. Craniopharyngioma (see Chapter 16)	b. Orbital
c. Leukemia	7. Tumor
d. Lymphoma	a. Cavernous sinus hemangioma
e. Metastases	b. Orbital tumors
f. Pineal region tumors	c. Sellar and parasellar tumors (see Chapter 16)
6. Vascular	d. Sphenoid sinus tumors
a. Arteriovenous malformation	8. Vascular
b. Hemorrhage	a. Aneurysm
c. Infarction	b. Carotid-cavernous fistula
d. Migraine	c. Cavernous sinus thrombosis
e. Vasculitis	d. Migraine
Nerve	**Neuromuscular Transmission**
1. Familial recurrent cranial neuropathies (see Chapter 17)	1. Botulism (see Chapter 7)
2. Increased intracranial pressure (see Chapter 4)	2. Myasthenia gravis
3. Infectious	**Myopathies**
a. Diphtheria	1. Fiber-type disproportion myopathies (see Chapter 6)
b. Gradenigo syndrome	2. Kearns-Sayres syndrome
c. Meningitis (see Chapter 4)	3. Mitochondrial myopathies (see Chapter 8)
d. Orbital cellulitis	4. Oculopharyngeal dystrophy (see Chapter 17)
4. Inflammatory	5. Orbital pseudotumor
a. Sarcoid	6. Thyrotoxicosis
b. Tolosa-Hunt syndrome	7. Vitamin E deficiency

personality change, and headache are early symptoms in occasional patients.

Brainstem gliomas carry the worst prognosis of any childhood tumor. The course is one of steady progression with median survival times of 9 to 12 months.

Diagnosis. The characteristic computed tomography (CT) appearance of most brainstem gliomas is isodense and enhanced with contrast medium. MRI delineates the tumor well and is preferable to CT (Figure 15–1).

Treatment. Radiation therapy is the treatment of choice. Several chemotherapeutic programs are undergoing trials, but none is established as beneficial.

Brainstem Stroke

The causes of stroke in children are summarized in Table 11–2. Small brainstem hemorrhages resulting from emboli, leukemia, or blood dyscrasias have the potential to cause isolated ocular motor nerve palsies, but this is not the rule. Other cranial nerves are also involved, and hemiparesis, ataxia, and decreased consciousness are typical associated features.

Cavernous Sinus Fistula

Clinical Features. Arteriovenous communications between the carotid artery and the cavernous sinus may be congenital but are usually caused by trauma. The injury may be closed or penetrating. The carotid artery or one of its branches ruptures into the cavernous sinus, increasing pressure in the venous system. The results are a pulsating proptosis, redness and swelling of the conjunctiva, and ophthalmoplegia. A bruit, heard over the eye, is reduced in volume by compression of the ipsilateral carotid artery.

Diagnosis. CT of the head and orbit scan is usually the first study in patients with the acute onset of proptosis. It often shows an enlarged superior ophthalmic vein. Intravenous digital sub-

Table 15-4 ◆ Causes of Acute Unilateral
Ophthalmoplegia

1. Aneurysm*†
2. Brain tumors
   a. Brainstem glioma
   b. Parasellar tumors (see Chapter 16)
   c. Tumors of pineal region (see Chapter 4)
3. Brainstem stroke*
4. Cavernous sinus fistula
5. Cavernous sinus thrombosis
6. Gradenigo syndrome
7. Idiopathic cranial nerve palsy*
8. Increased intracranial pressure (see Chapter 4)
9. Multiple sclerosis* (see Chapter 10)
10. Myasthenia gravis*
11. Ophthalmoplegic migraine*†
12. Orbital pseudotumor*†
13. Orbital tumor†
14. Recurrent familial* (see Chapter 17)
15. Tolosa-Hunt syndrome*†
16. Trauma
    a. Head
    b. Orbital

*May be recurrent.
†May be associated with pain.

traction angiography demonstrates early filling of the cavernous sinus and retrograde filling of the superior ophthalmic vein.

Treatment.   Several surgical procedures are recommended, including carotid ligation, injection of fibrin glue through the superior ophthalmic vein, transcavernous electrocoagulation, and intraarterial occlusion with a balloon catheter.

Cavernous Sinus Thrombosis

Cavernous sinus thrombosis may produce either unilateral or bilateral ophthalmoplegia. It is almost always caused by anterograde spread of infection from the mouth, face, or nose.

Clinical Features.   A typical history is the development of fever, malaise, and frontal headache following dental infection. These are followed by proptosis, orbital congestion, ptosis, external ophthalmoplegia, and sometimes pupillary paralysis and blindness (Harbour et al, 1984). The infection begins in one cavernous sinus and spreads to the other. If untreated, it may extend to the meninges. Even with vigorous antibiotic treatment the mortality rate is 15%.

Diagnosis.   The ocular signs may suggest orbital cellulitis or orbital pseudotumor. The cerebrospinal fluid is normal early in the course. A

mixed leukocytosis develops, and the protein concentration is moderately elevated even in the absence of meningitis. Once the meninges are involved, the pressure becomes elevated, the leukocytosis increases, and the glucose concentration falls.

CT of the head may show clouding of infected paranasal sinuses. Angiography shows attentuation or complete blockage of the cavernous portion of the carotid artery.

Treatment.   The infection must be vigorously treated with intravenous antibiotics as if the child had meningitis. Surgical drainage of infected paranasal sinuses is sometimes necessary.

Gradenigo Syndrome

Clinical Features.   The abducens nerve lies adjacent to the medial aspect of the petrous bone before entering the cavernous sinus. Infections of the middle ear sometimes extend to the petrous bone and cause thrombophlebitis of the inferior petrosal sinus. The infection involves not only the abducens nerve but also the facial nerve and the trigeminal ganglion. The resulting syndrome is characterized by ipsilateral paralysis of abduction, facial palsy, and facial pain.

Diagnosis.   The combination of unilateral abducens and facial palsy can also be seen after closed

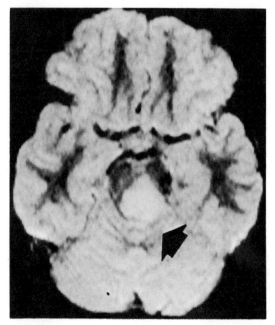

Figure 15-1   Brainstem glioma. T2-weighted magnetic resonance image demonstrates an area of increased signal in the brainstem.

head injuries. The diagnosis of Gradenigo syndrome requires the demonstration of middle ear infection. Radiographs of the mastoid bone and lumbar puncture are indicated in all patients in whom the syndrome is suspected.

Treatment. Antibiotic therapy must be initiated early to prevent permanent nerve damage.

Idiopathic Cranial Nerve Palsy

Clinical Features. The sudden onset of a single cranial neuropathy without apparent cause is frequently attributed to a viral infection occurring during the previous month. The condition is thought to be immunologically mediated. However, since the typical school-age child has an average of four to six viral infections a year, up to 50% of children with a cranial neuropathy may have a history of a preceding viral infection by chance alone.

The abducens nerve is more commonly affected than either the oculomotor or the trochlear nerve. Bilateral involvement is unusual. The complaints are of painless diplopia and paralytic strabismus. Full motility is restored within 6 months to a year. Recurrent abducens nerve palsy of unknown cause occurs in some children, especially girls (Afifi et al, 1990). The left side is affected far more often than the right.

Diagnosis. Other causes of isolated nerve palsy must be excluded. Examination of the cerebrospinal fluid and MRI of the head and orbit are warranted in every case to exclude tumor and infection. Tumors in and around the orbit are sometimes difficult to demonstrate, and if ophthalmoplegia persists, a repeat MRI may be necessary. Myasthenia gravis is always a consideration, and a Tensilon test should be performed even though myasthenia gravis is less likely when there is a fixed single nerve deficit.

Treatment. Corticosteroids are not recommended. Intermittent patching of the normal eye may be necessary if the affected eye is not used for fixation.

Myasthenia Gravis

Some neonatal forms of myasthenia are discussed in Chapter 6, congenital myasthenia is included in the section "Congenital Ophthalmoplegia" earlier in this chapter, and limb-girdle myasthenia is discussed in Chapter 7. This section describes the immune-mediated form of myasthenia that is encountered from late infancy through adult life. Two forms are recognized: *ocular myasthenia,* in which the eye muscles are primarily or exclusively affected but facial and limb muscles

may also be mildly involved, and *generalized myasthenia,* in which weakness of bulbar and limb muscles is moderate to severe.

The term *juvenile myasthenia* is sometimes used to denote myasthenia gravis in children, but since the nongenetic forms of myasthenia in children are no different from myasthenia in adults, the term should not suggest a separate disorder.

Clinical Features. The first symptoms do not appear until after 6 months of age; 75% of children first have symptoms after age 10. Prepubertal onset is associated with a slight male bias and only ocular symptoms, whereas postpubertal onset is associated with a strong female bias and generalized myasthenia (Batocchi et al, 1990). The initial features of both the ocular and the generalized form are usually ptosis, diplopia, or both. Myasthenia is the most common cause of both unilateral and bilateral acquired ptosis. Pupillary function is normal. Between 40% and 50% of patients demonstrate weakness of other bulbar muscles or limb weakness at the time of onset. Ocular motor weakness is generally not constant initially, and the specific muscles affected may change from examination to examination. Usually both eyes are affected, but one more than the other.

Children with ocular myasthenia may have mild facial weakness and easy fatigability of the limbs. However, they do not have respiratory distress or difficulty speaking or swallowing. Two subsequent courses of ocular myasthenia have been described. One is characterized by steady progression to complete ophthalmoplegia and the other by relapses and remissions. The relapses are of varying severity and last for weeks to years (Rollinson and Fenichel, 1981). Remissions as long as 14 years have been recorded. At least 20% of patients have permanent remissions.

Children with generalized myasthenia have generalized weakness within 1 year of the initial ocular symptoms. Dysarthria, dysphagia, difficulty chewing, and limb muscle fatigability are observed. Spontaneous remissions are unusual. As many as 40% of patients experience respiratory insufficiency, or *myasthenic crises,* if not treated.

Children with generalized myasthenia, but not those with ocular myasthenia, have a higher than expected incidence of other autoimmune disorders, especially thyroiditis and collagen vascular diseases. Thymoma is present in 15% of adults with generalized myasthenia but occurs in less than 5% of children (Lanska, 1991).

Diagnosis. The *Tensilon test* has been used as a standard of diagnosis for both the ocular and generalized forms of myasthenia gravis but has limitations. Tensilon (edrophonium chloride) is a short-acting anticholinesterase that is administered intravenously at a dose of 0.15 mg/kg. Before the test is initiated, an endpoint for the study must be determined. The best endpoint is the resolution of ptosis or the restoration of ocular motility. Ptosis generally responds better to Tensilon than does ocular motor paralysis. In the absence of ptosis or strabismus, the test results are difficult to evaluate (Daroff, 1986).

Some patients with myasthenia are supersensitive to Tensilon, and fasciculations and sometimes respiratory arrest develop when a full dose is administered. For this reason a test dose of one-tenth the full dose is injected first. Unfortunately, respiratory embarrassment sometimes develops in response to the test dose, and a hand ventilator should be readily available before any drug is given. Atropine is an effective antidote to the muscarinic side effects of Tensilon but does not counteract the nicotinic effects on the motor endplate that result in paralysis of the skeletal muscles.

After the test dose is given, the remainder should be injected one third at a time (approximately 0.05/mg/kg), with up to 1 minute allowed after each injection to test the response. Interpretation may be difficult. The judgment of improved strength is subjective and may be influenced by examiner bias. The test becomes more objective when combined with electrophysiologic studies.

Repetitive stimulation of the ulnar nerve is abnormal in 17% of patients with ocular myasthenia and in all patients with generalized myasthenia (Oh et al, 1982). In patients with mild myasthenia a decremental response is recorded at low rates of stimulation (2 to 5 per second) but not at high rates (50 per second). In severe myasthenia a decremental response is recorded at both low and high rates of stimulation.

The clinical manifestations of myasthenia gravis are attributed to the presence of antibodies against the acetylcholine receptor protein. Elevated concentrations of the antibody, greater than 10 nmol/L, are detected in the sera of 90% of patients with generalized myasthenia. Patients with ocular myasthenia have antibody concentrations up to 10 nmol/L.

Patients who have generalized myasthenia but do not have detectable concentrations of antibody against acetycholine receptor protein may have antibodies to another receptor site. The clinical characteristics and response to treatment of individuals with generalized myasthenia who are seronegative do not differ from those who are seropositive, except that seronegative patients are unlikely to show thymic abnormalities and show only a modest improvement after thymectomy (Soliven et al, 1988; Verma and Oger, 1992).

Treatment. The treatment program depends on whether the child has ocular or generalized myasthenia. Children with ocular myasthenia have a reasonable hope of spontaneous remission, but those with generalized disease do not. Anticholinesterase therapy is the treatment of choice for ocular myasthenia. The initial dose of neostigmine is 0.5 mg/kg every 4 hours in children younger than 5 years of age and 0.25 mg/kg in older children, not to exceed 15 mg for any child. The equivalent dose of pyridostigmine is four times greater. After treatment is initiated, the dose is slowly increased as tolerated. Diarrhea and gastrointestinal cramps are the usual limiting factors. Tensilon should not be administered to determine whether the child would benefit from higher oral doses of anticholinesterase. It is not an accurate guide and may cause cholinergic crisis in children with generalized myasthenia.

Ocular myasthenia is difficult to treat. The response to anticholinesterase is often transitory, and the addition of corticosteroids usually has no benefit. The efficacy of any drug regimen in ocular myasthenia is difficult to assess because of the fluctuating course of the disease.

Children with generalized myasthenia and increased concentrations of antibody against acetylcholine receptor protein should undergo thymectomy as quickly as possible after diagnosis. Thymectomy must be performed by thoracotomy and not by transcervical approach. Sixty-one percent of children have remission within 3 years of thymectomy if it is performed early in the course of disease (Rodriguez et al, 1983). Corticosteroids should be started immediately after surgery, preferably while the patient is still in the surgical intensive care unit. An equivalent dose to prednisone, 1.5 mg/kg/day (not to exceed 100 mg), is given parenterally until the patient can take oral medication. After 5 days an alternate-day regimen is used for the remainder of the month. The prednisone dose is then tapered by 10% each month until a dose is reached that keeps the patient symptom free. Withdrawal of prednisone should be attempted after the child has been free of symptoms for 1 year (Miano et al, 1991). High-dose corticosteroids may make the patient weaker at first. For this reason treatment is initiated while the patient is still in intensive care with ventilator support. Improvement usually begins after the first week and continues in the months that follow.

Anticholinesterase medication should not be given concurrently with corticosteroids at first but may be used later if the patient weakens on days that corticosteroids are not taken.

Plasmapheresis is useful as an acute intervention in patients who have respiratory insufficiency (myasthenic crisis) or are so weak that strength must be restored before thymectomy.

Ophthalmoplegic Migraine

Clinical Features. Transitory ocular motor palsy, lasting sometimes as long as 4 weeks, may occur as part of a migraine attack in children and adults. The palsy affects the oculomotor nerve alone in 83% of cases and all three nerves in the remainder (Vijayan, 1980). Ptosis usually precedes ophthalmoplegia. Partial or complete pupillary involvement is present in 60%. The average age at occurrence is 15 years, but the onset may be as early as infancy. In infants recurrent painless ophthalmoplegia or ptosis may be the only manifestation of the migraine attack (Durkan et al, 1981). In older children ophthalmoplegia usually occurs during the headache phase and is ipsilateral to the headache.

The mechanism of ophthalmoplegia is uncertain but has been attributed to either an ischemic neuropathy or compression of the nerve by a swollen carotid artery in the cavernous sinus. Although migraine is hereditary, the tendency for ophthalmoplegia is not.

Diagnosis. The diagnosis is obvious when ophthalmoplegia occurs during a typical migraine attack in a child previously known to have migraine. Diagnostic uncertainty is greatest when an infant has transitory strabismus or ptosis as an isolated sign. In such cases family history of migraine is essential for diagnosis. Even so, most infants with a first episode of ophthalmoplegia should be studied with MRI of the head and orbit to exclude other causes. The transitory nature of the palsy is comforting and indicates that a structural abnormality is unlikely.

Treatment. Children with ophthalmoplegic migraine should be treated in the same manner as other children with migraine (see Chapter 3).

Orbital Pseudotumor

The term "orbital pseudotumor" encompasses a group of nonspecific inflammatory conditions involving the orbit. Some experts include the Tolosa-Hunt syndrome as part of the spectrum of orbital pseudotumor. Inflammation may be diffuse or localized to specific tissues within the orbit *(orbital myositis).*

Clinical Features. The disorder is unusual in those under 20 years of age but has been recorded as early as 3 months of age (Grossniklaus et al, 1985). Males and females are affected equally. Acute and chronic forms are described.

The cardinal features of acute, diffuse orbital inflammation are pain, ophthalmoplegia, proptosis, and lid edema evolving over several days or weeks. One eye or both eyes may be involved. Ocular motility is disturbed in part by the proptosis, but mainly by myositis. Some patients have only myositis, whereas others have inflammation in other orbital structures. Vision is initially preserved, but loss of vision is a threat if the condition remains untreated. The chronic form has an insidious onset, progresses over several months, and results in complete ophthalmoplegia.

Diagnosis. The development of unilateral pain and proptosis in a child should suggest an orbital tumor. This possibility must be excluded by MRI or CT of the orbit. Bilateral proptosis suggests thyroid myopathy.

Imaging studies of the orbit demonstrate a soft tissue mass without sinus involvement or bone erosion. This radiographic appearance may also be seen with orbital involvement by lymphoma or leukemia. The extraocular muscles may appear enlarged (Mauriello and Flanagan, 1984).

Treatment. Orbital pseudotumor has a self-limited course but must be treated to prevent vision loss or permanent ophthalmoplegia. Prednisone, 1 mg/kg/day, should be administered for at least 1 month and then tapered. If the disorder recurs during the tapering, the full dose should be reinitiated.

Orbital Tumors

Clinical Features. The initial manifestation of intraorbital tumors is proptosis, ophthalmoplegia, or ptosis. When the globe is displaced forward, the palpebral fissure is widened and it may not be possible to close the eye fully. As a consequence, the exposed portion of the eye becomes erythematous and may suffer exposure keratitis. The direction of displacement of the globe is the best clue to the tumor's position. Ophthalmoplegia may occur because the globe is displaced or because of direct pressure on one or more ocular nerves.

Diagnosis. The differential diagnosis of proptosis in children includes infection and inflammation (30%), hemorrhage and other vascular disorders (19%), orbital tumors (16%), hyperthyroidism and other metabolic disorders (14%), developmental anomalies (9%), and Hand-Schuller-Christian disease and related disorders (7%); the remainder are idiopathic (Crawford, 1967). The most common orbital tumors are dermoid cyst, hemangioma, metastatic neuroblastoma, optic glioma, and rhabdo-myosarcoma (Youseffi, 1969).

Treatment. Treatment varies with tumor type. Surgical resection is indicated for many.

Tolosa-Hunt Syndrome

Tolosa-Hunt syndrome is a painful ophthalmo-plegia attributed to an idiopathic granulomatous disease of the cavernous sinus or superior orbital fissure. No other structure is involved.

Clinical Features. The pain is described as steady and penetrating, involving the entire hemi-cranium but centered around or behind the eye. It may precede the ophthalmoplegia by several days, may occur concurrently, or may appear later. The oculomotor nerve is ordinarily involved first and more severely than the two other ocular motor nerves, but all three, as well as the first and second divisions of the trigeminal nerve, may be affected. Vision may be diminished; the pupil is usually small and may be reactive or nonreactive. Symptoms last for days or months. Spontaneous remissions occur, but partial neurologic deficits may persist.

Diagnosis. Tolosa-Hunt syndrome is a diagnosis of exclusion. It is easily confused with ophthalmoplegic migraine (Kandt and Goldstein, 1985). The major clinical points of differentiation are that patients with ophthalmoplegic migraine also have nonophthalmoplegic migraine attacks, that they have a family history of migraine, and that the trigeminal nerve is not involved.

Tolosa-Hunt syndrome is differentiated from orbital pseudotumor by the absence of proptosis and the presence of trigeminal nerve involvement. Other diseases of the cavernous sinus, such as tumor or thrombosis, may resemble Tolosa-Hunt syndrome.

The erythrocyte sedimentation rate is elevated in most patients. Radiographs of the orbit may demonstrate bone erosion in the sellar and parasellar regions. Arteriography reveals irregular narrowing and displacement of the cavernous portion of the carotid artery, suggesting either vasculitis or a mass lesion.

Treatment. Prednisone, 1 mg/kg/day, is both diagnostic and therapeutic. If pain subsides within 2 days of initial administration, the diagnosis is likely but not certain. Other lesions in the cavernous sinus or orbit may also respond to corticosteroids. Ophthalmoplegia may subside but can take several days or weeks to clear completely. If prednisone has no effect on symptoms, Tolosa-Hunt syndrome can be excluded and another cause must be identified.

Trauma

Trauma is a common cause of isolated ocular motor nerve palsies and extraocular muscle damage (Baker and Epstein, 1991). Hemorrhage and edema into the nerves or muscles may occur from closed head injuries even in the absence of direct orbital injury. When orbital fracture is present, the nerves and muscles may be lacerated, avulsed, or entrapped by bone fragments.

Clinical Features. Superior oblique palsy, caused by trochlear nerve damage, is a relatively common consequence of closed head injuries. Usually the trauma is severe, often causing loss of consciousness, but it may be mild. The palsy is more often unilateral than bilateral. Patients with unilateral superior oblique palsy have a marked hypertropia in primary position and a compensatory head tilt to preserve fusion; 65% of cases resolve spontaneously. When bilateral involvement is present, the hypertropia is milder and alternates between the two eyes; spontaneous recovery occurs in only 25% of cases.

Transient lateral rectus palsy is rare in newborns and has been attributed to birth trauma (de Grauw and Rotteveel, 1983). The palsy is unilateral and clears completely within 6 weeks.

Diagnosis. Direct injuries to the orbit with associated hemorrhage and swelling do not pose a diagnostic dilemma. CT of the head with orbital views shows the extent of fracture so the need for surgical intervention can be determined. CT may also demonstrate a lateral midbrain hemorrhage as the cause of a trochlear nerve palsy.

A greater problem of diagnosis is caused by a delay between the time of injury and the onset of ophthalmoplegia. The possible mechanisms of delayed ophthalmoplegia following trauma to the head include progressive local edema in the orbit; progressive brainstem edema; progressive increased intracranial pressure; development of meningitis, mastoiditis, or petrous osteomyelitis; venous sinus or carotid artery thrombosis; and carotid cavernous fistula (Marmor et al, 1982).

Treatment. Local trauma and fracture of the orbit may require surgical repair. Permanent ocular motor nerve palsies following head injury are sometimes improved by surgery directed at rebalancing the extraocular muscles.

ACUTE BILATERAL OPHTHALMOPLEGIA

Many of the conditions that cause acute unilateral ophthalmoplegia (Table 15–4) may also cause acute bilateral ophthalmoplegia. The conditions listed in Table 15–5 are marked by a high incidence of bilateral involvement. Thyrotoxicosis could be added to this list, but it is discussed with the chronic conditions because progression of ophthalmoplegia is likely to occur over a period greater than 1 week.

Botulism

Botulism is caused by a toxin elaborated by several strains of the bacterium *Clostridium botulinum*. The infantile form of botulism causes ptosis but not ophthalmoplegia and is discussed in Chapter 6. This section deals with cases of later onset.

Clinical Features. Botulism is most often caused by ingestion of toxin in home-canned food. This is most likely when canning is done at high altitudes where the boiling temperature is too low to destroy spores (Cherrington, 1974). Because *C. botulinum* spores are ubiquitous in soil, infection may also follow burns and wounds. Blurred vision, diplopia, dizziness, dysarthria, and dysphagia begin 12 to 36 hours after ingestion of toxin. The pupillary response is usually normal. The early symptoms are followed by an ascending paralysis that suggests the Guillain-Barré syndrome and may lead to death from respiratory paralysis. Patients remain conscious and alert throughout. Most patients make a complete recovery within 2 to 3 months, but those with severe involvement may not return to normal for a year.

Diagnosis. The presence of ophthalmoplegia and normal findings of a spinal fluid examination distinguish botulism from the Guillain-Barré syndrome. EMG is useful in the diagnosis (Swift, 1981). The motor and sensory nerve conduction velocities are normal, evoked muscle action potentials are usually reduced in amplitude, and a decremental response is not ordinarily present at low rates of stimulation, although facilitation may be present at high rates of stimulation.

Definitive diagnosis requires demonstration of the organism or the toxin in food, stool, or wound.

Treatment. The administration of antitoxin, 20,000 to 40,000 units two to three times a day, is recommended. The stomach and intestines should be emptied. Guanidine, 35 mg/kg, is effective in some patients and should be used for those with potential respiratory failure. Mechanical respiratory support must be made available to every patient as soon as the diagnosis is suspected.

Intoxications

Clinical Features. Anticonvulsants, tricyclic antidepressants, and many other psychoactive drugs selectively impair ocular motility at toxic blood concentrations. The overdose may be accidental or intentional. A child is found unconscious and brought to the emergency room. The state of consciousness varies from obtundation to stupor, but the eyes cannot be made to move either by rapidly rotating the head laterally or with ice water irrigation of the ears. Complete ophthalmoplegia may be expected in a comatose child if other brainstem function is impaired (see Chapter 2), but if it occurs in a noncomatose child with otherwise intact brainstem function, ingestion of a drug that selectively impairs ocular motility should be suspected.

Diagnosis. The family should be questioned about drugs available in the household, and the blood and urine should be screened for toxic substances.

Treatment. Specific treatment depends on the drug ingested. In most cases supportive care is sufficient.

CHRONIC BILATERAL OPHTHALMOPLEGIA

The conditions responsible for bilateral ophthalmoplegia developing over a period longer than 1 week are listed in Table 15–6. Most are discussed in previous sections of this chapter or in other chapters.

Graves Ophthalmopathy

It is not clear whether the association of ophthalmopathy with hyperthyroidism is causal or the two are associated autoimmune diseases (Feldon, 1990). One hypothesis suggests the presence of a cross-reacting antigen in thyroid and orbital tissues.

Table 15–5 ♦ Causes of Acute Bilateral Ophthalmoplegia

1. Basilar meningitis (see Chapter 4)
2. Botulism
3. Brainstem encephalitis (see Chapter 10)
4. Carotid-cavernous fistula
5. Cavernous sinus thrombosis
6. Diphtheria
7. Intoxication
8. Miller-Fisher syndrome (see Chapter 10)
9. Myasthenia gravis
10. Polyradiculoneuropathy (see Chapter 7)
11. Subacute necrotizing encephalomyelopathy (see Chapter 5)
12. Tick paralysis (see Chapter 7)

Table 15–6 ◆ Causes of Chronic Bilateral Ophthalmoplegia

1. Brainstem glioma
2. Chronic meningitis (see Chapter 4)
3. Chronic orbital inflammation
4. Graves ophthalmopathy
5. Kearns-Sayres syndrome
6. Myasthenia gravis
   a. Congenital
   b. Juvenile
7. Myopathies
   a. Fiber-type disproportion myopathy (see Chapter 6)
   b. Mitochondrial myopathies (see Chapter 8)
   c. Myotubular myopathy (see Chapter 6)
8. Subacute necrotizing encephalomyelopathy (see Chapter 5)
9. Vitamin E deficiency

Clinical Features. Disorders of ocular motility are present in the majority of patients with hyperthyroidism and may precede systemic features of nervousness, heat intolerance, diaphoresis, weight loss, tachycardia, tremulousness, and weakness. The major pathologic condition in the orbit is a myopathy of the extraocular muscles. They become inflamed, swollen with interstitial edema, and finally fibrotic. If the two eyes are affected equally, the patient may not complain of diplopia despite considerable limitation of ocular motility. Staring or lid retraction (Dalrymple sign) occurs in more than 50% of cases, lid lag on downward gaze (von Graefe sign) in 30% to 50%, and proptosis (exophthalmos) in almost 90%. Severe exophthalmos is due to edema and infiltration of all orbital structures.

Diagnosis. Thyroid disease should be considered in any child with evolving ophthalmoplegia. CT of the orbit demonstrates enlargement of the extraocular muscles. This finding must be followed by direct measurement of plasma thyroxine, triiodothyronine, and thyroid-stimulating hormone concentrations. If these are normal but the diagnosis remains suspect, a thyroid-releasing hormone stimulation test and a measure of the concentration of thyroid-stimulating immunoglobulin may confirm the diagnosis.

Treatment. Meticulous control of hyperthyroidism provides the best relief of the ophthalmopathy but is not necessarily curative (Prummel et al, 1990). Hypothyroidism must be avoided. If the exophthalmos progresses even after the patient is euthyroid, corticosteroids may prevent further proptosis, but surgical decompression is indicated if optic nerve compression persists.

Kearns-Sayre Syndrome

Kearns-Sayre syndrome is caused by deletions of mitochondrial DNA (Moraes et al, 1989) and falls within the spectrum of mitochondrial disorders (see Chapter 8). Variability in the clinical syndrome reflects variability in the size of the deletion and the specific respiratory complex affected. Most cases are sporadic.

Clinical Features. The invariable features of the disease are onset before 20 years of age, progressive external ophthalmoplegia, and pigmentary degeneration of the retina. At least one of three other major manifestations must also be present for diagnosis: heart block, cerebrospinal fluid protein greater than 100 mg/dl, and cerebellar dysfunction.

Diagnosis. Diagnosis is based on the major clinical criteria. Electrocardiographic monitoring for cardiac arrhythmia and examination of the cerebrospinal fluid are essential.

Treatment. Treatment with vitamins or coenzyme Q, depending on the specific respiratory complex defect, may be beneficial in some patients (Phillips and Gosden, 1991). A cardiac pacemaker may be lifesaving.

◆ Gaze Palsies

This section deals with supranuclear palsies. To verify that a palsy is supranuclear and not due to an abnormality of the ocular motor nuclei or nerves, ocular muscles, or myasthenia, the examiner must demonstrate that the eyes move normally in response to brainstem reflexes, such as doll's head maneuver, caloric testing, and Bell phenomenon. The differential diagnosis of gaze palsies is listed in Table 15–7.

APRAXIA OF HORIZONTAL GAZE

Ocular motor apraxia is characterized by a deficiency in voluntary horizontal lateral fast eye movements (saccades) with retention of slow pursuit movements. Jerking movements of the head are used to bring the eyes to a desired position. The rapid phase of optokinetic nystagmus is absent.

Congenital Ocular Motor Apraxia

Clinical Features. Although ocular motor apraxia is present at birth, it is usually not detected until infancy. Blindness may be suspected because of failure of fixation. Instead, overshooting head thrusts, often accompanied by blinking of the eyes,

Table 15–7 ◆ Gaze Palsies

Apraxia of Horizontal Gaze
1. Ataxia-telangiectasia (see Chapter 10)
2. Ataxia–ocular motor apraxia (see Chapter 10)
3. Brainstem glioma
4. Congenital ocular motor apraxia
5. Huntington disease (see Chapter 5)

Internuclear Ophthalmoplegia (INO)
1. Brainstem stroke
2. Brainstem tumor
3. Exotropia (pseudo–INO)
4. Multiple sclerosis
5. Myasthenia gravis (pseudo-INO)
6. Toxic-metabolic

Vertical Gaze Palsy
1. Aqueductal stenosis (see Chapter 18)
2. Congenital vertical ocular motor apraxia
3. Gaucher disease (see Chapter 5)
4. Hydrocephalus (see Chapters 4 and 18)
5. Miller-Fisher syndrome (see Chapter 10)
6. Niemann-Pick disease, type C (see Chapter 5)
7. Tumor (see Chapter 4)
   a. Midbrain
   b. Pineal region
   c. Third ventricle
8. Vitamin B_{12} deficiency

Horizontal Gaze Palsy
1. Adversive seizures (see Chapter 1)
2. Brainstem tumors
3. Destructive lesions of the frontal lobe (see Chapter 11)
4. Familial horizontal gaze palsy

Convergence Paralysis
1. Head trauma
2. Idiopathic
3. Multiple sclerosis (see Chapter 10)
4. Pineal region tumors (see Chapter 4)

are used for refixation. When the head is held immobile, the child makes no effort at initiating horizontal eye movements.

Many children with ocular motor apraxia have other signs of cerebral abnormality, such as psychomotor retardation, learning disabilities, and clumsiness. When hypotonia is present, the child may have difficulty making the head movements needed for refixation. Agenesis of the corpus callosum and agenesis of the cerebellar vermis have been described in several patients with congenital ocular motor apraxia. These malformations are more likely to be associated with than responsible for ocular motor apraxia.

Diagnosis. The possibility of ocular motor apraxia must be considered in any infant referred for evaluation of blindness. Once the presence of apraxia is established, MRI is indicated to search for other cerebral malformations and tests for ataxia-telangiectasia (see Chapter 10) and lysosomal storage disease (see Chapter 5) should be performed.

Treatment. No treatment is available.

INTERNUCLEAR OPHTHALMOPLEGIA

The medial longitudinal fasciculus (MLF) contains fibers that connect the abducens nucleus to the contralateral ocular motor nucleus for the purpose of performing horizontal conjugate lateral gaze. Unilateral lesions in the MLF disconnect the two nuclei, so that when the patient attempts lateral gaze, the adducting eye ipsilateral to the normal MLF is unable to move medially but the abducting eye is able to move laterally. Nystagmus (actually *overshoot dysmetria*) is often present in the abducting eye. This symptom complex, which may be unilateral or bilateral, is called internuclear ophthalmoplegia (INO). Unilateral INO is most often caused by vascular occlusive disease. Bilateral INO usually results from demyelinating disease or toxic-metabolic causes.

Patients with myasthenia gravis sometimes have ocular motility dysfunction that resembles an INO except that nystagmus is usually lacking. This disorder is referred to as pseudo-INO because the MLF is intact. Pseudo-INO can also be caused by exotropia (Ellenberger and Daroff, 1984). When the normal eye is fixating in full abduction, there is no visual stimulus to bring the paretic eye into full adduction. Nystagmus is not present in the abducting eye.

The combination of an INO in one direction of lateral gaze and a complete gaze palsy in the other is called *one-and-a-half syndrome*. The syndrome is caused by a unilateral lesion in the dorsal pontine tegmentum affecting the pontine lateral gaze center and the adjacent MLF. It is most often due to multiple sclerosis but may be caused by brainstem glioma, infarction (Wall and Wray, 1980), or myasthenia gravis (Davis and Lavin, 1989).

Toxic-Metabolic

Clinical Features. Toxic doses of several drugs may produce the clinical syndrome of INO. The patient is usually found comatose and may have complete ophthalmoplegia that evolves into a bilateral INO, or a bilateral INO may be present at onset. The drugs reported to produce INO include amitriptyline, barbiturates, doxepin, phenothiazine, carbamazepine, and phenytoin. INO may also occur during hepatic coma.

Diagnosis. Drug intoxications are always a consideration in children who were previously well and then evidence decreased consciousness. The presence of an INO following drug ingestion limits the possibilities to anticonvulsant and psychotropic drugs.

Treatment. The INO resolves as the blood concentration of the drug falls.

VERTICAL GAZE PALSY

Children with supranuclear vertical gaze palsies are unable to look upward or downward fully, but they retain reflex eye movements such as the Bell phenomenon. Disorders of upward gaze in children are generally due to lesions in the region of the dorsal midbrain and are almost always caused by tumors in the pineal region or aqueductal stenosis. The usual features are impaired upward and downward gaze, eyelid retraction, occasional disturbances in horizontal movement, convergence, and skew deviation. Mydriasis with light-near dissociation is an early feature of extrinsic compression of the dorsal midbrain. Isolated paralysis of upward gaze may be the initial feature of the Miller-Fisher syndrome (Keane and Finstead, 1982) and of vitamin B_{12} or B_1 deficiency (Sandyk, 1984).

Isolated disturbances of downward gaze are caused by bilateral lesions in the midbrain reticular formation. They are rare in children but may occur in neurovisceral lipid storage disease.

Congenital Vertical Ocular Motor Apraxia

Clinical Features. Congenital vertical ocular motor apraxia is a rare syndrome similar to congenital horizontal ocular motor apraxia, except for the direction of gaze palsy. At rest the eyes are fixed in either an upward or a downward position

with little random movement. Head flexion or extension is used initially to fixate in the vertical plane; later the child learns to use head thrusts. The Bell phenomenon is present.

Diagnosis. Vertical gaze palsy suggests intracranial tumor, and MRI must be performed. Low-density lesions on both sides of the posterior third ventricle were demonstrated in one child (Ebner et al, 1990). However, the presence of a gaze palsy from birth without the development of other neurologic signs usually indicates a nonprogressive process. Bilateral restriction of upward eye movement resulting from muscle fibrosis must also be considered (Tychsen et al, 1986). However, in children with ocular motor apraxia the eyes can move upward reflexively or by forced ductions; in children with muscle fibrosis the eyes will not move upward by any means.

HORIZONTAL GAZE PALSY

Inability to look to one side is generally caused by a lesion in the contralateral frontal or ipsilateral pontine gaze center. With frontal lesions the eyes are tonically deviated toward the side of the lesion and contralateral hemiplegia is often present. The eyes can be made to move horizontally by stimulation of the brainstem gaze center with ice water caloric techniques.

In contrast, an irritative frontal lobe lesion, such as an epileptic seizure, generally causes the eyes to deviate in a direction opposite to the side with the seizure focus. Movements of the head and eyes during a seizure are called *adversive seizures* (see Chapter 1). The initial direction of eye movement reliably predicts a contralateral focus, especially if the movement is forced and sustained in a unilateral direction (Wyllie et al, 1986). Later movements that are mild and unsustained are not predictive.

CONVERGENCE PARALYSIS

Convergence paralysis, inability to adduct the eyes to focus on a near object in the absence of medial rectus palsies, can be caused by a pineal region tumor; in such cases, however, other signs of midbrain compression are usually present. Convergence paralysis is sometimes factitious or due to lack of motivation or attention; this can be identified by the absence of pupillary constriction when convergence is attempted.

Convergence insufficiency is frequently encountered after closed head injuries (Waltz and Lavin, in press). The head injury need not be severe to produce symptoms. Diplopia, headache, or eyestrain during reading or other close work is reported. Convergence insufficiency also occurs in the absence of prior head injury. The onset often follows a change in study time or intensity, poor lighting in the workplace, or the use of new contact lenses or eyeglasses. Treatment consists of convergence exercises or prisms.

◆ Nystagmus

Nystagmus is an involuntary, rhythmic oscillation of the eyes in which at least one phase is slow. With *pendular nystagmus* the movements in each direction are slow. The oscillations of pendular nystagmus are in the horizontal plane even on vertical gaze. On lateral gaze the oscillations may change to jerk nystagmus.

Jerk nystagmus is characterized by movements of unequal speed. There is first a slow component in one direction, then a fast component in the other. Oscillation may be horizontal or vertical. The direction of jerk nystagmus is named for the fast (saccadic) component. Nystagmus intensity increases in the horizontal plane when gaze is in the direction of the fast phase.

Table 15–8 describes other eye movements that cannot be classified as nystagmus but have diagnostic significance. *Opsoclonus* consists of conjugate, rapid, chaotic movements in all directions of gaze, often referred to as "dancing eyes." It occurs in infants with neuroblastoma or with idiopathic encephalopathy (see Chapter 10). *Ocular flutter* is a brief burst of conjugate horizontal saccadic eye movements that interrupt fixation. It may be seen in the recovery phase of opsoclonus or in association with cerebellar disease. *Ocular dysmetria* is either an overshoot of the eyes during refixation or an oscillation before the eyes come to rest on a new fixation target. *Ocular bobbing* is not downbeat nystagmus, but rather a sudden downward movement of both eyes with a slow drift back to midposition. It is most often seen in comatose patients with pontine dysfunction.

Congenital nystagmus and acquired nystagmus are discussed separately because their differential diagnoses are different (Table 15–9).

PHYSIOLOGIC NYSTAGMUS

A high-frequency (1 to 3 Hz), low-amplitude, pendular oscillation of the eyes occurs normally when lateral gaze is sustained to the point of fatigue. A jerk nystagmus, present at the endpoint of lateral gaze, is also normal. A few beats are usual, but even sustained nystagmus occurring at the endpoint should be considered normal unless it is associated with other signs of neurologic dysfunction or is distinctly asymmetric.

CONGENITAL NYSTAGMUS

Although congenital nystagmus is present at birth, it may not be noticed until infancy or childhood and then is misdiagnosed as acquired nystagmus. One reason that it may not be noticed is that the *null point,* the angle of ocular movement at which the nystagmus is minimal, may be very wide (Gresty et al, 1984). Often the nystagmus is observed but is mistaken for normal movement.

The cause of congenital nystagmus is thought to be a defect in the gaze-holding mechanism (Dell'Osso, 1988). In the past, it was thought that loss of visual acuity, regardless of cause, before the age of 2 could produce nystagmus and that the nystagmus could be reversed by correction of the visual disturbance. It is now accepted that the visual defect is not causal, but associated, and intensifies the underlying defect in neural control.

Congenital nystagmus is sometimes inherited. The pattern of inheritance may be autosomal recessive, autosomal dominant, or X linked.

Clinical Features. Congenital nystagmus is almost always horizontal in plane but may be either pendular or jerk in character. It is generally diminished by convergence and increased by fixation. Because a null zone exists where nystagmus is minimal, the head may be held to one side to

Table 15–8 ◆ Abnormal Eye Movements

Movement	Appearance	Pathology
Nystagmus	Rhythmic oscillation	Variable
Opsoclonus	Nonrhythmic, chaotic conjugate movements	Neuroblastoma, encephalitis
Ocular flutter	Intermittent bursts of rapid, horizontal, oscillations during fixation	Cerebellar or brainstem disease
Ocular dysmetria	Overshooting or oscillation on refixation	Cerebellar disease
Ocular bobbing	Intermittent, rapid downward movement	Pontine lesions

Table 15–9 ◆ Differential Diagnosis of Nystagmus

Physiologic

Congenital
1. Associated with blindness
2. Familial
3. Idiopathic

Spasmus Nutans
1. Idiopathic
2. Tumors of optic nerve and chiasm (see Chapter 16)

Acquired Nystagmus
1. Pendular
   a. Brainstem infarction
   b. Ictal nystagmus
   c. Multiple sclerosis (see Chapter 10)
   d. Oculopalatal syndrome
      (1) Brainstem infarction
      (2) Spinocerebellar degeneration
2. Jerk
   a. Horizontal
      (1) Drug induced
      (2) Ictal
      (3) Vestibular nystagmus
   b. Vertical
      (1) Downbeat
      (2) Upbeat
3. Dissociated
   a. Divergence
   b. Monocular
   c. See-saw

improve vision. Periodic head turning may accompany periodic alternating nystagmus.

Two forms of head oscillation may be associated with congenital nystagmus. One is involuntary and does not improve vision. The other, also seen in spasmus nutans, is opposite in direction to the nystagmus and improves vision. Many children have impaired vision from the nystagmus in the absence of a primary disturbance in visual acuity.

Diagnosis. Determination that the nystagmus was present at birth is important, but not always possible. The eyes must be carefully examined for abnormalities in the sensory system that may be accentuating nystagmus. If the neurologic findings are otherwise normal, CT is unnecessary.

Treatment. Nystagmus may be reduced by correcting a visual defect and by the use of prisms or surgery to move the eyes into the null zone without the head's turning.

SPASMUS NUTANS

Spasmus nutans is difficult to classify as either a congenital or an acquired nystagmus. It is prob-

ably never present at birth; the onset is early in infancy. The clinical entity of spasmus nutans is characterized by nystagmus, head nodding, and abnormal head positioning.

Clinical Features. Onset typically occurs between 6 and 12 months of age. Nystagmus is characteristically binocular (but may be monocular), has a high frequency and a low amplitude, and can be horizontal, vertical, or torsional in direction. The head is held in a tilted position and titubates in a manner that resembles nodding. Head tilt and movement may be more prominent than nystagmus, and torticollis is often the first complaint (see Chapter 14). The syndrome usually lasts 1 to 2 years, sometimes as long as 5, and then resolves spontaneously.

Diagnosis. Spasmus nutans is ordinarily a transitory, benign disorder of unknown cause. On rare occasions the syndrome may be mimicked by a glioma of the anterior visual pathways (Newman, 1990) or by subacute necrotizing encephalopathy (see Chapter 10). Tumor should be considered if the nystagmus is monocular, the optic nerve is pale, or the onset is after 1 year of age. I do not image the head and orbit in typical cases, although others have recommended this (Gottlob et al, 1990).

Treatment. Treatment is not needed.

ACQUIRED NYSTAGMUS
Pendular Nystagmus

Pendular nystagmus may be either congenital or acquired. In adults the usual causes of acquired pendular nystagmus are brainstem infarction or multiple sclerosis. In children pendular nystagmus in the absence of other neurologic signs is either congenital or the first sign of spasmus nutans. However, the development of optic atrophy in a child with pendular nystagmus indicates a glioma of the anterior visual pathway (Lavery et al, 1984).

Vertical pendular nystagmus is unusual and sometimes occurs in association with rhythmic vertical oscillations of the palate (palatal myoclonus or tremor). This syndrome of oculopalatal oscillation is encountered in some spinocerebellar degenerations and ischemic disorders of the deep cerebellar nuclei and central tegmental tract.

Jerk Nystagmus
Drug-Induced Nystagmus

Clinical Features. Many psychoactive drugs, including tranquilizers, antidepressants, anticonvulsants, and alcohol, produce nystagmus at high therapeutic or toxic blood concentrations. The nystagmus is horizontal or horizontal-rotary and is augmented by lateral gaze. Vertical nystagmus may be present on upward, but rarely on downward, gaze. Phenytoin and carbamazepine occasionally produce primary position downbeat nystagmus.

Diagnosis. Drug-induced nystagmus is common and should be considered in any patient taking psychoactive drugs. Drug overdose should be suspected in patients with nystagmus and decreased consciousness. A drug screen and measurement of drug blood concentrations are indicated.

Treatment. Nystagmus resolves when the blood concentration of the drug falls.

Ictal Nystagmus

Clinical Features. Nystagmus as a seizure manifestation can be binocular or monocular (Jacome and FitzGerald, 1982); it can be jerk, pendular, or rotary; and it may occur alone or in association with other ictal manifestations. Pupillary oscillations synchronous with the nystagmus may be observed (Lavin, 1986). As a rule, concurrent epileptiform discharges are focal, contralateral to the fast phase of nystagmus, and frontal, parietooccipital, or occipital. However, there are individual case reports of nystagmus accompanying generalized 3 Hz spike-wave discharges, ipsilateral focal discharges, and periodic lateralized epileptiform discharges.

Diagnosis. Other seizure manifestations that identify the nature of the nystagmus are usually present. The electroencephalogram confirms the diagnosis by the presence of epileptiform activity concurrent with nystagmus.

Treatment. Ictal nystagmus responds to anticonvulsant drug therapy (see Chapter 1).

Vestibular Nystagmus

Vestibular nystagmus may occur with disorders of the labyrinth, vestibular nerve, vestibular nuclei of the brainstem, or cerebellum.

Clinical Features. Labyrinthine disease (especially labyrinthitis) is usually associated with severe vertigo, nausea, and vomiting (see Chapter 17). Deafness or tinnitus is often present as well. All symptoms and signs are enhanced by movement of the head, and motion may be more critical to the mechanism of nystagmus than the position obtained. Nystagmus is usually horizontal and torsional, with an initial linear slow phase followed by a rapid return. It is worse when gaze is in the direction of the fast phase. Fixation reduces nystagmus and vertigo.

Vertigo and nausea are mild when nystagmus is of central origin. Nystagmus is constantly present and not affected by head position. It may be horizontal or vertical and does not improve with fixation. Other neurologic disturbances referable to the brainstem or cerebellum are frequently associated features.

Diagnosis. Vestibular nystagmus is readily identified by observation and is identical to the nystagmus provoked by caloric stimulation or rotation. Labyrinthine disorders in children are almost always infectious, sometimes viral, and sometimes a result of otitis media. Central causes of vestibular nystagmus include spinocerebellar degeneration, brainstem glioma or infarction, subacute necrotizing encephalomyelitis, and demyelinating disorders.

Treatment. Vertigo and nausea associated with labyrinthine disease are appreciably improved by several different classes of drugs. Diazepam is especially effective. Other useful drugs include scopolamine, antihistamines, and tranquilizers.

Downbeat Nystagmus

Clinical Features. In primary position the eyes drift slowly upward and then spontaneously beat downward. The intensity of the nystagmus is usually greatest when the eyes are directed slightly downward and laterally. Downbeat nystagmus should be distinguished from *downward beating nystagmus* in which the nystagmus is present only on downward gaze. Downward beating nystagmus is usually caused by toxic doses of anticonvulsant and sedative drugs, while downbeat nystagmus indicates a structural abnormality of the brainstem, especially the cervicomedullary junction or cerebellum.

Patient complaints include dizziness, oscillopsia, blurred vision, or difficulty reading. Approximately one third of patients are asymptomatic. Cerebellar ataxia is present in about half of patients and usually is the only associated neurologic sign (Halmagyi et al, 1983).

Diagnosis. Cerebellar degenerations, both congenital and acquired, are the most common identifiable cause. The Chiari malformation must be considered as well. Metabolic disturbances include thiamine deficiency, phenytoin toxicity, and hypomagnesemia resulting from either dietary depletion or the use of lithium salts.

A congenital hereditary downbeat nystagmus was described in a mother and son (Bixenman, 1983). It was noted in the boy at birth, and by infancy he needed to keep his chin down to look at people. He had no other neurologic abnormalities, but the nystagmus caused difficulty in learning to read. His mother had a subclinical downbeat nystagmus evident only in oblique downward gaze.

Treatment. Oscillopsia and acuity can be improved in some individuals by the use of clonazepam (Currie and Matsuo, 1986). A single test dose of 1 to 2 mg can be tried to determine whether long-term therapy will be useful. Trihexyphenidyl may prove effective when clonazepam fails. Prisms that increase convergence may also be useful.

Upbeat Nystagmus

Clinical Features. In primary position the eyes drift slowly downward and then spontaneously beat upward. Upward gaze accentuates the nystagmus. A large- and a small-amplitude type are described (Fisher et al, 1983). Large-amplitude nystagmus increases in intensity during upward gaze and indicates a lesion in the anterior vermis of the cerebellum or an abnormality in the anterior visual pathway (Good et al, 1990). Anterior visual pathway abnormalities include Leber congenital amaurosis (see Chapter 16), bilateral optic nerve hypoplasia, and congenital cataract. Small-amplitude nystagmus decreases in intensity during upward gaze and indicates an intrinsic lesion of the medulla.

Diagnosis. Upbeat nystagmus is usually an acquired disorder caused by vascular lesions or tumors of the brainstem or cerebellum. Therefore cranial MRI is indicated in every child with a normal anterior visual pathway. Upbeat nystagmus is also reported with impairment of smooth pursuit movements in a familial cerebellar vermian atrophy transmitted by autosomal dominant inheritance (Furman et al, 1986).

Treatment. No specific treatment is available.

Dissociated Nystagmus
Divergence Nystagmus

Divergence nystagmus is a rare condition in which each eye beats outward simultaneously. The mechanism is poorly understood, but the condition suggests an abnormality in the posterior fossa and may be seen with spinocerebellar degenerations.

Monocular Nystagmus

Monocular nystagmus may be congenital or acquired. The most important diagnostic considerations in children are spasmus nutans and chiasmal tumors (Farmer and Hoyt, 1984). Although no clinical feature consistently differentiates the two groups, optic nerve abnormalities, especially optic

hypoplasia, are sometimes found in children with tumors but not in those with spasmus nutans.

A coarse pendular vertical nystagmus may develop in an amblyopic eye years after the visual loss (Smith et al, 1982). The nystagmus is noted in the blind eye when distance fixation is attempted with the sighted eye and is inhibited by convergence.

See-Saw Nystagmus

See-saw nystagmus is the result of two different oscillations. One is a pendular vertical oscillation, the other a torsional movement in which one eye rises and intorts while the other falls and extorts. It may be congenital or acquired. The congenital form is sometimes associated with a horizontal pendular nystagmus. Acquired cases are usually due to tumors of the sellar and parasellar regions and are associated with bitemporal hemianopia.

References

Afifi AK, Bell WE, Bale JF, et al: Recurrent lateral rectus palsy in childhood. Pediatr Neurol 6:315, 1990.
Apt L, Axelrod RN: Generalized fibrosis of the extraocular muscles. Am J Ophthalmol 85:822, 1978.
Baker RS, Epstein AD: Ocular motor abnormalities from head trauma. Surv Ophthalmol 35:245, 1991.
Batocchi AP, Evoli A, Palmisani MT, et al: Early-onset myasthenia gravis: Clinical characteristics and response to therapy. Eur J Pediatr 150:66, 1990.
Bixenman WW: Congenital hereditary downbeat nystagmus. Can J Ophthalmol 18:344, 1983.
Cherrington M: Botulism: Ten-year experience. Arch Neurol 30:432, 1974.
Crawford JS: Disease of the orbit. In Toronto Hospital for Sick Children, Department of Ophthalmology: The Eye in Childhood, Year Book, Chicago, 1967, p 331.
Currie JN, Mutsuo V: The use of clonazepam in the treatment of nystagmus-induced oscillopsia. Ophthalmology 93:924, 1986.
Daroff RB: The office Tensilon test for myasthenia gravis. Arch Neurol 43:843, 1986.
Davis TL, Lavin PJM: Pseudo one-and-a-half syndrome with ocular myasthenia. Neurology 39:1553, 1989.
de Grauw AJC, Rotteveel JJ: Transient sixth cranial nerve paralysis in the newborn infant. Neuropediatrie 14:164, 1983.
Dell'Osso LF: Nystagmus and other ocular motor oscillations and intrusions. In Lessell S, van Dalen JTW, eds: Current Neuro-ophthalmology, Vol 1. Year Book, Chicago, 1988.
Durkan GP, Troost BT, Slamovits TL, et al: Recurrent painless oculomotor palsy in children: A variant of ophthalmoplegic migraine? Headache 21:58, 1981.
Ebner R, Lopez L, Ochoa S, et al: Vertical ocular motor apraxia. Neurology 40:712, 1990.
Ellenberger C, Daroff RB: Neuro-ophthalmic aspects of multiple sclerosis. In Poser CM, ed: The Diagnosis of Multiple Sclerosis. Grune & Stratton, New York, 1984, p 49.
Farmer J, Hoyt CS: Monocular nystagmus in infancy and early childhood. Am J Ophthalmol 98:504, 1984.

Feldon SE: Graves' ophthalmopathy: Is it really a thyroid disease? Arch Intern Med 150:948, 1990.

Fisher A, Gresty M, Chambers B, et al: Primary position upbeat nystagmus: A variety of congenital positional nystagmus. Brain 106:949, 1983.

Furman JMR, Baloh RW, Yee RD: Eye movement abnormalities in a family with cerebellar vermian atrophy. Acta Otolaryngol (Stockh) 101:371, 1986.

Good WV, Bradsky MC, Hoyt CS, et al: Upbeating nystagmus in infants: A sign of anterior visual pathway disease. Binocular Vis Q 5:13, 1990.

Gottlob I, Zubcov A, Catalano RA, et al: Signs distinguishing spasmus nutans (with and without central nervous system lesions) from infantile nystagmus. Ophthalmology 97:1166, 1990.

Gresty ME, Page N, Barratt H: The differential diagnosis of congenital nystagmus. J Neurol Neurosurg Psychiatry 47:936, 1984.

Grossniklaus HE, Lass JH, Abramowsky CR, et al: Childhood orbital pseudotumor. Ann Ophthalmol 17:372, 1985.

Halmagyi GM, Rudge P, Gresty MA, et al: Downbeating nystagmus: A review of 62 cases. Arch Neurol 40:777, 1983.

Harbour RC, Trobe JD, Ballinger WE: Septic cavernous sinus thrombosis associated with gingivitis and parapharyngeal abscess. Arch Ophthalmol 102:94, 1984.

Hickey WF, Wagoner MD: Bilateral congenital absence of the abducens nerve. Virchows Arch 402:91, 1983.

Hoyt CS, Mousel DK, Weber AA: Transient supranuclear disturbances of gaze in healthy neonates. Am J Ophthalmol 89:708, 1980.

Jacome DE, FitzGerald R: Monocular ictal nystagmus. Arch Neurol 39:653, 1982.

Kandt RS, Goldstein GW: Steroid-responsive ophthalmoplegia in a child: Diagnostic considerations. Arch Neurol 42:589, 1985.

Keane JR, Finstead BA: Upward gaze paralysis as the initial sign of Fisher's syndrome. Arch Neurol 39:781, 1982.

Kissel JT, Burde RM, Klingele TG, et al: Pupil-sparing oculomotor palsies with internal carotid-posterior communicating artery aneurysms. Ann Neurol 13:149, 1983.

Langmoen IA, Lundar T, Storm-Mathisen I, et al: Management of pediatric pontine gliomas. Child Nerv Syst 7:13, 1991.

Lanska DJ: Diagnosis of thymoma in myasthenics using antistriated muscle antibodies: Predictive value and gain in diagnostic certainty. Neurology 41:520, 1991.

Lavery MA, O'Neill JF, Chu FC, et al: Acquired nystagmus in early childhood: A presenting sign of intracranial tumor. Ophthalmology 91:425, 1984.

Lavin PJM: Pupillary oscillations synchronous with ictal nystagmus. Neuro-ophthalmology 6:113, 1986.

Magoon E, Scott AB: Botulinum toxin chemodenervation in infants and children: An alternative to incisional strabismus surgery. J Pediatr 110:719, 1987.

Marmor M, Wertenbaker C, Berstien L: Delayed ophthalmoplegia following head trauma. Surv Ophthalmol 27:126, 1982.

Mauriello JA, Flanagan JC: Management of orbital inflammatory disease: A protocol. Surv Ophthalmol 29:104, 1984.

Miano MA, Bosley TM, Heiman-Patterson TD, et al: Factors influencing outcome of prednisone dose reduction in myasthenia gravis. Neurology 41:919, 1991.

Misulis KE, Fenichel GM: Genetic forms of myasthenia gravis. Pediatr Neurol 5:205, 1989.

Moraes CT, DiMauro S, Zeviani M, et al: Mitochondrial DNA deletions in progressive external ophthalmoplegia and Kearns-Sayre syndrome. N Engl J Med 320:1293, 1989.

Nelson LB: Diagnosis and management of strabismus and amblyopia. Pediatr Clin North Am 30:1003, 1983.

Newman SA: Spasmus nutans—or is it? Surv Ophthalmol 34:453, 1990.

Oh SJ, Eslami N, Nishihira T, et al: Electrophysiological and clinical correlation in myasthenia gravis. Ann Neurol 12:348, 1982.

Palace J, Wiles CM, Newsom-Davis J: 3, 4-Diaminopyridine in the treatment of congenital (hereditary) myasthenia. J Neurol Neurosurg Psychiatry 54:1069, 1991.

Phillips CI, Gosden CM: Leber's hereditary optic neuropathy and Kearns-Sayre syndrome: Mitochondrial DNA mutations. Surv Ophthalmol 35:463, 1991.

Prakash P, Menon V, Ghosh G: Congenital fibrosis of superior rectus and superior oblique: A case report. Br J Ophthalmol 69:57, 1985.

Prummel MF, Wiesinga WM, Mourits MP, et al: Effect of abnormal thyroid function on the severity of Graves' disease. Arch Intern Med 150:1098, 1990.

Rodriguez M, Gomez MR, Howard FM, et al: Myasthenia gravis in children: Long-term follow-up. Ann Neurol 13:504, 1983.

Rollinson RD, Fenichel GM: Relapsing ocular myasthenia. Neurology 31:325, 1981.

Sandyk R: Paralysis of upward gaze as a presenting symptom of vitamin B12 deficiency. Eur Neurol 23:198, 1984.

Smith JL, Flynn JT, Spiro HJ: Monocular vertical oscillations of amblyopia: The Hermann-Bielschowsky phenomenon. J Clin Neuro-ophthalmol 2:85, 1982.

Soliven BC, Lange DJ, Penn AS, et al: Seronegative myasthenia gravis. Neurology 38:514, 1988.

Swift TR: Disorders of neuromuscular transmission other than myasthenia gravis. Muscle Nerve 4:334, 1981.

Tachibana M, Hoshino A, Nishimura H, et al: Duane's syndrome associated with crocodile tear and ear malformation. Arch Otolaryngol 110:761, 1984.

Tychsen L, Imese RK, Hoyt WF: Bilateral congenital restriction of upward eye movement. Arch Neurol 43:95, 1986.

Verma PD, Oger JJ-F: Seronegative generalized myasthenia gravis: Low frequency of thymic pathology. J Neurology 42:586, 1992.

Victor DI: The diagnosis of congenital unilateral third-nerve palsy. Brain 99:711, 1976.

Vijayan N: Ophthalmoplegia migraine: Ischemic or compressive neuropathy? Headache 20:300, 1980.

von Noorden GK, Murray E, Wong SY: Superior oblique paralysis: A review of 270 cases. Arch Ophthalmol 104:1771, 1986.

Wall M, Wray SH: The one-and-a-half syndrome: A unilateral disorder of the pontine tegmentum; A study of twenty cases and review of the literature. Neurology 33:971, 1980.

Waltz K, Lavin PJM: Accommodative insufficiency. In Margo

CE, Hamed RN, eds: Diagnostic Problems in Clinical Ophthalmology. WB Saunders, Philadelphia, in press.

Wang FM, Wertenbaker C, Behrens MM, et al: Acquired Brown's syndrome in children with juvenile rheumatoid arthritis. Ophthalmology 91:23, 1984.

Wyllie E, Luders H, Morris HM, et al: The lateralizing significance of versive head and eye movements during epileptic seizures. Neurology 36:606, 1986.

Youssefi B: Orbital tumors in children: A clinical study of 62 cases. J Pediatr Ophthalmol 6:177, 1969.

Disorders of the Visual System

Congenital blindness and acquired visual loss in childhood are frequently associated with neurologic disorders. In newborns and infants, visual loss may be brought to neurologic, rather than ophthalmologic, attention because of nystagmus or abnormal development. Ophthalmologic abnormalities such as clouding of the cornea and cataracts are often the first clue to neurologic or systemic disorders. In older children loss of visual acuity may be brought to attention because of strabismus, declining school performance, withdrawal and irritability, or clumsiness. The terms used in reference to disturbed vision are defined in Table 16–1 (Martyn, 1983).

◆ Assessment of Visual Acuity

The assessment of visual acuity in preverbal children is difficult. Although no universally accepted tests or norms of visual acuity are available for children under 6 years of age, many pediatric ophthalmologists use a preferential looking test, the Teller Card Visual Acuity Testing System (Sebris et at, 1987). Clinical assessment requires careful observation of the way an infant or young child interacts with the environment.

CLINICAL ASSESSMENT

The pupillary light reflex is an excellent test of the functional integrity of the afferent and efferent pathways and is reliably present after 31 weeks' gestation. A blink response to light develops at about the same time, and the lid may remain closed for as long as light is present *(dazzle reflex)*. The blink response to threat may not be present until 5 months of age. These responses are integrated in the brainstem and do not provide information on the cognitive (cortical) aspects of vision.

Fixation and following are the principal means to assess visual function in newborns and infants. The human face, at a distance of approximately 30 cm, is the best target for fixation. After fixation is obtained, the examiner slowly moves from side to side to test the *following response*. The child's head should be held to avoid eliciting a vestibulo-ocular reflex.

Visually directed grasping is present in normal children by 3 months of age. It is difficult to test before 6 months of age, however, and its absence may indicate motor rather than visual disturbances.

Optokinetic nystagmus can demonstrate fixation in infants when observation alone is inconclusive. The stimulus must be compelling, filling the visual field. Small hand-held tapes or drums may not be satisfactory. When such small stimuli are used, the demonstration of optokinetic nystagmus is clear evidence of visual function, but its absence does not establish that an abnormality is present.

Visual fields can be evaluated in infants and young children by eliciting a refixation reflex when a stimulus is moved in the peripheral field.

VISUAL EVOKED RESPONSE

The visual evoked response to strobe light is an excellent technique for demonstrating the anatomic integrity of subcortical visual pathways without patient cooperation. A positive "cortical" wave with a peak latency of 300 ms is first demonstrated at 30 weeks' gestation. The latency linearly declines at a rate of 10 ms each week throughout the last 10 weeks of gestation (Hybek et al, 1973). In the newborn the morphology of the visual evoked response is variable during wakefulness and active sleep and is best studied just after the child goes to sleep. By 3 months of age the morphology and latency of the visual evoked response are mature.

Table 16–1 ◆ Definitions

Amaurosis	Partial or total loss of vision not caused by ocular disease.
Amblyopia	Defective visual acuity despite correction of refractive error; customarily reserved for developmental visual loss associated with strabismus.
Cortical blindness	Visual loss caused by cerebral disease uncomplicated by abnormalities of the orbit or anterior visual pathways.
Obscurations	Transitory episodes of visual loss or blurring lasting seconds or minutes.
Photopsias	Abnormal visual sensations (hallucinations) such as flashing lights.
Scotoma	A visual field defect. *Central scotoma* involves the point of fixation and indicates macular or optic nerve disease. *Cecocentral scotoma* also involves the blind spot and suggests optic nerve disease. *Arcuate scotoma* follows the pattern of the retinal fiber bundles and indicates segmental optic nerve disease.

◆ Congenital Blindness

Cortical blindness is the most common cause of congenital blindness, especially among children referred to a neurologist. The causes are numerous and include prenatal and perinatal disturbances. Optic nerve dysplasia, with or without other ocular malformations, is second in frequency, followed by congenital cataracts and corneal opacities. Corneal abnormalities usually do not cause visual loss unless clouding is extensive. Such extensive clouding may occur in the mucopolysaccharidoses and Fabry disease. Table 16–2 lists conditions in which corneal clouding is present during childhood.

Congenital Cataract

For the purpose of this discussion, congenital cataract includes cataracts discovered within the first 3 months. The differential diagnosis is listed in Table 16–3 (Kohn, 1976).

Approximately one third of congenital cataracts are caused by intrauterine infection, one third are hereditary, and in one third the cause cannot be determined (Pike et al, 1989). When cataract is the

Table 16–2 ◆ Causes of Corneal Clouding in Childhood

1. Cerebrohepatorenal syndrome (Zellweger syndrome)
2. Congenital lues
3. Fabry disease (ceramide trihexosidosis)
4. Familial high-density lipoprotein deficiency (Tangier disease)
5. Generalized gangliosidosis GM₁
6. Juvenile metachromatic dystrophy
7. Marinesco-Sjogren disease
8. Mucolipidosis
9. Mucopolysaccharidoses
10. Pelizaeus-Merzbacher disease

only hereditary abnormality, genetic transmission is usually by autosomal dominant inheritance; when hereditary cataracts are associated with other features composing a syndrome, the mode of genetic transmission varies. In many hereditary syndromes cataracts can be either congenital or delayed in appearance until infancy, childhood, or even adulthood. Several of these syndromes are associated with dermatoses: incontinentia pigmenti (irregular skin pigmentation), Marshall syndrome (anhidrotic ectodermal dysplasia), Schafer syndrome (follicular hyperkeratosis), congenital ichthyosis, and Siemens syndrome (cutaneous atrophy).

Congenital cataracts are present in approximately 10% of children with trisomy 13 and trisomy 18. Cataracts develop in the majority of children with Down syndrome, but they are not ordinarily present at birth. In up to 40% of children with Turner syndrome, cataracts develop by puberty.

Clinical Features. Small cataracts do not impair vision and may be difficult to detect by direct ophthalmoscopy. Large cataracts appear as a white mass in the pupil and, if left in place, lead to loss of vision. The initial size of a cataract does not predict its course; congenital cataracts may remain stationary or become more dense, but they never improve spontaneously.

Other congenital ocular abnormalities, such as aniridia, coloboma, and microphthalmos, occur in 40% to 50% of newborns with congenital cataracts.

Diagnosis. Large cataracts are obvious on inspection. Smaller cataracts distort the normal red reflex when the direct ophthalmoscope is held at a distance from the eye and a plus 12 to 20 lens is used.

Genetic disorders and maternal drug exposure should be considered when cataracts are the only abnormality. Intrauterine disturbances, such as maternal illness and fetal infection, are usually as-

Table 16–3 ◆ Lens Abnormalities in Childhood

Congenital Cataract

1. Chromosomal aberrations
   a. Down syndrome*
   b. Trisomy 13
   c. Trisomy 18
   d. Turner syndrome*
2. Drug exposure during pregnancy
   a. Chlorpromazine
   b. Corticosteroids
   c. Sulfonamides
3. Galactosemia
   a. Galactokinase deficiency
   b. Galactose-1-phosphate uridyltransferase deficiency
4. Genetic
   a. Autosomal dominant inheritance
      (1) Hereditary spherocytosis*
      (2) Incontinentia pigmenti*
      (3) Marshall syndrome*
      (4) Myotonic dystrophy*
      (5) Schafer syndrome*
      (6) Without other anomalies
   b. Autosomal recessive inheritance
      (1) Congenital ichthyosis*
      (2) Congenital stippled epiphyses (Conradi disease)
      (3) Marinesco-Sjogren syndrome*
      (4) Siemens syndrome*
      (5) Smith-Lemli-Opitz syndrome
   c. X-linked inheritance (oculocerebrorenal syndrome*
5. Idiopathic
6. Intrauterine infection*
   a. Mumps
   b. Rubella
   c. Syphilis
7. Maternal factors
   a. Diabetes
   b. Radiation
   c. Malnutrition
8. Prematurity
9. Syndromes of uncertain etiology
   a. Hallerman-Streiff syndrome
   b. Pseudo-Turner syndrome*
   c. With oxycephaly
   d. With polydactyly

Acquired Cataract

1. Drug induced
   a. Corticosteroids
   b. Long-acting miotics
2. Genetic
   a. Autosomal dominant inheritance (Alport syndrome)
   b. Autosomal recessive inheritance
      (1) Cockayne disease
      (2) Hepatolenticular degeneration (Wilson disease)
      (3) Laurence-Moon-Biedl syndrome
      (4) Rothmund-Thompson syndrome
      (5) Werner syndrome
   c. X-linked inheritance (pseudo-pseudohypoparathyroidism)
   d. Chromosomal (Prader-Willi syndrome)
3. Metabolic disorders
   a. Cretinism
   b. Hypocalcemia
   c. Hypoparathyroidism
   d. Juvenile diabetes
   e. Pseudohypoparathyroidism
4. Trauma
5. Varicella (postnatal)

Dislocated Lens

1. Crouzon syndrome
2. Ehlers-Danlos syndrome
3. Homocystinuria
4. Hyperlysinemia
5. Marfan syndrome
6. Sturge-Weber syndrome
7. Sulfite oxidase deficiency

*Cataracts may not be noted until infancy or childhood.

sociated with growth retardation and other malformations. Chromosome analysis should be performed for all children with dysmorphic features. Galactosemia is suspected in children with hepatomegaly and milk intolerance (see Chapter 5), but cataracts may be present even before the development of systemic features.

Treatment. Early recognition and removal of cataracts in infants is important to prevent devel-opmental amblyopia. Urgent referral to a pediatric ophthalmologist is warranted.

CONGENITAL OPTIC NERVE HYPOPLASIA

Optic nerve hypoplasia is a developmental defect in the number of optic nerve fibers and may result from excessive regression of retinal ganglion cell axons (Zeki and Dutton, 1990). Hypoplasia may be bilateral or unilateral and varies in severity. It may occur as an isolated defect and cause astigmatism (Zeki, 1990), or it may be associated with other congenital anomalies. The most common association is with midline defects of the septum pellucidum and hypothalamus, *septo-optic dysplasia*.

Clinical Features.   When hypoplasia is severe, the child is blind and attention is drawn to the eyes at birth because of strabismus and nystagmus. Ophthalmoscopic examination reveals a small, pale nerve head (Figure 16–1). A pigmented area surrounded by a yellowish mottled halo is sometimes present at the edge of the disk margin, giving the appearance of a double ring.

The degree of hypothalamic-pituitary involvement varies (Costello and Gluckman, 1988). Possible symptoms include neonatal hypoglycemia and seizures, recurrent hypoglycemia in childhood, growth retardation, diabetes insipidus, and sexual infantilism. Some combination of mental retardation, cerebral palsy, and epilepsy is often present and indicates malformations in other portions of the brain.

Diagnosis.   Magnetic resonance imaging (MRI) or computed tomography (CT) of the head and an assessment of endocrine status should be performed on all infants with ophthalmoscopic evidence of optic nerve hypoplasia. The most common finding in imaging studies is absence of the septum pellucidum, but other malformations may also be present. Endocrine studies should include

assays of growth hormone, antidiuretic hormone, and the integrity of hypothalamic-pituitary control of the thyroid, adrenal, and gonadal systems. Infants with hypoglycemia usually have growth hormone deficiency.

Treatment.   No treatment is available for optic hypoplasia, but endocrine abnormalities respond to replacement therapy.

OTHER DISK ANOMALIES

Morning glory disk is an enlarged dysplastic disk with a white excavated center surrounded by an elevated annulus of pigmentary change. Retinal vessels enter and leave at the margin of the disk, giving the appearance of a morning glory flower. The cause is unknown, and no familial tendency has been established. In most cases visual acuity is decreased in one eye. The anomaly is sometimes associated with basal encephalocele, retinal detachment, esotropia, and hyaloid membrane (Steinkuller, 1980).

Congenital coloboma is a defect in embryogenesis that may affect only the disk or may include the retina, iris, ciliary body, and choroid. Colobomas isolated to the nerve head appear as deep excavations. They may be unilateral or bilateral and sometimes are transmitted as an autosomal dominant trait (Savall and Cook, 1976). Retinochoroidal colobomas are glistening white or yellow defects inferior or inferior-nasal to the disk. The margins are distinct and surrounded by pigment. The anomaly is sometimes inherited but more often sporadic. It may be associated with some chromosomal disorders and with Aicardi syndrome.

LEBER CONGENITAL AMAUROSIS

Leber congenital amaurosis is a hereditary generalized retinal degeneration that is present at birth or in early infancy and is transmitted by autosomal recessive inheritance. The term was used in the past to include some peroxisomal disorders, and for that reason the disorder was thought to have genetic heterogeneity (Lambert et al, 1989).

Clinical Features.   Blindness is present at birth or shortly thereafter. The child may have pendular nystagmus, upbeat nystagmus, and photophobia. Ophthalmoscopy of the retina shows no abnormality in infancy and early childhood, but with time, progressive retinal stippling and pallor of the disk appear. Mental retardation and epilepsy are often associated features.

Diagnosis.   The disease is seldom diagnosed in infancy because the retina appears normal. Electroretinography is the primary method for detecting

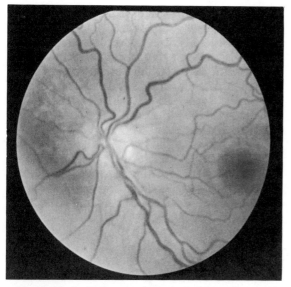

Figure 16–1   Optic nerve hypoplasia. The optic nerve is small and pale, but the vessels are of normal size.

the widespread retinal degeneration. Other disorders that may be mistaken for Leber congenital amaurosis are Zellweger syndrome, infantile Refsum disease, and several varieties of infantile-onset progressive retinal degeneration.

Treatment.   No treatment is available.

◆ Acute Monocular or Binocular Blindness

The differential diagnoses of acute and progressive blindness show a considerable overlap. Although older children recognize sudden visual loss, slowly progressive ocular disturbances may provide an asymptomatic decline until vision is severely disturbed. When finally noticed, the child's loss of visual acuity seems to be recent. Slowly progressive visual disturbances are often noted first by a teacher or parent rather than by the child. Table 16–4 lists conditions in which visual acuity is normal and then suddenly lost. Table 16–5 lists disorders in which the underlying pathologic process is progressive; in most of these conditions the patient quickly perceives the visual loss.

Table 16–4 ◆ Causes of Acute Loss of Vision

Carotid Dissection (see Chapter 11)

Cortical Blindness
1. Anoxic encephalopathy (see Chapter 2)
2. Benign occipital epilepsy (see Chapter 1)
3. Hypoglycemia
4. Hypotension
5. Migraine (see Chapter 3)
6. Occipital metastatic disease
7. Posttraumatic transient cerebral blindness

Hysteria

Optic Neuropathy
1. Demyelinating
   a. Idiopathic optic neuritis
   b. Multiple sclerosis (see Chapter 10)
   c. Neuromyelitis optica (see Chapter 12)
2. Ischemic
3. Toxic
4. Traumatic

Pituitary Apoplexy

Pseudotumor Cerebri (see Chapter 4)

Retinal Disease
1. Central retinal artery occlusion
2. Measles retinitis
3. Migraine
4. Trauma

Therefore both tables should be consulted in the differential diagnosis of "acute blindness."

The duration of transient monocular blindness suggests the underlying cause: seconds indicates disk swelling, minutes emboli, hours migraine, and days optic neuritis.

CORTICAL BLINDNESS

Cortical blindness in children may be permanent or transitory depending on the cause (Wong, 1991). Transitory cortical blindness in childhood may be caused by migraine (see Chapter 3), mild head trauma, brief episodes of hypoglycemia or hypotension, and benign occipital epilepsy (see Chapter 1). Acute and sometimes permanent blindness may occur following anoxia; as a result of massive infarction of, or hemorrhage into, the visual cortex; and when multifocal metastatic tumors or abscesses are located in the occipital lobes.

The salient feature of cortical blindness is loss of vision with preservation of the pupillary light reflex. The results of ophthalmoscopic examination are normal.

Hypoglycemia

Repeated episodes of acute cortical blindness occurred in two children with different glycogen storage diseases at the time of mild hypoglycemia (Garty et al, 1987). Similar episodes may occur following insulin overdose in diabetic children.

Clinical Features.   Sudden blindness is associated with clinical evidence of hypoglycemia (sweating and confusion). Ophthalmoscopic and neurologic findings are normal. Recovery is complete in 2 to 3 hours.

Diagnosis.   During an episode of cortical blindness caused by hypoglycemia, electroencephalography (EEG) shows high-voltage slowing over both occipital lobes. Afterward the EEG returns to normal.

Treatment.   Glucose can be given during the attack, but treatment may not be needed.

Transient Posttraumatic Cerebral Blindness

Clinical Features.   Transient posttraumatic cerebral blindness is a benign syndrome that most often occurs in children with a history of migraine or seizures (Greenblatt, 1982). The spectrum of visual disturbance is broad, but a juvenile and an adolescent pattern have been delineated. In children younger than 8 years, the precipitating trauma is usually associated with either a brief loss of consciousness or a report that the child was

Table 16–5 ◆ Causes of Progressive Loss of Vision

Amblyopia-Strabismus (see Chapter 15)	**Tapetoretinal Degenerations**
	1. Abnormal carbohydrate metabolism
Compressive Optic Neuropathies	a. Mucopolysaccharidosis (see Chapter 5)
1. Aneurysm (see Chapters 4 and 15)	b. Primary hyperoxaluria
2. Arteriovenous malformations (see Chapters 4, 10, and 11)	2. Abnormal lipid metabolism
3. Craniopharyngioma	a. Abetalipoproteinemia (see Chapter 10)
4. Hypothalamic and optic tumors	b. Hypobetalipoproteinemia (see Chapter 10)
5. Pituitary adenoma	c. Multiple sulfatase deficiency (see Chapter 5)
6. Pseudotumor cerebri (see Chapter 4)	d. Neuronal ceroid lipofuscinosis (see Chapter 5)
	e. Niemann-Pick disease (see Chapter 5)
Disorders of the Lens (see Table 16–3)	f. Refsum disease (see Chapter 7)
1. Cataract	3. Aminoacidopathies
2. Dislocation of the lens	a. Cystinosis
	b. Cystinuria
Hereditary Optic Atrophy	c. Gyrate atrophy of choroid and retina
1. Dominant optic neuropathy	4. Other syndromes of unknown etiology
2. Infantile Refsum disease	a. Cockayne syndrome
3. Leber optic neuropathy	b. Laurence-Moon-Biedl syndrome (see Chapter 17)
4. Wolfram syndrome	c. Refsum disease (see Chapter 7)
	d. Usher syndrome (see Chapter 17)
Intraocular Tumors	
Progressive Optic Neuritis	

"stunned." Blindness is noted almost immediately on recovery of consciousness and lasts for an hour or less. During the episode the child may be lethargic and irritable but is usually coherent. Recovery is complete, and the child may not recall the event.

In older children the syndrome is characterized by blindness, confusion, and agitation several minutes or hours after trivial head trauma. Consciousness is not lost. All symptoms resolve after several hours, and the child has complete amnesia for the event. These episodes share many features with acute confusional migraine and are probably a variant of that disorder (see Chapter 2).

Diagnosis. All children with blindness following head trauma, no matter how trivial the injury, should be studied by CT to exclude injury to the occipital lobes. In this condition CT results are normal. EEG findings within the first 24 hours are usually abnormal and may include occipital intermittent rhythmic delta (see Figure 10–2), diffuse slowing, or epileptiform activity that may be generalized or restricted to the occipital region.

Recognition of the syndrome can spare the trouble and expense of other studies. Family history should be scrutinized for migraine or epilepsy. The rapid and complete resolution of symptoms confirms the diagnosis.

Treatment. Treatment is not needed. Symptoms resolve spontaneously.

HYSTERICAL BLINDNESS

A claim of complete binocular blindness is easily identified as spurious. A pupillary response to light indicates that the anterior pathway is intact and only cerebral blindness is a possibility. Visual function can be assessed by using a full-field optokinetic stimulus tape or by moving a large mirror in front of the patient to stimulate matching eye movements. When monocular blindness is claimed, the same tests can be performed with a patch covering the good eye.

Spurious claims of partial visual impairment are more difficult to challenge. Helpful tests include failure of acuity to improve linearly with increasing test size, inappropriate ability to detect small test objects on tangent screen, constricted (tunnel) visual fields to confrontation, and normal results on testing stereoscopic visual acuity or color perception (Keane, 1982; Thompson, 1985).

OPTIC NEUROPATHIES
Demyelinating Optic Neuropathy

Demyelination of the optic nerve (optic neuritis) may occur as an isolated finding affecting one or both eyes, or it may be associated with demyelination in other portions of the nervous system. *Neuromyelitis optica* (Devic syndrome), the syndrome combining optic neuritis and transverse myelitis, is discussed in Chapter 12 and multiple sclerosis in Chapter 10. MRI is a useful technique for surveying the central nervous system for demyelinating lesions (see Figure 10–3). The incidence of later multiple sclerosis among children with optic neuritis is 15% or less if the child has no evidence of more diffuse involvement when brought to medical attention (Kriss et al, 1988), but the incidence of multiple sclerosis is almost 100% when diffuse involvement is present or when relapse of optic neuritis occurs within 1 year (Riikonen et al, 1988). Unilateral optic neuritis has a higher incidence of later multiple sclerosis than does bilateral optic neuritis.

Clinical Features. Monocular involvement is the rule in adults, but binocular involvement occurs in more than half of children (Riikonen et al, 1988). Binocular involvement may be concurrent or sequential, sometimes occurring over a period of weeks. The initial symptom in some children is pain in the eye, but for most it is blurred vision, progressing within hours or days to partial or complete blindness. Visual acuity is reduced to less than 20/200 in almost all patients within 1 week. A history of a preceding "viral" infection or immunization is often presented, but no evidence has shown a cause-and-effect relationship between optic neuritis and either of these events.

Results of ophthalmoscopic examination may be normal at the onset of symptoms if neuritis is primarily retrobulbar. However, most children have papillitis rather than retrobulbar neuritis, and the nerve head is swollen and hemorrhagic, resembling papilledema. The two are readily distinguished because optic neuritis is characterized by early and severe visual loss with afferent pupillary defect and papilledema is not.

Optic neuritis that spreads to the peripapillary nerve fiber layer of the retina is called *neuroretinitis*. Ophthalmoscopic examination reveals disk swelling, peripapillary retinal detachment, and a macular star (Figure 16–2). Neuroretinitis suggests the possibility of conditions other than idiopathic optic neuritis (Table 16–6).

In the absence of myelitis the prognosis in children with bilateral optic neuritis is good; complete recovery occurs in 90%.

Diagnosis. Optic neuritis must be considered when monocular or binocular blindness develops suddenly in a child. The diagnosis is often established by ophthalmoscopic or slitlamp examination. Further confirmation, when necessitated by the suspicion of malingering or hysteria, can be accomplished by testing the visual evoked response. In children with optic neuritis the latency of the major negative wave that ordinarily appears at 100 ms is invariably prolonged. Once optic neu-

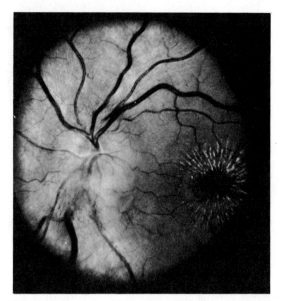

Figure 16–2 Neuroretinitis. The optic disk is swollen with peripapillary nerve fiber layer opacification. Exudates surround the macula in a star pattern. (Courtesy of Patrick Lavin, M.D.)

ritis is confirmed, MRI of the head is indicated to search for diffuse encephalomyelitis or paranasal sinusitis because these findings influence therapy. Peroneally stimulated somatosensory evoked responses and MRI of the spine are indicated if the history or physical findings suggest spinal dysfunction.

Examination of the cerebrospinal fluid is unnecessary. Such examination sometimes reveals leukocytosis and an increased concentration of protein but does not provide information about etiology or prognosis.

Treatment. Until recently, oral corticosteroids were widely used in the treatment of optic neuritis, but a controlled study in adults has shown that intravenous methylprednisolone, 1 mg/kg/

Table 16–6 ◆ Causes of Neuroretinitis*

1. Cat scratch disease
2. Erysipelas
3. Herpes simplex encephalitis
4. Human immunodeficiency virus infection
5. Mycoses
6. Psittacosis
7. Sarcoid
8. Syphilis
9. Toxoplasma
10. Tuberculosis
11. Viral infections (mumps, influenza, zoster)

*Courtesy of Patrick Lavin, M.D.

day for 14 days, followed by oral prednisone, 1 mg/kg/day for 14 days, speeds the recovery of visual loss, while oral prednisone alone is ineffective and increases the risk of recurrence (Beck et al, 1992).

Ischemic Optic Neuropathy

Infarction of the anterior portion of the optic nerve is rare in children and usually associated with systemic vascular disease or hypotension.

Clinical Features. Ischemic optic neuropathy usually occurs as a sudden segmental loss of vision in one eye, but slow or stepwise progression over several days is possible. Recurrent episodes are unusual except with migraine and some idiopathic cases (Dutton and Burde, 1983).

Diagnosis. Altitudinal visual field defects are present in 70% to 80% of patients. Color vision loss is roughly equivalent in severity to visual acuity loss, whereas in demyelinating optic neuritis, color vision is affected more than visual acuity. Ophthalmoscopic examination reveals diffuse or partial swelling of the optic disk. When swelling is diffuse, it gives the appearance of papilledema, and flame-shaped hemorrhages may be present adjacent to the disk margin. After acute swelling subsides, optic atrophy follows.

Treatment. Treatment depends on the underlying disease that causes the ischemia.

Toxic-Nutritional Optic Neuropathies

Toxic optic neuropathies may be due to drugs (Spiteri and James, 1983) or nutritional deficiency (Knox et al, 1982).

Clinical Features. Implicated drugs include barbiturates, antibiotics (chloramphenicol, isoniazid, streptomycin, sulfonamides), chemotherapeutic agents, chlorpropamide, digitalis, ergot, halogenated hydroxyquinolines, penicillamine, and quinine. Nutritional deficiencies that may cause toxic optic neuropathy include folic acid and vitamins B_1, B_2, B_6, and B_{12}.

Symptoms vary with the specific drug, but progressive loss of central vision is typical. In some cases visual loss is rapid and develops as acute binocular blindness that may be asymmetric at onset, suggesting monocular involvement. Many of the drugs produce optic neuropathy by interfering with the action of folic acid or vitamin B_{12} and thereby causing a nutritional deficiency.

Diagnosis. Drug toxicity should be suspected whenever central and paracentral scotomas develop during the course of drug treatment. Optic nerve hyperemia may be an early feature with small

paracentral hemorrhages. Later the disk becomes pale.

Treatment. Drug-induced optic neuropathy is dose related. Dosage reduction may be satisfactory in some cases, especially if concurrent treatment with folic acid or B_{12} reverses the process. Some drugs must be discontinued completely.

Traumatic Optic Neuropathies

Trauma to the head may cause an indirect optic neuropathy in one or both eyes (Wolin and Lavin, 1990). The nerve is tethered along its course, not free to move, and subject to shearing forces with sudden acceleration or deceleration of the skull. Possible consequences include acute swelling, hemorrhage, or tear.

Clinical Features. Loss of vision is immediate. Traumatic optic neuropathy is readily distinguished from cortical blindness because the pupillary response is diminished or absent. Prognosis for recovery is best if there is a brief delay between the time of injury and the onset of blindness.

Diagnosis. The loss of vision and pupillary light response immediately following a head injury should suggest the diagnosis. Ophthalmoscopic examination may reveal peripapillary hemorrhages.

Treatment. Corticosteroids and surgical decompression of the nerve are suggested.

PITUITARY APOPLEXY

Pituitary apoplexy is a rare, life-threatening condition caused by hemorrhagic infarction of the pituitary gland (Reid et al, 1985).

Clinical Features. Pituitary infarction occurs most often when there is a preexisting pituitary tumor but may also occur in the absence of tumor. Predisposing factors are summarized in Table 16–7.

Depending on the structures affected by the swollen gland, a variety of clinical manifestations are possible. These include any of the following, alone or in combination: monocular or binocular blindness, visual field defects, proptosis, ophthalmoplegia, ptosis, facial paresthesias, and hemiplegia. Leakage of blood and necrotic material into the subarachnoid space causes a chemical meningitis associated with headache, meningismus, and loss of consciousness.

Diagnosis. MRI of the head with views of the pituitary gland establishes the diagnosis. Endocrine testing may show a deficiency of all pituitary hormones.

Treatment. Patients deteriorate rapidly and may die within a few days if corticosteroids are

Table 16–7 ◆ Predisposing Factors in Pituitary Apoplexy

1. Acromegaly
2. Adrenalectomy
3. Anticoagulation
4. Bleeding disorders
5. Carotid angiography
6. Cushing syndrome
7. Diabetes
8. Increased intracranial pressure
9. Mechanical ventilation
10. Pituitary radiation
11. Pituitary tumor
12. Pregnancy
13. Sickle cell trait
14. Upper airway obstruction

not administered promptly. Other hormones must also be replaced but are not lifesaving. Patients who continue to do poorly, as evidenced by loss of consciousness, hypothalamic instability, or loss of vision, require urgent surgical decompression of the expanding pituitary mass.

RETINAL DISEASE
Central Retinal Artery Occlusion

In one series of retinal artery obstruction in children and young adults (Brown et al, 1981), a history of migraine was present in one third and coagulopathy in another third. The remaining third had a variety of etiologic factors, including sickle cell disease, cardiac disorders, vasculitis, and pregnancy. No cause could be determined in 15%. Congenital heart disease is the usual condition causing emboli to the central retinal artery in young people. Mitral valve prolapse is a potential cause but is more likely to produce transient cerebral ischemia than transient monocular blindness (Jackson et al, 1984). Coagulopathies, especially when combined with other risk factors such as pregnancy or migraine, are more frequently associated with retinal artery obstruction than embolic disease. The more common coagulopathies are increased factor VIII and increased platelet coagulant activity.

Clinical Features. Most patients have an abrupt loss of monocular vision of variable intensity without premonitory symptoms. Occasional patients describe spots, a shadow, or a descending veil before the loss of vision. Bilateral retinal artery occlusion is uncommon in children.

Diagnosis. The diagnosis of retinal artery obstruction is usually based on the clinical history and ophthalmoscopic examination. The posterior pole of the retina becomes opacified except in the

foveal region, where a cherry-red spot is seen. The peripheral retina appears normal. Visual field examination and fluorescein angiography help confirm the diagnosis in some cases. Once the diagnosis is established, the underlying cause must be found. Evaluation should include auscultation of the heart, radiographs of the chest, echocardiography in selected cases, complete blood cell count with sedimentation rate, cholesterol and triglyceride screening, coagulation studies, hemoglobin electrophoresis, and lupus anticoagulant and antiphospholipid antibodies (Brey et al, 1990).

Treatment. Treatment is determined by underlying cause. The management of idiopathic occlusion of the retinal artery in adults is controversial, with some authorities recommending the use of corticosteroids. In children, giant cell arteritis is not a consideration and corticosteroids are not indicated. Visual acuity is more likely to improve when the obstruction is in a branch artery than in the central retinal artery.

Measles Retinitis

Retinitis is a known complication of natural measles infection, subacute sclerosing panencephalitis, and immunization with live-attenuated measles vaccine (Marshall et al, 1985).

Clinical Features. Sudden blindness occurs 6 to 12 days after appearance of the measles exanthem. Ophthalmoscopic examination reveals a diffuse chorioretinitis with perivascular retinal edema, mild papilledema, and a stellate macular configuration. In the following days a "salt-and-pepper" pigmentary pattern develops along the retinal veins. Recovery occurs over several months but is frequently incomplete.

Diagnosis. The diagnosis is based on characteristic retinitis in temporal sequence with measles infection.

Treatment. No treatment is available.

Retinal Migraine

Clinical Features. Visual symptoms are relatively common during an attack of classic migraine (see Chapter 3). The typical scintillating scotomas, or "fortification spectra," are field defects caused by altered neuronal function in the occipital cortex. The affected field is contralateral to the headache.

Transient monocular blindness (amaurosis fugax) is caused by retinal ischemia. It is not associated with stroke in children, who usually have migraine as the underlying cause (Tippin et al, 1989). The visual loss is sudden in most cases, may be partial or complete, and often precedes and is ipsilateral to the headache (Appleton et al, 1988). Recurrences are usually in the same eye, and attacks may occur without headache.

Patients typically have a long history of classic migraine in which field defects and monocular blindness are experienced separately or together. The visual aberrations are often described as a mosaic or jigsaw pattern of scotomas that clear within minutes. Permanent monocular blindness is unusual and occurs mainly in adolescent and adult women (Coppeto et al, 1986). Many patients with persistent blindness have other risk factors for vascular disease, such as the use of oral contraceptives or vasculitis.

Diagnosis. The diagnosis can be considered only in patients with classic migraine. Ophthalmoscopic findings may be normal initially and then include retinal edema with scattered hemorrhages. Several patterns of retinal vaso-occlusive disease may be observed by fluorescein angiography: branch retinal artery, central retinal artery, central retinal vein, and cilioretinal artery.

Treatment. Children who have retinal ischemia during migraine attacks should be treated with agents that prevent further episodes. Propranolol remains the most effective drug against migraine despite the theoretical, but unproven, fear that it might enhance vasospasm.

Retinal Trauma

Direct blunt injury to the orbit may produce visual impairment by retinal contusion, tear, or detachment. All three are characterized by diminished pupillary response. Contusion is associated with retinal edema. Although visual loss is immediate, the retina appears normal for the first few hours and only later becomes white and opaque. The severity of visual loss varies, but complete recovery is the rule.

Retinal tear is often associated with vitreous hemorrhage. Visual loss is usually immediate and easily diagnosed by ophthalmoscopic appearance. Recovery is spontaneous unless there is detachment, for which cryotherapy is required.

◆ Progressive Loss of Vision
COMPRESSIVE OPTIC NEUROPATHY

Compression of one or both optic nerves often occurs in the region of the chiasm. Visual loss may be confined to one eye or to a visual field. In children with tumors in and around the diencephalon, the most constant feature is growth failure. This may not be recognized until other symptoms develop.

Craniopharyngioma

Clinical Features. The common initial features are growth retardation and visual disturbances in children and failure of sexual maturation in adolescents. Field defects are frequently asymmetric or unilateral. Bitemporal hemianopsia is present in 50% of children and homonymous hemianopsia in 10% to 20%. Visual acuity is diminished in one or both eyes in every child (Hoffman et al, 1977).

Approximately 25% of children have hydrocephalus that causes headache and papilledema. Hypothalamic involvement may produce diabetes insipidus or the *hypodipsia-hyponatremia syndrome* characterized by lethargy, confusion, and hypotension. Other features depend on the direction of tumor growth. Anterior extension may compress the olfactory tract, causing anosmia, whereas lateral extension may compress the third and fifth nerves.

Diagnosis. Craniopharyngiomas are readily visualized by MRI.

Treatment. Subtotal resection followed by radiation therapy is the accepted standard of treatment. The extent of resection remains an issue, but total resection is discouraged (Baskin and Wilson, 1986; Fischer et al, 1985).

The recommended dosage of local radiation is 5,000 rad with the dose per fraction not to exceed 200 rad per day. Hormone replacement therapy is needed.

Hypothalamic and Optic Gliomas

Gliomas of the hypothalamus and optic nerves are difficult to distinguish by histologic criteria and share many clinical features. Optic gliomas represent 3% to 5% of childhood brain tumors. Approximately half of children with optic gliomas have neurofibromatosis type 1 (Alvord et al, 1988; Wright et al, 1989). The clinical symptoms and subsequent course are similar whether or not neurofibromatosis is present, except that recurrences are more common in children with neurofibromatosis.

Clinical Features. Initial symptoms depend on location, but hypothalamic tumors eventually affect the optic chiasm and optic chiasm tumors affect the hypothalamus. In children under the age of 3, tumors of the hypothalamus or optic chiasm are frequently manifested as the *diencephalic syndrome*.

The diencephalic syndrome is characterized by

marked loss of subcutaneous fat and total body weight with maintenance or acceleration of long bone growth. Despite the appearance of cachexia the infant is mentally alert and does not seem as sick as the appearance suggests. Pendular nystagmus is often present. The precise endocrine mechanism of the diencephalic syndrome has never been clarified. Precocious puberty, rather than the diencephalic syndrome, can be the initial manifestation of hypothalamic tumors in infants and children. Hamartomas of the tuber cinereum, astrocytomas, ependymomas, ectopic pinealomas, and craniopharyngiomas have all been associated with the diencephalic syndrome.

Slowly progressive loss of vision is the most common early feature. Monocular visual loss suggests optic nerve involvement but also may occur with tumors of the chiasm. Binocular involvement suggests involvement of the optic chiasm or tract. Visual field deficits vary. Tumors in or near the orbit may produce proptosis, optic disk swelling in which blurring of the disk resembles papilledema, and central loss of vision. Ophthalmoplegia is unusual.

Increased intracranial pressure suggests extension of tumor from the chiasm to the hypothalamus. When this is the initial feature, the site of tumor origin is difficult to determine.

Diagnosis. MRI with an eye coil is the preferred imaging modality because it permits visualization of the hypothalamus in several different planes and identification of brainstem extension of tumor (Figure 16–3).

Optic nerve gliomas usually produce an enlarged, tubular appearance of the nerve and chiasm. Sometimes the tumors are globular and suprasellar and appear to compress the chiasm.

Intrinsic gliomas of the hypothalamus are identified by MRI as high-density signals on T2-weighted studies.

Treatment. Stereotaxic guided biopsy of hypothalamic tumors should be performed before treatment to identify histologic type. The combination of radiation therapy and chemotherapy provides 5- and 10-year survivals of 93% and 74% respectively (Rodriguez et al, 1990).

Management of optic gliomas is a greater problem. Half of these tumors grow slowly and have a relatively benign course. Unfortunately, slow-growing tumors are difficult to differentiate from aggressive tumors at the onset.

Biopsy of tumors to identify tissue type is recommended. Several other tumors may mimic optic nerve gliomas at both the orbit and the chiasm. Children with hydrocephalus require ventricular shunt to relieve symptoms of hydrocephalus. Sur-

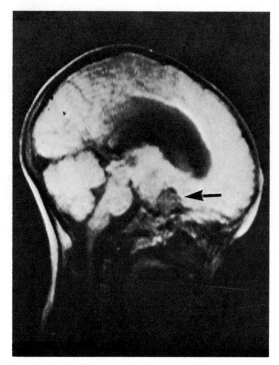

Figure 16–3 Optic nerve glioma identified by magnetic resonance image *(arrow).*

gical excision of the optic nerve to remove the tumor completely should be considered if vision is already negligible. This is most easily accomplished when the tumor is intraorbital. Patients with chiasmatic tumors causing hypothalamic dysfunction require partial excision and radiation therapy with doses greater than 4,500 rad (Alvord et al, 1988).

Because radiation has serious adverse effects on the developing brain, progressive chiasmatic and hypothalamic tumors in children less than 5 years of age have been treated with chemotherapy (actinomycin D and vincristine) without radiation therapy (Packer et al, 1988). Chemotherapy may prevent disease progression without shrinking tumor size and delay radiation therapy until the child is older.

Pituitary Adenoma

Pituitary adenomas represent only 1% to 2% of intracranial tumors of childhood. The sexes are affected equally.

Clinical Features. The initial diagnosis is usually during adolescence (Mukai et al, 1986). Amenorrhea is usually the first symptom in girls with prolactin-secreting tumors. Galactorrhea may also be present. In boys the initial features are growth retardation, delayed puberty, and headache.

Papilledema is rare, but optic atrophy is present in 10% to 20% of cases. Visual field defects may be unilateral temporal, bitemporal, or homonymous.

Diagnosis. Visualization of the tumor and identification of its extrasellar extent are best accomplished by MRI. Measurement of hormone production is useful in distinguishing tumor type. Increased concentration of prolactin is recorded in 60% of adenomas, growth hormone in 15%, and adrenocorticotropic hormone in 12%; 12% of adenomas are nonfunctioning.

Treatment. The tumor can be totally resected when restricted to the sella. In such cases the outcome is generally good, the recurrence rate is low, and hormone replacement therapy is not always required. Radiation therapy should be used in patients with partial excision or recurrence.

HEREDITARY OPTIC ATROPHY

Several hereditary optic neuropathies have been described. Some affect only the visual system, others involve the visual system and central nervous system, and still others cause multisystem disease (Neetens and Martin, 1986). These disorders may produce acute, subacute, or chronic decline in visual acuity. Diagnosis relies heavily on family history.

Dominant Optic Neuropathy

Clinical Features. The onset of symptoms is insidious, but most patients date the beginning of visual disturbances to the first decade, usually 4 to 8 years of age (Glaser, 1990). The progressive reduction in visual acuity occurs equally in both eyes and may be mild, with vision remaining between 20/30 and 20/70 and considerable asymmetry between the eyes. In some cases the disease is identified only because other family members are affected.

Visual fields show central, paracentral, or cecocentral scotomas, which are best delineated with red test objects. Optic atrophy primarily affects the temporal portion of the disk, which appears pale. Additional neurologic abnormalities are unusual.

Diagnosis. A family history of the defect is critical for diagnosis. It is easily distinguished from Leber optic neuropathy by the absence of microangiopathy.

Treatment. No treatment is available.

Infantile Refsum Disease

Infantile Refsum disease is a generalized peroxisomal disorder that is closely related to the oculocerebrorenal syndrome and neonatal adrenoleukodystrophy (see Chapter 6). It is probably different from the later onset Refsum disease described in Chapter 7. Autosomal recessive inheritance is suspected.

Clinical Features. The initial features are early acquired blindness and deafness, which are usually detected during infancy and may be congenital. These are followed by slow neurologic deterioration characterized by dementia, ataxia, hypotonia, and nystagmus (Torvik et al, 1988). Hepatomegaly and growth retardation are common features. Death ordinarily occurs in the second decade.

Diagnosis. The concentration of protein in the spinal fluid is elevated, and EEG may demonstrate epileptiform activity. Liver transaminase levels are elevated, as is the serum concentration of bile acids. An elevated concentration of serum phytanic acid is essential to the diagnosis.

Treatment. No treatment is available.

Leber Optic Neuropathy (Neuroretinopathy)

Leber optic neuropathy is a multisystem mitochondrial disease transmitted by mitochondrial DNA (Singh et al, 1989). Intrafamily phenotypic variability may be caused by the ratio of mutant to normal mitochondrial DNA within an individual, but interfamily variability is probably caused by alternative mutations (Vikki et al, 1989).

Clinical Features. The characteristic early symptom is rapid loss of vision in young, otherwise healthy men. Onset is most frequent between 18 and 23 years, but children younger than 10 years of age may be affected. Age at onset may vary by several decades within a kindred.

The initial complaint is usually painless blurred central vision in one eye, described as fogging of vision or central fading of color. The other eye ordinarily shares the symptom within days or weeks but may remain unimpaired for several years. Examination of the visual fields reveals first central and then cecocentral scotomas.

The characteristic changes in the ocular fundus include circumpapillary telangiectatic microangiopathy, edema of the nerve fiber layer around the disk, and absence of peripapillary staining on fluorescein angiography. Telangiectatic microangiopathy is the earliest feature and may be observed in presymptomatic family members (Lopez and Smith, 1986; Nikoskelainen et al, 1982). As the patient's symptoms develop, the nerve fiber layer becomes swollen; retinal vessels on and around the disk become dilated, tortuous, and telangiectatic; and hemorrhages appear in the nerve fiber layer (Nikoskelainen et al, 1983). Atrophy first appears in the papillomacular bundle and then involves the rest of the retina. The vascular bed involutes, leaving a pale retina and optic atrophy.

Visual improvement occurs in perhaps 20% of patients 1 to 5 years after vision is lost. Ten percent are reported to regain full vision. Once vision is restored, relapses do not occur.

Although visual loss is the only symptom in most families, neurologic impairment may be an associated feature in some kindreds. Commonly associated disturbances include dystonia, spastic paraplegia, and ataxia. Some family members may have neurologic impairment without atrophy, and some have optic atrophy with neurologic impairment.

Diagnosis. Leber optic neuropathy should be suspected in every kindred with optic neuropathy or with progressive neurologic impairment in which transmission is restricted to the maternal line. The optic fundus changes, especially the microangiopathy, are the basis for diagnosis in the context of a compatible family history. Fluorescein angiography definitively demonstrates the development and involution of the telangiectatic microangiopathy and is useful in the diagnosis before symptoms occur (Nikoskelainen et al, 1984).

Treatment. No effective treatment is available.

Wolfram Syndrome

The major features of Wolfram syndrome are juvenile diabetes mellitus, optic atrophy, and bilateral hearing loss (Aldenhovel HB et al, 1991). The pattern of genetic transmission is uncertain, but autosomal recessive inheritance is presumed.

Clinical Features. The onset of diabetes usually occurs in the first decade. Insulin therapy is required soon after diagnosis. Visual loss progresses rapidly in the second decade but does not lead to complete blindness. The sensorineural hearing loss affects high frequencies first and progresses slowly, rarely leading to severe hearing loss. Features reported in some patients include anosmia, autonomic dysfunction, ptosis, external ophthalmoplegia, tremor, ataxia, nystagmus, seizures, central diabetes insipidus, and endocrinopathies.

Diagnosis. Diagnosis depends on the combination of juvenile-onset diabetes mellitus and optic atrophy. Wolfram syndrome is distinguished from infantile Refsum disease by the concurrence of diabetes mellitus and a later age at onset. A family history of the syndrome is not always present. Diabetes is not thought to cause optic atrophy. It is more likely that all features result from a progressive neurodegenerative process.

Treatment. Each of the clinical features is treated symptomatically.

INTRAOCULAR TUMORS

Although retro-orbital tumors generally cause strabismus and proptosis, intraocular tumors always diminish visual acuity. Retinoblastoma is the most common malignant intraocular tumor. Its prompt recognition can be lifesaving.

The typical features of intraocular tumor in a young child are an abnormal appearance of the eye, loss of vision, and strabismus. Monocular blindness is usually unrecognized by parents. Older children may complain of visual blurring and floaters. Ocular pain in uncommon.

Leukokoria, a white pupillary reflex, is the initial feature in most children with retinoblastoma. This is first noted in bright sunlight or in a flash photograph; the pupil does not constrict and has a white color. Strabismus occurs when visual acuity is impaired. The sighted eye is used for fixation, and the other remains deviated outward in all directions of gaze.

Most children with intraocular tumors are referred directly to an ophthalmologist. A neurologist may be the primary consulting physician when the tumor is part of a larger syndrome that includes mental retardation. Such syndromes include retinoblastoma associated with chromosome 13 long arm deletion, retinal astrocytoma associated with tuberous sclerosis, choroidal hemangioma associated with Sturge-Weber disease, and optic nerve glioma in children with neurofibromatosis.

PROGRESSIVE OPTIC NEURITIS

Optic neuritis is generally regarded as an acute process with sudden onset of blindness in one eye and then the other (see "Demyelinating Optic Neuropathy" earlier in this chapter). Occasionally patients have a slowly progressive optic neuritis (Roseman and Ellenberger, 1982). Those with adult onset usually have multiple sclerosis, but this may not be the case in children.

Clinical Features. Onset occurs in adolescence or later. Initial symptoms may be transitory monocular blindness or blurring of vision during strenuous exercise. Disturbed color discrimination is an early feature. Vision worsens over a period of years, usually stepwise. Some patients report deterioration of vision in bright light. Recovery is unusual.

Diagnosis. Any possibility of compressive optic neuropathy must be excluded. MRI is needed both for this purpose and to determine the presence of other foci of demyelination. Visual evoked response should demonstrate a prolonged latency of the major positive wave.

Treatment. There is no established treatment for this disorder, but the regimen of corticosteroids suggested for acute demyelinating optic neuropathy should be tried.

TAPETORETINAL DEGENERATIONS

Most tapetoretinal degenerations are hereditary and due to inborn errors of lipid or carbohydrate metabolism. These disorders also cause dementia, peripheral neuropathy, and ataxia as initial features and are discussed in several chapters (see Table 16–5). The conditions discussed here are less common, but other neurologic features are not prominent initial complaints.

Aminoacidopathies

Cystinuria is transmitted as a recessive trait. Intestinal absorption and renal tubular reabsorption of cystine, lysine, arginine, and ornithine are impaired. The most common feature is renal stones, but retinal degeneration may be an associated feature.

Cystinosis is a lysosomal storage disease transmitted by autosomal recessive inheritance. Cystine is stored in the viscera, bone marrow, and eyes. The major clinical features are dwarfism, renal tubulopathy, vitamin-resistant renal rickets, and hepatosplenomegaly. In addition to having cystine storage in the cornea, conjunctiva, and iris, the child has pigmentary degeneration of the retina. Neurologic dysfunction may be present.

Gyrate atrophy of the choroid and retina is probably a disorder of ornithine metabolism (Francois, 1982). It may be the homozygote form of the *Alder anomaly,* in which azurophilic granules are present in the cytoplasm of leukocytes. Visual function is adequate for many years, but eventually the patient becomes blind.

Cockayne Syndrome

Cockayne syndrome is transmitted by autosomal recessive inheritance with a male-to-female bias of 3:1. It is probably an inborn error of lipid metabolism and produces a leukodystrophy.

Clinical Features. Primary pigmentary de-

generation of the retina occurs during infancy. Affected children appear cachectic, and a disproportionate dwarfism develops in which the limbs are large compared with the trunk. The characteristic facies includes lack of subcutaneous fat with prominence of facial bones, enophthalmos, a beaklike nose, and large ears. Mental deficiency and microcephaly are constant features. Neurologic signs may include cerebellar ataxia, involuntary movements, spasticity, peripheral neuropathy, and sensorineural hearing loss.

Diagnosis. The constellation of clinical signs suggests the diagnosis. Hyperbetaglobulinemia, hyperinsulinemia, and hyperlipoproteinemia are present in some cases.

Treatment. No treatment is available.

Laurence-Moon-Biedl Syndrome

Laurence-Moon-Biedl syndrome comprises a heterogeneous group of disorders that share ocular and systemic features. It is transmitted by autosomal recessive inheritance.

Clinical Features. Pigmentary retinopathy usually is manifested in the second decade. It may be characterized by salt-and-pepper retinopathy, macular pigmentation, or macular degeneration. In some patients the retina appears normal, but the electroretinogram always shows abnormalities. Other cardinal features include hypogenitalism, obesity, polydactyly, and mental retardation. Less common associated features are sensorineural deafness, cataract, external ophthalmoplegia, and diabetes mellitus.

Diagnosis. Diagnosis depends on recognition of the constellation of symptoms and signs.

Treatment. No treatment is available for the underlying defect.

◆ Disorders of the Pupil

In the awake state, the size of the pupil is constantly changing in response to light and autonomic input. This pupillary unrest is called *hippus*. An isolated disturbance of pupillary size is *not* evidence of intracranial disease.

ESSENTIAL ANISOCORIA

Between 20% and 30% of healthy people have an observable difference in the size of their pupils. Like congenital ptosis, it may go unnoticed until late in childhood or adult life and then be thought to be a new finding. The difference is constant at all levels of illumination. The absence of other pupillary dysfunction or disturbed ocular motility suggests essential anisocoria, but old photographs are invaluable to confirm the diagnosis.

TONIC PUPIL SYNDROME (ADIE SYNDROME)

Clinical Features. Tonic pupil syndrome is caused by a defect in the orbital ciliary ganglion. The onset usually occurs after childhood but has been reported as early as 5 years. Women are affected more often than men.

The defect is usually monocular and is manifested as anisocoria or photophobia. The abnormal pupil is slightly larger in bright light but changes little, if at all, with alteration in illumination. In a dark room the normal pupil dilates and then is larger than the tonic pupil. With attempted accommodation, which may also be affected, the pupil constricts slowly and incompletely and redilates slowly afterward.

Binocular tonic pupils are seen in children with dysautonomia and are also seen in association with diminished tendon reflexes *(Holmes-Adie syndrome)*.

Diagnosis. The tonic pupil is supersensitive to parasympathomimetic agents; constriction is achieved with 0.125% pilocarpine.

Treatment. The condition is benign and seldom needs treatment.

FIXED DILATED PUPIL

Clinical Features. A fixed dilated pupil is an ominous sign in unconscious patients because it suggests transtentorial herniation (see Chapter 4). However, a dilated pupil that does not respond to light or accommodation in a child who is otherwise well and has no evidence of ocular motor dysfunction can result only from the application of a pharmacologic agent or from a ruptured sphincter. The application may be accidental, as when a drug or chemical is inadvertently wiped from hand to eye. Many cosmetics contain chemicals that can induce mydriasis. A careful history must be obtained.

Factitious application of mydriatics is a relatively common attention-seeking device, and convincing parents that the problem is self-inflicted may be difficult.

Diagnosis. Pilocarpine 1% should be instilled in both eyes using the normal eye as a control. Parasympathetic denervation produces prompt constriction. A slow or incomplete response indicates pharmacologic dilation.

Treatment. Most pharmacologic agents are long acting, and their effects cannot be rapidly reversed.

HORNER SYNDROME

Horner syndrome is characterized by sympathetic denervation and may be congenital or acquired. When acquired, it may occur at birth as part of a brachial plexus injury, during infancy from neuroblastoma, or in childhood from tumors or injuries affecting the superior cervical ganglion or the carotid artery.

Clinical Features. Unilateral Horner syndrome consists of the following ipsilateral features: mild to moderate ptosis; miosis, which is best appreciated in dim light so that the normal pupil dilates; and anhidrosis of the face. Enophthalmos and heterochromia are apparent when the syndrome is congenital.

Diagnosis. Horner syndrome may be caused by disruption of the sympathetic system anywhere from the hypothalamus to the eye. Brainstem disturbances from stroke are common in adults, but peripheral lesions are more common in children. Topical instillation of dilute norepinephrine produces immediate pupillary dilation when postganglionic denervation is present. Ten percent cocaine solution produces little or no dilation regardless of the site of abnormality.

Treatment. Treatment depends on the underlying cause.

ARGYLL ROBERTSON PUPIL

Argyll Robertson pupil is associated with tertiary syphilis and is almost never seen in children. Both pupils are irregularly shaped and miotic. Iris atrophy may be present. The pupils respond poorly to light, but response to near is present (light-near dissociation).

ANIRIDIA

Hypoplasia of the iris may occur as a solitary abnormality or may be associated with mental retardation, genitourinary abnormalities, and Wilm tumor. In some cases the short arm of chromosome 11 is abnormal.

References

Aldenhovel HBG, Gallenkamp U, Suelemana CA: Juvenile onset diabetes mellitus, central diabetes insipidus and optic atrophy (Wolfram syndrome)—neurological findings and prognostic implications. Neuropediatrics 22:103, 1991.

Alvord EC, Lofton S: Gliomas of the optic nerve or chiasm:

Outcome by patient's age, tumor site, and treatment. J Neurosurg 68:85, 1988.

Appleton R, Farrell K, Buncie R, et al: Amaurosis fugax in teenagers: A migraine variant. AJDC 142:331, 1988.

Baskin DS, Wilson CB: Surgical management of craniopharyngiomas: A review of 74 cases. J Neurosurg 65:22, 1986.

Beck RW, Cleary PA, Anderson MM, et al: A randomized controlled trial of corticosteroids in the treatment of acute optic neuritis. N Engl J Med 326:581, 1992.

Brey RL, Hart RG, Sherman DG, et al: Antiphospholipid antibodies and cerebral ischemia in young people. Neurology 40:1190, 1990.

Brown GC, Magaral LE, Shields JA, et al: Retinal artery obstruction in children and young adults. Ophthalmology 88:18, 1981.

Coppeto JR, Lessell S, Sciarra R, et al: Vascular retinopathy in migraine. Neurology 36:267, 1986.

Costello JM, Gluckman PD: Neonatal hypopituitarism: A neurological perspective. Dev Med Child Neurol 30:190, 1988.

Dutton JJ, Burde RM: Anterior ischemic optic neuropathy of the young. J Clin Neuro-ophthalmol 3:137, 1983.

Fischer EG, Welch K, Belli JA, et al: Treatment of craniopharyngiomas in children: 1972-1981. J Neurosurg 62:496, 1985.

Francois J: Metabolic tapetoretinal degenerations. Surv Ophthalmol 26:293, 1982.

Garty B-Z, Dinari G, Nitzan M: Transient acute cortical blindness associated with hypoglycemia. Pediatr Neurol 3:169, 1987.

Glaser JS: Topical diagnosis: Prechiasmal visual pathways. In Glaser JS (ed): Neuro-ophthalmology, 2nd edition. JB Lippincott, Philadelphia, 1990, p 108.

Greenblatt SH: Posttraumatic transient cerebral blindness: Association with migraine and seizure diathesis. JAMA 225:1073, 1982.

Hoffman HJ, Hendrick EB, Humphreys RP, et al: Management of craniopharyngioma in children. J Neurosurg 47:218, 1977.

Hrbek A, Karlberg P, Olsson T: Development of visual and somatosensory evoked responses in pre-term newborn infants. Electroencephalogr Clin Neurophysiol 34:225, 1973.

Jackson AC, Boughner DR, Barnett HJM: Mitral valve prolapse and cerebral ischemic events in young patients. Neurology 34:784, 1984.

Keane JR: Neuro-ophthalmic signs and symptoms of hysteria. Neurology 32:757, 1982.

Knox DL, Chen MF, Guilarte TR, et al: Nutritional amblyopia: Folic acid, vitamin B_{12}, and other vitamins. Retina 2:288, 1982.

Kohn BA: The differential diagnosis of cataracts in infancy and childhood. AJDC 130:184, 1976.

Kriss A, Francis DA, Cuendet F, et al: Recovery after optic neuritis in childhood. J Neurol Neurosurg Psychiatry 51:1253, 1988.

Lambert SR, Kriss A, Taylor D, et al: Follow-up and diagnostic reappraisal of 75 patients with Leber's congenital amaurosis. Am J Ophthalmol 107:624, 1989.

Lopez PF, Smith JL: Leber's optic neuropathy: New observations. J Clin Neuro-ophthalmol 6:144, 1986.

Marshall GS, Wright PF, Fenichel GM, et al: Diffuse retinopathy following measles, mumps, and rubella vaccination. Pediatrics 76:989, 1985.

Martyn LJ: Pediatric neuro-ophthalmology. Pediatr Clin North Am 30:1103, 1983.

Mukai K, Seljeskog EL, Dehner LP: Pituitary adenomas in patients under 20 years old: A clinicopathological study of 112 cases. J Neuro-oncol 4:79, 1986.

Neetens A, Martin JJ: The hereditary optic atrophies. Neuro-ophthalmology 6:277, 1986.

Nikoskelainen E, Hoyt WF, Nummelin K: Ophthalmoscopic findings in Leber's hereditary optic neuropathy. I. Fundus findings in asymptomatic family members. Arch Ophthalmol 100:1597, 1982.

Nikoskelainen E, Hoyt WF, Nummelin K: Ophthalmoscopic findings in Leber's hereditary optic neuropathy. II. The fundus finding in the affected family members. Arch Ophthalmol 101:1059, 1983.

Nikoskelainen E, Hoyt WF, Nummelin K: Ophthalmoscopic findings in Leber's hereditary optic neuropathy. III. Fluorescein angiographic findings. Arch Ophthalmol 102:981, 1984.

Packer RJ, Sutton LN, Bilaniuk LT, et al: Treatment of chiasmatic/hypothalamic gliomas of childhood with chemotherapy: An update. Ann Neurol 23:79, 1988.

Pike MG, Jan JE, Wong PKH: Neurological and developmental findings in children with cataracts. AJDC 143:706, 1989.

Reid RL, Quigley ME, Yen SSC: Pituitary apoplexy: A review. Arch Neurol 42:712, 1985.

Riikonen R, Donner M, Erkkila H: Optic neuritis in children and its relationship to multiple sclerosis: A clinical study of 21 children. Dev Med Child Neurol 30:349, 1988.

Rodriguez LA, Edwards MSB, Levin VA: Management of hypothalamic gliomas in children: An analysis of 33 cases. Neurosurgery 26:242,1990.

Roseman R, Ellenberger C Jr: Slowly progressive optic neuritis. Neuro-ophthalmology 2:183, 1982.

Savall J, Cook JR: Optic nerve colobomas of autosomal dominant heredity. Arch Ophthalmol 94:395, 1976.

Sebris SL, Dobson V, McDonald MA, et al: Acuity cards for visual acuity assessment of infants and children in clinical settings. Clin Visual Sci 2:45, 1987.

Singh G, Lott MT, Wallace DC: A mitochondrial DNA mutation as a cause of Leber's hereditary optic neuropathy. N Engl J Med 320:1300, 1989.

Spiteri MA, James DG: Adverse ocular reactions to drugs. Postgrad Med J 59:343,1983.

Steinkuller PG: The morning glory disc anomaly: Case report and literature review. J Pediatr Ophthalmol 17:81, 1980.

Thompson HS: Functional visual loss. Am J Ophthalmol 100:209, 1985.

Tippin J, Corbett JJ, Kerber RE, et al: Amaurosis fugax and ocular infarction in adolescents and young children. Ann Neurol 26:69, 1989.

Torvik A, Torp S, Kase BF, et al: Infantile Refsum's disease: A generalized peroxisomal disorder; Case report with post-mortem examination. J Neurol Sci 85:39, 1988.

Vikki J, Savontaus M-J, Nikoskelainen EK: Genetic heterogeneity in Leber optic neuroretinopathy revealed by mitochondrial DNA polymorphism. Am J Hum Genet 45:206, 1989.

Wolin MJ, Lavin PJM: Spontaneous visual recovery from traumatic optic neuropathy after blunt head injury. Am J Ophthalmol 109:430, 1990.

Wong VCN: Cortical blindness in children: A study of etiology and prognosis. Pediatr Neurol 7:178, 1991.

Wright JE, NcNab AA, McDonald WI: Optic nerve glioma and the management of optic nerve tumors in the young. Br J Ophthalmol 73:967, 1989.

Zeki SM: Optic nerve hypoplasia and astigmatism: A new association. Br J Ophthalmol 76:297, 1990.

Zeki SM, Dutton GH: Optic nerve hypoplasia in children. Br J Ophthalmol 76:300, 1990.

Lower Brainstem and Cranial Nerve Dysfunction

This chapter considers disorders causing dysfunction of the seventh through twelfth cranial nerves. Many such disorders also disturb extraocular motility and are discussed in Chapter 15. This assignment may seem arbitrary, but it is based on the most common early manifestation. For example, myasthenia gravis is discussed in Chapter 15 because diplopia is a much more common initial complaint than dysphagia.

An acute isolated cranial neuropathy, such as facial palsy, is usually a less ominous sign than multiple cranial neuropathies and is likely to have a self-limited course. However, an isolated cranial neuropathy may be the first sign of progressive cranial nerve dysfunction. Therefore conditions causing isolated and multiple cranial neuropathies are discussed together because they may not be separable at first.

◆ Facial Weakness and Dysphagia
ANATOMIC CONSIDERATIONS
Facial Movement

The motor nucleus of the facial nerve is a column of cells in the ventrolateral tegmentum of the pons. Nerve fibers leaving the nucleus take a circuitous path in the brainstem before emerging close to the pontomedullary junction, where they enter the internal auditory meatus with the acoustic nerve. After bending forward and downward around the inner ear, the facial nerve traverses the temporal bone in the facial canal and exits the skull at the stylomastoid foramen. Extracranially, the facial nerve passes into the parotid gland, where it divides into several branches and is distributed to all muscles of facial expression except the levator palpebrae superioris.

Sucking and Swallowing

The sucking reflex requires the integrity of the trigeminal, facial, and hypoglossal nerves. Stimulation of the lips produces coordinated movements of the face, jaw, and tongue. The automatic aspect of the reflex disappears after infancy but returns in bilateral disease of the cerebral hemispheres.

The afferent arc of the swallowing reflex is formed by fibers of the trigeminal and glossopharyngeal nerves that end in the nucleus solitarius. The efferent arc is formed by the motor root of the trigeminal nerve, glossopharyngeal and vagus fibers from the nucleus ambiguus, and the hypoglossal nerves. A swallowing center that coordinates the reflex is located in the lower pons and upper medulla. A bolus of food stimulates the pharyngeal wall or back of the tongue, and food is moved into the esophagus by action of the tongue, palatine arches, soft palate, and pharynx.

APPROACH TO DIAGNOSIS

Weakness of facial muscles may be caused by supranuclear palsy (pseudobulbar palsy), intrinsic brainstem disease, or disorders of the motor unit: facial nerve, neuromuscular junction, and facial muscles (Tables 17–1 and 17–2). The differential diagnosis of dysphagia is similar (Table 17–3) except that isolated dysfunction of the nerves that enable swallowing is uncommon.

Pseudobulbar Palsy

Because the corticobulbar innervation of most cranial nerves is bilateral, pseudobulbar palsy occurs only when hemispheric disease is bilateral. Children with pseudobulbar palsy are likely to have

Table 17–1 ◆ Causes of Congenital Facial Weakness

1. Aplasia of facial muscles
2. Birth injury
3. Congenital myotonic dystrophy (see Chapter 6)
4. Fiber-type disproportion myopathies (see Chapter 6)
5. Myasthenic syndromes
   a. Congenital myasthenia (see Chapter 15)
   b. Familial infantile myasthenia (see Chapter 6)
   c. Transitory neonatal myasthenia (see Chapter 6)

cerebral palsy or a progressive degenerative disorder of gray or white matter. Most of these disorders are discussed in Chapter 5 because dementia is usually the initial feature. In some disorders, such as the juvenile form of Alexander disease, pseudobulbar palsy may be an early manifestation (Borrett and Becker, 1985). Bilateral stroke, simultaneous or in sequence, is a common cause of pseudobulbar palsy in adults but not in children.

The usual causes of bilateral stroke in children are coagulation defects, leukemia, and trauma (see Chapter 11).

Pseudobulbar palsy is characterized by inability to use bulbar muscles in voluntary effort, whereas reflex movements initiated at a brainstem level are performed normally. Extraocular motility is unaffected. The child can suck, chew, and swallow but is unable to smile or make facial movements on command. Severe dysarthria is often present (van Dongen et al, 1987). Affected muscles do not show atrophy or fasciculations. The gag reflex and jaw jerk are usually exaggerated, and emotional volatility is often an associated feature.

Newborns with familial dysautonomia have difficulty in feeding, despite normal sucking and swallowing, because they fail to coordinate the two reflexes (see Chapter 6). The differential diagnosis of feeding difficulty in an alert newborn is summarized in Table 6–8. Children with cerebral palsy often have a similar disturbance in the coordination of chewing and swallowing, and feeding is impaired.

Table 17–2 ◆ Causes of Postnatal Facial Weakness

Autoimmune and Postinfectious
1. Bell palsy
2. Idiopathic cranial polyneuropathy
3. Miller-Fisher syndrome (see Chapter 10)
4. Myasthenia gravis (see Chapter 15)

Genetic
1. Muscular disorders
   a. Facioscapulohumeral syndrome, infantile form
   b. Facioscapulohumeral syndrome (see Chapter 7)
   c. Fiber-type disproportion myopathies (see Chapter 6)
   d. Myotonic dystrophy (see Chapter 7)
   e. Oculopharyngeal dystrophy
2. Myasthenic syndromes
   a. Congenital myasthenia (see Chapter 15)
   b. Familial infantile myasthenia (see Chapter 6)
3. Recurrent facial palsy
   a. Melkersson syndrome
   b. Multiple cranial neuropathies

Hypertension

Infectious
1. Diphtheria
2. Herpes zoster oticus
3. Infectious mononucleosis
4. Lyme disease (see Chapter 2)
5. Otitis media
6. Sarcoidosis
7. Tuberculosis

Juvenile Progressive Bulbar Palsy (Fazio-Londe Disease)

Metabolic Disorders
1. Hyperparathyroidism
2. Hypothyroidism
3. Osteopetrosis (Albers-Schönberg disease)

Multiple Sclerosis (see Chapter 10)

Syringobulbia

Toxins

Trauma
1. Delayed
2. Immediate

Tumor
1. Glioma of brainstem (see Chapter 15)
2. Histiocytosis X
3. Leukemia
4. Meningeal carcinoma
5. Neurofibromatosis

Table 17–3 ◆ Neurologic Causes of Dysphagia

Autoimmune and Postinfectious 1. Dermatomyositis (see Chapter 7) 2. Guillain-Barré syndrome (see Chapter 7) 3. Idiopathic cranial polyneuropathy 4. Myasthenia gravis (see Chapter 15) 5. Transitory neonatal myasthenia gravis (see Chapter 6) **Congenital or Perinatal** 1. Aplasia of brainstem nuclei 2. Cerebral palsy (see Chapter 5) 3. Chiari malformation (see Chapter 10) 4. Syringobulbia	**Genetic** 1. Degenerative disorders (see Chapter 5) 2. Familial dysautonomia (see Chapter 6) 3. Familial infantile myasthenia (see Chapter 6) 4. Fiber-type disproportion myopathies (see Chapter 6) 5. Myotonic dystrophy (see Chapters 6 and 7) 6. Oculopharyngeal dystrophy **Glioma of Brainstem** **Infectious** 1. Botulism (see Chapters 6 and 7) 2. Diphtheria 3. Poliomyelitis (see Chapter 7) **Juvenile Progressive Bulbar Palsy**

Motor Unit Disorders

Disorders of the facial nuclei and nerves always produce ipsilateral facial weakness and atrophy, but associated features vary with site of abnormality:

1. Motor nucleus: Hyperacusis is present, but taste, lacrimation, and salivation are normal.
2. Facial nerve between the pons and the internal auditory meatus: Taste is spared, but lacrimation and salivation are impaired and hyperacusis is present.
3. Geniculate ganglion: Taste, lacrimation, and salivation are impaired, and hyperacusis is present.
4. Facial nerve from the geniculate ganglion to the stapedius nerve: Taste and salivation are impaired and hyperacusis is present, but lacrimation is normal.
5. Facial nerve from the stapedius nerve to the chorda tympani: Taste and salivation are impaired, hyperacusis is not present, and lacrimation is normal.
6. Facial nerve below the exit of the chorda tympani nerve: Only facial weakness is present.

Disturbances of cranial nerve nuclei seldom occur in isolation; they are often associated with other features of brainstem dysfunction (bulbar palsy). Usually some combination of dysarthria, dysphagia, and diplopia is present. Examination may reveal strabismus, facial diplegia, loss of gag reflex, atrophy of bulbar muscles, and fasciculations of the tongue.

The weakness of myasthenia gravis and facial myopathies is almost always bilateral, whereas brainstem disorders usually begin on one side but eventually cause bilateral impairment. Facial nerve palsies are usually unilateral. The differential di-

agnosis of recurrent facial palsy or dysphagia is limited to disorders of the facial nerve and neuromuscular junction (Table 17–4).

CONGENITAL FACIAL ASYMMETRY

Not all facial asymmetries observed at birth are traumatic in origin; some are due to congenital aplasia of muscle. Facial diplegia, whether complete or incomplete, suggests the Möbius syndrome or other congenital muscle aplasia. Complete unilateral palsies are likely to be traumatic in origin, whereas partial unilateral palsies may be either traumatic or aplastic. The term *neonatal facial asymmetry* is probably more accurate than *facial nerve palsy* to denote partial or complete unilateral facial weakness in the newborn and emphasizes the difficulty in differentiating traumatic nerve palsies from congenital aplasias.

Aplasia of Facial Muscles

Clinical Features. The Möbius syndrome is the best-known congenital aplasia of facial nerve nuclei and facial muscles. Whether nerve or muscle aplasia is the primary event has not been established. Facial diplegia may occur alone, with bi-

Table 17–4 ◆ Causes of Recurrent Cranial Neuropathies and Palsy

1. Familial
   a. Isolated facial palsy
   b. Melkersson syndrome
2. Hypertensive facial palsy
3. Myasthenia gravis
4. Sporadic multiple cranial neuropathies
5. Toxins

lateral abducens palsies, or with involvement of several cranial nerves (Sudarshan and Goldie, 1985). Congenital malformations elsewhere in the body—dextrocardia, talipes equinovarus, absent pectoral muscle, and limb deformities—may be associated features. Unilateral facial weakness is unusual in the Möbius syndrome but has been reported with documented evidence of nuclear hypoplasia (Richter, 1960).

Diagnosis. Congenital facial diplegia is by definition a Möbius syndrome. Imaging studies of the brain are indicated in all such cases to determine whether other cerebral malformations are present. Causes other than primary malformation must be considered as well. Some cases are due to intrauterine toxins or structural disturbances of the brainstem, such as vascular malformation or infarction (Sudarshan and Goldie, 1985).

Electromyography (EMG) can help determine the timing of injury. Denervation potentials are present only if the facial nuclei or nerves were injured 2 to 6 weeks before the study. Facial muscles that are aplastic as a result of Möbius syndrome or nerve injury occurring early in gestation do not demonstrate active denervation.

Treatment.   No treatment is available.

Depressor Anguli Oris Muscle Aplasia

Clinical Features.   Isolated unilateral weakness of the depressor anguli oris muscle (DAOM) is the most common cause of facial asymmetry at birth (Nelson and Eng, 1972). One corner of the mouth fails to move downward when the child cries. All other facial movements are symmetric. The lower lip on the paralyzed side feels thinner to palpation, even at birth, suggesting antepartum hypoplasia.

Diagnosis.   Traumatic lesions of the facial nerve would not selectively injure nerve fibers to the DAOM and spare all other facial muscles. Electrodiagnostic studies aid in differentiating aplasia of the DAOM from traumatic injury. In aplasia the conduction velocity and latency of the facial nerve are normal. Fibrillations are not present at the site of the DAOM. Instead, motor unit potentials are absent or decreased in number.

Treatment.   No treatment is available or needed. The DAOM is not a significant component of facial expression in older children and adults, and its absence is not noticed.

Birth Injury

The overall incidence of partial or complete facial paralysis in newborns is approximately 0.3 per 1000 live births (McHugh et al, 1969). The incidence is 60 per 1000 live births when premature infants and breech deliveries are excluded (Hepner, 1951). These data suggest that facial palsy is most often encountered in full-term newborns delivered from cephalic presentation. The 6% incidence of facial nerve palsy among this group remains constant regardless of whether a forceps was applied. The relationship between the side of the facial palsy and the obstetric position is remarkably constant. Fetuses who lie in left occipital positions have left facial palsies; fetuses who lie in right occipital positions have right facial palsies (Hepner, 1951). The implication of this relationship is that traumatic facial nerve palsies in the newborn are the result of nerve compression against the sacrum during labor and not of misapplication of the forceps. Although the site of nerve compression is generally believed to be extracranial, beyond the point of emergence from the stylomastoid foramen, evidence suggests that the segment of nerve within the facial canal, without fracture of the thin overlying bone, can also sustain a compression injury (McHugh, 1963). Facial nerve injuries within the facial canal are often associated with hemotympanum.

Clinical Features.   The clinical expression of complete unilateral facial palsy in the newborn can be subtle and may not be apparent immediately after birth. Failure of eye closure on the affected side is the first noticeable sign of weakness. Only when the child cries does flaccid paralysis of all facial muscles become obvious. The eyeball rolls up behind the open lid, the nasolabial fold remains flat, and the corner of the mouth droops during crying. The normal side, which appears to pull and distort the face, may be thought to be paralyzed and the paralyzed side normal.

When paralysis of the facial nerve is partial, the orbicularis oculi is the muscle most frequently spared. In these injuries the compression site is usually over the parotid gland with sparing of nerve fibers that course upward just after leaving the stylomastoid foramen.

Diagnosis.   Facial asymmetry is diagnosed by observation of the crying newborn. The facial skin must be carefully examined for laceration. Otoscopic examination is useful to establish the presence of hemotympanum, and EMG demonstrates the severity of involvement of the facial nerve.

Treatment.   Prospective studies regarding the natural outcome of perinatal facial nerve injuries are not available. Most authors are optimistic and indicate a high rate of spontaneous recovery. The optimism may be warranted, but it is based on anecdotal experience alone. In the absence of data on long-term outcome, the efficacy of suggested therapeutic measures cannot be evaluated. Most newborns should not be subjected to surgical intervention unless the nerve is lacerated. In that event the best response is to reconstitute the nerve if possible or at least to allow the proximal stump a clear pathway toward regeneration by debridement of the wound.

CONGENITAL DYSPHAGIA

Congenital dysphagia is usually associated with infantile hypotonia and is therefore discussed in Chapter 6. Because the neuroanatomic substrates of swallowing and breathing are contiguous, congenital dysphagia and dyspnea are often concurrent (Alvord and Shaw, 1989). Isolated aplasia of cranial nerve nuclei subserving swallowing has not been documented, but I have seen one infant in whom the clinical syndrome was consistent with isolated aplasia.

AUTOIMMUNE AND POSTINFECTIOUS DISORDERS

Most cases of acute unilateral facial neuritis (Bell palsy) or bilateral facial neuritis (Guillain-Barré syndrome) are attributed to postinfectious demyelination of the nerve. The distinction between Bell palsy and the Guillain-Barré syndrome is not clear; 75% of patients with Bell palsy are found to have electrophysiologic evidence of neuritis on the clinically unaffected side (Safman, 1971). The Guillain-Barré syndrome (acute inflammatory demyelinating polyneuropathy) is discussed in Chapter 7.

Bell Palsy

Bell palsy is an acute idiopathic paralysis of one side of the face and is due to dysfunction of the facial nerve. In adults the pathogenesis is considered to be autoimmune demyelination or vascular insufficiency. Childhood cases are almost always considered to be immune mediated. The annual incidence is 2.7 per 100,000 in the first decade and 10.1 per 100,000 in the second (Katusic et al, 1986).

Clinical Features. A history of viral infection, usually upper respiratory, is recorded in many cases, but the frequency is not significantly greater than expected by chance. The initial feature of neuritis is often pain or tingling in the ear canal ipsilateral to the subsequent facial palsy. Sensory symptoms, when present, are usually mild and do not demand medical attention.

The palsy has an explosive onset and becomes maximal within hours. It may be noticed first by the child or the parents. The palsy affects all muscles on one side of the face. Half the face sags, enlarging the palpebral fissure. Weakness of the levator palpebrae muscle prevents closure of the lid. Efforts to use muscles of expression cause the face to pull to the normal side. Eating and drinking become difficult, and the dribbling of liquids from the weak corner of the mouth causes embarrassment.

The most commonly affected portion of the nerve is within the temporal bone; taste, lacrimation, and salivation are impaired, and hyperacusis is present. However, examination of all facial nerve functions in small children is difficult and precise localization is not critical to diagnosis or prognosis.

The muscles remain weak for 2 to 4 weeks, and then strength returns spontaneously. There are no prospective studies on the natural history of Bell palsy in children, but experience indicates that almost all patients recover completely.

Diagnosis. Every child with acute unilateral facial weakness must be fully examined to determine whether the palsy is an isolated abnormality. Mild facial weakness on the other side or the absence of tendon reflexes in the limbs suggests the possibility of Guillain-Barré syndrome. In such a case the child must be watched carefully for the development of progressive limb weakness.

Possible underlying causes (e.g., hypertension, infection, trauma) of facial nerve palsy should be excluded before the diagnosis of Bell palsy is considered satisfactory. The ear ipsilateral to the facial palsy should be examined for herpetic lesions (see later discussion of herpes zoster oticus). Computed tomography (CT) of the head is not indicated for every child with acute, isolated facial palsy. A more reasonable approach is to watch the child and recommend an imaging study if other neurologic disturbances develop or if the palsy does not begin to resolve within 1 month.

Treatment. If the blink reflex is absent, the cornea must be protected. The eye should be patched when the child is outside the home or at play, and artificial tears should be applied several times a day to keep the cornea moist.

The use of corticosteroids has been advocated on the basis of several controlled trials in adults (Brown, 1982; May et al, 1976; Wolf et al, 1978), but all of these trials were flawed by faulty study design (Burgess et al, 1984). The use of corticosteroids in children has no scientific basis, since their prognosis for complete spontaneous recovery is excellent. The clinician who elects to use corticosteroid therapy must first exclude hypertension or infection as an underlying cause of the disorder.

Idiopathic Cranial Polyneuropathy

As the name implies, idiopathic cranial neuropathy is of uncertain nosology. It is presumed to be a postinfectious syndrome, and some consider it to be an abortive form of the Guillain-Barré syndrome (Ropper, 1986).

Clinical Features.   Onset usually occurs in adulthood (Juncos and Beal, 1987). Most childhood cases occur in adolescence. Similar cases have been described in infants, but in many of these limb weakness subsequently developed and the disorder may actually have been infant botulism.

Constant, aching facial pain precedes weakness by hours or days in most cases. The pain is usually localized to the temple or frontal region but can be anywhere in the face. The weakness may develop all in a day or may evolve over several weeks. Extraocular motility is usually affected. Facial and trigeminal nerve disturbances occur in half of cases, but lower cranial nerve involvement is uncommon. Occasional patients have transitory visual disturbances, ptosis, pupillary abnormalities, and tinnitus. Tendon reflexes in the limbs remain active.

Recurrences, even multiple, of idiopathic cranial neuropathies are reported in adults (Kansu et al, 1983). These are sporadic cases. Recurrent cranial neuropathies with childhood onset are more likely to be familial.

Diagnosis.   The differential diagnosis includes the Guillain-Barré syndrome, infant and childhood forms of botulism, brainstem glioma, juvenile progressive bulbar palsy, pontobulbar palsy with deafness, and the Tolosa-Hunt syndrome. Preservation of tendon reflexes in idiopathic cranial polyneuropathy is the major feature distinguishing it from the Guillain-Barré syndrome. Botulism can be separated clinically by its prominent autonomic dysfunction and limb weakness (see Chapters 6 and 7). Cranial nerve dysfunction in patients with brainstem glioma, juvenile progressive bulbar palsy, and pontobulbar palsy with deafness usually evolves over a longer period. The Tolosa-Hunt syndrome of painful ophthalmoplegia and idiopathic cranial polyneuropathy shares many features and may be a variant of the same disease process (see Chapter 15).

All laboratory findings are normal. Magnetic resonance imaging (MRI) of the brainstem should be performed in all cases to exclude the possibility of a brainstem glioma. Examination of the cerebrospinal fluid occasionaly reveals a mild elevation of protein concentration and a lymphocyte count of 5 or 6/mm^3.

Treatment.   The disease is self-limited, and full recovery is expected 2 to 4 months from onset. Corticosteroids are used routinely and are believed to relieve facial pain and shorten the course. The relief of pain may be dramatic, but evidence documenting a shortened course is lacking.

GENETIC DISORDERS
Facioscapulohumeral Syndrome

The facioscapulohumeral (FSH) syndrome, which is discussed in Chapter 7, has a rare infantile form. All forms of the disease are transmitted by autosomal dominant inheritance.

Clinical Features.   Onset of infantile FSH syndrome occurs usually during infancy and no later than age 5 (Bailey et al, 1986). Facial diplegia, the first symptom, may be misdiagnosed as a congenital aplasia of facial muscles when the onset is in infancy. Later, nasal speech and sometimes ptosis develop. Progressive proximal weakness begins 1 to 2 years after onset, first affecting the shoulders and then the pelvis. Pseudohypertrophy of the calves may be present. Tendon reflexes are depressed and then absent in weak muscle. Progression of weakness is rapid and unrelenting, leading to disability and death from respiratory insufficiency before age 20.

Coates syndrome (retinal telangiectasia) and hearing impairment may be associated with infantile FSH dystrophy (Taylor et al, 1982; Voit et al, 1986). In such cases children have the triad of hearing loss, visual impairment, and facial weakness.

Diagnosis.   The diagnosis should be suspected in any child with progressive facial diplegia. A family history of FSH dystrophy cannot always be obtained because the defect may be only minimally expressed in the affected parent.

Myasthenia gravis and brainstem glioma are the major entities that produce progressive facial diplegia in infants. The serum concentration of creatine kinase is helpful in differentiating these disorders. It is usually five to ten times the upper limit of normal in infantile FSH dystrophy and is normal in myasthenia gravis and brainstem glioma.

Electrophysiologic studies reveal brief, small-amplitude polyphasic potentials in weak muscles and a normal response to repetitive nerve stimulation.

Treatment.   No treatment is available.

Oculopharyngeal Muscular Dystrophy

Oculopharyngeal muscular dystrophy is transmitted by autosomal dominant inheritance and is often described in families of French-Canadian descent (Little and Perl, 1982), although it is not restricted to any ethnic group. Many cases of oculopharyngeal muscular dystrophy will prove to be mitochondrial myopathies (Pauzner et al, 1991).

Clinical Features.   Onset usually occurs in the fourth decade but may take place as early as adolescence. The initial features are ptosis and dysphagia, followed by proximal weakness in the legs and external ophthalmoplegia. Eventually all skeletal muscle is affected, but smooth muscle and cardiac muscle are spared.

Childhood cases are more likely to begin as ptosis and external ophthalmoplegia without dysphagia (Bray et al, 1965). Facial weakness may be present as well. It is not clear whether early-onset cases with pure ocular myopathy are genetically distinct from late-onset cases of oculopharyngeal dystrophy.

Diagnosis.   Myasthenia gravis must be excluded by an edrophonium chloride (Tensilon) test and repetitive nerve stimulation. Serum concentration of creatine kinase is normal, but EMG of affected muscles demonstrates brief, small-amplitude polyphasic potentials. The presence of ragged-red fibers on muscle biopsy indicates an underlying mitochondrial myopathy.

Treatment.   Therapy is directed at the symptoms. Ptosis can be corrected by levator palpebrae shortening, and dysphagia may be helped by constrictor or cricopharyngeal myotomy.

Melkersson Syndrome

At least 2% of facial palsies are recurrent (Yanagihara et al, 1984). Autosomal dominant inheritance with variable expression is suspected in most cases. Some members of a kindred may have only recurrent facial nerve palsy, whereas others have recurrent neuropathies of the facial and ocular motor nerves (Aldrich et al, 1984).

The Melkersson syndrome may be genetically distinct from other recurrent facial palsies but could also represent the concurrence of several linked genetic errors such as recurrent facial palsy, lingua plicata (deeply furrowed tongue), and migraine.

Clinical Features.   Melkersson syndrome is a rare disorder characterized by the triad of recurrent facial palsy, lingua plicata, and facial edema (Levenson et al, 1984). Attacks of facial palsy usually begin in the second decade, but the deeply furrowed tongue is present from birth.

The first attack of facial weakness is indistinguishable from Bell palsy except that it may be preceded by a migrainelike headache. Subsequent attacks are associated with facial edema, which is soft, painless, nonerythematous, and nonpruritic. The edema is most often asymmetric, involving only the upper lip on the paralyzed side, but may affect the cheek and eyelid of one or both sides. Attacks of facial swelling may be precipitated by cold weather or emotional stress and are not coincident with attacks of facial palsy.

Lingua plicata is present in 30% to 50% of cases. Furrowing and deep grooving on the dorsal surface of the tongue are permanent from birth. This feature is transmitted by autosomal dominant inheritance and occurs as an isolated finding in some families.

Diagnosis.   Melkersson syndrome can be diagnosed when two features of the triad are present. It should be considered in any child with a personal or family history of recurrent facial palsy or recurrent facial edema. The presence of lingua plicata in any member of the kindred confirms the diagnosis.

Treatment.   This disease has no established treatment. Corticosteroids have not proved beneficial.

HYPERTENSION

Unilateral facial palsy may be a feature of malignant hypertension in children (Lloyd et al, 1966). The palsy is caused by swelling and hemorrhage into the facial canal.

Clinical Features.   The course of the facial paralysis is indistinguishable from that in Bell palsy. The nerve is compressed in its proximal segment, impairing lacrimation, salivation, and taste. The onset coincides with a rise in blood pressure to greater than 120 mm Hg, and recovery begins when pressure is reduced. The duration of palsy varies from days to weeks. Recurrences are associated with repeated episodes of hypertension.

Diagnosis.   The occurrence of facial palsy in a child with known hypertension suggests that the hypertension is out of control. Blood pressure should be measured in every child thought to have Bell palsy.

Treatment.   Control of hypertension is the only effective treatment.

INFECTION

The facial nerve is sometimes involved when bacterial infection spreads from the middle ear to the mastoid. External otitis may lead to facial nerve involvement by spread of infection from the tympanic membrane to the chorda tympani.

Diphtheria may cause single or multiple cranial neuropathies from a direct effect of its toxin. Facial palsy, dysarthria, and dysphagia are potential complications.

Basilar meningitis, from tuberculosis or other bacterial infections, causes inflammation of cranial nerves as they leave the brain and enter the skull. Multiple and bilateral cranial nerve involvement is usually progressive.

Herpes Zoster Oticus (Ramsay Hunt Syndrome)

Herpes zoster oticus is a rare disorder caused by herpes zoster infection of the geniculate ganglion.

Clinical Features.   The initial feature is pain in and behind the ear. This pain is more severe and persistent than that expected with Bell palsy. Unilateral facial palsy, which cannot be distinguished from Bell palsy by appearance, follows. However, examination of the ipsilateral ear, especially in the fossa of the helix and behind the lobule, shows a vesicular eruption characteristic of herpes zoster (Aleksic et al, 1973).

Diagnosis.   The only historical feature distinguishing herpes zoster oticus from Bell palsy is the severity of ear pain. Examination of the ear for vesicles is critical to the diagnosis. Herpes zoster is uncommon in childhood, and the possibility of an immunosuppressed state must be considered.

Treatment.   Herpes zoster infections are self-limited but painful. Oral acyclovir, 800 mg five times a day, has been found beneficial in adults to shorten the course of disease and reduce pain (Huff et al, 1988).

Sarcoidosis

Cranial nerve dysfunction with sarcoidosis is usually due to basilar meningitis, but the facial nerve may also be involved when parotitis is present.

Clinical Features.   Onset is usually in the third decade but may be as early as adolescence. Neurologic manifestations develop in only 5% of patients with sarcoidosis but when present are often an early feature of the disease. Facial nerve palsy, unilateral or bilateral, is the single most common manifestation (Stern et al, 1985). Visual impairment or deafness is next in frequency. Single cranial neuropathies are present in 73% and multiple cranial neuropathies in 58%. Any cranial nerve except the accessory nerve may be involved. Systemic features of sarcoidosis are demonstrable in almost every case: intrathoracic involvement is present in 81%, and ocular involvement is present in 50%.

Uveoparotitis is an uncommon manifestation of sarcoidosis. The patient ordinarily comes to medical attention because of visual impairment and a painful eye. The mouth is dry and the parotid gland swollen. Facial nerve compression and palsy are present in 40% of cases.

Diagnosis.   Sarcoidosis should be considered in any patient with single or multiple cranial neuropathies. The suspicion is confirmed by documentation of multisystem disease. Radiographs of the chest establish the diagnoses or at least are compatible with it in 94% of patients with neurologic manifestations. The Kveim skin test is positive in almost all cases, but the antigen is not always readily available and interpretation requires experience (Sharma, 1983). Increased concentrations of serum angiotensin-converting enzyme are detected in approximately 75% of patients with active pulmonary disease. Biopsy of lymph nodes or other affected tissues provides histologic confirmation.

Treatment.   Prednisone, 0.5 to 1 mg/kg/day, should be maintained until a clinical response is evident and then tapered at a slow enough rate to prevent relapse. The prognosis for neurologic complications of sarcoidosis is good without treatment, but corticosteroids appear to hasten recovery.

JUVENILE PROGRESSIVE BULBAR PALSY

Juvenile progressive bulbar palsy, also known as *Fazio-Londe disease,* is a motor neuron disease limited to bulbar muscles. Most cases are sporadic, but heredofamilial cases have been reported (Albers et al, 1983). No specific genetic mode of transmission has been identified.

Clinical Features.   Age at onset is usually in the second decade. The initial feature may be facial weakness, dysphagia, or dysarthria. Eventually all the lower motor cranial nerve nuclei are affected, but the ocular motor nerve nuclei are spared. Fasciculations and atrophy of the arms are reported in some cases, but these patients may have a different disease. In most patients bulbar atrophy is severe but limb muscles are spared and tendon reflexes are normal.

Diagnosis.   The major diagnostic considerations are myasthenia gravis and brainstem glioma. These must be excluded with a Tensilon test and

MRI of the brainstem. EMG is useful to demonstrate active denervation of facial muscles with sparing of the limbs and normal repetitive stimulation of nerves.

Children with rapidly progressive motor neuron disease affecting the face and limbs should be considered to have a childhood form of amyotrophic lateral sclerosis.

Treatment. The disorder is often devastating. A previously normal child is no longer able to speak intelligibly or swallow. Feeding gastrostomy is soon required. The child needs considerable psychologic support. No treatment is available for the underlying disease.

METABOLIC DISORDERS
Hyperparathyroidism

The most common neurologic manifestations of primary hyperparathyroidism are headache and confusion (see Chapter 2). Occasionally a syndrome that is similar to amyotrophic lateral sclerosis and includes ataxia and internuclear ophthalmoplegia may develop (Patten and Pages, 1984). Dysarthria and dysphagia are prominent features.

Hypothyroidism

Cranial nerve abnormalities are unusual in hypothyroidism. Deafness is the most common manifestation, but acute facial nerve palsy resembling Bell palsy is occasionally described.

Osteopetrosis (Albers-Schönberg Disease)

Osteopetrosis is a genetic disease transmitted by autosomal recessive inheritance. The calvarium becomes thickened, and cranial nerves are compressed and compromised as they pass through the bone. Deafness and facial diplegia are common manifestations.

SYRINGOBULBIA

Syringobulbia is usually the medullary extension of a cervical syrinx (see Chapter 12) but may also originate in the medulla. In most cases it involves the nucleus ambiguus and the spinal tract and the motor nucleus of the trigeminal nerve. Swallowing and chewing are impaired.

TOXINS

Most neurotoxins produce either diffuse encephalopathy or peripheral neuropathy. Only eth-ylene glycol, trichlorethylene, and chlorocresol have been associated with selective toxicity to cranial nerves.

Ethylene glycol is used as an antifreeze. Ingestion produces facial diplegia, hearing impairment, and dysphagia (Mallya et al, 1986). Trichlorethylene intoxication may produce multiple cranial neuropathies but has a predilection for the trigeminal nerve (Feldman et al, 1970) and was previously used in the treatment of tic douloureux.

Chlorocresol, a compound used in the industrial production of heparin, produced recurrent unilateral facial palsy in an exposed worker (Dossing et al, 1986). Inhalation of the compound caused tingling of one side of the face followed by weakness of the muscles. The neurologic disturbance was brief, relieved by exposure to fresh air, and could be reproduced experimentally.

TRAUMA

Facial palsy following closed head injury is usually associated with bleeding from the ear and fracture of the petrous bone (Maiman et al, 1985; Puvanendren et al, 1977).

Clinical Features. The onset of palsy may be immediate or may be delayed for as long as 3 weeks after injury. In most cases the interval is between 2 and 7 days. The mechanism of delay is unknown.

Diagnosis. Electrophysiologic studies are helpful in prognosis. If the nerve is intact but demonstrates a conduction block, recovery usually begins within 5 days and is complete. The majority of patients with partial denervation recover full facial movement but have evidence of aberrant reinnervation. Full recovery is not expected when denervation is complete.

Treatment. The management of traumatic facial palsy is controversial. Some authors have recommended surgical decompression and corticosteroids, but no evidence supporting either mode of therapy is available.

TUMORS

Tumors of the facial nerve are rare in children. The major neoplastic cause of facial palsy is brainstem glioma (see Chapter 15), followed by tumors that infiltrate the meninges, such as leukemia, meningeal carcinoma, and histiocytosis X. Acoustic neuromas are unusual in childhood and are limited to children with neurofibromatosis type 2. These neuromas cause hearing impairment before facial palsy and are discussed in the next section.

◆ Hearing Impairment and Deafness

ANATOMIC CONSIDERATIONS

Sound is funneled through the external auditory canal to the tympanic membrane, causing it to vibrate. The vibrations are transmitted by ossicles to the oval window of the cochlea, the sensory organ of hearing. The air-filled space from the tympanic membrane to the cochlea is the middle ear. The membranous labyrinth within the osseous labyrinth is the principal structure of the inner ear. It contains the cochlea, the semicircular canals, and the vestibule. The semicircular canals and vestibule are the sensory organs of vestibular function. The cochlea consists of three fluid-filled canals wound into a snail-like configuration.

The organ of Corti is the transducer within the cochlea that converts mechanical to electrical energy. Impulses are transmitted in the auditory portion of the eighth nerve to the ipsilateral cochlear nuclei of the medulla. The cochlear nuclei on each side transmit information to both superior olivary nuclei, causing bilateral representation of hearing throughout the remainder of the central pathways. From the superior olivary nuclei, impulses are transmitted by the lateral lemniscus to the inferior colliculus. Further cross-connections occur in collicular synapses. Rostrally directed fibers from the inferior colliculi ascend to the medial geniculate and auditory cortex of the temporal lobe.

SYMPTOMS OF AUDITORY DYSFUNCTION

The major symptoms of disturbance in the auditory pathways are hearing impairment, tinnitus, and hyperacusis. Hearing impairment is characterized in infants by failure to develop speech (see Chapter 5) and in older children by inattentiveness and poor school performance.

Fifty percent of infants use words with meaning by 12 months and join words into sentences by 21 months. Failure to accomplish these tasks by 21 months and 3 years, respectively, is always abnormal (Neligan and Prudham, 1969).

Hearing Impairment

Hearing impairment is classified as conductive, sensorineural (perceptive), or central. *Conductive hearing impairment* results from disturbances in the external or middle ear; the mechanical vibrations that make up the sensory input of hearing are not faithfully delivered to the inner ear because the external canal is blocked or the tympanic membrane or ossicles are abnormal. The major defect in hearing is sound amplification. Patients with conductive hearing impairment are better able to hear loud speech in a noisy background than soft speech in a quiet background.

Sensorineural hearing impairment results from disturbances of the cochlea or auditory nerve. The frequency content of sound is improperly analyzed and transduced. High frequencies may be selectively lost. Individuals with sensorineural hearing impairment have difficulty discriminating speech when there is background noise.

Central hearing impairment results from disturbance of the cochlear nuclei or their projections to the cortex. With lesions in the brainstem, hearing impairment is usually bilateral. Cortical lesions lead to difficulty in processing information. Pure tone audiometry is normal, but speech discrimination is impaired by background noise or competing messages.

Thirty percent of childhood deafness is clearly genetic in origin, 40% is acquired, and the remaining 30% is idiopathic. Probably many of the idiopathic cases are also genetic (Beighton, 1990).

Tinnitus

Tinnitus is the illusion of noise in the ear. The noise is usually high pitched and constant. In most cases tinnitus is caused by disturbances of the auditory nerve, but it may occur as a simple partial seizure originating from the primary auditory cortex. Sounds generated by the cardiovascular system (heartbeat and bruit) are sometimes audible, especially while a person is lying down, but should not be confused with tinnitus.

Hyperacusis

The term "hyperacusis" is sometimes used to denote an exaggerated startle response, but I believe that its use should be reserved for failure of the stapedius muscle to dampen sound by its effect on the ossicles. This occurs when the chorda tympani branch of the facial nerve is damaged (see the discussion of Bell palsy earlier in this chapter).

APPROACH TO THE PATIENT

Hearing assessment in the office is satisfactory for severe hearing impairment but is unsatisfactory for detecting loss of specific frequency bands. The speech and hearing handicap generated by a high-frequency hearing impairment should not be underestimated.

When testing an infant the physician should stand behind the patient and provide interesting sounds to each ear. Such sounds could be produced by bells, chimes, rattles, or a tuning fork. Dropping a large object and watching the infant and parents startle from the noise is not a test of hearing. Once the infant sees the source of the interesting sound or hears it several times, interest is lost. Therefore different high-frequency and low-frequency sounds should be used for each ear. The normal responses of the infant are to become alert and to look for the source of the sound.

Older children can be tested by observing their response to spoken words at different intensities and with tuning forks that provide pure tones of different frequencies. The *Rinne test* compares air conduction (conductive plus sensorineural hearing) with bone conduction (sensorineural hearing). A tuning fork is held against the mastoid process until the sound fades and is then held 1 inch from the ear. Normal children hear the vibration produced by air conduction twice as long as that produced by bone conduction. Impaired air conduction with normal bone conduction indicates a conductive hearing loss.

The *Weber test* compares bone conduction in the two ears. A tuning fork is placed at the center of the forehead, and the patient is asked whether sound is perceived equally in both ears. A normal response is to hear the sound in the center of the head. If bone conduction is normal in both ears, sound is localized to an ear with impaired air conduction because the normal blocking response of air conduction is lacking. If a sensorineural hearing impairment is present in one ear, bone conduction is perceived in the good ear.

Otoscopic examination is imperative in every child with hearing problems or tinnitus. The cause may be seen through the speculum in the form of impacted wax, otitis media, perforated tympanic membrane, or cholesteatoma.

TESTS OF HEARING
Pure Tone Audiometry

Selected frequencies are presented by earphones (air conduction) or by a vibrator applied to the mastoid (bone conduction), and the subject is asked to determine the minimum level perceived for each frequency. Normal hearing levels are defined by an international standard. The test can be performed adequately only in children old enough to cooperate. With conductive hearing impairment, air conduction is abnormal and bone conduction is normal; with sensorineural hearing impairment, both are abnormal; and with central hearing impairment, both are normal.

Speech Tests

The *speech reception threshold* measures the intensity at which a subject can repeat 50% of presented words. The *speech discrimination test* measures the subject's ability to understand speech at normal conversational levels. Both tests are abnormal out of proportion to pure tone loss with auditory nerve disease, abnormal in proportion to pure tone loss with cochlear disease, and normal with conductive and central hearing loss.

Special Tests

Cochlear lesions may produce *diplacusis* and *recruitment*. Auditory nerve lesions produce *tone decay*. Diplacusis is a distortion of pure tones so that the subject perceives a mixture of tones. With recruitment the sensation of loudness increases at an abnormally rapid rate as the intensity of sound is increased. Tone decay is diminished perception of a suprathreshold tone with time.

Brainstem Auditory Evoked Response

The brainstem auditory evoked response (BAER) is used to test hearing and the integrity of the brainstem auditory pathways in infants and small children. No cooperation is required, and sedation improves the accuracy of results.

When each ear is stimulated with repetitive clicks and simultaneous recordings are made from an electrode over the ipsilateral mastoid referenced to the forehead, five waves are recorded (Figure 17–1). Wave I is generated by the acoustic nerve, wave II by the cochlear nerve, wave III by the superior olivary complex, wave IV by the lateral lemniscus, and wave V by the inferior colliculus. Several authors have published normal values for the absolute latency of waves I and V; the values of Despland and Galambos (1980) are summarized in Table 17–5.

The BAER first appears at a conceptional age of 26 to 27 weeks. The absolute latencies of waves I and V and the V-I interpeak interval decline progressively with advancing conceptional age. The latency of wave V bears an inverse relationship to the intensity of the stimulus and can be used to test hearing.

An initial test is performed with a stimulus intensity of 70 dB. If wave V is not produced, hearing is impaired and the test should be repeated at higher

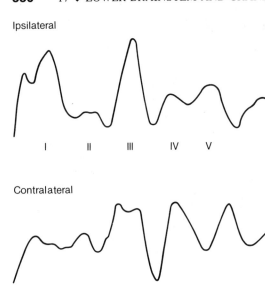

Ipsilateral

Contralateral

1.2 ms

Figure 17–1 Normal brainstem auditory evoked responses. The generators of the five positive waves are: I, acoustic nerve; II, cochlear nucleus; III, superior olivary complex; IV, lateral lemniscus; and V, inferior colliculus. (From Fenichel GM: Neonatal Neurology, 3rd edition. Churchill Livingstone, New York, 1990. By permission.)

intensities until a response threshold is found. If wave V is present, the test is repeated at sequential reductions of 10 dB until the lowest intensity capable of producing wave V—the hearing threshold—is established. Because the latency of wave V is proportional to the intensity of the stimulus, a latency-intensity curve can be drawn (Figure 17–2). In normal newborns the latency of wave V decreases by 0.24 to 0.44 ms for each 10 dB in sound intensity between 70 and 110 dB (Stockard et al, 1983).

In children with conductive hearing impairment the time required to transmit sound across the middle ear and activate the cochlea is prolonged and the total amount of sound energy is reduced. As a consequence the latency of wave I is prolonged and the latency-intensity curve of wave V shifts to the right by an amount equivalent to the hearing impairment, without any alteration in the slope of the curve.

In children with sensorineural hearing impairment the latency-intensity curve of wave V is shifted to the right because of the hearing impairment and in addition the slope of the curve becomes steeper, exceeding 0.55 ms/dB.

CONGENITAL DEAFNESS

Congenital deafness is often missed in the newborn unless there is an obvious deformity of the external ear or a family history of genetic hearing loss. Congenital ear malformations are present in approximately 2% of newborns with congenital deafness (Fraser, 1964), and genetic factors are responsible for 35% of cases (Konigsmark and Gorlin, 1976). If profound deafness of early onset is included, genetic causes account for 50%.

Table 17–5 ◆ Brainstem Auditory Evoked Response Latencies

Conceptional Age (weeks)		Wave I (ms)	Wave V (ms)	V-I Interval (ms)
30-31	Mean	3.50	9.10	5.60
	±3 SD	5.09	10.06	7.25
32-33	Mean	2.78	8.36	5.62
	±3 SD	3.44	9.98	6.52
34-35	Mean	2.56	8.00	5.44
	±3 SD	3.31	9.41	6.41
36-37	Mean	2.53	7.80	5.27
	±3 SD	3.10	9.42	6.41
38-39	Mean	2.30	7.42	5.09
	±3 SD	3.02	8.71	6.06
40-41	Mean	2.28	7.35	5.07
	±3 SD	3.09	8.73	6.30
42-43	Mean	2.28	7.17	4.89
	±3 SD	2.88	7.47	5.49

Stimulus intensity is 60 dB above adult threshold, and stimulus frequency is 10 per second.
SD, Standard deviation.

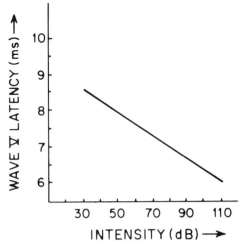

Figure 17–2 Wave V latency-intensity curve. In full-term newborns the latency of wave V decreases about 0.3 ms for each intensity increase of 10 dB. (From Fenichel GM: Neonatal Neurology, 3rd edition. Churchill Livingstone, New York, 1990. By permission.)

Aplasia of Inner Ear

Inner ear aplasia is always associated with auditory nerve abnormalities. There are three main types:

1. Michel defect, complete absence of the otic capsule and eighth cranial nerve
2. Mondini defect, incomplete development of the bony and membranous labyrinths and dysgenesis of the spiral ganglion
3. Scheibe defect, dysplasia of the membranous labyrinth and atrophy of the eighth nerve

Chromosome Disorders

Hearing impairment is relatively uncommon in children with chromosomal disorders. Abnormalities of chromosome 18 are often associated with profound sensorineural hearing loss and malformations of the external ear.

Genetic Disorders
Isolated Deafness

Isolated deafness in newborns and infants is usually genetic and may be transmitted by autosomal dominant, autosomal recessive, or X-linked inheritance. In many sporadic cases the hearing loss proves to be transmitted by autosomal recessive inheritance.

The association of congenital deafness and external ear deformities is often caused by genetic disorders transmitted by autosomal dominant inheritance, but chromosomal disorders and fetal exposure to drugs and toxins must be considered as well. Maternal use of heparin during pregnancy produces an embryopathy characterized by skeletal deformities, flattening of the nose, cerebral dysgenesis, and deafness (Hall et al, 1980).

In the absence of external malformation, a sporadic case of deafness may not be suspected until the infant fails to develop speech. Intrauterine infection with cytomegalovirus is an important cause of congenital deafness (see Chapter 5). Nearly 1% of newborns in the United States are infected with cytomegalovirus, and sensorineural hearing loss develops in approximately 10% (Bale, 1984). In the past, rubella embryopathy was an important cause, but it has been almost eliminated in the United States by mass vaccination.

Pendred Syndrome

Pendred syndrome is a genetic defect in thyroxine synthesis transmitted by autosomal recessive inheritance (Konigsmark and Gorlin, 1976). It is characterized by goiter and sensorineural hearing impairment.

Clinical Features. Sensorineural hearing impairment is present at birth and is severe in 50% of cases. Milder hearing impairment may not be detected until the child is 2 years of age. Vestibular function may also be impaired.

A diffuse, nonnodular goiter becomes apparent during the first decade, often in infancy. No clinical signs of hypothyroidism are present. Growth and intelligence are usually normal.

Diagnosis. The laboratory method for assessing iodide organification is the perchlorate discharge test. It is a measure of thyroidal radioactive iodine content following the administration of potassium perchlorate. A decline of 10% or more from baseline levels of thyroidal radioactive iodine is considered a positive result.

Treatment. Goiter is best treated medically and not surgically. Exogenous hormone decreases production of thyroid-stimulating hormone with subsequent reduction in goiter size. Hearing loss is not reversible.

Usher Syndrome

The Usher syndrome, characterized by congenital deafness and retinitis pigmentosa, is believed to be transmitted by autosomal recessive inheritance, but there is probably genetic heterogeneity (McLeod et al, 1971).

Clinical Features. Bilateral severe sensorineural deafness is present at birth. Slowly progressive loss of vision caused by retinitis pigmentosa begins during the second decade and leads to blindness in the fifth decade or later. Vestibular responses to caloric testing are absent, and mild ataxia may be present. Mental retardation is present in 25% of cases.

Diagnosis. The combination of retinitis pigmentosa and hearing impairment is also present in other syndromes: *Alström syndrome*, obesity and diabetes mellitus; *Cockayne syndrome* (see Chapter 16); *Laurence-Moon-Biedl syndrome*, mental deficiency, hypogonadism, obesity; and *Refsum disease* (see Chapter 7). Usher syndrome is the only one in which profound deafness is present at birth.

Treatment. Deafness is too profound to be corrected with hearing aids. No treatment is available.

ACQUIRED HEARING IMPAIRMENT
Drug-Induced Impairment

Antibiotics are the most commonly used class of drugs with potential ototoxicity in children (Snavely and Hodges, 1984). The incidence of toxic reactions is greatest with amikacin, furosemide, and vancomycin and only a little less with kanamycin and neomycin. Permanent damage is unusual with any of these drugs. The characteristic syndrome consists of tinnitus and high-frequency hearing impairment. Vancomycin produces hearing loss only when blood concentrations exceed 45 μg/ml.

By contrast, aminoglycosides may produce irreversible cochlear toxicity, which begins as tinnitus, progresses to vertigo and high-frequency hearing impairment, and finally impairs all frequencies. This is of special concern in sick preterm newborns who are given aminoglycosides for 15 days or longer (Pettigrew et al, 1988).

Beta-adrenoceptor blocking drugs are a rare cause of hearing impairment and tinnitus (Faldt et al, 1984). Cessation of therapy reverses symptoms. Cisplatin, an anticancer drug, has ototoxic effects in 30% of recipients (Rozencweig et al, 1977). Tinnitus is the major feature. Hearing impairment occurs at frequencies above those used for speech.

Salicylates tend to concentrate in the perilymph of the labyrinth and are ototoxic. Tinnitus and high-frequency hearing impairment result from long-term exposure to high doses.

Genetic Neurologic Disorders

Several of the disorders listed in Table 17–6 are discussed in other chapters. Sensorineural hearing impairment occurs as part of several spinocerebellar degenerations, hereditary motor sensory neuropathies, and sensory autonomic neuropathies. It is a major feature of Refsum disease (hereditary motor sensory neuropathy type IV) and can be controlled by dietary measures to reduce serum concentrations of phytanic acid (Djupesland et al, 1983).

Pontobulbar Palsy with Deafness

A rare motor neuron disorder transmitted by autosomal recessive inheritance, pontobulbar palsy with deafness shares many clinical features with juvenile progressive bulbar palsy, and some cases may be variant expressions of the same genetic error (Brucher et al, 1981).

Clinical Features. Onset most often occurs during the second decade. Progressive sensorineural hearing loss is the initial symptom and may affect first one ear and then the other. Deafness is accompanied or quickly followed by facial weakness and dysphagia. Tongue atrophy occurs in most cases, but masseter and ocular motor nerve palsies are uncommon.

Approximately half of patients have evidence of pyramidal tract dysfunction, such as extensor plantar responses, and half have atrophy and fasciculations of limb muscle. Loss of tendon reflexes is an early feature of most cases.

Respiratory insufficiency is a common feature and a frequent cause of death.

Diagnosis. The presence of deafness and areflexia distinguishes pontobulbar palsy from juvenile progressive bulbar palsy but can also suggest a hereditary motor sensory neuropathy if symptoms of bulbar palsy are delayed. The diagnosis depends on the clinical features and cannot be confirmed by laboratory tests. MRI of the brainstem should be performed to exclude the possibility of tumor.

Treatment. A feeding gastrostomy is needed in most patients. No treatment is available for the underlying disease.

Infectious Diseases

Otitis media is a common cause of reversible conductive hearing impairment in children, but only rarely does suppurative infection spread to the inner ear (see "Vertigo" later in this chapter). Hearing impairment is a relatively common symptom of viral encephalitis (see Chapter 2) and may be an early feature (Rosenberg, 1984). Sudden hearing loss may also accompany childhood exanthems (chickenpox, mumps, measles), and in such cases

Table 17-6 ◆ Hearing Impairment and Deafness

Congenital
1. Aplasia of inner ear
   a. Michel defect
   b. Mondini defect
   c. Scheibe defect
2. Chromosome disorders
   a. Trisomy 13
   b. Trisomy 18
   c. 18q − syndrome
3. Genetic disorders
   a. Isolated deafness
   b. Pendred syndrome
   c. Usher syndrome
4. Intrauterine viral infection (see Chapter 5)
5. Maternal drug use

Drugs
1. Antibiotics
2. Beta-blockers
3. Chemotherapy

Genetic Neurologic Disorders
1. Facioscapulohumeral dystrophy (see Chapter 7)
2. Familial spastic paraplegia (see Chapter 12)
3. Hereditary motor sensory neuropathies (see Chapter 7)
4. Hereditary sensory autonomic neuropathies (see Chapter 9)
5. Infantile Refsum disease (see Chapter 16)
6. Neurofibromatosis type 2 (see "Acoustic Neuroma")
7. Pontobulbar palsy with deafness
8. Mitochondrial disorders (see Chapter 8)
9. Spinocerebellar degenerations (see Chapter 10)
10. Xeroderma pigmentosum (see Chapter 5)

Infectious Diseases
1. Bacterial meningitis
2. Otitis media (see "Vertigo")
3. Sarcoidosis (see "Facial Weakness")
4. Viral encephalitis (see Chapter 2)
5. Viral exanthems

Metabolic Disorders
1. Hypothyroidism
2. Ménière disease (see "Vertigo")

Skeletal Disorders
1. Apert acrocephalosyndactyly
2. Cleidocranial dysostosis
3. Craniofacial dysostosis (Crouzon disease)
4. Craniometaphyseal dysplasia (Pyle disease)
5. Klippel-Feil syndrome
6. Mandibulofacial dysostosis (Treacher Collins syndrome)
7. Osteogenesis imperfecta
8. Osteopetrosis (Albers-Schönberg disease)

Trauma (see "Vertigo")

Tumor
1. Acoustic neuroma
2. Cholesteatoma (see "Vertigo")

---

virus can be isolated from the cochlear and auditory nerves.

The overall incidence of persistent unilateral or bilateral hearing loss in children with acute bacterial meningitis is 10% (Dodge et al, 1984). The risk can be reduced by early treatment with dexamethasone (see Chapter 4). *Streptococcus pneumoniae* meningitis is also associated with a 20% incidence of persistent dizziness, gait ataxia, and other neurologic deficits (Bohr et al, 1984).

The site of disease is probably the inner ear or auditory nerve. Organisms may gain access to the inner ear from the subarachnoid space. Otitis media is the source of meningitis in many children and produces a transitory conductive hearing loss, but it has not been proved to cause permanent sensorineural hearing loss.

Toward the end of their hospitalization, all children with acute bacterial meningitis should undergo BAER audiometry to screen for hearing loss.

Metabolic Disorders

Ménière disease is characterized by vertigo, tinnitus, and hearing impairment. Vertigo is often the first feature (see later discussion of vertigo).

Tinnitus and decreased hearing are common features of hypothyroidism and are reversible by thyroid replacement therapy (Swanson et al, 1981).

Skeletal Disorders

The combination of hearing impairment and skeletal deformities almost always indicates a genetic disease. Skeletal disorders may be limited, usually to the face and digits, or generalized. The partial list in Table 17–6 highlights the more common syndromes. Almost all are transmitted by autosomal dominant inheritance with variable expression. The exceptions are osteopetrosis, which is transmitted by autosomal recessive inheritance;

craniometaphyseal dysplasia, which has both a dominant and a recessive form; and the Klippel-Feil anomaly, for which the pattern of transmission is uncertain.

Trauma

Acute auditory and vestibular injuries occur with fractures of the petrous portion of the temporal bone. Vestibular function is more likely to be impaired than auditory function (see "Vertigo" later in this chapter).

Tumor

Acoustic neuroma and cholesteatoma are the tumors most likely to impair children's hearing. Other cerebellopontine angle tumors are extremely rare before the third or fourth decade. Cholesteatoma is discussed in the section on vertigo.

Acoustic Neuroma

Acoustic neuromas are more properly classified as schwannomas of the eighth nerve. Only 6% of acoustic neuromas come to medical attention in the second decade, and even fewer are seen in the first decade. Children with acoustic neuroma almost always have *neurofibromatosis type 2 (NF2)*, a genetic disease distinct from neurofibromatosis type 1 (see Chapter 5), NF2 is transmitted by autosomal dominant inheritance with the locus on chromosome 22 (Wertelecki et al, 1988). NF2 is characterized by bilateral acoustic neuromas and the later development of other cerebral tumors such as meningioma, glioma, schwannoma, and juvenile posterior subcapsular lenticular opacity. Café au lait spots may be present on the skin but are fewer than five in number (Listernick and Charrow, 1990).

Clinical Features. Deafness or tinnitus is the usual first complaint. Approximately one third of patients have nonaudiologic symptoms, such as facial numbness or paresthesia, vertigo, headache, and ataxia (Hart et al, 1983). Hearing impairment is present in almost every patient; ipsilateral diminished corneal reflex occurs in half; and ataxia, facial hypesthesia or weakness, and nystagmus are found in 30% to 40%. Large tumors produce obstructive hydrocephalus with symptoms of increased intracranial pressure and brainstem compression.

Diagnosis. Every child with progressive hearing impairment or tinnitus should be carefully examined for café au lait spots on the skin. The family history should be explored for acoustic neuroma or other neurologic disturbance.

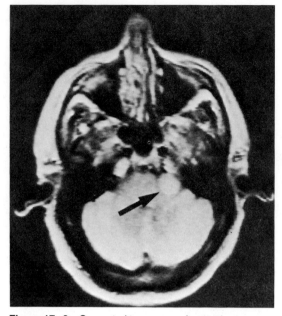

Figure 17–3 Computed tomogram of acoustic neuroma. A large tumor *(arrow)* is pressing on and displacing the brainstem.

Abnormalities in pure tone audiometry and in the BAER are present in almost every patient. Audiometry is consistent with a sensorineural hearing impairment. Small tumors produce ipsilateral prolongation of the V-I interval or absence of wave I of the BAER; large tumors cause absence of waves on the ipsilateral side and prolongation of the V-III interval on the contralateral side as a result of brainstem compression.

CT provides excellent visualization of tumors larger than 1.5 cm (Figure 17–3). The important CT findings are enlargement and erosion of the internal auditory canal and the presence of a mass in the cerebellopontine angle that is isodense with brain but that demonstrates contrast enhancement. Large tumors shift the brainstem and cause obstructive hydrocephalus.

Treatment. Acoustic neuromas must be resected, either by surgery or the photon (gamma ray) knife. Surgery sacrifices residual hearing and sometimes causes a facial palsy. Both functions can be preserved when the photon knife is used.

◆ Vertigo

Vertigo is the sensation of rotation or spinning. It can terrify small children. Balance is lost, and posture is difficult to maintain, giving the appearance of ataxia (see Chapter 10). Nausea and nystagmus are often associated features. When nystagmus is present, the fast phase is in the same direction as the perceived rotation. All symptoms are exacerbated by movement of the head.

ANATOMIC CONSIDERATIONS

The semicircular canals and the vestibule, within the labyrinth, are the sensory organs of the vestibular system. The stimulus for excitation of the semicircular canals is rotary motion of the head; for the vestibule it is gravity. Information from the sensory organs is transmitted by the vestibular portion of the eighth cranial nerve to the vestibular nuclei in the brainstem and the cerebellum. From the vestibular nuclei there are extensive connections to the cerebellum and medial longitudinal fasciculus. Cortical projections terminate in the superior temporal gyrus and frontal lobe.

APPROACH TO VERTIGO
History and Physical Examination

Patients complaining of dizziness or lightheadedness must be carefully questioned about the sensation of rotation. Whether the subject or the environment is perceived to rotate is irrelevant. The illusion of rotation separates vertigo from presyncope, ataxia, and other disturbances of balance and localizes the disturbance to the vestibular system. Vertigo implies dysfunction of the labyrinth or vestibular nerve (peripheral vertigo) or the brainstem or temporal lobe (central vertigo).

Important historical points to document include the course of vertigo (acute, recurrent, chronic), precipitating events (trauma, infection, position change), association of hearing impairment and tinnitus, drug exposure, cardiovascular disease, and family history of migraine.

Acute, episodic attacks of vertigo, not induced by motion, are most often caused by migraine or epilepsy, with migraine as the more common of the two. A single, prolonged attack of vertigo, especially when combined with nausea and vomiting, is usually due to infection of the labyrinth or vestibular nerve. Chronic vertigo often waxes and wanes and may seem intermittent rather than chronic. Both central and peripheral causes must be considered (Table 17–7), but the two are readily distinguished by their clinical and laboratory features (Table 17–8).

Special Tests

Caloric and audiometric testing is indicated for most children with chronic vertigo. Caloric testing

Table 17–7 ◆ Causes of Vertigo

1. Drugs and toxins
2. Epilepsy
   a. Complex partial seizures
   b. Simple partial seizures
3. Infectious
   a. Otitis media
   b. Vestibular neuronitis
4. Ménière disease
5. Migraine
   a. Benign paroxysmal vertigo (see Chapter 10)
   b. Benign recurrent vertigo
6. Motion sickness
7. Multiple sclerosis (see Chapter 10)
8. Psychogenic (hyperventilation syndrome) (see Chapter 1)
9. Trauma
   a. Migraine
   b. Posttraumatic neurosis
   c. Temporal bone fracture
   d. Vestibular concussion
   e. Whiplash injury

is described in this section and audiometric testing in the section on hearing impairment. The Nylen-Hallpike test is useful to define position-induced vertigo.

Caloric Testing

The simplest method of caloric testing is to instill small quantities of cool water into the external auditory canal with a rubber-tipped syringe. The canal must first be inspected to determine whether there is clear passage to an intact tympanic membrane. A sufficient quantity of water is used, depending on the child's size, to keep the tympanic membrane cooled for 20 seconds. The eyes are then observed for nystagmus. A normal response is slow deviation of the eyes to the side stimulated, followed by a fast component to the opposite side. If stimulation with cool water fails to produce a response, the procedure is repeated with ice water. Absence of nystagmus indicates absence of peripheral vestibular function. Partial dysfunction of one vestibular apparatus results in asymmetry of response (*directional preponderance*).

Electronystagmography

Electronystagmography is a technique that allows better quantification of caloric testing. A standard caloric stimulus is delivered into the ear, and the duration and velocity of nystagmus are recorded on paper by a machine designed for this purpose.

Table 17–8 ◆ Distinguishing Peripheral and Central Vertigo

Peripheral Vertigo	**Central Vertigo**
Clinical Features	***Clinical Features***
1. Hearing loss, tinnitus, and otalgia may be associated features.	1. Cerebellar and cranial nerve dysfunction are frequently associated.
2. Past pointing and falling in direction of unilateral disease occur.	2. Hearing is intact.
3. Ataxia occurs with eyes closed in bilateral disease.	3. Loss of consciousness may be associated.
4. Vestibular and positional nystagmus is present.	***Laboratory Features***
Laboratory Features	1. Pure tone audiometry and speech discrimination are normal.
1. Caloric testing reveals vestibular paresis, directional preponderance, or both.	2. Comprehension of competing messages is impaired.
2. Pure tone audiometry reveals sensorineural hearing loss.	3. Caloric testing may reveal directional preponderance but not vestibular paresis.
3. Recruitment is present with end organ disease and tone decay with nerve disease.	4. Brainstem evoked response, electroencephalography, computed tomography, or magnetic resonance imaging may be abnormal.

Nylen-Hallpike Test

In the Nylen-Hallpike test the patient is tilted backward from the sitting position to the supine position so that the head hangs down below the level of the examining table. The head is then turned 45 degrees to the right, and the eyes are observed for position-induced nystagmus. Several minutes later the maneuver is repeated with the head turned 45 degrees to the left, then repeated again with the head tilted 45 degrees backward.

CAUSES OF VERTIGO
Drugs

Many drugs that disturb vestibular function also disturb auditory function. This section deals only with drugs affecting vestibular function more than auditory function. Toxic doses of anticonvulsants and neuroleptics produce ataxia, incoordination, and measurable disturbances of vestibular function, but patients do not ordinarily complain of vertigo.

Antibiotics are the major class of drugs producing vestibular toxicity (Snavely and Hodges, 1984). Streptomycin, minocycline, and aminoglycosides are associated with a high incidence of toxic reactions, sulfonamides with a low incidence.

Streptomycin disturbs vestibular function but has little effect on hearing. A milligram-per-kilogram dose that produces toxic effects cannot be stated because of variation in individual susceptibility. However, the vestibular toxicity of streptomycin is so predictable at high doses that the drug

has been used to destroy vestibular function in patients with severe Ménière disease. Dihydrostreptomycin affects auditory function and spares vestibular function. It is so ototoxic that its use has been abandoned.

Minocycline produces nausea, vomiting, dizziness, and ataxia at standard therapeutic doses. Symptoms begin 2 to 3 days after initiation of therapy and cease 2 days after therapy is discontinued.

Gentamicin and other aminoglycosides have an adverse effect on both vestibular and auditory function. Some disturbance is noted in 2% of patients treated with gentamicin. Vestibular dysfunction, either alone or in combination with auditory dysfunction, occurs in 84% of cases, whereas auditory dysfunction alone occurs in only 16%. Ototoxic effects develop when the total dose exceeds 17.5 mg/kg (Gailiunas et al, 1978).

Epilepsy

Vertigo may be the only manifestation of a simple partial seizure or an initial feature of a complex partial seizure. Between 10% and 20% of patients with complex partial seizures experience vertigo as an aura (Currie et al, 1971; Deonna et al, 1986).

Clinical Features.   When vertigo is followed by a complex partial seizure, it is readily recognized as an aura. Diagnosis becomes a problem when vertigo is the solitary manifestation of a simple partial seizure. The child ceases activity, becomes pale, appears frightened, and then recovers. Unsteadiness and nausea may be associated features.

Diagnosis.   Electroencephalography (EEG) is

indicated in children with unexplained brief attacks of vertigo, especially when vestibular and auditory function is normal between attacks. Ambulatory EEG or 24-hour video monitoring may be needed to capture an attack if interictal EEG is normal.

Treatment. Management of simple and complex partial seizures is discussed in Chapter 2.

Infections
Bacterial Infection

Otitis media and meningitis are leading causes of vestibular and auditory impairment in children. Syphilis is no longer the important cause it was before the antibiotic era.

Acute suppurative labyrinthitis resulting from extension of bacterial infection from the middle ear has become uncommon since the introduction of antibiotics. However, even without direct bacterial invasion, bacterial toxins may cause serous labyrinthitis.

Chronic otitic infections cause labyrinthine damage by the development of *cholesteatoma*. A cholesteatoma is a sac containing keratin, a silvery-white debris shed by squamous epithelial cells. Such cells are not normal constituents of the middle ear but gain access from the external canal when the eardrum is repeatedly perforated by infection. Cholesteatomas erode surrounding tissues, including bone, and produce a fistula between the perilymph and the middle ear.

Clinical Features. Acute suppurative or serous labyrinthitis is characterized by the sudden onset of severe vertigo, nausea, vomiting, and unilateral hearing loss. Meningismus may also be present. Chronic otitis produces similar symptoms. Fistula formation is identified when severe vertigo is provoked by sneezing, coughing, or merely applying pressure on the external canal.

Otoscopic examination reveals evidence of otitis media and tympanic membrane perforation and allows visualization of cholesteatoma.

Diagnosis. When vestibular dysfunction develops in children with otitis media, radiographs or CT scans of the skull are needed to visualize erosion of bone or mastoiditis. The presence of meningismus or increased intracranial pressure (see Chapter 4) necessitates CT to exclude the possibility of abscess and then examination of cerebrospinal fluid to exclude meningitis.

Treatment. Vigorous antibiotic therapy and drainage of the infected area are required in every case. Myringotomy and mastoidectomy may be needed for drainage. Cholesteatomas are progressive and must be surgically excised.

Viral Infections

Viral infections may affect the labyrinth or vestibular nerve. The two are difficult to differentiate by clinical features, and the term "vestibular neuritis" or "neuronitis" is used to describe acute peripheral vestibulopathies. Vestibular neuritis may be part of a systemic viral infection, such as mumps, measles, and infectious mononucleosis, or it may occur in epidemics without an identifiable viral agent. In many patients vestibular neuritis may be part of a postinfectious cranial polyneuritis (Adour et al, 1981).

Clinical Features. The major feature is the acute onset of vertigo. Any attempt to move the head is met with severe exacerbation of vertigo, nausea, and vomiting. Nystagmus is present on fixation and increased by head movement (Brandt, 1985). The patient is unable to maintain posture and lies motionless in bed. Recovery begins after 3 days. Spontaneous nausea diminishes, and nystagmus on fixation ceases. During the second week, vertigo decreases in severity but positional nystagmus is still present. Recovery is usually complete within 3 weeks.

Diagnosis. The diagnosis is often established on the basis of clinical features alone. Caloric testing reveals unilateral vestibular paresis, and hearing is normal.

Treatment. During the acute phase the patient must be kept in bed and provided with vestibular sedation. Diazepam or dimenhydrinate is given orally. Transdermal scopolamine should not be used in children but may be administered to adolescents. As recovery progresses, activity is gradually increased and sedation reduced.

Ménière Disease

Ménière disease is believed to be an overaccumulation of endolymph resulting in rupture of the labyrinth. It is uncommon in children.

Clinical Features. The clinical features of hearing impairment, tinnitus, and vertigo are attributed to rupture of the labyrinth. Hearing impairment fluctuates and may temporarily return to normal when the rupture heals. Tinnitus may be ignored, but vertigo demands attention and is often the complaint that brings the disorder to attention.

A typical attack consists of disabling vertigo and tinnitus lasting 1 to 3 hours. The vertigo may be preceded by tinnitus, fullness in the ear, or increased loss of hearing. Tinnitus becomes worse during the attack. Pallor, sweating, nausea, and vomiting are often associated features. Afterward the patient is tired and sleeps. Attacks occur at unpredictable intervals for years and then subside, leaving the patient with permanent hearing loss. Bilateral involvement is present in 20% of cases (Baloh and Honrubia, 1979).

Nystagmus is present during an attack. At first the fast component is toward the abnormal ear (irritative); later, as the attack subsides, the fast component is away (paralytic). Between attacks the results of examination are normal with the exception of unilateral hearing impairment.

Diagnosis. Pure tone audiometry demonstrates threshold fluctuation. Speech discrimination is preserved, and recruitment is present on the abnormal side. Caloric stimulation demonstrates unilateral vestibular paresis or directional preponderance.

Treatment. The underlying disease cannot be reversed. Treatment is directed at management of the acute attack and attempts to increase the interval between attacks. The acute attack is treated with bed rest, sedation, and antiemetics. Maintenance therapy usually consists of a low-salt diet and diuretics; neither provides substantial benefit.

Migraine

Seventeen percent of migraineurs report vertigo at the time of an attack (Kayan and Hood, 1984). Such individuals have no difficulty in recognizing vertigo as a symptom of migraine. Another 10% experience vertigo in the interval between attacks and may have difficulty relating vertigo to migraine.

Brief (minutes), recurrent episodes of vertigo in infants and small children are recognized as a migraine equivalent, despite the absence of headache, because the attacks evolve into classic migraine. Affected children appear ataxic, and for this reason the disorder is discussed in Chapter 10 (see "Benign Paroxysmal Vertigo").

Benign Recurrent Vertigo

Benign recurrent vertigo is similar to benign paroxysmal vertigo and is also believed to be a migraine equivalent (Slater, 1979).

Clinical Features. Children and adults are affected. The onset of vertigo is severe and without warning. Posture cannot be maintained. After a variable interval of minutes to hours the spontaneous vertigo resolves, but positional vertigo persists for hours to days. Some attacks are associated with unilateral throbbing headache.

Diagnosis. Many patients have a family history of either benign recurrent vertigo or migraine.

Between attacks audiometric and vestibular function is normal. Permanent positional vertigo develops in some patients.

Treatment. No treatment has been established as beneficial, but prophylactic treatment with propranolol is suggested (see Chapter 3).

Motion Sickness

Motion sickness is induced by unfamiliar body accelerations or a mismatch in information provided by the visual and vestibular systems to the brain on acceleration of the body (Brandt and Daroff, 1980). It is inhibited when motion in the visual field is in opposition to actual body movement. Therefore looking out the window when driving reduces motion sickness. Small children in the back seat, where the only visual input is the car interior, are at the greatest risk for motion sickness.

The incidence of motion sickness depends on how violent the movement is and approaches 100% in the worst case (Money, 1970). Twenty-five percent of a ship's passengers become sick during a 2- to 3-day Atlantic crossing, and 0.5% of commercial airline passengers are affected.

The first symptom is pallor, which is followed by nausea and vomiting. Because nausea usually precedes vomiting, there is time to prevent vomiting in some situations. Stopping the motion is the best way to abort an attack. Early attacks may be inhibited by watching the environment move opposite the direction of body movement. Individuals with known susceptibility to motion sickness should take an antihistamine, diazepam, or scopolamine before travel.

Trauma

Fifty percent of children complain of dizziness and headache during the first 3 days after a closed head injury, with or without loss of consciousness (Eviatar et al, 1986). One third have persistent vertigo without hearing loss. This group may be separated into patients with direct trauma to the labyrinth *(vestibular concussion)* and those in whom the vestibular apparatus is not injured (whiplash injury, migraine, and vertiginous seizures). Children with posttraumatic neurosis complain of dizziness or giddiness but do not experience the illusion of rotation.

Vestibular Concussion

Clinical Features. Vestibular concussion follows blows to the parieto-occipital or temporoparietal region of the skull. Severe vertigo is present immediately after injury. The child is unsteady and sways toward the affected side. Symptoms persist for several days and then resolve completely, but recurrent episodes of vertigo and nausea lasting 5 to 10 seconds are precipitated by specific movements of the head *(paroxysmal positional vertigo)*.

Diagnosis. Radiography of the skull is indicated for all children with vertigo following head injury. Special attention should be paid to fractures through the petrous pyramid. Bleeding from the ear or a facial palsy should raise suspicion of such a skull fracture.

Positional nystagmus is induced by the Nylen-Hallpike technique when the injured ear is moved down. Caloric testing or electronystagmography demonstrates a reduced response from the injured ear.

Treatment. Immediately after injury the patient should be treated with an antihistamine and diazepam until the acute phase is over.

Individuals with paroxysmal positional vertigo are treated with *fatigue therapy*. The patient is tilted to a position that reproduces symptoms. The patient remains in that position until the vertigo subsides for at least 30 seconds, then sits up for 30 seconds. The procedure is repeated four times. This exercise is performed several times each day until the patient is no longer sensitive to positional change.

Whiplash Injury

Whiplash injuries are frequently associated with vestibular and auditory dysfunction. Symptoms are probably caused by basilar artery spasm.

Clinical Features. Vertigo may be present immediately after injury and subsides within a few days. Brief attacks of vertigo and tinnitus, sometimes associated with headache or nausea, may develop months later in children who appear fully recovered from the injury. Many features of the attacks suggest basilar artery migraine (see Chapter 10) and probably represent posttraumatic migraine.

Diagnosis. During the acute phase, vertigo may be induced by the Nylen-Hallpike technique and unilateral dysfunction is documented by caloric testing. Vestibular function may also be abnormal in children who are experiencing basilar artery migraine, especially at the time of attack. EEG often demonstrates occipital intermittent rhythmic delta activity (see Figure 10–2).

References

Adour KK, Sprague MA, Hilsinger RL Jr: Vestibular vertigo: A form of polyneuritis? JAMA 246:1564, 1981.

Albers JW, Zimnowodski S, Lowrey CM, et al: Juvenile progressive bulbar palsy: Clinical and electrodiagnostic findings. Arch Neurol 40:351, 1983.

Aldrich MS, Beck RW, Albers J: Familial recurrent facial and ocular motor palsies. Neurology 34(suppl 1):165, 1984.

Aleksic SN, Budzilovich GN, Lieberman AN: Herpes zoster oticus and facial paralysis (Ramsay Hunt syndrome): Clinico-pathologic study and review of literature. J Neurol Sci 20:149, 1973.

Alvord EC, Shaw C-M: Congenital difficulties with swallowing and breathing associated with maternal polyhydramnios: Neurocristopathy or medullary infarction? J Child Neurol 4:299, 1989.

Bailey RO, Marzulo DC, Hans MB: Infantile facioscapulohumeral muscular dystrophy: New observations. Acta Neurol Scand 74:51, 1986.

Bale JF Jr: Human cytomegalovirus infection and disorders of the nervous system. Arch Neurol 41:310, 1984.

Baloh RW, Honrubia V: Clinical Neurophysiology of the Vestibular System. Contemporary Neurology Series. FA Davis Co, Philadelphia, 1979, p 203.

Beighton P: Hereditary deafness. In Emery AE, Rimoin DA (eds): Principles and Practice of Medical Genetics, 2nd edition. Churchill Livingstone, London, 1990, p 733.

Bohr V, Paulson OB, Rasamussen N: Pneumococcal meningitis: Late neurological sequelae and features of prognostic impact. Arch Neurol 41:1045, 1984.

Borrett D, Becker LE: Alexander's disease: A disease of astrocytes. Brain 108:367, 1985.

Brandt T: Episodic vertigo. In Rakel RE (ed): Conn's Current Therapy. WB Saunders, Philadelphia, 1985, p 741.

Brandt T, Daroff RB: The multisensory physiological and pathological vertigo syndromes. Ann Neurol 7:195, 1980.

Bray GM, Kaarsoo M, Ross RT: Ocular myopathy with dysphagia. Neurology 15:678, 1965.

Brown JS: Bell's palsy: A 5-year review of 174 consecutive cases: An attempted double-blind study. Laryngoscope 92:1369, 1982.

Brucher JM, Dom R, Lombaert A, et al: Progressive pontobulbar palsy with deafness: Clinical and pathological study of two cases. Arch Neurol 38:186, 1981.

Burgess LPA, Yim DWS, Lepore LM, et al: Bell's palsy: The steroid controversy revisited. Laryngoscope 94:1472, 1984.

Currie S, Heathfield KWG, Henson RA, et al: Clinical course and prognosis of temporal lobe epilepsy: A survey of 666 patients. Brain 94:173, 1971.

Deonna T, Ziegler A-L, Despland P-A, et al: Partial epilepsy in neurologically normal children: Clinical syndromes and prognosis. Epilepsia 27:241, 1986.

Despland PA, Galambos R: Use of the auditory brainstem responses by prematures and newborn infants. Neuropediatrics 11:99, 1980.

Dodge PR, Davis H, Feigen RD, et al: Prospective evaluation of hearing impairment as a sequela of acute bacterial meningitis. N Engl J Med 311:869, 1984.

Djupesland G, Flottorp G, Refsum S: Phytanic acid storage disease: Hearing maintained after 15 years of dietary treatment. Neurology 33:237, 1983.

Dossing M, Wulff CH, Olsen PZ: Repeated facial palsies after chlorocresol inhalation. J Neurol Neurosurg Psychiatry 49:1452, 1986.

Eviatar L, Bergtraum M, Randel RM: Post-traumatic vertigo in children: A diagnostic approach. Pediatr Neurol 2:61, 1986.

Faldt R, Liedholm H, Aurnes J: Beta blockers and loss of hearing. Br Med J 289:1490, 1984.

Feldman RG, Mayer RM, Taub A: Evidence for a peripheral neurotoxic effect of trichlorethylene. Neurology 20:599, 1970.

Fraser GR: Profound childhood deafness. J Med Genet 1:118, 1964.

Gailiunas P, Dominguez-Moreno M, Lazarus M, et al: Vestibular toxicity of gentamicin. Arch Intern Med 138:1621, 1978.

Hall JG, Pauli RM, Wilson KM: Maternal and fetal sequelae of anticoagulation during pregnancy. Am J Med 68:122, 1980.

Hart RG, Gardner DP, Howieson J: Acoustic tumors: Atypical features and recent diagnostic tests. Neurology 33:211, 1983.

Hepner WR Jr: Some observations on facial paresis in the newborn infant: Etiology and incidence. Pediatrics 8:494, 1951.

Huff JC, Bean B, Balfour HH Jr, et al: Therapy of herpes zoster with oral acyclovir. Am J Med 85(suppl 2A):84, 1988.

Juncos JL, Beal MF: Idiopathic cranial polyneuropathy: A fifteen year experience. Brain 110:197, 1987.

Kansu T, Us O, Sarpel G, et al: Recurrent multiple cranial nerve palsies (Tolosa-Hunt plus?). J Clin Neuro-ophthalmol 3:263, 1983.

Katusic S, Beard CM, Wiederholt WC, et al: Incidence, clinical features, and prognosis in Bell's palsy, Rochester, Minnesota, 1968–1982. Ann Neurol 20:622, 1986.

Kayan A, Hood JD: Neuro-otological manifestations of migraine. Brain 107:1123, 1984.

Konigsmark BW, Gorlin RJ: Genetic and Metabolic Deafness. WB Saunders, Philadelphia, 1976.

Levenson MJ, Ingerman M, Grimes C, et al: Melkersson-Rosenthal syndrome. Arch Otolaryngol 110:540, 1984.

Listernick R, Charrow J: Medical progress: Neurofibromatosis type 1 in childhood. J Pediatr 116:845, 1990.

Little BW, Perl DP: Oculopharyngeal muscular dystrophy: An autopsied case from the French-Canadian kindred. J Neurol Sci 53:145, 1982.

Lloyd AVC, Jewitt DE, Lloyd-Still JD: Facial paralysis in children with hypertension. Arch Dis Child 41:292, 1966.

Maiman DJ, Cusick JF, Anderson AJ, et al: Nonoperative management of traumatic facial nerve palsy. J Trauma 25:644, 1985.

Mallya KB, Mendis T, Guberman A: Bilateral facial paralysis following ethylene glycol ingestion. Can J Neurol Sci 13:340, 1986.

May M, Wette R, Hardin WB, et al: The use of steroids in Bell's palsy: A prospective controlled study. Laryngoscope 86:1111, 1976.

McHugh HE: Facial paralysis in birth injury and skull fractures. Arch Otolaryngol 78:445, 1963.

McHugh HE, Sowden KA, Levitt MH: Facial paralysis and muscle agenesis in the newborn. Arch Otolaryngol 89:157, 1969.

McLeod AC, McConnell F, Sweeney A, et al: Clinical variation in Usher syndrome. Arch Otolaryngol 94:321, 1971.

Money KE: Motion sickness. Physiol Rev 50:1, 1970.

Neligan G, Prudham D: Norms for four standard developmental milestones by sex, social class and place in family. Dev Med Child Neurol 11:413, 1969.

Nelson KB, Eng GD: Congenital hypoplasia of the depressor anguli oris muscle: Differentiation from congenital facial palsy. J Pediatr 81:16, 1972.

Patten BM, Pages M: Severe neurological disease associated with hyperparathyroidism. Ann Neurol 15:453, 1984.

Pauzner R, Blatt I, Mouallem M, et al: Mitochondrial abnormalities in oculopharyngeal muscular dystrophy. Muscle Nerve 14:947, 1991.

Pettigrew AG, Edwards DA, Henderson-Smart DJ: Perinatal risk factors in preterm infants with moderate-to-profound hearing deficits. Med J Aust 148:174, 1988.

Puvanendran K, Vitharana M, Wong PK: Delayed facial palsy after head injury. J Neurol Neurosurg Psychiatry 40:342, 1977.

Richter RB: Unilateral congenital hypoplasia of the facial nucleus. J Neuropathol Exp Neurol 19:33, 1960.

Ropper AH: Unusual clinical variants and signs of Guillain-Barré syndrome. Arch Neurol 43:1150, 1986.

Rosenberg NL: Hearing loss as an initial symptom of the opsoclonus-myoclonus syndrome. Arch Neurol 41:998, 1984.

Rozencweig M, Von Hoff DD, Slavik M, et al: Cis-diamminedichloroplatinum (II): A new anticancer drug. Ann Intern Med 86:803, 1977.

Safman BL: Bilateral pathology in Bell's palsy. Arch Otolaryngol 93:55, 1971.

Sharma OP: Diagnosis of sarcoidosis. Arch Intern Med 143:1418, 1983.

Slater R: Benign recurrent vertigo. J Neurol Neurosurg Psychiatry 42:363, 1979.

Snavely SR, Hodges GR: The neurotoxicity of antibacterial agents. Ann Intern Med 101:92, 1984.

Stern BJ, Krumholz A, Johns C, et al: Sarcoidosis and its neurological manifestations. Arch Neurol 42:909, 1985.

Stockard JE, Stockard JJ, Kleinberg F, et al: Prognostic values of brainstem auditory evoked responses in newborns. Arch Neurol 40:360, 1983.

Sudarshan A, Goldie WD: The spectrum of congenital facial diplegia (Möbius syndrome). Pediatr Neurol 1:180, 1985.

Swanson JW, Kelly JJ Jr, McConahey WM: Neurologic aspects of thyroid dysfunction. Mayo Clin Proc 56:504, 1981.

Taylor DA, Carroll JE, Smith ME, et al: Facioscapulohumeral dystrophy associated with hearing loss and Coats syndrome. Ann Neurol 12:395, 1982.

van Dongen HR, Arts WFM, Yousef-Bak E: Acquired dysarthria in childhood: An analysis of dysarthric features in relation to neurologic deficits. Neurology 37:296, 1987.

Voit T, Lamprecht H-G, Goebel HH: Hearing loss in facioscapulohumeral dystrophy. Eur J Pediatr 145:280, 1986.

Wertelecki W, Rouleau GA, Superneau DW, et al: Neurofibromatosis 2: Clinical and DNA linkage studies of a large kindred. N Engl J Med 319:278, 1988.

Wolf SM, Wagner JH Jr, Davidson S, et al: Treatment of Bell's palsy with prednisone: A prospective-randomized study. Neurology 28:158, 1978.

Yanagihara N, Mori H, Kozawa T, et al: Bell's palsy: Nonrecurrent v recurrent and unilateral v bilateral. Arch Otolaryngol 110:374, 1984.

Disorders of Cranial Volume and Shape

During infancy the size of the skull is determined by the volume of its contents: brain, cerebrospinal fluid, and blood. These three compartments fill the calvarium. Expansion of one compartment is at the expense of another so that intracranial volume and pressure remain constant (see Chapter 4). The extracerebral spaces (epidural, subdural, and subarachnoid) may expand with blood and significantly affect cranial volume. Less important factors contributing to head size are the thickness of the skull bones and the rate of their fusion.

The skull's shape is determined in part by its content, but external forces on the skull and the rate at which individual skull bones fuse are even more important factors.

◆ Measuring Head Size

Head circumference is a time-honored and relatively accurate measure of cranial volume. It is determined by measuring the greatest occipitofrontal circumference. Two variables, fluid in and beneath the scalp and head shape, influence the accuracy of using head circumference to estimate cranial volume.

The scalp can be thickened from edema or blood following a prolonged and difficult delivery, and cephalohematoma may be present as well. Fluid that infiltrates from a scalp infusion can markedly increase head circumference.

A round head has a larger intracranial volume than an oval head of equal circumference. A head with a relatively large occipitofrontal diameter has a larger volume than a head with a relatively large biparietal diameter.

Head circumference measurements are most in-

formative when plotted over time. The head sizes of male and female infants are different, and head growth charts that provide median values for both sexes should not be used. The rate of head growth in premature infants is considerably faster than in full-term newborns (Figure 18–1). For this reason head circumference must always be charted by conceptional age and not by postnatal age.

◆ Macrocephaly

Macrocephaly means a large head, larger than 2 standard deviations from the normal distribution. Thus 2% of the "normal" population has macrocephaly. Investigation of such individuals usually reveals some abnormality that causes them to be in the top 2% for head size. However, some are normal, often with a familial tendency for a large head.

The causes of a large head include *hydrocephalus,* or excessive volume of cerebrospinal fluid in the skull; *megalencephaly,* or enlargement of the brain; thickening of the skull; and hemorrhage into the subdural or epidural spaces.

Hydrocephalus is traditionally *communicating* (nonobstructive) or *noncommunicating* (obstructive), depending on whether cerebrospinal fluid communicates between the ventricles and subarachnoid space (Table 18–1). Hydrocephalus is the only cause of macrocephaly at birth associated with increased intracranial pressure.

Megalencephaly has been divided into two major categories: *anatomic* and *metabolic* (DeMyer, 1986). Anatomic disorders include primary megalencephaly and neurocutaneous disorders (Table 18–2). Children with anatomic megalencephaly often have macrocephaly at birth, but intracranial

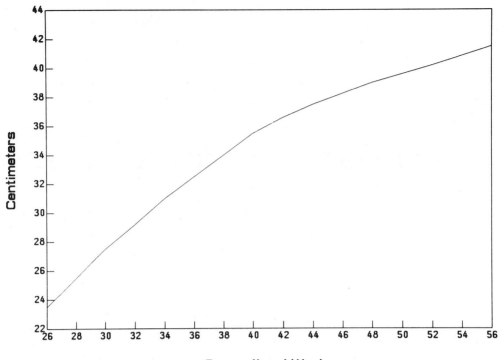

Figure 18–1   Normal growth of head circumference in boys. The rate of growth in premature infants is greater than that in full-term infants.

Table 18–1 ◆ Causes of Hydrocephalus

Communicating
1. Achondroplasia
2. Basilar impression (see Chapter 10)
3. Benign enlargement of subarachnoid space
4. Choroid plexus papilloma (see Chapter 4)
5. Meningeal malignancy
6. Meningitis (see Chapter 4)
7. Posthemorrhagic (see Chapter 4)

Noncommunicating
1. Aqueductal stenosis
   a. Infectious
   b. X-linked
2. Chiari malformation (see Chapter 10)
3. Dandy-Walker malformation
4. Klippel-Feil syndrome
5. Mass lesions
   a. Abscess (see Chapter 4)
   b. Hematoma (see Chapters 1 and 2)
   c. Tumors and neurocutaneous disorders
   d. Vein of Galen malformation
6. Warburg syndrome

Hydranencephaly
1. Holoprosencephaly
2. Massive hydrocephalus
3. Porencephaly

pressure is not increased. Those with metabolic megalencephaly have normal head size at birth, but cerebral edema and macrocephaly develop during the neonatal period.

Macrocephaly caused by increased thickness of the skull bones is not present at birth or in the newborn period but develops during infancy. The conditions associated with increased skull growth are summarized in Table 18–3 but are not discussed in the text.

Intracranial hemorrhage in the newborn is discussed in Chapter 1; intracranial hemorrhage in older children is detailed in Chapter 2.

COMMUNICATING HYDROCEPHALUS

Communicating hydrocephalus is usually caused by impaired absorption of cerebrospinal fluid secondary to meningitis or subarachnoid hemorrhage. Meningeal malignancy, usually resulting from leukemia or primary brain tumor, is a less common cause. The excessive production of cerebrospinal fluid by a choroid plexus papilloma rarely causes communicating hydrocephalus because the potential rate of cerebrospinal reabsorption far exceeds the productive capacity of the cho-

Table 18–2 ◆ Causes of Megalencephaly

Anatomic Megalencephaly	Metabolic Megalencephaly
1. Genetic megalencephaly	1. Alexander disease (see Chapter 5)
2. Megalencephaly with achondroplasia	2. Canavan disease (see Chapter 5)
3. Megalencephaly with gigantism (Sotos syndrome)	3. Galactosemia: transferase deficiency (see Chapter 5)
4. Megalencephaly with neurologic abnormality	4. Gangliosidosis (see Chapter 5)
5. Neurocutaneous disorders	5. Globoid leukodystrophy (see Chapter 5)
a. Hypomelanosis of Ito	6. Glutaric aciduria type I (see Chapter 14)
b. Incontinentia pigmenti (see Chapter 1)	7. Maple syrup urine disease (see Chapter 1)
c. Linear nevus sebaceus syndrome	8. Metachromatic leukodystrophy (see Chapter 5)
d. Neurofibromatosis (see Chapter 5)	9. Mucopolysaccharidoses (see Chapter 5)
e. Tuberous sclerosis (see Chapter 5)	

roid plexus (see Chapter 4). Such tumors more commonly cause hydrocephalus by obstructing one or more ventricles.

Achondroplasia

Achondroplasia is a genetic disorder, transmitted as an autosomal dominant trait, that produces skeletal deformities resulting in dwarfism.

Clinical Features. The major features of achondroplasia are macrocephaly and rhizomelic shortening of the limbs: the proximal portion of the limbs is shorter than the distal portion. Enchondral bone formation at the skull base and in the face is stunted, causing the typical recessed facial appearance.

Affected newborns have megalencephaly but do not have hydrocephalus (Mueller, 1980). The ventricles begin to enlarge during infancy because of impaired reabsorption of cerebrospinal fluid as a result of increased venous pressure (Mueller and Reinertson, 1980). Venous return from the brain is probably obstructed because of narrowed venous sinuses in the small posterior fossa.

Despite considerable, and sometimes alarming,

Table 18–3 ◆ Conditions with a Thickened Skull Causing Macrocephaly

1. Anemia
2. Cleidocranial dysostosis
3. Craniometaphyseal dysplasia of Pyle
4. Epiphyseal dysplasia
5. Hyperphosphatemia
6. Leontiasis ossea
7. Orodigitofacial dysostosis
8. Osteogenesis imperfecta
9. Osteopetrosis
10. Pyknodysostosis
11. Rickets
12. Russell dwarfism

Modified from DeMyer W: Pediatr Neurol 2:321, 1986.

enlargement of head circumference, achondroplastic dwarfs seldom show clinical evidence of increased intracranial pressure or progressive dementia.

Respiratory disturbances occur in 85% of children with achondroplasia (Reid et al, 1987). In 35% of these the difficulties are caused by cervicomedullary compression, but in the majority they result from primary pulmonary problems, such as a small thoracic cage or an obstructed airway. Other features of cervicomedullary compression include hyperreflexia, spasticity, and sensory abnormalities of the limbs.

Diagnosis. The diagnosis of achondroplasia is established by clinical examination. Because of a high mutation rate, the family may not have a history of the disorder. Computed tomography (CT) reveals a small posterior fossa and enlargement of the sphenoid sinuses. Basilar impression is sometimes present. Ventricular size varies from normal in newborns and young infants to moderate or severe dilation in older children and adults.

Treatment. Ventricular size, after initial dilation, usually remains stable, and surgical diversion of cerebrospinal fluid is rarely required. Decompressive surgery is required in children with evidence of progressive cervicomedullary compromise.

Benign Enlargement of Subarachnoid Space

Benign enlargement of the subarachnoid space is described under several names in the literature: *external hydrocephalus, extraventricular hydrocephalus, benign subdural effusions,* and *benign extracerebral fluid collections* (Hamza et al, 1987). It is a relatively common cause of macrocephaly in infants (16%), a fact not fully appreciated before the widespread use of CT to investigate large head size (Nickel and Gallenstein, 1987). A genetic cause for this condition is likely in some cases, with the infant's father often having a large head.

Clinical Features.   The condition occurs more commonly in males than females. A large head circumference is the only feature. An otherwise normal infant is brought to medical attention because serial head circumference measurements show an enlarging head size. Circumference is usually above the 90th percentile at birth, grows to exceed the 98th percentile, and then parallels the normal curve (Figure 18–2). The anterior fontanelle is large but soft. Neurologic findings and developmental status are normal.

Diagnosis.   Cranial CT shows an enlarged frontal subarachnoid space, widening of the sylvian fissures and other sulci, and normal or minimally enlarged ventricular size (Figure 18–3). Normal ventricular size distinguishes this condition from cerebral atrophy. In infants the upper limit of normal size for the frontal subarachnoid space is 5.7 mm and for the sylvian fissure is 7.6 mm (Fukuyama et al, 1979).

Treatment.   Most affected infants develop normally and do not require ventricular shunts. Head circumference measurements should be plotted monthly for the 6 months after diagnosis to be certain that growth is paralleling the normal curve. Repeat CT is not needed unless head growth deviates upward from the normal curve, neurologic findings become abnormal, or development is delayed.

Meningeal Malignancy

Tumors that infiltrate the meninges and subarachnoid space impair the reabsorption of cerebrospinal fluid and may produce communicating hydrocephalus. The primary site of tumor is usually established before its meningeal spread, but hydrocephalus may be the initial feature of diffuse meningeal gliomatosis (Whelan et al, 1987).

Clinical Features.   Tumors that infiltrate the meninges are usually aggressive, causing a rapid progression of symptoms. Headache and vomiting are the initial features and are followed by lethargy and personality change. Examination often reveals meningismus and papilledema, which suggest bacterial meningitis. Multifocal neurologic disturbances may be present.

Diagnosis.   Cranial CT shows dilation of the

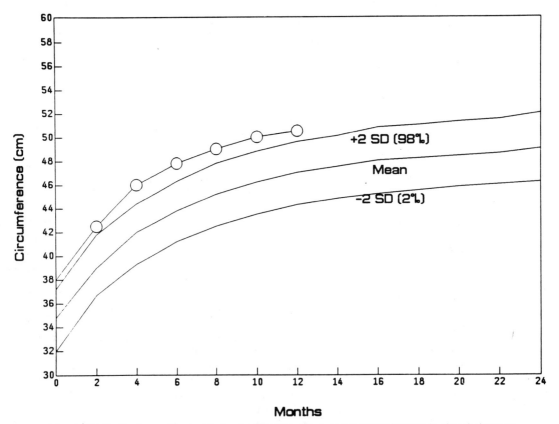

Figure 18–2 Benign enlargement of subarachnoid space. Head circumference is already large at birth, grows to exceed the 98th percentile, and then parallels the curve.

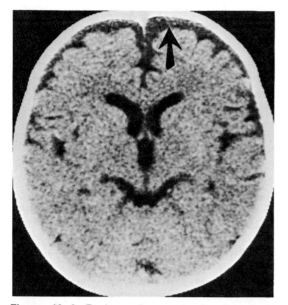

Figure 18–3 Benign enlargement of subarachnoid space. Computed tomography reveals an enlarged frontal subarachnoid space, prominent sulci, and normal ventricular size.

entire ventricular system but not of the subarachnoid space, which may appear obliterated. Some tumors cause contrast enhancement of the meninges (Jaeckle et al, 1985).

Examination of the cerebrospinal fluid demonstrates an increased pressure and protein concentration. The glucose concentration may be depressed or normal. Tumor cell identification in the cerebrospinal fluid is essential for early diagnosis and treatment, although it is rarely accomplished unless large volumes are examined. Meningeal biopsy is required for tissue diagnosis in many cases.

Treatment. A ventricular shunt is necessary to relieve symptoms of increased intracranial pressure. Radiation therapy and chemotherapy provide palliation and extend life in some cases, but the outcome is generally poor.

NONCOMMUNICATING HYDROCEPHALUS

Complete obstruction of the egress of cerebrospinal fluid from the ventricles to the subarachnoid space causes increased pressure and dilation of all ventricles proximal to the obstruction.

Noncommunicating hydrocephalus is the most common form of hydrocephalus in fetuses, with aqueductal stenosis accounting for 20% of congenital hydrocephalus without other malformations

(Burton, 1977). It becomes less common during infancy but increases in frequency again during childhood. Childhood onset is usually caused by mass lesions.

Aqueductal Stenosis

The mean length of the cerebral aqueduct at birth is 12.8 mm (Friede, 1975). At its smallest cross-sectional diameter the cerebral aqueduct of normal newborns is usually 0.5 mm. The small lumen of the cerebral aqueduct, in relation to its length, makes it especially vulnerable to internal compromise from infection and hemorrhage and external compression by tumors and venous malformations.

Congenital atresia or stenosis of the cerebral aqueduct can occur as a solitary malformation, but a familial form transmitted by X-linked inheritance accounts for 2% of all cases of congenital hydrocephalus.

Clinical Features. Hydrocephalus is present at birth. Head circumference ranges from 40 to 50 cm and may cause cephalopelvic disproportion and poor progress of labor. The forehead is bowed, the scalp veins are dilated, the skull sutures are widely separated, and the fontanelles are large and tense. These signs are exaggerated when the child cries but are also present in the quiet state. The eyes are deviated downward so that the sclera shows above the iris *(setting-sun sign),* and abducens palsies may be present.

Adduction and flexion of the thumbs are noted in approximately 20% of newborns with X-linked aqueductal stenosis (Kuzniecky et al, 1986). This phenomenon was thought to be an associated malformation but probably represents a nonspecific sign of corticospinal tract compression by the dilated lateral ventricles.

Diagnosis. Antenatal diagnosis has been made possible by intrauterine sonography. When macrocephaly is present in the fetus, alpha-fetoprotein should be assayed in the amniotic fluid for the detection of neural tube defects (see Chapter 12) and chromosomal analysis should be performed. Information concerning the integrity of the fetal nervous system is needed to develop a management plan.

The postpartum diagnosis of aqueductal stenosis is readily accomplished with CT. The lateral and third ventricles are markedly enlarged, as is the cephalic end of the cerebral aqueduct. The remainder of the cerebral aqueduct and the fourth ventricle cannot be visualized (Figure 18–4).

Treatment. Congenital hydrocephalus caused by aqueductal stenosis is severe, does not

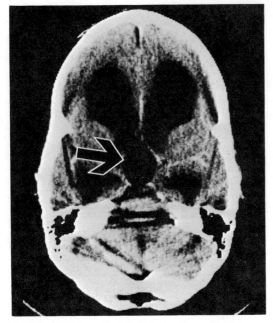

Figure 18–4 Aqueductal stenosis. Computed tomography demonstrates marked enlargement of the third ventricle *(arrow)* and the lateral ventricles.

respond to medical therapy directed at decreasing the volume of cerebrospinal fluid, and progresses to a stage that harms the brain. Diversion of the cerebrospinal fluid from the venticular system to an extracranial site is the only effective method of management.

The management of fetal hydrocephalus depends on the presence of other malformations. Between 70% and 80% of patients have other abnormalities, usually spina bifida (Chervenak et al, 1985; Vintzileos et al, 1987). Many pregnancies with an affected fetus are terminated voluntarily.

Ventriculoperitoneal shunt is generally considered the procedure of choice for newborns and small infants with aqueductal stenosis. It is easier to revise and better tolerated than ventriculoatrial shunt. Mechanical obstruction and infection are the most common complications of shunt placement in infancy (see Chapter 4).

The relief of hydrocephalus increases the potential for normal development even when the cerebral mantle appears very thin preoperatively (Kovnar et al, 1984) but does not necessarily result in a normal child. The growth of intelligence is often uneven, with better development of verbal than of nonverbal skills (Dennis et al, 1981). Associated anomalies may cause motor deficits and seizures.

Dandy-Walker Malformation

The Dandy-Walker malformation consists of partial or complete agenesis of the cerebellar vermis, cystic dilation of the posterior fossa communicating with the fourth ventricle, and hydrocephalus (Bordarier and Aicardi, 1990). The hydrocephalus may not be present at birth but more often develops during childhood or even later. The size of the lateral ventricles does not correlate with the size of the cyst in the fourth ventricle. Other malformations are present in 68% of patients. The most common associated malformation is agenesis of the corpus callosum. Others include heterotopia, abnormal gyrus formation, dysraphic states, aqueductal stenosis, and congenital tumors.

Clinical Features. The diagnosis is made at birth in only 25% of cases and by 1 year in 75% (Pascual-Castroviejo et al, 1991). Macrocephaly is the usual initial feature. Bulging of the skull, when present, is more prominent in the occipital than in the frontal region. The rapidity of head growth is considerably slower than with aqueductal stenosis. Compression of posterior fossa structures leads to neurologic dysfunction: apneic spells, nystagmus, truncal ataxia, cranial nerve palsies, and hyperreflexia in the legs.

Diagnosis. A CT scan is usually ordered because of macrocephaly or ataxia. Cystic dilation of the posterior fossa and partial or complete agenesis of the cerebellar vermis are readily visualized (Figure 18–5). Magnetic resonance imaging (MRI) is useful to identify other cerebral abnormalities such as heterotopia. Incomplete vermian agenesis may be difficult to differentiate from an enlarged cisterna magna.

Treatment. Decompression of the cyst alone provides immediate relief of symptoms; however, hydrocephalus recurs and ventricular shunting is required in two thirds of affected children. Shunting of the lateral ventricle alone provides immediate relief of hydrocephalus but fails to relieve brainstem compression. The procedure of choice is a dual shunt of both the lateral ventricle and the posterior fossa cyst.

Even after successful shunt placement, many children have transitory episodes of lethargy, personality change, and vomiting. Shunt failure is suspected but cannot be substantiated. The mechanism of such episodes, which may prove fatal, is unknown.

Klippel-Feil Syndrome

Klippel-Feil syndrome is a malformation of the craniocervical skeleton that may be associated with

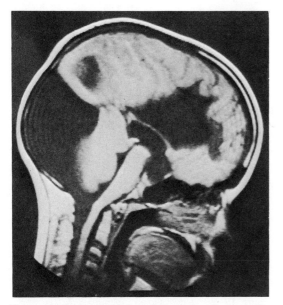

Figure 18–5 Dandy-Walker malformation. Computed tomography demonstrates cystic dilation of the fourth ventricle and partial agenesis of the cerebellar vermis. (From Fenichel GM: Neonatal Neurology, 2nd edition. Churchill Livingstone, New York, 1985. By permission.)

the Chiari malformation and basilar impression. Hydrocephalus is produced by obstruction of the egress of cerebrospinal fluid from the fourth ventricle to the subarachnoid space. The malformation is classified into three types: I, extensive fusion of thoracic and upper cervical vertebrae; II, one or two interspace fusions with hemivertebrae and occipitoatlantal fusion; and III, cervical and lower thoracic or lumbar fusion. Type II is the most common form.

Clinical Features. The essential features of Klippel-Feil syndrome are a low posterior hairline, short neck, and limitation of neck movement (Nagib et al, 1985). Head asymmetry, facial asymmetry, and scoliosis are common. Unilateral or bilateral failure of downward migration of the scapula (Sprengel deformity) is present in 25% to 35% of patients. Mirror movements of the hands are noted in the majority of patients. Malformations of the genitourinary system and deafness are associated features.

Hydrocephalus affects the fourth ventricle first and then the lateral ventricles. This results in symptoms of posterior fossa compression: ataxia, apnea, and cranial nerve dysfunction.

Diagnosis. Radiographs of the spine reveal the characteristic fusion and malformations of vertebrae. MRI may demonstrate an associated Chiari malformation and dilation of the ventricles.

Treatment. Children with unstable cervical vertebrae require cervical fusion to prevent myelopathy. Those with symptoms of obstructive hydrocephalus require ventriculoperitoneal shunt to relieve pressure in the posterior fossa.

Congenital Brain Tumors

There is considerable concurrence between congenital brain tumors and congenital brain malformations. Both are disorders of cellular proliferation, and a noxious agent active during early embryogenesis might stimulate either or both abnormalities. The relative oncogenicity or teratogenicity depends on the virulence of the agent, the timing of the insult, the duration of exposure, and the genetic background and health of the fetus.

The tumors most common during infancy are astrocytoma, medulloblastoma, teratoma, and choroid plexus papilloma (Jellinger and Sunder-Plassman, 1973; Tomita and McLone, 1985).

Clinical Features. Congenital tumors are more often supratentorial than infratentorial and more often in the midline than placed laterally. Newborns with hemispheric gliomas and teratomas may have intrauterine hydrocephalus, or hydrocephalus may develop in the first days or weeks post partum. The point of obstruction is usually at the cerebral aqueduct (see Chapter 4). Choroid plexus papillomas are usually located in one lateral ventricle and are more likely to be manifested during infancy than in the perinatal period. They produce hydrocephalus either by obstruction of the foramen of Monro or by excessive production of cerebrospinal fluid (see Chapter 4). Medulloblastomas are located in the posterior fossa and obstruct the fourth ventricle and cerebral aqueduct (see Chapter 10).

The clinical features of all congenital tumors are those of increasing intracranial pressure: enlarging head size, separation of the sutures, lethargy, irritability, difficult feeding, and vomiting. Seizures are unusual. Because of its posterior fossa location, medulloblastoma also produces nystagmus, downward deviation of the eyes, opisthotonos, and apnea.

Diagnosis. All congenital tumors are readily visualized by CT or MRI performed to investigate hydrocephalus. Fetal teratoma has been identified by uterine sonography (Lipman et al, 1985).

Treatment. Complete resection of congenital brain tumors is unusual with the exception of choroid plexus papilloma. The management of individual tumors is discussed in Chapters 4 and 10.

Vein of Galen Malformation

Various arteriovenous malformations of the cerebral circulation may be present during infancy and childhood (see Chapters 4 and 10), but the one associated with congenital hydrocephalus is the vein of Galen malformation (Lasjaunias et al, 1989). The vein of Galen is just above the quadrigeminal plate and, when dilated, compresses the cerebral aqueduct and causes dilation of the lateral ventricles. The increased blood volume in the skull also causes macrocrania.

Clinical Features. Eighty percent of newborns with vein of Galen malformation are males. The usual manifestation is either high-output cardiac failure or an enlarging head. Hemorrhage is almost never an initial feature. A cranial bruit is invariably present. Unexplained, persistent hypoglycemia has been noted in some children.

Large midline arteriovenous malformations produce a hemodynamic stress in the newborn because of the large quantities of blood shunted from the arterial to the venous system. The heart enlarges in an effort to keep up with the demands of the shunt, but high-output cardiac failure ensues. Affected newborns often come to the attention of a pediatric cardiologist because congenital heart disease is suspected. The intracranial malformation is then diagnosed during cardiac catheterization.

When the hemodynamic stress is not severe and cardiac compensation is possible, symptoms are delayed until infancy or early childhood. In such a case the malformation becomes manifest by direct compression of the tegmentum and aqueduct, causing obstructive hydrocephalus. Symptoms usually begin before age 5 and always before age 10. The lateral ventricles enlarge, causing headache, lethargy, and vomiting. In infants the head enlarges and the fontanelle feels full.

Diagnosis. Vein of Galen malformations are readily visualized by contrast-enhanced CT (Figure 18–6). The lateral and third ventricles are dilated behind the compressed cerebral aqueduct. Radiographs of the chest in newborns with high-output cardiac failure show an enlarged heart that has a normal shape.

Treatment. The overall results of direct surgical approaches are poor; the mortality rate is high, as is neurologic morbidity in survivors. Embolization has become the treatment of choice, but the long-term results are not known.

Warburg Syndrome

The Warburg syndrome is characterized by cerebral and ocular abnormalities (Bordarier et al,

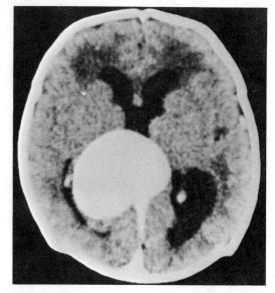

Figure 18–6 Vein of Galen malformation. The malformation is visible on a contrast-enhanced computed tomogram as a large aneurysmal sac compressing the midbrain and producing obstructive hydrocephalus.

1984; Williams et al, 1984). Hydrocephalus is a constant feature. The combination of Warburg syndrome and congenital muscular dystrophy is called cerebro-ocular dysplasia (see Chapter 6).

The risk of recurrence among siblings exceeds 50%, but the syndrome is not transmitted from one generation to the next. Some believe that this is a genetic disease transmitted by autosomal recessive inheritance; others think that it is caused by an acquired agent transmitted transplacentally through consecutive pregnancies.

Clinical Features. Hydrocephalus is usually present at birth. It may be caused by aqueductal stenosis or the Dandy-Walker malformation. Most cases of Dandy-Walker malformation with ocular abnormalities are probably cases of the Warburg syndrome. Some children are born with microcephaly yet have enlarged ventricles.

Severe neurologic abnormalities are caused by partial or total agyria (lissencephaly) resulting from failure of neuronal migration. The pattern of architectural abnormalities throughout the neuraxis suggests a disruption of cerebral maturation in the fourth conceptional month.

Several ocular abnormalities may be present, usually in combination: hypoplasia of the iris, abnormal anterior chamber, microphthalmos, cataracts, persistence of primary vitreous, optic disk coloboma, retinal detachment, retinal dysplasia, and hypoplasia of the optic nerve.

In addition to having hydrocephalus and blindness, affected infants are hypotonic and have difficulty feeding. Seizures are uncommon. Most children with Warburg syndrome die during the neonatal period or early infancy.

Diagnosis. The diagnosis is based on the characteristic combination of cerebral and ocular abnormalities. Congenital infections may produce similar disturbances and must be excluded, but multisystem disease (visceromegaly and disturbed hematopoiesis), an expected feature of most intrauterine infections, is lacking in the Warburg syndrome.

Cerebro-ocular abnormalities at birth are also encountered in septo-optic dysplasia (see Chapter 16) and oculocerebrorenal syndrome (see Chapter 6), but hydrocephalus is not a component of either syndrome.

Treatment. Hydrocephalus can be managed by ventricular shunt, but the outcome is poor because of the severe cerebral malformations.

HYDRANENCEPHALY

The term "hydranencephaly" encompasses several conditions that result in the extensive replacement of brain by cerebrospinal fluid. This may result from failure of normal brain development or from an intrauterine disorder that destroys the brain parenchyma. Progressive obstructive hydrocephalus may cause hydranencephaly if left untreated. Excessive pressure within the lateral ventricles destroys the midline structures and reduces the cerebral mantle to a thin membrane.

Head circumference at birth is large when hydranencephaly is caused by obstructive hydrocephalus, is small when the condition is caused by intrauterine diseases, and may be large or small with primary malformations.

PORENCEPHALY

Porencephaly is a term used loosely in the literature. Originally it was used to describe defects in the final stage of prosencephalization resulting in a hemispheric cyst that communicated with the subarachnoid space and the lateral ventricle. The term is now used broadly for any hemispheric cyst; most are caused by intrauterine or perinatal infarction or trauma. The injured immature brain loses neurons, glia, and supporting structures. A fluid-filled cyst is formed in the injured area and may not communicate with either the ventricular system or the subarachnoid space. Pressure within the cyst often becomes excessive, causing compression of adjacent structures and macrocrania.

Congenital Midline Porencephaly

Congenital midline porencephaly is a distinct malformation characterized by congenital hydrocephalus, alopecia or encephalocele in the parietal midline, and a midline defect in the posterior cerebral mantle (Yokota and Matsukado, 1979). Midline porencephaly differs from holoprosencephaly because the forebrain divides into two separate hemispheres. It may be caused by early hydrocephalus with upward outpouching and destruction of adjacent structures: corpus callosum, cerebral mantle, skull, and scalp.

Clinical Features. The head is large in utero and may cause cephalopelvic disproportion. Possible defects in the parietal midline range from a small round area of alopecia to encephalocele. Affected children are severely retarded and blind. Most die during infancy or early childhood.

Diagnosis. A large dorsal cyst that has destroyed the septum pellucidum and corpus callosum is seen on CT or MRI. The cyst communicates with enlarged lateral ventricles and extends through a skull defect to produce an encephalocele.

Treatment. Shunting the cyst may ease child care by reducing the size of the head or encephalocele, but it does not prevent severe neurologic impairment from the underlying cerebral malformation.

ANATOMIC MEGALENCEPHALY

Anatomic megalencephaly includes conditions in which the brain is enlarged because the number or size of cells increases. There is no evidence of metabolic disease or acute encephalopathy.

Genetic Megalencephaly

Clinical Features. The term "genetic megalencephaly" describes a familial condition in which neurologic and mental function is normal but head circumference is larger than the 98th percentile. Head circumference may not be large at birth but increases during infancy, usually to between 2 and 4 cm above the 98th percentile (Lorber and Priestly, 1981). Body size is normal, and there are no physical deformities.

Diagnosis. The enlargement is indistinguishable by examination from benign enlargement of the subarachnoid space, but they can be differentiated by CT, the results of which are normal in genetic megalencephaly.

Treatment. No treatment is required.

Megalencephaly With Neurologic Disorder

The term "megalencephaly with neurologic disorder" is used to encompass all disorders, other than neurocutaneous syndromes, that are manifested as megalencephaly and evidence of cerebral dysfunction.

Clinical Features. Head circumference may be large at birth or may become large during infancy. It is generally 2 to 4 cm greater than the 98th percentile. Results of neurologic tests are normal, but the children have learning disabilities, mental deficiency, or seizures. Neurologic status remains stable.

Diagnosis. The skin of the patient and other family members must be carefully examined with a Wood light to exclude the possibility of a neurocutaneous disorder. Ophthalmoscopic examination of family members should be carried out.

Results of CT or MRI may be normal or may reveal mild dilation of the ventricular system. Agenesis of the corpus callosum is the only abnormality found in some families with macrocrania and borderline intelligence (Lynn et al, 1980).

Treatment. Seizures often respond to anticonvulsant therapy. Special education is usually required. No treatment is available for the underlying disorder.

Megalencephaly With Gigantism

Megalencephaly with gigantism is also termed *cerebral gigantism* or *Sotos syndrome*. It probably encompasses several disorders, most of them sporadic and some clearly genetic, transmitted by autosomal recessive or dominant inheritance (Winship, 1985). Chromosome studies are normal.

Clinical Features. Affected children are large at birth (75th to 90th percentile) and demonstrate excessive growth with advanced height, weight, head circumference, and bone age up to the age of 3 (Sotos and Cutler, 1977). Afterward the rate of growth is normal. All children with the syndrome are large as adults, but they are not usually giants.

Prominent forehead, high-arched palate, and hypertelorism are present in almost every case. Several other dysmorphic features are reported in small numbers of patients. Approximately 80% of patients have some degree of mental retardation.

Diagnosis. Cranical CT is usually normal except for mild ventricular widening. Extensive studies of endocrine function have failed to reveal a consistent abnormality other than glucose intolerance. Plasma somatomedin levels are elevated during the first year in some infants and fall below normal during early childhood (Wit et al, 1985).

Treatment. Girls may benefit from high doses of estrogens to curtail excessive growth, but no treatment is available for the underlying disorder.

Neurocutaneous Disorders

Seizures (see Table 1–8) and mental retardation (see Chapter 5) are the common features of most neurocutaneous disorders. Some are present at birth (incontinentia pigmenti) or during infancy (neurofibromatosis, tuberous sclerosis) with macrocrania caused by either hydrocephalus or megalencephaly. Hemimegalencephaly, hemihypertrophy of the body, or hypertrophy of a single limb should always suggest the possibility of a neurocutaneous disorder.

Hypomelanosis of Ito

Hypomelanosis of Ito, also called *incontinentia pigmenti achromians,* is a rare syndrome believed to be transmitted by autosomal dominant inheritance. Some patients have been reported to have chromosomal abnormalities: trisomy 18 and a balanced translocation between chromosomes 2 and 8.

Clinical Features. The cutaneous manifestation is a large hypopigmented area that has a whorled or streaked appearance. It is a negative image of the hyperpigmented lesions of incontinentia pigmenti (see Chapter 1). Other cutaneous manifestations include café au lait spots, angiomatous nevi, heterochromia of the iris or hair, and other nevi. Mental capacity is retarded or borderline in 80%, and seizures are present in half (Pascual-Castroviejo et al, 1988). Spastic diplegia may also be present. These symptoms are caused by disturbances of neuronal migration. Megalencephaly occurs in approximately 25% of cases.

About one third of patients have skeletal and eye anomalies: limb hypertrophy or atrophy, facial hemiatrophy, poorly formed ears, dysplastic teeth, hypertelorism, strabismus, and corneal opacities.

Diagnosis. The characteristic cutaneous lesions are critical to the diagnosis and should be sought in the parents and siblings as well as the child. Chromosome studies are indicated in the child and parents.

Treatment. No treatment is available.

Linear Nevus Sebaceus Syndrome

Linear nevus sebaceus syndrome is sporadic and is also called the *organoid nevus syndrome* (Clancy et al, 1985), and the *epidermal nevus syndrome* (Pavone et al, 1991).

Clinical Features.   The cutaneous manifestation is a unilateral linear nevus, usually on the face or scalp, that may not be visible at birth but darkens during infancy and becomes verrucous. Hemihypertrophy of the face, head, and limbs ipsilateral to the nevus may be present at birth or may develop during infancy.

The spectrum of neurologic disability is considerable. Most affected children experience developmental delay and seizures. The head may be enlarged generally or unilaterally. Focal neurologic deficits, such as hemiplegia and hemianopia, contralateral to the nevus are relatively common. Eye abnormalities such as microphthalmia and coloboma occur in one third of children.

Diagnosis.   Diagnosis relies on recognition of the dermatologic manifestations. Electroencephalography (EEG) frequently reveals unilateral slowing and epileptiform discharges ipsilateral to the nevus. Hypsarrhythmia is present when infantile spasms are the first manifestation (see Chapter 1). Hemihypsarrhythmia has been described as well (Tjiam et al, 1978).

CT reveals asymmetry of the cranial vault with enlargement of one hemisphere. The abnormal hemisphere may have porencephaly or an enlarged lateral ventricle and a simplified convolutional pattern.

Treatment.   Seizures may respond to standard anticonvulsant therapy (see Chapter 1), but no treatment is available for the underlying cerebral malformation.

METABOLIC MEGALENCEPHALY

Several inborn errors of metabolism produce megalencephaly by storage of abnormal substances or by producing cerebral edema (Table 18–2). They are discussed elsewhere in the text because they usually are manifested as developmental regression (see Chapter 5) or seizures (see Chapter 1). Most affected infants have a normal head circumference at birth. Head enlargement parallels neurologic regression and clinical evidence of increased intracranial pressure. The ventricles are often small.

◆ Microcephaly

Microcephaly means a head circumference that is smaller than 2 standard deviations below the normal distribution. A small head circumference indicates a small brain. Most full-term newborns whose head circumferences are smaller than 2 standard deviations but who are neurologically normal will have normal intelligence at 7 years of age, but head circumferences smaller than 3 standard deviations usually indicate later mental retardation (Dolk, 1991).

A small head circumference at birth establishes the antepartum timing of brain damage but does not distinguish primary from secondary microcephaly (Table 18–4). *Primary microcephaly* encompasses conditions in which the brain is small and never formed properly because of genetic or chromosomal abnormality. *Secondary microcephaly* implies that the brain was forming normally but a disease process impaired further growth. Normal head circumference at birth, followed by failure of normal head growth, usually indicates a secondary microcephaly. Chromosomal disorders are an exception to that rule unless they produce defective prosencephalization or cellular migration.

Perinatal brain damage does not cause a recognizable decrease of head circumference until 3 to 6 months post partum. Failure of normal brain growth removes the force keeping the cranial bones separated, and they fuse prematurely. A primary disorder of the skull (craniostenosis) may cause premature closure of the cranial sutures even though the brain is attempting to grow normally. The distinction between the two is relatively simple: craniostenosis is always associated with an abnormal skull shape and heaping up of bone along the cranial sutures; failure of brain growth produces a relatively normal-shaped skull with some overlapping of skull bones.

Cranial CT may be informative in distinguishing primary from secondary microcephaly (Jaworski et al, 1986). In most children with primary microcephaly, either CT results are normal or a recognizable pattern of cerebral malformation is present. In those with secondary microcephaly, CT results are usually abnormal, characterized by one or more of the following features: ventricular enlargement, cerebral atrophy, and porencephaly.

PRIMARY MICROCEPHALY

Many cerebral malformations are of uncertain cause and cannot be classified as primary or secondary. Morphogenetic errors, although lacking in the traditional stigmata of tissue injury, could result from exposure of the embryo to a noxious agent during the first weeks after conception. At this early stage the delicate sequencing of neuronal development could be disorganized at a time when the brain is incapable of generating a cellular response.

Table 18–4 ◆ Conditions Causing Microcephaly

Primary Microcephaly	Secondary Microcephaly
1. Microcephaly vera (genetic)	1. Intrauterine disorders
2. Chromosomal disorders	a. Infection
3. Defective neurolation	b. Toxins
a. Anencephaly	c. Vascular
b. Encephalocele	2. Perinatal brain injuries
4. Defective prosencephalization	a. Hypoxic-ischemic encephalopathy
a. Agenesis of the corpus callosum	b. Intracranial hemorrhage
b. Holoprosencephaly (arhinencephaly)	c. Meningitis and encephalitis
5. Defective cellular migration	d. Stroke
	3. Postnatal systemic diseases
	a. Chronic cardiopulmonary disease
	b. Chronic renal disease
	c. Malnutrition

Microcephaly Vera (Genetic)

Microcephaly vera is a term applied to genetic defects that decrease bulk growth of the brain. Autosomal dominant and autosomal recessive transmissions are described (Haslam and Smith, 1979).

Clinical Features. The autosomal dominant form is less disabling than the recessive form. Intelligence ranges from normal to mildly retarded (Rossi et al, 1987). Learning disabilities are a common feature. The face is not usually dysmorphic, although some children have a receding forehead, upslanting of the palpebral fissures, and large prominent ears. Physical stature is normal. Seizures may be present during childhood but tend to disappear by adult life.

Children with the autosomal recessive form of microcephaly vera are usually short and have a characteristic disproportion in size between the face and the skull. The forehead slants backward, and the reduced size of the skull causes the scalp to wrinkle in the occipital region. The chin is small, and the ears and nose are prominent. Mental retardation is moderate to severe, and other neurologic abnormalities, such as spastic diplegia and seizures, may be present.

Diagnosis. A family history of microcephaly is critical to the diagnosis in the autosomal dominant form but is often lacking in the autosomal recessive form. Results of brain imaging are normal.

Treatment. No treatment is available.

Chromosomal Disorders

Chromosomal disorders are unlikely to be manifested as microcephaly at birth unless cerebral aplasia, such as holoprosencephaly, is part of the syndrome. Hypotonia and dysmorphism are the prominent features of the chromosomal disorders in the newborn (see Chapter 5), and microcephaly becomes evident during infancy.

Defective Neurulation

At the end of the first week a rostrocaudal axis appears on the dorsal aspect of the embryo. This axis is responsible for the subsequent induction of a neural plate, the anlage of the nervous system. The neural plate is converted into a closed neural tube during the third and fourth weeks. Defects in closure are called dysraphic states. The most rostral portion of the neural tube, the anterior neuropore, closes at about the twenty-fourth day.

Anencephaly

Anencephaly is the result of defective closure of the anterior neuropore, just as myelomeningocele is the result of defective closure of the posterior neuropore (see Chapter 12). The rate of each is declining. The cause of the malformations and the reason for their decline in prevalence are unknown.

Clinical Features. Less than half of anencephalics are born alive, and those who are rarely survive the first month (Raven et al, 1983). The scalp is absent, and the skull is open from the vertex to the foramen magnum. The brain, appearing hemorrhagic and fibrotic, is exposed to view. It consists mainly of the hindbrain and parts of the diencephalon; the forebrain is completely lacking.

The orbits are shallow, and the eyes protrude. The neck is held in retroflexion, and the proximal portion of the arms seems overgrown compared with the legs. The overall appearance of the anencephalic newborn is grotesque and described as "toadlike."

Diagnosis. Following the birth of a child with a neural tube defect, the chance of anencephaly or myelomeningocele in subsequent pregnancies increases twofold to fivefold. After two affected children have been born, the chance of having another affected child doubles again (McBride, 1979). The prenatal diagnosis of dysraphic states is discussed in the section on myelomeningocele (see Chapter 12).

Treatment. No effort to prolong life should be made.

Encephalocele

An encephalocele is a protrusion of cortex and meninges, covered by skin, through a defect in the skull. Encephaloceles may occur in any location; however, most are midline-occipital, except in Asians, in whom the defects are usually midline-frontal.

Clinical Features. The size of the encephalocele may range from a small protrusion to a cyst as big as the skull. When the protrusion is large, the skull is likely to be microcephalic. No conclusion can be drawn concerning the contents of the mass by its size, but an encephalocele with a sessile base is more likely to contain cerebral tissue than is one with a pedunculated base.

Encephaloceles rarely occur as a solitary cerebral malformation and are usually associated with abnormalities of the cerebral hemispheres, cerebellum, and midbrain (Friede, 1975).

Diagnosis. Cranial CT is reasonably accurate in defining the contents of the encephalocele. Despite its midline location, the protruded material is usually derived from one hemisphere that is smaller than the other and is displaced across the midline by the larger hemisphere.

Treatment. The desire to remove the encephalocele surgically should be tempered by its contents and the extent of associated anomalies. Occipital meningocele, in which the sac contains no neural tissue, should be surgically removed, and the outcome is often excellent. Children with protruded brain material and associated malformations usually die during infancy.

Defective Prosencephalization

The forebrain develops between 25 and 30 days' gestation from a midline vesicle that is generated from the closed anterior neuropore. Between 30 and 40 days' gestation, bilateral cerebral vesicles are formed by the cleavage and outpouching of the midline vesicle. The midline vesicle is the primordium of the third ventricle, and the bilateral cerebral vesicles are the primordia of the lateral ventricles.

Holoprosencephaly

A spectrum of malformations has been described as resulting from defective cleavage of the embryonic forebrain. The term *arhinencephaly* is often used for the full spectrum of abnormalities (Kobori et al, 1987), but holoprosencephaly is a more accurate term.

Total failure of cleavage produces a small brain with a midline vesicle covered by a horseshoe of limbic cortex. With less severe defects the third ventricle and diencephalon differentiate, and the hemispheres are partially cleaved in the occipital lobe. The corpus callosum is hypoplastic or absent. The minimal defect (arhinencephaly) is the unilateral or bilateral absence of the olfactory bulbs and tracts associated with some degree of rhinic lobe aplasia. Hemispheric cleavage is complete, the ventricles are normal, and the corpus callosum is present in part or in total.

Chromosomal abnormalities are often demonstrable in newborns with holoprosencephaly. Trisomy, deletions, and rings of chromosome 13 account for most of the chromosomal abnormalities. The remainder are composed of trisomy, deletions, and rings of chromosome 18 and partial trisomy of chromosome 7.

Clinical Features. Holoprosencephaly is associated with craniofacial dysplasia in 93% of cases and with malformations in other organs in 53% to 67% (Jellinger et al, 1981). The facial deformities are primarily in the midline (cyclopia or ocular hypotelorism, flat nose, cleft lip, cleft palate), and their severity is often predictive of the severity of the brain malformation. Associated malformations include congenital heart defects, clubbing of the hands or feet, polydactyly and syndactyly, hypoplasia of the genitourinary system, accessory spleen and liver, and malrotation of the intestine.

Most children with severe defects in cleavage of the forebrain are stillborn or die in the neonatal period. Microcephaly, hypotonia, apnea, and seizures are prominent features. Hypotonia is especially severe when the defect is associated with a chromosomal abnormality. Infants who survive have severe intellectual, motor, and sensory impairment.

Children with only arhinencephaly may appear physically normal and may display minor disturbances in neurologic function such as learning disabilities and seizures.

Diagnosis. Holoprosencephaly should be suspected in every child with midline facial deformities, especially when malformations are present in other organs. Excellent visualization of the malformation is provided by CT or MRI.

Treatment. Considering the multiplicity of malformations, measures to extend life are inappropriate.

Agenesis of the Corpus Callosum

Anomalous development of the three telencephalic commissures—the corpus callosum, the anterior commissure, and the hippocampal commissure—is an almost constant feature of defective prosencephalization, but it also occurs in association with many other malformations and as a solitary genetic defect (see "Megalencephaly" earlier in this chapter).

Solitary agenesis of the corpus callosum is clinically inapparent except for subtle disturbances in the interhemispheric transfer of information, for which special testing is needed.

Defective Cellular Migration

When neurons that should form the superficial layers of the cerebral cortex are unable to pass through the already established deeper layers of neurons, the results are a simplification of the cortical convolutional pattern *(agyria)* and an abnormal accumulation of neurons in the white matter *(heterotopia)*. Complete absence of gyri causes a smooth cerebral surface *(lissencephaly)*, whereas incomplete gyral formation causes the existing convolutions to be reduced in number and large in size *(pachygyria)*.

Most cases are sporadic, and the cause is probably multifactorial but must be operative early in gestation. Several neurocutaneous disorders are characterized by disturbances of neuronal migration.

Clinical Features. Most children are referred for evaluation because of developmental delay or intractable myoclonic seizures. Microcephaly is present in only half of patients, but all are mentally retarded (Gastaut et al, 1987). Many infants have an infiltrated and swollen appearance of the face and palmar skin, but only a few have dysmorphic features: high forehead, dolichocephaly, anteverted nostrils, polydactyly, and syndactyly. Axial hypotonia is constant.

Diagnosis. EEG findings are characteristic but not specific. Fast, high-voltage dysrhythmic activity dominates the background. It does not react to eye opening or photic stimulation and resembles a fast hypsarrhythmia.

The diagnosis is based on MRI abnormalities:

a smooth cortical surface except for rudimentary sulci (agyria) may be limited to the parietal or frontal regions or encompass the whole brain; the Sylvian fissure is broad and triangular; the interhemispheric fissure is widened; and nests of gray matter are present within the white matter. The ventricles may be enlarged and the corpus callosum absent (Barkovich et al, 1991).

Treatment. Seizures are usually intractable but may be partially controlled by standard drugs for the management of infantile spasms or myoclonic seizures (see Chapter 1). Death often occurs during infancy, but long survival is possible.

SECONDARY MICROCEPHALY
Intrauterine Disorders

Intrauterine infection is an established cause of microcephaly. Cytomegalovirus infection (see Chapter 5) can be manifested as microcephaly, without any features of systemic disease. Because maternal infection is asymptomatic, such cases are difficult to identify as being caused by cytomegalovirus disease. However, surveys of cytomegalovirus antibody demonstrate a higher rate of seropositive individuals among microcephalic than normocephalic children (Hanshaw, 1966). This suggests that such cases do exist.

Efforts to identify environmental toxins that produce cerebral malformation have had only limited success (Kalter and Warkany, 1983). Drugs of abuse and several pharmaceutical agents have been implicated, but the evidence is rarely compelling. The only absolute conclusion that can be derived from an abundance of studies is that a negative impact occurs on fetuses of women whose life-style includes some combination of heavy alcohol or drug use, poor nutrition, and inadequate health care. This negative impact is usually expressed as intrauterine growth retardation, dysmorphic features, and microcephaly.

Aplasia of major cerebral vessels is a rare malformation of unknown cause. Brain tissue that should have been supplied by the aplastic vessels either never forms or is infarcted and replaced by calcified cystic cavities. The cavities are present at birth, and the CT appearance suggests an intrauterine infection except that the cysts conform to a vascular distribution.

Perinatal Brain Injuries

Perinatal brain injuries are an important cause, but not the only cause, of failure of brain growth during infancy when head circumference is normal at birth. This group of disorders generally is manifested as neonatal seizures (see Chapter 1). Children with microcephaly and mental retardation from perinatal brain injuries always have cerebral palsy and often have epilepsy. Microcephaly and mental retardation in the absence of motor impairment are always of prenatal origin.

Postnatal Systemic Disease

Infants who are chronically ill and malnourished fail to thrive. All growth is retarded; however, as a rule, head circumference is maintained better than length and weight. Therefore, if body size is below the third percentile, head circumference might be at the fifth or tenth percentile. If the systemic disturbance is not corrected, brain injury generally occurs, brain growth slows, and head circumference falls into the microcephalic range.

◆ Abnormal Head Shape

Whereas the size of the skull is determined almost exclusively by its contents, the shape of the skull is the result of forces acting from within and without, and of the time of closure of the cranial sutures.

INTRACRANIAL FORCES

The shape of the brain contributes to the shape of the skull by influencing the time of closure of cranial sutures. Temporal lobe agenesis results in a narrower calvarium, and cerebellar agenesis results in a small posterior fossa. Hydrocephalus produces characteristic changes in skull shape. Large lateral ventricles cause bowing of the forehead, and the Dandy-Walker malformation causes bowing of the occiput. In infants with subdural hematomas, bitemporal widening may be seen because of separation of the sagittal suture.

EXTRACRANIAL FORCES

Head shape may be influenced in utero by constricting forces, such as a bicornuate uterus or multiple fetuses. Physical constraint of the skull in utero may contribute to premature closure of a cranial suture (Graham and Smith, 1980; Graham et al, 1980), but perinatal and postnatal constraints do not. Molding of the skull is common during a prolonged vaginal delivery, but the closure of cranial sutures is unaffected and eventual head shape is not influenced by the molding.

In premature infants *scaphocephaly* (Table 18–5) often develops because the poorly miner-

Table 18–5 ◆ Terms That Describe Head Shapes

Acrocephaly	High, towerlike head with vertical forehead
Brachycephaly	Broad head with recessed lower forehead
Oxycephaly	Pointed head
Plagiocephaly	Flattening of one side of head
Scaphocephaly (dolicocephaly)	Abnormally long and narrow head
Trigonocephaly	Triangular head with prominent vertical ridge in midforehead

alized skull becomes flattened on one side and then the other as the child is turned back and forth. The shape of the skull becomes normal with maturity.

Plagiocephaly or occipital flattening is a frequent finding in hypotonic infants. This is caused by constantly lying in the same position. The hair over the flattened portion of skull is usually sparse from rubbing against the bed surface. A normal head shape is resumed if the infant's lying position can be changed.

CRANIOSTENOSIS

Craniostenosis and *craniosynostosis* are terms for premature closure of one or more cranial sutures that results in an abnormal skull shape. These terms should be applied only to infants in whom the sutures close while the brain is growing. Early closure of sutures in infants with microcephaly is not premature because the intracranial pressure required to keep sutures apart is lacking.

Most cases of craniostenosis are sporadic and of uncertain etiology. Autosomal dominant and recessive forms of single-suture closure are reported (Cohen et al, 1990). Autosomal dominant inheritance is more common than autosomal recessive inheritance but is also more easily identified as hereditary. Many sporadic cases could represent autosomal recessive inheritance.

Craniostenosis may be one feature of a larger recognized syndrome of chromosomal or genetic abnormality. Genetic disorders are often associated with syndactyly or polydactyly (see "Acrocephalosyndactyly" later in this chapter), whereas chromosomal disorders are characterized by other limb malformations and growth retardation.

Craniostenosis is also reported in association with other disorders (Table 18–6). Some of these associations are coincidental, but a cause-and-effect relationship probably does exist with metabolic disorders of bone.

Table 18–6 ◆ Disorders Associated with Craniostenosis

1. Ataxia-telangiectasia
2. Familial hypophosphatemia
3. Hyperthyroidism
4. Idiopathic hypercalcemia
5. Mucopolysaccharidoses
6. Polycythemia vera
7. Rickets
   a. Renal rickets
   b. Vitamin D deficient
   c. Vitamin D resistant
8. Sickle cell disease
9. Thalassemia major

Clinical Features. The first, and usually the only, symptom is an abnormal head shape. Normal bone growth is impaired in a plane perpendicular to the fused suture but is able to grow in a parallel plane. Scaphocephaly is caused by premature fusion of the sagittal suture, brachycephaly by fusion of both coronal sutures, plagiocephaly by fusion of one coronal or one lambdoid suture, trigonocephaly by fusion of the metopic suture, and oxycephaly by fusion of all sutures.

When several sutures close prematurely, the growing brain is constricted and symptoms of increased intracranial pressure develop. Hydrocephalus occurs more frequently in children with craniostenosis than in normal children (Whittle et al, 1984). Several forms of communicating and noncommunicating hydrocephalus are described. It seems more likely that both are caused by a common underlying factor rather than one causing the other.

Sagittal synostosis accounts for almost 60% of cases of craniostenosis and occurs primarily in males. Coronal synostosis accounts for approximately 20% of cases and occurs primarily in females.

Diagnosis. Visual inspection of the skull and palpation of the sutures are sufficient for diagnosis in most cases of single-suture craniostenosis. Radiographs of the skull demonstrate a band of increased density at the site of the prematurely closed suture. CT is indicated in all children with craniostenosis of multiple sutures and in children with craniostenosis of a single suture if hydrocephalus is suspected.

Treatment. The two indications for surgery to correct craniostenosis are to improve the appearance of the head and to relieve increased intracranial pressure (Winston, 1985). The cosmetic indication should be used sparingly and only to make severe deformities less noticeable.

Crouzon Disease (Craniofacial Dysostosis)

Crouzon disease is the combination of premature closure of any or all cranial sutures and maldevelopment of facial bones. It is transmitted by autosomal dominant inheritance.

Clinical Features. The facial deformity is present at birth and becomes worse during infancy. The skull is usually widened anteriorly as a result of premature closure of the coronal suture. The eyes are widely separated and prominent, but the lower face appears recessed because of maxillary hypoplasia and prognathism. Adding to the deformity are a beaklike nose and a large protuberant tongue. Intracranial pressure is often increased because several cranial sutures are usually involved.

Diagnosis. The typical facies and genetic pattern of inheritance are diagnostic. Cranial CT is indicated in every case to follow the progression of cerebral compression.

Treatment. A sequential neurosurgical and plastic surgical approach has been successful in opening the sutures to relieve intracranial pressure and in advancing the facial bones forward to improve cosmetic appearance.

Acrocephalosyndactyly

Acrocephalosyndactyly is characterized by the combination of craniostenosis and fusion of fingers and toes. Some degree of mental retardation is often present. Several different syndromes with this basic combination have been described (Cohen et al, 1990).

Apert syndrome is characterized by syndactyly and premature closure of the coronal suture resulting in brachycephaly. The forehead is high and prominent, and the face is similar to, but less severely deformed than, the face in Crouzon disease. Most cases are sporadic, but autosomal dominant inheritance is suspected. Agenesis of the corpus callosum and limbic structures may be an associated feature (de Leon et al, 1987).

Carpenter syndrome differs from Apert syndrome because it is transmitted by autosomal recessive inheritance and the patient has polydactyly as well as syndactyly, premature closure of all sutures, obesity, and hypogonadism.

Chotzen syndrome is similar to Carpenter syndrome but is transmitted by autosomal dominant inheritance and also is marked by a low-set frontal hairline, ptosis, and a deviated nasal septum.

References

Barkovich AJ, Koch TK, Carrol CL: The spectrum of lissencephaly: Report of ten patients analyzed by magnetic resonance imaging. Ann Neurol 30:139, 1991.

Bordarier C, Aicardi J: Dandy-Walker syndrome and agenesis of the cerebellar vermis: Diagnostic problems and genetic counselling. Dev Med Child Neurol 32:285, 1990.

Bordarier C, Aicardi J, Goutieres F: Congenital hydrocephalus and eye abnormalities with severe developmental brain: Warburg's syndrome. Ann Neurol 16:60, 1984.

Burton B: Recurrence risks for congenital hydrocephalus. Clin Genet 16:47, 1977.

Chervenak FA, Berkowitz RL, Tortora M, et al: The management of fetal hydrocephalus. Am J Obstet Gynecol 151:933, 1985.

Clancy RR, Kurtz MB, Baker D, et al: Neurologic manifestations of the organoid nevus syndrome. Arch Neurol 42:236, 1985.

Cohen MM Jr, Fraser FC, Gorlin RJ: Craniofacial disorders. In Emery AE, Rimoin DA (eds): Principles and Practice of Medical Genetics, 2nd edition. Churchill Livingstone, London, 1990, p 749.

de Leon GA, de Leon G, Grover WD, et al: Agenesis of the corpus callosum and limbic malformation in Apert syndrome (type I acrocephalosyndactyly). Arch Neurol 44:979, 1987.

DeMyer W: Megalencephaly: Types, clinical syndromes, and management. Pediatr Neurol 2:321, 1986.

Dennis M, Fitz CR, Netley CT, et al: The intelligence of hydrocephalic children. Arch Neurol 38:607, 1981.

Dolk H: The predictive value of microcephaly during the first year of life for mental retardation at seven years. Dev Med Child Neurol 33:974, 1991.

Friede RL: Developmental Neuropathology. Springer-Verlag, New York, 1975, p 315.

Fukuyama Y, Miyao M, Ishizu, et al: Developmental changes in normal cranial measurements by computed tomography. Dev Med Child Neurol 21:425, 1979.

Gastaut H, Pinsard N, Raybaud C, et al: Lissencephaly (agyriapachygyria): Clinical findings and serial EEG. Dev Med Child Neurol 29:167, 1987.

Graham JM Jr, Badura RJ, Smith DW: Coronal craniostenosis: Fetal head constraint as one possible cause. Pediatrics 65:995, 1980.

Graham JM Jr, Smith DW: Metopic craniostenosis as a consequence of fetal head constraint: Two interesting experiments of nature. Pediatrics 65:1000, 1980.

Hamza M, Bodensteiner JB, Noorani PA, et al: Benign extracerebral fluid collections: A cause of macrocrania in infancy. Pediatr Neurol 3:218, 1987.

Hanshaw JB: Cytomegalovirus complement-fixing antibodies in microcephaly. N Engl J Med 275:476, 1966.

Haslam RHA, Smith DW: Autosomal dominant microcephaly. J Pediatr 95:701, 1979.

Jaeckle KA, Krol G, Posner JB: Evolution of computed tomographic abnormalities in leptomeningeal metastases. Ann Neurol 17:85, 1985.

Jaworski M, Hersh JH, Donat J, et al: Computed tomography of the head in the evaluation of microcephaly. Pediatrics 78:1064, 1986.

Jellinger K, Gross H, Kaltenback E, et al: Holoprosencephaly and agenesis of the corpus callosum: Frequency of associated malformations. Acta Neuropathol 55:1, 1981.

Jellinger K, Sunder-Plassman M: Connatal intracranial tumors. Neuropediatrie 4:46, 1973.

Kalter H, Warkany J: Congenital malformations. N Engl J Med 308:491, 1983.

Kobori JA, Herrick MK, Urich H: Arhinencephaly: The spectrum of associated malformations. Brain 110:237, 1987.

Kovnar EH, Coxe WS, Volpe JJ: Normal neurologic development and marked reconstitution of cerebral mantle after postnatal treatment of intrauterine hydrocephalus. Neurology 34:840, 1984.

Kuzniecky RI, Watters GV, Watters L, et al: X-linked hydrocephalus. Can J Neurol Sci 13:344, 1986.

Lasjaunias P, Rodesch G, Pruvost P, et al: Treatment of vein of Galen malformation. J Neurosurg 70:746, 1989.

Lipman SP, Pretorius H, Rumack CM, et al: Fetal intracranial teratoma: US diagnosis of three cases and a review of the literature. Radiology 157:491, 1985.

Lorber J, Priestly BL: Children with large heads: A practical approach to diagnosis in 577 children, with special reference to 109 children with megalencephaly. Dev Med Child Neurol 23:494, 1981.

Lynn RB, Buchanan DC, Fenichel GM, et al: Agenesis of the corpus callosum, Arch Neurol 37:444, 1980.

McBride ML: Sib risks of anencephaly and spina bifida in British Columbia. Am J Med Genet 3:377, 1979.

Mueller SM: Enlarged cerebral ventricular system in infant achondroplastic dwarf. Neurology 30:767, 1980.

Mueller SM, Reinertson JE: Reversal of emissary vein blood flow in achondroplastic dwarfs. Neurology 30:769, 1980.

Nagib MG, Maxwell RE, Chou SN: Klippel-Feil syndrome in children: Clinical features and management. Child Nerv Syst 1:255, 1985.

Nickel RE, Gallenstein JS: Developmental prognosis for infants with enlargement of the subarachnoid spaces. Dev Med Child Neurol 29:181, 1987.

Pascual-Castroviejo I, Lopez-Rodriquez L, de la Cruz Medina M, et al: Hypomelanosis of Ito: Neurological complications in 34 cases. Can J Neurol Sci 15:124-129, 1988.

Pascual-Castroviejo I, Velez A, Pascual-Pascual SI, et al: Dandy-Walker malformation: Analysis of 38 cases. Child Nerv Syst 7:88, 1991.

Pavone L, Curatolo P, Rizzo R, et al: Epidermal nevus syndrome: A neurologic variant with hemimegalencephaly, gyral malformation, mental retardation, seizures, and facial hemihypertrophy. Neurology 41:226-271, 1991.

Raven RH, Schoenberg BS, Bharucha NE, et al: Geographic distribution of anencephaly in the United States. Neurology 33:1243, 1983.

Reid CS, Pyeritz RE, Kopits SE, et al: Cervicomedullary compression in young patients with achondroplasia: Value of comprehensive neurologic and respiratory evaluation. J Pediatr 110:522, 1987.

Rossi LN, Candini G, Scarlatti G, et al: Autosomal dominant microcephaly without mental retardation. Am J Dis Child 141:655, 1987.

Sotos JF, Cutler EA: Cerebral gigantism. Am J Dis Child 131:625, 1977.

Tjiam AT, Stefanko S, Schenk VW, et al: Infantile spasms associated with hemihypsarrhythmia and hemimegalencephaly. Dev Med Child Neurol 20:779, 1978.

Tomita T, McLone DG: Brain tumors during the first twenty-four months of life. Neurosurgery 17:913, 1985.

Vintzileos AM, Campbell WA, Weinbaum PJ, et al: Perinatal

management and outcome of fetal ventriculomegaly. Obstet Gynecol 69:5, 1987.

Whelan HT, Sung JH, Mastri AR: Diffuse leptomeningeal gliomatosis: Report of three cases. Clin Neuropathol 6:164, 1987.

Whittle IR, Johnston IH, Besser M: Intracranial pressure changes in craniostenosis. Surg Neurol 21:367, 1984.

Williams RS, Swisher CN, Jennings M, et al: Cerebro-ocular dysgenesis (Walker-Warburg syndrome): Neuropathologic and etiologic analysis. Neurology 34:1531, 1984.

Winship IG: Sotos syndrome—autosomal dominant inheritance substantiated. Clin Genet 28:243, 1985.

Winston KR: Craniosynostosis. In Wilkins RH, Rengachary SS (eds): Neurosurgery. McGraw-Hill, New York, 1985, p 2171.

Wit JM , Beemer FA, Barth PG, et al: Cerebral gigantism (Sotos syndrome): Compiled data of 22 cases; Analysis of clinical features, growth and plasma somatomedin. Eur J Pediatr 144:131, 1985.

Yokota A, Matsukado Y: Congenital midline proencephaly: A new malformation associated with scalp anomaly. Child Brain 5:380, 1979.

Index

Note: Page numbers in *italics* refer to illustrations; page numbers followed by t refer to tables.